Rehabilitation Nursing
Perspectives and Applications

Rehabilitation Nursing

Perspectives and Applications

Victor A. Christopherson
Chairman, Division of Child Development/Family Relations
University of Arizona

Pearl Parvin Coulter
Dean and Professor Emeritus of Nursing
University of Arizona

Mary Opal Wolanin
Associate Professor of Nursing
University of Arizona

McGRAW-HILL BOOK COMPANY
A Blakiston Publication

New York St. Louis San Francisco
Düsseldorf Johannesburg Kuala Lumpur
London Mexico Montreal New Delhi Panama
Rio de Janeiro Singapore Sydney Toronto

Rehabilitation Nursing:
Perspectives and Applications

Copyright © 1974 by McGraw-Hill, Inc. All rights reserved.
Printed in the United States of America. No part of this
publication may be reproduced, stored in a retrieval system,
or transmitted, in any form or by any means, electronic,
mechanical, photocopying, recording, or otherwise, without
the prior written permission of the publisher.

1 2 3 4 5 6 7 8 9 0   KPKP   7 9 8 7 6 5 4 3

Library of Congress Cataloging in Publication Data

Christopherson, Victor A   1923-   comp.
    Rehabilitation nursing.

"A Blakiston publication."
1. Rehabilitation—Addresses, essays, lectures.
2. Sick—Psychology—Addresses, essays, lectures.
3. Nurse and patient—Addresses, essays, lectures.
I. Coulter, Pearl Parvin, joint comp. II. Wolanin,
Mary Opal, 1910-   joint comp. III. Title.
[DNLM: 1. Nursing care—Collected works. 2. Rehabilitation—Collected works. 3. Rehabilitation—Nursing
texts. WY156 C556r 1974]
RT120.R4C45   610.73   73-8922
ISBN 0-07-010815-3

This book was set in Times Roman by Rocappi, Inc.
The editors were Cathy Dilworth and Annette Hall;
the designer was Anne Canevari Green;
and the production supervisor was Joe Campanella.
The drawings were done by John Cordes, J & R Technical Services, Inc.
The printer and binder was Kingsport Press, Inc.

Contents

		List of Contributors	ix
		Preface	xiii
PART ONE **Perspectives**	**A**	**CULTURAL CONSIDERATIONS**	3
		1 Perspectives in Rehabilitation	6
		2 Disability Viewed in Its Cultural Context	8
		3 Cultural Influences on Patient Behavior	13
		4 Territoriality in Man: A Comparison of Behavior in Home and Hospital	21
		5 The Patient and the Family	26
	B	**PSYCHOLOGICAL CONSIDERATIONS**	40
		6 Role Modifications of the Disabled Male	43
		7 Body Image and Self-esteem	49
		8 Sexual Problems in Rehabilitation	56
		9 The Psychology of Illness	60
		10 Sexual Adjustments in Relation to Pregnancy, Illness, Surgery, Physical Handicaps, and Other Unusual Circumstances	69
		11 The Doctor-Nurse Game	84
PART TWO **Teaching** **and** **Prevention**	**A**	**THE ROLE OF THE NURSE AS A TEACHER**	97
		12 The Role of the Nurse in the Prevention of Illness and in Health Teaching	99
		13 What Is Experiential Teaching?	106
	B	**THE ROLE OF THE NURSE IN DISABILITY PREVENTION**	114
		14 Exercises for Bedfast Patients	117
		15 Effects on Cardiovascular Function	122
		16 Effects on Gastrointestinal Function	126
		17 Effects on Respiratory Function	132
		18 Effects on Motor Function	136
		19 Effects on Urinary Function	141
		20 Effects on Metabolic Equilibrium	145
		21 Effects on Psychosocial Equilibrium	148

PART THREE
Rehabilitation Nursing Care in Non-Life-Threatening Conditions

A NEUROLOGICAL DEFICITS — 155
- 22 Nursing Care of the Patient with a Stroke — 158
- 23 Listen: The Patient — 167
- 24 Infancy to Adolescence: Habilitation of Children with Meningomyelocele — 171
- 25 Dysphasia: The Patient, His Family, and the Nurse — 181
- 26 Rehabilitation Nursing in Non-Life-Threatening Problems — 191

B ARTHRITIC CONDITIONS — 195
- 27 Arthritis: A Patient's View — 201
- 28 The Rehabilitation Process—As Viewed from the Inside — 205
- 29 Rehabilitation of Patients with Rheumatoid Arthritis — 209

C BOWEL AND BLADDER DISORDERS — 217
- 30 Achieving Bladder Control — 220
- 31 The Myelodysplastic Child—Bowel and Bladder Control — 227
- 32 Learning Colostomy Control — 237

D AMPUTATION CONDITIONS — 252
- 33 Amputee Needs, Frustrations, and Behavior — 256
- 34 Battle Casualty: Amputee — 269
- 35 Stump Hygiene — 279

E SIGHT AND HEARING DISORDERS — 294
- 36 Understanding Your Blind Patient — 298
- 37 Caring for the Blind Patient — 302
- 38 The Needs of the Visually Handicapped — 306
- 39 Available Training Opportunities for Deaf People — 313
- 40 Rehabilitation for Irreversible Deafness — 321
- 41 Deaf Patients Learn to Listen on a New Wave Length — 328
- 42 A Guide for Nurses in a Hearing Conservation Program — 330

F PAIN — 339
- 43 Nursing Intervention for Bodily Pain — 341
- 44 Sociocultural Correlates of Pain Response — 347
- 45 Phantom Limbs — 354

CONTENTS

PART FOUR
Rehabilitation Nursing Care in Life-Threatening Conditions

A CARDIOVASCULAR DISORDERS — 363

46 The Nurse's Role in Rehabilitation of the Myocardial Infarction Patient — 367
47 Move That Cardiac Early — 377
48 Teaching Patients about Pacemakers — 384

B PULMONARY DISORDERS — 392

49 Physical and Muscular Reconditioning — 395
50 Rehabilitation of Chronic Obstructive Lung Disease — 398
51 Rehabilitation of Patients with COLD — 408

C MALIGNANCY CONDITIONS — 421

52 Cancer: The Emotional Component — 426
53 What Can I Say to the Cancer Patient — 434
54 Adaptation of the Spouse and Other Family Members to the Colostomy Patient — 440
55 A Dynamic Approach to the Ileal Conduit Patient — 446
56 Early Carcinoma of the Breast — 454
57 Psychological Impact of Cancer and Its Treatment IV—Adaption to Radical Mastectomy — 463
58 Laryngectomy — 467
59 Speech after Laryngectomy — 479
60 Milieu Design for Adolescents with Leukemia — 485

D GERIATRIC CONDITIONS — 490

61 Environmental Aids for the Aged Patient — 500
62 Give the Older Person Time — 503
63 Outstanding Characteristics of Older Patients — 507
64 Remotivation: Toward Reality for the Aged — 514
65 Nursing the Patient with Internal Hip Fixation — 520
66 The Nurse's Role in Preventing Circulatory Complications in the Patient with a Fractured Hip — 524
67 Using Crutches, Canes, and Walkers — 529
68 It's Not Age That Interferes with Nutrition of the Elderly — 537

PART FIVE
Alcoholism and Drug Abuse

A ALCOHOLISM — 545

69 The Nurse's Role: In the Prevention and Control of Problem Drinking — 547
70 Nursing the Alcoholic — 550
71 Adjusting Nursing Techniques to the Treatment of Alcoholic Patients — 557

B DRUG ABUSE — 565

72 Treatment of Youthful Drug Abusers — 567
73 Help for the Addict — 570
74 Methadone Maintenance in Heroin Addiction: The Program at Beth Israel Medical Center — 580

List of Contributors

Sol Adler, B.A., M.A., Ph.D. Professor, Department of Audiology and Speech Pathology, University of Tennessee Hospital Branch, Knoxville, Tennessee.

Immaculata M. Alba, B.S., M.S. Assistant Professor, School of Nursing, Southern Connecticut State College, New Haven, Connecticut.

M. A. Aliapoulios, M.D. Associate Professor of Surgery, Harvard Medical School, Boston, Massachusetts.

Julian S. Ansell, M.D. School of Medicine, Department of Urology, University of Washington, Seattle, Washington.

Virginia Barckley, B.S., M.S. American Cancer Society, New York, New York.

Morton Bard, B.A., M.A., Ph.D. Professor of Psychology, City University of New York, New York, New York.

Gilbert H. Barnes, M.D. School of Medicine, Division of Dermatology, University of California, San Francisco, California.

Helen K. Branson, A.B., M.A. Mendota Research Group, Englewood, New Jersey.

H. Bryce Brooks, B.A. Executive Director, Awareness House Training Center, Berkeley, California, and Far West Regional Training and Research Center, U.S. Office of Education.

McKenzie Buck, B.A., M.A., Ph.D. Associate Professor of Otalaryngology, University of Oregon Medical School, Portland, Oregon.

Douglas G. Carroll, M.D. Editorial Office, Maryland Medical Journal, Baltimore, Maryland.

Warren H. Chapman, M.D. School of Medicine, Department of Urology, University of Washington, Seattle, Washington.

Don C. Charles, B.A., M.A., Ph.D. Professor of Psychology, Iowa State University, Ames, Iowa.

Victor A. Christopherson, B.S., M.A., Ed.D. Chairman, Division of Child Development/Family Relations, School of Home Economics, University of Arizona, Tucson, Arizona.

Arthur D. Coleman, M.D. Psychiatrist, San Francisco Medical Center, School of Medicine, Department of Psychology, University of California, San Francisco, California.

Pearl Parvin Coulter, A.B., M.S. Dean Emeritus, College of Nursing, University of Arizona, Tucson, Arizona.

LIST OF CONTRIBUTORS

Pamela Culbert, B.S., M.S. Clinical Nurse Specialist, North Shore Hospital, Manhasset, New York.

Lorraine Delehanty, B.S., M.S. Department of Physical Medicine and Rehabilitation, University of Minnesota Hospitals, Minneapolis, Minnesota.

Pauline I. Amburgey Dunn, R.N. 2413 Lynn Street, Bellingham, Washington.

Ruth B. Dyk, B.A., M.S. 275 Clinton Avenue, Brooklyn, New York.

Ruth E. Edmonds, B.S., M.S. Associate Professor, Department of Nursing, School of Medicine and Dentistry, University of Rochester, Rochester, New York.

Mary Lane Epp, R.N. Director of Nursing, The Bell Clinic, Willowdale, Ontario, Canada.

Gloria M. Francis, B.S., M.S. Doctoral Student in Sociology, University of Pennsylvania, Philadelphia, Pennsylvania.

Sister Maria Francis, B.S. Supervisor, Surgical Specialties, Good Samaritan Hospital, Cincinnati, Ohio.

Alan Frankel, Ph.D. Department of Psychology, University of Portland, Portland, Oregon.

Sister M. Agnes Clare Frenay, B.S., M.S. Associate Professor of Nursing, Department of Nursing, St. Louis University, St. Louis, Missouri.

Carol A. Gribbons, B.S. Nurse Consultant-BUMC, Regional Cancer Program, Coordinating Nurse, Tumor Service, Peter Brent Brigham Hospital, Boston, Massachusetts.

Margaret L. Hill, R.N., P.H.N., M.N. Assistant Professor in Nursing, Lecturer in Pediatrics, Division of Congenital Defects, School of Medicine, Department of Pediatrics, University of Washington, Seattle, Washington.

Eric Hodgins. Deceased.

Francis Hoffman, Ph.D., P.T. Department of Health and Physical Education, Queens College, City University of New York, Flushing, New York.

George D. Jackson, B.A., M.S. Clinical Psychologist, Essex County Penitentiary, Caldwell, New Jersey.

Bonnie Jean Johnson, B.S., M.S. Associate Professor, Department of Nursing, School of Medicine and Dentistry, University of Rochester, Rochester, New York.

Elizabeth Katona, B.S., M.A. Instructor of Inservice Education, Veteran's Administration Hospital, New York, New York.

Mary M. Kelly, B.S.N., M.N.Ed. Assistant Professor, University of Michigan School of Nursing, Ann Arbor, Michigan.

Marjorie Kinney, B.S., M.S. Assistant Professor, Medical-Surgical Nursing, Michigan State University, School of Nursing, East Lansing, Michigan.

Sandra Kirkpatrick, B.S. Lieutenant, U.S.N., U.S. Naval Hospital, Guam.

Barbara A. Kos, B.S., M.S., A.A.S. Professor, Medical-Surgical Nursing, Adelphi University, School of Nursing, Garden City, New York.

S. William Levy, M.D. Biomechanics Laboratory, University of California, Berkeley and San Francisco, Division of Dermatology, University of California, School of Medicine, San Francisco, California.

Janet L. Lunceford, B.S., M.S. Head Nurse, Cancer Nursing Unit, National Cancer Institute.

LIST OF CONTRIBUTORS

Gracia S. McCabe, B.S., M.S. Instructor, Virginia Polytechnic Institute and State University, College of Home Economics, Blacksburg, Virginia.

Margo McCaffery, B.S., M.S. Assistant Professor, School of Nursing, The Center for the Health Sciences, University of California at Los Angeles, Los Angeles, California.

Joyce A. McCarthy, B.S., M.S. Associate Professor, Department of Nursing, School of Medicine and Dentistry, University of Rochester, Rochester, New York.

Ronald Melzack, B.S., M.S., Ph.D. Professor, Department of Psychology, McGill University, Montreal, Quebec, Canada.

Fay Moss, B.S., M.S. Clinical Research Nurse, City of Hope Medical, Duarte, California.

Anne J. Murphy, R.N. Scott Paper Company, Philadelphia, Pennsylvania.

Edith V. Olson, B.S., M.S. Associate Professor in Nursing, Nursing Coordinator for the Rochester Regional Medical Program, Department of Nursing, School of Medicine, University of Rochester, Rochester, New York.

Paul C. O'Neill, M.A., CPRS Acc. Director of Public Relations, Canadian National Institute for the Blind, Toronto, Ontario, Canada.

Janice Papeika, B.S., M.S. Assistant Professor, Department of Nursing, University of Connecticut, Storrs, Connecticut.

Barbara A. Pearson, B.S.N. Master's Student in Adult Psychiatric Nursing Program at New York University.

Hildegard E. Peplau, B.A., M.A., Ed.D. President, American Nurses' Association, New York, New York.

Elizabeth Ford Pitorak, B.S., M.S. Assistant Professor, Medical-Surgical Nursing, Case Western Reserve University, Cleveland, Ohio.

Helen L. Potter, R.N., B.S., M.S. Director, Inservice Education, Memorial Hospital of Joy.

Alyce Quiros, B.S. Chief Psychiatric Nurse, Adult Guidance Center, San Francisco, California.

Efren Ramirez, M.D. Psychiatric Center-Research, State Psychiatric Hospital, Box 61, Rio Piedras Station, Puerto Rico.

Isadore Rubin. Deceased.

Reva Rubin, M.N., M.S., certificate in midwifery. Professor and Chairman, Department of Obstetrical and Gynecological Nursing, School of Nursing, University of Pittsburgh, Pittsburgh, Pennsylvania.

Lois M. Schroeder, B.S., M.S. Associate Professor, Department of Nursing, School of Medicine and Dentistry, University of Rochester, Rochester, New York.

Lucie C. M. Schultz, R.N. Associate Professor, Texas Women's University, Houston, Texas.

Franklin E. Scott, Colonel, U.S.A., retired, 642 Weatherly Drive, San Antonio, Texas.

W. Henry Sebrell, Jr., M.D. Director of the Institute of Human Nutrition at Columbia University, College of Physicians and Surgeons, New York, New York.

David B. Shurtleff, M.D. Associate Professor, Department of Pediatrics, School of Medicine, University of Washington, Seattle, Washington.

S. Richard Silverman, B.A., M.S., Ph.D. Director-Professor, Department of Otolaryngology, Washington University School of Medicine, St. Louis, Missouri.

Susan Mary Sink, R.N. Harborview Medical Center, Seattle, Washington.

Sydney R. Smith, Ph.D. The Menninger Foundation, Topeka, Kansas.

Shirley Steele, R.N., B.S., M.A., Ph.D. Associate Professor, Child Health Nursing, The State University of New York at Buffalo, New York, and Main Advisor and Project Director, Graduate Program in Child Health Nursing.

Virginia Stone, B.S., M.S., Ph.D. Professor of Nursing and Director, Department of Graduate Studies, Duke University Medical Center, School of Nursing, Durham, North Carolina.

Vincent Stravino, M.D. Department of Physical Medicine and Rehabilitation, University of Minnesota Hospitals, Minneapolis, Minnesota.

Arthur H. Sutherland, M.D. Department of Obstetrics, Clinical Instructor in Obstetrics and Gynecology, Vanderbilt University, Nashville, Tennessee.

Frank M. Swartz. Assistant to the Director of the Rehabilitation Center, University of Arizona, College of Education, Tucson, Arizona.

Lida F. Thompson, B.S., M.S. Associate Professor, Department of Nursing, School of Medicine and Dentistry, University of Rochester, Rochester, New York.

Richard W. Thoreson, Ph.D. Assistant Director, Rehabilitation Counselor Training Program, University of Wisconsin, Madison, Wisconsin.

L. L. Trigiano, M.D. Temple University School of Medicine, Philadelphia, Pennsylvania. Chief of Rehabilitation, Medicine Lee Hospital, Johnstown, Pennsylvania.

Wilson Van Dusen, Ph.D. Associate Director and Director, Awareness House Training Program, Berkeley, California.

Joel Vernick, M.S.W. Children's Diagnostic and Study Unit, National Institute of Child Health and Human Development, U.S. Public Health Service, Bethesda, Maryland.

McCay Vernon, B.A., M.S., M.A., Ph.D. Professor of Psychology, Western Maryland College, Westminster, Maryland.

Mildred Wade, B.S., M.S. Associate Professor, Department of Nursing, School of Medicine and Dentistry, University of Rochester, Rochester, New York.

Mary Opal Wolanin, B.A., M.P.A. Associate Professor of Nursing, College of Nursing, University of Arizona, Tucson, Arizona.

Preface

The volume of literature concerned with rehabilitation and rehabilitation nursing has expanded rapidly during the past decade. It appears in a broad spectrum of periodicals and is directed toward the various members of the health team as well as the general public. New material is appearing constantly, and both an extensive library and an unlimited amount of reading time are required for the practitioner who wishes to read widely in the field.

The purpose of this collection of readings is to make readily available significant, carefully selected, and representative articles assembled in a compact and accessible form. Personnel practicing in isolated areas without library resources, and those with limited time for reading, should find it valuable.

The objectives listed below are related, but considered separately they help to explain the ways in which this book is useful to the various groups involved in patient care both within and associated with nursing:

1 To enlarge the reader's appreciation of the broad scope of rehabilitation as an integral component of patient care
2 To present patient care as a series of interactions between and among individuals which in toto constitute, control, or contribute to the patient's therapeutic environment
3 To consider nursing as a broad-gauge service, utilizing workers with skills ranging from professional to technical which touch other disciplines with both discrete and interlocking practices

While emphasis is given to professional leadership, including the assessment and planning of nursing care, the actualization of the care plan includes technical modalities which are essential to the patient's comfort and well-being. Thus it would be hard to imagine a student preparing for any type of nursing—or any member of the patient care team—who would not find much of the content helpful. Most of the articles were written by nurses, physicians, or physical therapists, although contributors from the social science areas have not been neglected. Familiarity with the knowledge contained in these readings should result in a better understanding of the contributions of the various patient-care disciplines as well as their coordinated efforts in behalf of the patient. The organization of the book is as follows:

Part One, "Perspectives," deals with philosophical, cultural, and psychological considerations. Each practitioner must practice within a philosophical framework, and his relationship with patients and coworkers will be derived from his philosophical posture. Much of the practitioner's effectiveness, moreover, will be related to his grasp and utilization of the cultural and psychological forces at work.

Part Two, "Teaching and Prevention," stresses the all-important but frequently neglected roles of patient care personnel—teaching and prevention—which help the patient achieve his full restorative potential.

Part Three, "Rehabilitation Nursing Care in Non-Life-Threatening Conditions," includes neurological and sensory deprivation which demand major adjustments in life style even though they do not offer escape by means of death. These losses may offer a greater challenge to the nurse's ingenuity and creativity than some of the more dramatic life-threatening conditions.

Part Four, "Rehabilitation Nursing Care in Life-Threatening Conditions," presents the nursing roles and concerns in the illnesses which can be and often are terminal, such as cancer and heart disease. Geriatric problems are also included.

Part Five, "Rehabilitation Nursing in Alcoholism and Drug Abuse," illuminates the nurse's role in dealing with alcoholism and drug addiction.

Most of the articles selected for the book were published within the last ten years. The few exceptions are the result of quality's triumph over recency.

Victor A. Christopherson
Pearl Parvin Coulter
Mary Opal Wolanin

Rehabilitation Nursing
Perspectives and Applications

Part One

Perspectives

Section A

Cultural Considerations

There are many potential causes of disability, and it should be noted that not all of them have to do with physical limitation or impairment. However, even when there is a strong physical component, the likelihood is almost certain that the manifestation of or reaction to the physical component is significantly modified by a cultural component. Unless the cultural background of the individual is taken into account, the nurse will often find unexplainable resistance or passivity on the part of the patient in relation to prescribed therapeutic procedures. The first-generation Eastern European woman who becomes physically handicapped, for example, may view her disability as a legitimate excuse to step out of a lifelong work routine which is her accepted cultural role otherwise. She may actively resist every effort to restore her physical capacity to the point where she can resume her former duties. The rehabilitation nurse who says in effect that "nursing is nursing, and the techniques can be applied willy-nilly to all patients regardless of their backgrounds," is a nurse who will enjoy only a modicum of the success that might be hers were she to understand and employ the cultural basis of behavior as a tool in her therapeutic endeavors.

Rehabilitation, as pointed out by Christopherson, is the product of cultural evolution—in fact, it is a deliberate reversal of life's natural processes. The first essay helps set the stage by characterizing the meaning and nature of rehabilitation, and then specifying its application through the nursing profession. A strong case can be made, of course, for the argument that all nursing is rehabilitation nursing. On the other hand, the recent emphasis on rehabilitation in comprehensive centers, special areas in hospitals, and specialization in the medical sciences seems to lend support to the assertion that rehabilitation nursing is a highly significant and bona fide specialization in its own right within the field of nursing.

Thoreson touches on the cultural bases for resistance to rehabilitative efforts. He points out some of the sociocultural variables (such as social class) that might serve as a perceptual lens for the nurse in order that her interpretation of behavior can be more relevant. Unless each other's value system or motivational basis is understood and taken into account, the patient and the nurse may in fact work at cross purposes. Thoreson also discusses the relation of personality structure in the patient's reaction to disability. He characterizes the counselor's role in maximizing rehabilitation potential from the standpoint of both patient and community resistance. The rehabilitation nurse would do well to follow this discussion carefully, for the observation that any but the most perfunctory therapeutic contact with the patient is in fact a counseling situation has long since been accorded the status of a truism.

McCabe's article is significant not only for the excellent and timely content it provides but also in terms of its implications. Our nation has been referred to as a melting pot—an amalgamation of many races, ethnic groups, and cultures. This notion has a basis in fact, but it is also an exaggeration; while our national society provides patterns and guidelines in which we all share and by which we govern and are governed, there are still many different traditions and approaches to the problems of day-to-day life. In short, we are a nation of subcultures—relatively small or circumscribed homogeneous societies within the large heterogeneous society. These subcultures are organized or stratified according to a number of different bases—race, nationality, rural or urban dwelling place, social class, religion, and possibly region. Moreover, these variables frequently combine to yield further refinements. McCabe, for example, illustrates the special orientation to illness on the part of the Southern rural black.

The main thrust of McCabe's article—the necessity for the nurse to become knowledgeable concerning the culture of the individuals with whom she is likely to come in contact—is very effectively illustrated. The article suggests that concepts of disease, health, pain, causality, alternatives to poor health, and other matters which affect patient care may be served best by careful attention to the cultural background of the individual and particularly to the sensitive interpretation of the cues provided by the patient within this context.

One of the largely neglected areas of study in which the family plays a prominent part is human ecology—or man's relationship to his environment. There is little question that some of the highly significant determinants of behavior are environmental in nature. Assumptions based upon this concept are to be seen in everything from justifications for urban renewal programs and theories of delinquent behavior to design of clinical approaches to family therapy.

Colman has emphasized an aspect of ecology that may prove to be highly significant in rehabilitation. His discussion of territoriality in man should provide fruitful, if largely uncharted, pathways to a better understanding of patient and family behavior in the rehabilitation process.

The last article in the section draws attention to the nature and significance of the relationship between patient and family. Christopherson suggests several dimensions of disability and discusses their significance. Examples of the kinds of family-patient interactions that tend to infantilize the patient are given.

Christopherson also suggests four stages of disability, namely, the acute stage, the reconstruction stage, the plateau stage, and the deteriorative stage. The patient's goals and the significance for the family are discussed for each stage. He points out that we cannot assume necessarily that the families of rehabilitation patients will automatically have the intelligence, values, motivation, or resources to proceed independently toward the goals of rehabilitation. The nurse may have to perceive the family as a patient as well as the primary patient if the maximum rehabilitation is to be realized.

Reading 1
Perspectives in Rehabilitation
Victor A. Christopherson

Rehabilitation is in a sense the reversal of the natural order of things. Without the intervention of concerned individuals—in our day, trained and skilled professionals—those with poor health or acquired disability would deteriorate and become casualties of various kinds in a disproportionately short time. Indeed, as Robert Straus[1] points out: "Throughout our history, persons disabled by problems for which little could be done or which appeared only remotely related to the broader social need, have usually been subjected to a variety of harsh and hideous treatments. These have included death, torture, ostracism, imprisonment, slavery, relegation to a caste-like separate society, and, as a minimum, living under a cloud of stigma and chronic awareness of being abhorrent to fellow man."

Until fairly recent times the process which Charles Darwin labeled "survival of the fittest" has been a strong force in shaping human destiny, if not history. Darwin, of course, applied the principle to the forms of life further down the phylogenetic scale than humans, and while the phylogeny of humans may or may not have been affected, there is little doubt that the ontogeny of afflicted individuals was deeply modified. The natural selective process in recent times has been replaced by a higher principle—one dedicated to the proposition that all individuals have a right to health and to pursue goals in life reasonably congruent with their aspirations. In the interest of serving this principle the health sciences have evolved—not least among them, that body of knowledge and its applications referred to as rehabilitation.

Rehabilitation has meant different things at different times. In the earlier phases rehabilitation was seen principally in terms of dealing with the disabling entity as such, whether disease, accident, etc. As Jerome Myers[2] points out, the reparation of the physical damage or insufficiency does not necessarily bring about maximal functional restoration. Rehabilitation has been broadened accordingly to include social and vocational functioning, and in recent times, it has reached out to begin to include the patient's principal life space, particularly the family and the community.

Modern rehabilitation is not based entirely on humanitarian considerations; for those whose bent is more pragmatic, there is indisputable evi-

---

[1] Robert Straus, "Social Change and the Rehabilitation Concept," in Marvin Sussman (ed.), *Sociology and Rehabilitation*, American Sociological Association, 1965, p. 3.

[2] Jerome K. Myers, "Consequences and Prognoses of Disability," in ibid., pp. 35-36.

dence that rehabilitation is an economically feasible undertaking. One of the sources of investment return is the tax dollars provided to the economy by rehabilitated workers. This highly visible and ever dramatic aspect of rehabilitation should not be permitted to eclipse an equally valuable result, namely, restoring the individual's capacity to the point where he or she can reassume roles not specifically designed to provide income but are sometimes capable of providing many social, emotional, and psychological returns. An example of such a role for the handicapped woman is that of homemaker.[3]

Fortunately, great advances have been made in medical science at the same time that the base of rehabilitation has been broadened to include social and vocational aspects. Developing apace, these two aspects of rehabilitation have facilitated rapid advancement. The great advancement in medical science, however, has helped to create some of the problems it is called upon to solve. The survival capacity of individuals has been dramatically increased, with the result that many people with various kinds of congenital anomalies, diseases, and injuries who otherwise would have succumbed to these conditions continue to live and become rehabilitation clients. It may be that the unquestioned valuation of human life and the problem in the broadest sense of economics—population, medical priorities, use of facilities, etc.—are traveling on a collision course. For the time, however, rehabilitation is perceived as having intrinsic value in all dimensions, and it is with this view of things that we proceed.

History has long since witnessed the passing of the age of encyclopedic man, or the time when anyone could claim to have a more or less universal understanding of even one branch of knowledge. In medical science alone we have seen increasing and necessary specialization. Sometimes we see a specialty that provides competence for a number of conditions of illness, and sometimes a condition that requires a number of specialties. The latter has come to be known as the team approach. As a field of therapy and medicine that is concerned with the many aspects of restoration, function, and well-being of the person suffering from some sort of debilitating condition, rehabilitation seems ideally suited to the team approach.

One of the most recent specialties to function both independently and as a member of the rehabilitation team is that of the rehabilitation nurse. In a sense, as pointed out by Kendell,[4] rehabilitation nursing is good nursing care with the rehabilitation philosophy added to it. In another sense, however, rehabilitation nursing places a good deal more emphasis on certain

---

[3] Victor A. Christopherson, "Role Modifications of the Handicapped Homemaker," *Rehabilitation Literature,* vol. 21, no. 4, April 1960.
[4] H. Worley Kendell, "Rehabilitation—A Doctor's Viewpoint," *Hospitals,* vol. 30, pp. 39-43, 124, March 1956.

modes or categories of disability than other kinds of nursing, and it presupposes rather specialized knowledge of theory of rehabilitation along with the specialized appropriate techniques for the amelioration of each disabling condition. To the extent that good nursing is good nursing in any or all situations, rehabilitation nursing is and should be properly included in the education and training of all nurses. Those who plan to work specifically in the rehabilitation setting should continue to acquire the more specialized knowledge. This book provides both the orientation for nursing in general into the rehabilitation nursing specialty and the kinds of background and specialized knowledge required for rehabilitation practice.

Rehabilitation, perhaps even more than other branches of medical science, involves the taking into account of the total social-cultural configuration of the patient and his life space. One of the reasons for this is that most patients who are ministered to by nurses and physicians occupy the role of patient for relatively short periods. They soon recover, as from illness or surgery. The rehabilitation patient, however, often faces a permanent and/or chronic form of handicap. His task is essentially to learn to overcome, compensate, and adjust in such ways as to approach as nearly as possible the optimum level of functioning. Within his life space are his family, friends, resources, his own perception of modified roles and circumstances, and the various other social and cultural components which have gone into the fashioning of his phenotypic and constitutional makeup.

It is particularly appropriate for the nurse to have a broad base of knowledge concerning these matters. She may well be in the most strategic of roles with regard to the potential for influencing the thought, efforts, understanding, and morale of the patient. The effectiveness of the therapeutic transactions between nurse and patient may well depend upon how completely she understands and functions in terms of the sometimes elusive fact that the patient is a product of his culture.

Reading 2
Disability Viewed in Its Cultural Context
Richard W. Thoreson

The principle of rehabilitation which recognizes the worth of the handicapped person as a valuable human resource is a well-established one in our society.

Reprinted from *The Journal of Rehabilitation*, vol. 30, pp. 12–13, January–February 1964.

In rehabilitation the practical objective of restoring the individual to productive employment deftly intertwines with the humanitarian concern for the handicapped person's movement from abasing helplessness to a position of dignity and self-respect. Thus, it is not surprising that rehabilitation has captured the imagination—and financial support—of state and federal as well as numerous private agencies.

What, perhaps, appears less understandable is the stubborn reluctance displayed by a number of the handicapped to accept the help which is offered and take their first step away from helplessness toward a more constructive independent life. It is this paradoxical feature in disability toward which this paper will give its attention and in doing so suggest factors operative in the psychosocial meaning of disability.

BASIC SUPPOSITIONS

1 Illness (physical and mental) operates as a cultural safety valve: i.e., it gives the individual a socially acceptable reason for his withdrawal from the multiplicity of problems experienced in living [5]. Through this withdrawal, and the constructive effects of regression, the ego is protected from disintegration.

2 Social class differences prevail in the role that disability plays in binding anxiety. For example, many mental patients from the lower social class have been found to perceive the hospital as a place to "get their nerves fixed" [3]. These phenomena of significant and stable differences in kinds of symptoms utilized by mental patients from different social class levels appear to have been convincingly demonstrated.

3 Both physical and emotional disability can serve as a tangible focal point for the organization of anxieties and hostilities which the disabled person harbors toward himself, and those anxieties and hostilities often carried by parents and "important others" in his life space. For those with acquired disabilities, this implies the need to search for the meaning of illness or injury in the total life sphere of the individual. In the case of the congenitally disabled, there is need to be sensitive to the anxieties and hostilities of the client, and of family members, which permeate the disability configuration.

4 The disabled serve as a reference group for gauging the dimensions of normality and in this way assist the "normal" in maintaining his sense of identity and personal integrity. We can expect some attempt at enforcement of this dichotomy by "normals" (such as employers) to "magically" ward off threat to their status.

5 Rehabilitation of the disabled person, a culture-bound concept, is rooted in the middle-class Protestant ethic: work is good, and man should strive continuously for self-improvement [8]. The rehabilitation counselor who is aware of this phenomenon will understand why a less than optimal (in the counselor's eyes) solution may sometimes be selected by a given

individual, or indeed why the organization of a handicapped person's life within a disability could represent a meaningful solution to his dilemma of coping with problems of existence.

6 The individual's choice of disability, its nature and temporal significance in the life of the disabled, has distinct implications for rehabilitation. Wittkower [9] has suggested that emotionally disturbing events precede the onset of symptoms in tuberculosis. Menninger [4] found physical illness to be a common substitute reaction among patients scheduled to enter therapy.

Parenthetically, the nature and site of the disability or disease appears to bear a predictable relationship to overall personality organization. Fisher and Cleveland [1] found that a particular aspect of body image, "the manner in which an individual perceives his body boundaries"—either as sharply bounded or permeable—relates to particular physiological patterns. Patients with such diseases as rheumatoid arthritis, neurodermatitis, and conversion symptoms involving the musculature have higher "barrier" and lower "penetration" scores than patients with stomach ulcers or spastic colitis. "Hard shell" responses appear to denote a higher level of ego integration, suggesting greater ability to be independent, to formulate goals, and to exhibit forceful action in approaching tasks.

Thus, for the disabled, the greater the extent of perceptual diffuseness, i.e., boundary vagueness, the greater the likelihood of limited personality integration and fragmentation under stress.

7 Barely hidden from conscious awareness by members of our culture is the view of disability as a symbolic representation of their unacceptable, fear-evoking impulses. Imbedded in this view appears to be a catastrophic reaction to vaguely defined threats to body integrity and an infantile fear of the return to a dependency status. The inadequate handling of hostility in our middle-class culture appears to make its members particularly vulnerable to intense guilt over and concomitant fear of retribution for their covert hostility.

IMPLICATIONS FOR THE REHABILITATION COUNSELOR

1 The rehabilitation counselor should be familiar with the constructive effect of illness and/or disability for both the individual and society. For any given person, disability may well represent his best means of extracting minimal satisfactions from living. Pause to consider whether we really should expect a quadraplegic to suffer "the slings and arrows of outrageous fortune" which are inevitably bound to his independent life outside the hospital. Could we rather accept his decision to live within the hospital comfortably fulfilling the demands of the "sick role"?

The rehabilitation counselor, quite justifiably, feels a certain vested interest in maximum rehabilitation; however, his enthusiasm should not shield him from the understanding that each human being is entitled to make his own unique transaction with the external world. It must be the client's transaction, not the counselor's.

2   Class differences in attitudes prevail toward physical health or illness, toward work and long-range goals, and, indeed, toward the overall concept of rehabilitation.

For the lower-class client, damage to the physical self represents a severe blow to ego integration. Consequently, the counselor who expects a rapid and smooth adjustment to a severe loss of physical prowess by such a client is likely to experience recurrent disappointment. Nor is the counselor likely to find among lower-class members the elegant insight into psychological dynamics that is found among middle- and upper-class clients.

The counselor who unwittingly imposes his own middle-class value system onto such a client clearly risks communication of disrespect for the client's values in such a way that the client may be driven into sullen defiance. Parenthetically, this defiance can serve to confirm the counselor's "self-fulfilling prophecy" to the effect that such a client has "low rehabilitation potential."

Obviously, the middle-class client suffering from cortical damage presents a quite different, but equally difficult rehabilitation problem.

3   Separation of the physically, mentally, or emotionally handicapped from society proper—independent of humanitarian motives—carries with it a possible "ghetto" effect in which the handicapped in toto take on the stereotypal features of their most extreme deviates. We infer from this that any large, well-publicized community program for severely disabled persons has the potentiality of mobilizing prejudice against the handicapped, and must be handled with delicacy.

4   The rehabilitation counselor's "hard sell" of the disabled qua handicapped to community groups, prospective employers, etc., must be carefully executed. The counselor must remember that "protesting too much" can serve to rigidify the normal-handicapped schism in the community and to enhance the probability of further sensitization to the disabled's deviation from normality.

5   In the instance of acquired disability or disease there is a critical need for the counselor to tease out the relationship between the specific encounter of disability and personality in the life space of the handicapped. To what extent does the disability represent a fear-engulfed relinquishment of active engagement with a hostile world by the encounter in the family configuration of the handicapped?

Only in his sophisticated understanding of the purposefulness of the disability can the counselor effect maximum rehabilitation.

6   As disability is defined in terms of its deviation from a social-ethical norm [8] it follows that the greater the tendency for the counselor to view his role as helping the disabled person because he is disabled (and handicapped), the greater the potential danger of the counselor's promoting the dichotomy between the normal and disabled. (Help is defined here as a guilt-ridden reaction of a societal member toward a debased, piteous creature.)

Conversely, the greater the tendency on the part of the rehabilitation counselor to view his role as helping the disabled person because he is another human being, the greater the potentialities for melting the rigid role barriers between the disabled and normal. As Garrett so aptly states, "Treat the individual, not the disability" [2].

SUMMARY

There are a number of forces operative within the client and within the culture proper which magnify the rehabilitation problem. In the complex interplay of forces, the counselor's contribution to his handicapped clients involves, in large measure, his communicating to them that they are human beings worthy of respect. The counselor's is a catalytic function in which an attempt is made to trigger the clients' inner forces toward growth, and to neutralize the operative regressive forces toward helplessness and dependency.

What the counselor comes to mean to his clients, his warmth, caring, respect, his overall meanings are more important than what he says or even what he does for them [6]. Should the counselor perform flawlessly all phases of his counseling techniques and rehabilitation plan and yet communicate disdain for his handicapped client, he may well "chalk up" another rehabilitation, but he will have done a basic disservice to a fellow human being and will have provided an impetus to the client to cling more rigidly to the handicapped role.

On the other hand, if the counselor conveys to his handicapped client clearly and honestly that the latter is a person worthy of dignity and respect, he may make errors in counseling strategy, but he will have initiated a richly productive human relationship and provided a service that can lead to a more fulfilling and personally gratifying life for a fellow human being.

REFERENCES

1. Fisher, S., and Cleveland, E. Body Image and Personality. Princeton: Van Nostrand, 1958.
2. Garrett, J. F. (ed.). Psychological Aspects of Physical Disability. Washington, D.C.: OVR, Government Printing Office, Rehabilitation Service Series 210, 1952.
3. Hollingshead, A. B., and Redlich, F. C. Social Class and Mental Illness. New York: Wiley and Sons, 1958.
4. Menninger, K. A. Man against Himself. New York: Harcourt, Brace and Co., 1938.
5. Parsons, T. Illness and the role of the physician: A sociological perspective. *Amer. J. Ortho-Psychiat.*, 1951, **21**:452-460.
6. Snyder, W. U. The psychotherapy research program at the Pennsylvania State University. *J. Counsel. Psychol.*, 1957, **4**:9-13.
7. Szasz, T. S. The myth of mental illness. *Amer. Psychologist*, 1960, **15**:113-118.

8 Vineberg, S. E. Concerning job readiness. *J. of Rehab.*, 1958, **6**:9.
9 Wittkower, E. A. A Psychiatrist Looks at Tuberculosis. London: National Assoc. for the Prevention of Tuberculosis, 1949.

Reading 3
Cultural Influences on Patient Behavior
Gracia S. McCabe

When the cultural backgrounds of the nurse and patient differ, some common ground of understanding must be established in order for communication and better nursing care to take place.

We accept quite readily that members of any subgroup, either racial or cultural, in our society present differing problems and behavior in connection with their health care. One example, difference in response to pain by members of Jewish, Italian, and "Old American" groups, has been pointed out by Zborowski [1]. These differences may logically be expected to become evident in the hospital adjustment of representatives of these groups.

As a nurse in a southern hospital I have been interested in the cultural heritage of Negro patients and uncomfortably aware of the fact that my lack of knowledge of their perceptions of illness and hospitalization markedly interfered with my ability to provide adequate nursing care.

A fairly exhaustive search of nursing literature, however, revealed a virtual absence of information on the nursing care of such patients. This paper attempts to narrow this gap by reporting a brief, exploratory study of Negro patients in a southern hospital where the patients observed were predominantly rural people.

For several weeks I had observed student nurses caring for such Negro patients on one hospital ward. Subsequently, I returned to this ward for more detailed observations on the nursing care of these patients, and worked as a general duty nurse for a five-week period—four weeks of day duty and one of evening duty. Although assigned to a nursing team, the number of patients I cared for was reduced to half that of other nurses in the ward. This

Reprinted from *American Journal of Nursing*, vol. 60, pp. 1101–1104, August 1960.
The author wishes to express her appreciation to Dr. Harry W. Martin for his help in the writing of this paper, and to Mary V. Cheek, director of nursing service at the North Carolina Memorial Hospital, and her staff for their excellent cooperation in carrying out this study.
This investigation was part of a study concerned with the application of social science and psychiatric concepts in nursing. The larger study was supported by training grant 2M-6157, National Institute of Mental Health, United States Public Health Service.

allowed time for a wider range of observations on the ward and more prolonged contact with individual patients. The focus of the study was limited to the patient and his adjustment to illness and hospitalization. No attempt was made to compare these observations with patients from other groups.

THE WARD SITUATION

The ward was a combined medical and surgical unit and one of the busiest in the hospital. Its busyness was a compound of several factors: the patients were usually quite ill; medical and surgical doctors were on the floor much of the time; medical and nursing students were assigned on rotation; and personnel from auxiliary services were frequently present. Thus, the number of personnel who were present gave the ward an atmosphere of intense activity during the day.

A rather marked change occurred in the ward atmosphere in the evening. The most obvious change was a decrease in numbers of nursing service personnel and doctors. Medical and nursing students were usually absent. The reduction of personnel reflected itself in working relationships; rates of interaction were reduced and the interactions themselves became less formal. Informality in working relationships increased among nursing personnel and also between medical and nursing personnel. The exercise of authority was less evident and cooperative effort increased.

THE PATIENTS AND HOSPITAL ADJUSTMENT

Most of the patients were of low economic status and poorly educated. They were generally considered sicker than patients in other areas of the hospital and usually had multiple diagnoses. Their conditions suggested that they did not seek hospitalization here until seriously and often critically ill.

It is important to recognize that these patients came to the hospital from a segregated society. Although the situation is changing, "the significant point is that in the rural South segregation is fairly generally accepted, either unconsciously as an unquestioned matter-of-fact or consciously, as a matter of expediency" [2].

CONCEPTS OF ILLNESS

No attempt was made in this study to explore patients' concepts of the causes of illness; however, generally they did not understand their illnesses and often described their symptoms in folk terms. Frazier, in his discussion of the psychological factors influencing Negro health, states:

... It is not surprising to find comparatively few Negroes ascribing disease to physical causes. When the writer [Frazier] has inquired of many Negroes the cause of disease, they have seemed puzzled. "People just get sick," was the extent of their insight in many cases [3].

A similar lack of understanding of the causes of illness was evident in most of the patients observed. Their concept of the body and its organ system was generally vague. Pain was identified in general terms as "the miseries." Many patients conceived of their illnesses as results of "something got in there"; this was particularly true of patients with head pain. There were also suggestions from some patients that their diseases were associated with powers of witchcraft, especially among older patients with diseases of the sensory organs.

These vague perceptions of the body and its diseases created difficulty for nurses. It was hard, sometimes almost impossible, to explain the purpose and procedure of treatments to patients who did not hold the usual concepts of illness. Furthermore, the lack of understanding of simple biophysiological functions made it difficult for some patients to grasp the significance of their medical regimes; they often appeared to cooperate in order to please the doctors and nurses rather than from an understanding of their conditions and the purposes of their treatments which apparently had little meaning for them.

Nurses were frequently frustrated by such behavior and by feelings of inadequacy in dealing with the situation. Personnel were particularly distressed by patients whose illnesses were not responsive to treatment. They sought to guide and support patients in understanding their illnesses and health care. Patients would listen, but their comments and subsequent behavior indicated that many persisted in clinging to their own interpretations of their illness. In despair one nurse explained, "They don't want to know what's wrong, they're happier with their own ideas."

ACCEPTANCE OF NURSING CARE

Despite the degree of illness present many patients tended to display a reluctance to accept complete nursing care from nurses. Whenever possible they helped themselves—assuming their personal care, making their bed, or tidying their rooms. If physically unable to do any of these things, patients often made apologies for having to accept assistance. Ambulant patients frequently took pride in helping sicker, bedridden patients; they seemed more content when they could be of service by feeding other patients, assisting those who needed help, calling for aid for those who needed help, calling for aid for those who needed attention. Women were inclined to do this more than men.

Many patients expressed feelings of being unworthy of the care and attention received. Though seriously ill, they were frequently hesitant to ask for relief of pain, even at times when pain was evidently severe. In some cases patients denied pain even when nurses had sound reasons for suspecting its existence. A frequent comment heard in nursing reports and in general conversation was "they suffer in silence." One nurse said, "They just hurt and hurt. They seem to think they're supposed to."

REQUESTING NURSING CARE

Many patients were obviously hesitant to ask for nursing service. Some never made requests of nurses; in such instances fellow patients would sometimes solicit nursing care for these patients. On occasions patients who were otherwise quite verbal were noted to have difficulty making requests and often fell into stuttering speech when asking for specific care. Some patients sought help through indirect means, for example, beseeching looks. If nurses responded to this cue with the slightest indication of recognizing the need patients were likely to verbalize their requests.

COMMUNICATING DISSATISFACTION

Direct expressions of dissatisfaction were very infrequent. It may be suggested, however, that one fairly frequent mode of expressing dissatisfaction was through joking and humorous behavior [4]. By use of this technique patients may give vent to feelings without jeopardizing themselves. A problem of the nursing staff is that of understanding the function of this behavior in order to avoid the error of thinking of such behavior only as interesting and "cute." For example:

> An elderly patient recovering from a prostatectomy was observed while being ambulated by a nursing aide and an orderly. When the aide swung his feet off the bed, the patient drew his face up in an expression of pain. He put up his hand and said, "Hold on there! I know I look hard and tough but I'm not today." The attendants laughed and continued their work in a more gentle manner. They related the incident to other staff members as an example of the patient's humor. Later the patient voluntarily recalled this incident and expressed anger because of the "rough treatment" he had received.

A mode of concealing expression of feelings, similar to the humorous approach, needing closer examination but deserving report, is the use of terms of address. Elderly Negro patients often used the term "nursey" in referring to their nurses; this was strongly resented by the people so addressed. Endearing terms such as "honey" or "sweetie," frequently used by women, created little resentment. Although many nurses may disagree, it can be hypothesized that such terms can be used to express hostility—particularly when patients are under stress. Again, it is important that the nurse recognize the function of this behavior for the patient. If she works in terms of this hypothesis, she should guard against reacting negatively to the underlying implications. One experience illustrates the general point:

> I approached a middle-aged woman who had recently been admitted. The patient required complete nursing care to which she submitted quietly. She spoke very little; her conversation was limited to replies to direct questions. The relationship continued for several days. On some occasions the patient would turn away from me, pull her curtain, or close the door to her room; when it was necessary for her to speak, her voice was pleasant, and she consistently called me "sweetie." During this period the doctor recommended a liver biopsy; the patient became upset and angry, refused the test and threatened to leave the hospital. I talked with her, encouraged her to discuss the matter with her husband and interpreted the procedure to both patient and husband. As the relationship progressed the patient began to talk about her fear of pain; this was relayed to the doctor; arrangements were made for special anesthesia to be used. The patient became less apprehensive and agreed to undergo the procedure. During the remainder of her hospitalization she was less seclusive; she opened her door and curtains and conversed more freely with staff. She had periods of pain and anxiety but at such times she asked for me and was apparently afforded relief by this relationship. Noteworthy, she stopped calling me "sweetie" and addressed me as Mrs. McCabe.

Patients often gave evidence of being frightened people. Three major fears were identified—fear of death, fear of the dark, and fear of being left alone. These appeared to be closely associated. Many patients were afraid of the dark, particularly if they were in a room alone. Some patients screamed from fear of being alone, others withdrew into lighted bathrooms or under bed covers to get away from whatever threat they envisioned. The primary fear seemed to be death though patients seldom expressed more than an apologetic, "I'm just scared of the dark." Some would reach out physically and hold nurses at the bedside. One patient, clutching my arm, pleaded, "Don't leave me alone to die." Fear of personal death was present among patients who were critically ill. There also seemed to be a prevalent fear of the hospital as a place where one dies, particularly evident among uneducated patients. Such fear may have been exaggerated beyond realistic limits because many patients had been referred from smaller hospitals for more specialized or intensive medical care. Patients frequently interpreted this as an indication of impending death—expressed in comments that, "People are sent here to die."

Patients freely resorted to religion for solace and comfort. The religious activities on the ward were one of its most outstanding characteristics; patients frequently chanted, prayed, sang hymns, preached, and encouraged one another to "trust in the Lord" [5]. Women patients engaged in religious activities openly. Men, particularly older ones, expressed faith in God and sought comfort from religion, but their supplications were generally less public.

Religious activity was most pronounced in a 10-bed ward of women. Ambulatory patients from other rooms frequently visited this ward and took part in the "services"; similar activities were seldom initiated in smaller rooms. Preaching was rather common but it did not always result in solace or improved relationships among patients. Verbal, and on one occasion physical, aggression occurred among patients competing to prove their "good works" and favor in the sight of God. In a majority of instances, the aggressive patients had terminal illnesses, though it was not clear whether these patients were aware of their prognoses. The observations suggest that resort to religion may be a fairly reliable index to nursing needs of many Negro patients. It may be that although religious expression appeared to be a communication from the patient to his God, these verbalizations were employed by some patients as an indirect method of expressing nursing needs to personnel.

Whether the source of discomfort was physical pain or emotional stress, many patients implied that only God was interested in their troubles. Personnel often responded to these religious demonstrations by withdrawing or jesting about them. A few attempts at responding differently to some of these situations resulted in better understanding of patients and provided information for helping them in their distress. For example:

An elderly Negro woman was admitted with metastatic carcinoma. She made many demands upon the staff and her constant calls for attention soon resulted in a general pattern of avoidance by the staff. She disturbed other patients with her constant talking. Several patients advised her to cease complaining and "pray to God"; she then began periodical singing and chanting, often accompanied by other patients. I approached this patient during one period of particularly loud and excited chanting. After watching me for several minutes the patient lowered her voice and then stopped chanting. She started talking to me about God and His concern for her (the patient); she then expressed loneliness and a feeling that everyone disliked her. Thereafter the patient talked frequently with me, telling me about her daughter living in a distant city who "doesn't care about me any more."

She often asked me to talk with her and expressed fear of being alone. Her demands decreased; she could accept time limits and wait for personnel. She became generally quieter and made fewer demands of the staff.

THE NURSE AND THE NEGRO PATIENT

The attitudes and behavior of the nurses working on the ward indicated a strong motivation to give optimal nursing care to these Negro patients. However, their comments also revealed feelings of frustration and hopelessness associated with their work. These nurses were busy but conversations suggested that the frequent sense of incomplete performance which they experienced resulted from something more than limitations of time. Technically, they provided competent nursing care; personally, they were interested and concerned for their patients. Still, problems existed which prevented fulfillment of the nurses' goals in patient care.

Nurses, like most other people, sometimes find it difficult to understand and accept forms of behavior which differ from their own. With respect to these patients, the nursing approach was sometimes based on preconceptions not always relevant to the situation. Negro patients were not infrequently viewed as poor, uneducated, superstitious people who believed more in witch doctors than in medicine. There was evidence to support some of these opinions; however, error can result from overgeneralization and dependence upon stereotypes of Negro patients [6]. For example, many patients who were employed by whites exhibited behavior indicating a reluctance to accept ministrations from nurses, even ordinary nursing procedures willingly administered. Since it was necessary for these patients to receive care from nursing personnel, they were forced to adapt in some manner. One adaptive pattern identified was complete submission expressed by childlike behavior. Nurses came to expect this behavior from all Negro patients and tended to deal with them as children rather than as adults. This was reinforced and perpetuated by the usual behavior between rural Negroes and "white folk." When patients failed to respond as anticipated nurses sometimes regarded them as problems.

The "busyness" of the nurse was a factor separating nurse and patient. It seemingly provided a rational explanation to patients for their reluctance to "bother" the staff. They were quite aware that nurses were busy people and seldom made requests or engaged nurses in more than brief conversation until assured they were not imposing upon their time. The separation of nurse from patients was increased when patients became aware that nurses had specific patient assignments. With this knowledge some patients hesitated to seek aid from nurses to whom they were not assigned. Although such assignments were made, they were not so rigidly adhered to as patients seemed to think. To exemplify the barrier created by the patient's interpretation:

> A nurse assigned to one of 10 patients in a ward stopped to help a paraplegic man (not assigned to her) who obviously needed assistance moving; later, she stopped to help him arrange his tray for lunch. He shyly thanked her after each of these instances. The following day this nurse was assigned to the patient. When she went in to him he said, "Are you my nurse today? I'm glad; now I can ask you to help me. Were you mad with me for calling you yesterday?"

There was evidence of lack of understanding in many nurse-patient situations. The patient was frequently unable to understand his own situation and unable to understand the situation of the nurse. The problem facing many nurses seemed to result not from disinterest but from a lack of understanding of the sociocultural aspects of the lives of many Negro patients and ineffective communication with these patients. The staff nurse in this environment was often uncomfortable. Frustration occurred at two levels: nurses were sometimes unable to identify patients' needs even though they recognized that "something was wrong"; nurses, having identified patients' needs, were not always able to institute effective nursing measures because of seeming lack of cooperation from the patient. In either case, nurses were left with the frustration of providing incomplete nursing care and were deprived of full nursing satisfaction.

CONCLUSION

Some tentative conclusions may be warranted on the basis of this exploration. It seems necessary to understand something of the larger society which contributes to the general patterns of thought and behavior of both nurses and these Negro patients in order to understand the behaviors observed during illness and hospitalization. Patterns of racial etiquette are changing; nevertheless, the expectations and behavior of many Negro patients are largely based on adjustment to segregation. Patients from rural backgrounds come to the hospital with definite expectations regarding the behavior of white people. The ". . . axiom that 'white folks is white folks' . . . implies a set of expectations and proscriptions with respect to behavior . . ." [7]. Similarly, the nurse has expectation regarding the behavior of Negroes [8].

Preconceptions of behavior as they exist in the mind of patient and nurse can present complications in the medical setting because illness, by its very nature, presents a stress situation which may exaggerate feelings and behavior. Also, hospitalization often brings about a reversal of roles in those hospital situations where Negro patients receive the professional services of white nurses; neither party may be prepared for this.

It would seem that the nurse plays a crucial part in the adjustment of the Negro patient to the hospital. If so, it is reasonable to assume that understanding the social and cultural backgrounds of these patients in relation to nursing situations would help correct misconceptions, remove some communication barriers, and improve nursing care. The hospital experience could become a more complete therapeutic experience for the patient while being more satisfying for the nurse.

REFERENCES

1 Zborowski, Mark. Cultural components in response to pain. *Journal of Social Issues,* **8**:16-30, 1952.
2 Johnson, Charles S. *Patterns of Negro Segregation.* New York, Harper & Bros., 1943, p. 249.
3 Frazier, E. Franklin. Psychological factors in Negro health. *Journal of Social Forces,* 3:488-490, March 1925, p. 488.
4 Johnson, op. cit., p. 284.
5 Rose, Arnold. *The Negro in America.* New York, Harper & Bros., 1948, pp. 296-297.
6 Simpson, George, and Yinger, J. Milton. *Racial and Cultural Minorities: An Analysis of Prejudice and Discrimination.* New York, Harper & Bros., 1953, pp. 239-241.
7 Lewis, Hylan. *Blackways of Kent.* Chapel Hill, N.C., University of North Carolina Press, 1955, p. 313.
8 Simpson and Yinger, op. cit.

Reading 4
Territoriality in Man: A Comparison of Behavior in Home and Hospital
Arthur D. Colman

Until recently, the emotionally disturbed were almost always diagnosed and treated in an environment familiar and "natural" to the examiner but unfamiliar and "artificial" to the examinee, despite 50 years of evidence that behavior is best understood when viewed as a function of the environment in which it is performed.

Ethologists such as Lorenz [7], Tinbergen [12], and Scott [11], who study animals in the field rather than in the laboratory, have developed the con-

Reprinted from *American Journal of Ortho-Psychiatry,* vol. 38, pp. 464-468, April 1968.

cept of territoriality, "the taking possession, use and defense of a territory on the part of a living organism." A male stickleback fish presents a clear illustration of the phenomenon. He easily drives away another male stickleback when attacked on his own territory (the area around his nest), but may lose his fighting dominance if the attack occurs a few centimeters away [13]. Similarly, a small, weak dog will routinely attack a larger, stronger dog if the meeting is on his own territory. But while territoriality has been investigated most thoroughly in fish and birds, it also holds true for mammals and primates [1,8].

The role of territoriality in humans is less well understood, perhaps because it is difficult to separate from factors of social organization. Hall [5] used territoriality as one of the "primary message systems" helpful in defining varieties of human culture. Horowitz [6] has experimented with changing dimensions of "personal space" in man for normals and schizophrenics. On the family level, the frequent designation of various rooms or individual pieces of furniture as "father's" or "mother's" and our desire to give each child a room of his own reflect human territorial needs. Many of us can only work or relax in one part of the home or library, or have one area, perhaps a bar stool, where we feel secure. Children often have their own "secret place" even after they have given up their security blanket or their favorite doll.

HOME VISITS:
A SHIFT OF TERRITORIES

Reports on observation and treatment of the disturbed family in the home setting have been increasingly frequent [3,9], and home visits have even been used to prevent hospitalization [4]. All reports comment that behavior which appears maladaptive in the doctor's office or hospital often makes sense when viewed in the home.

During the past year I observed "normal" families in both artificial and natural group settings as part of a study of pregnant women who had no history of physical or mental disorder. The women met in a group once a week from the second trimester of pregnancy to six weeks post partum. Each was seen with her husband in the clinic, in the labor and delivery suite, on the maternity floor, and during a home visit post partum. I was struck by the different psychological pictures obtained of the same people in different settings. Although the group allowed standard diagnostic appraisals of individual personality and interpersonal communication modes, it provided less useful information on adaptational mechanisms more relevant to the mothering adjustment I was studying. Even more striking was the disparity between the appearance of the husbands in the hospital setting and in their own homes. My first impressions of the "weak ineffectual husband" on hospital sighting (the common stereotype of the man of the family seen in clinic or office) simply did not hold up when he sat in his own easy chair.

I found that the physical home setting, the peculiar arrangement of family life space, was a most valuable aid in understanding the form of the couple's adjustment. The couples in which one or both members appeared emotionally disturbed away from home had rigid, constricted, yet personally significant home environments which seemed to be an important factor in maintaining the family equilibrium. A case history focused on the husband of one of the women in my group will illustrate this point.

USE OF HOME FOR SECURITY: TERRITORIAL DOMINANCE

Mrs. Pond was still working as a secretary when she began coming to the group in her fourth month of pregnancy. She talked about her husband frequently as an unsuccessful harpsichordist who had little use for the conventional ways of making a living. She was bitter that his musical talents should be atrophying, yet she expressed anxiety about their financial insecurity, particularly in relation to the expected child. Mr. Pond had recently begun training as a computer programmer, but she had little faith that he would last. She was intent on involving her husband in the pregnancy and took him with her to natural childbirth classes. At first he resisted, but eventually he became a natural-childbirth afficionado, probably motivated by his avowed dislike of doctors.

In the seventh month of the pregnancy, a close friend of Mr. Pond's became acutely paranoid and was hospitalized on a ward which emphasized involvement of family and friends in the treatment process. The Ponds participated in biweekly meetings of patients and their families. Mr. Pond characteristically remained silent even when spoken to, except for unprovoked outbursts against the staff. His relationship with the patient was considered "pathological." Both of them spoke of feeling a communion in their music which shut out everything and everyone else. Quotes from the staff refer to Mr. Pond as "disturbed," "irrational," "schizophrenic."

My first contact with Mr. Pond was during his wife's labor. He was extremely attentive and remained in constant physical touch with her. He would not leave the labor room when the doctor came to do a pelvic examination or when the nurse came to "prep" her. The medical staff was so angered they threatened to call the police. Mrs. Pond suggested to her husband that they needed the doctors and perhaps should compromise their "togetherness," but Mr. Pond refused to obey any of the rules. My contacts with Mr. Pond were marked by the sparseness of verbal communication, although there was much angry, suspicious glaring on his part. He did not want to talk about himself, his wife, or the baby.

The home visit took place three weeks post partum. The house was an old, three-story Victorian structure sandwiched between commercial buildings in a slum area. No light or life was visible from the street, for the window shades were pulled to the sill. Mr. Pond greeted me in a warm, gracious manner and asked me to call him by his first name. He led me one flight up to a spacious living room almost entirely bare of furniture. Only an old stuffed chair and a mattress covered by an embroidered blanket provided seats. Unpacked and half-opened cartons and a scattering of books lay on the bare wood floor. The white walls seemed to have occasional doodles on them. An adjoining room was totally bare except for an impressive double-keyboard harpsichord and a viola da gamba with a music stand.

I was offered coffee and sat down in the chair; but Mr. Pond pressed me to sit with his wife on the mattress. He then took the stuffed chair and stretched out his legs so that I could not straighten mine from their cramped position without touching his. The next hour was spent in conversation controlled by Mr. Pond. The Ponds were at ease and calm in contrast to my own anxiousness in the unfamiliar and provocative surroundings. He talked about his home and "his rooms" (the ones we were in) with pride, referring to their present state as "being what I want—I have the feeling that I will never grow out of this house—that I will never get too big for it." Mrs. Pond explained that the living and music rooms were "his," while the bedroom and adjacent baby's room were "hers." Toward the end of the visit, Mr. Pond talked of the open-house musicals they had on Saturdays, when people came to listen or to play without needing to tell who they were or to commit themselves to future weeks.

At no time during the visit was Mr. Pond's relaxed and confident tone lost. Nor did I see any signs of the disturbed behavior that had characterized his outside-home contacts. His needs for situational control, which made his behavior so unpleasant and even bizarre in the hospital, were satisfied by the aggressive seating arrangement and the security he felt in his self-styled rooms.

DISCUSSION

This case is an extreme example of behavioral shifts which can be fruitfully viewed as being modulated by "territorial" concerns. Most individuals are capable of maintaining reasonably appropriate and consistent behavior in a majority of environments and interpersonal situations. Yet for some who find personal relationships particularly difficult, territoriality and idiosyntonic territorial structuring may provide useful personality support. Mr. Pond used the barren, doodled walls, the half-opened packing boxes, and the contrasting magnificent musical instruments to construct a highly personalized living space, an externalization of poorly integrated and conflicting aspects of his own personality, but nevertheless a place where he felt comfortable and secure. Its very lack of completeness and harmony in a conventional sense freed him from a constricting and demanding world. "I have the feeling I will never grow out of this—that I will never get too big for it."

Horowitz [6] has shown that the "body buffer zone" of schizophrenics is larger than that of normals. His experiments were done in a laboratory situation, that is, the territory was unfamiliar to the people being examined. It would be interesting to see if the individual's "buffer zone" diminished in his own environment where the territory itself could offer protection. In Mr. Pond's case, the entire house in a sense acted as a "buffer zone," allowing him to feel secure within its protective confines. Furthermore, inside its territory he was able to use spatial relationships as interpersonal control measures, as illustrated by the inhibiting and provocative seating arrangement he skillfully manipulated during my visit. A shift in dominance with territoriality, alluded to earlier in dogs and sticklebacks, certainly was evident in the changed relationship with Mr. Pond when we were in my territory (the hospital) versus his.

It is striking how often the hospitalized mental patient and the prisoner do not have a home of their own. If it is true that these people with least potential for social adaptation are in most need of territorial strengths, then not having a home is a circular dilemma. They have lost (or never had) the skills to build one, yet its absence deprives them of the supporting structure they need. Perhaps some of the success of the halfway house and other more "natural" community treatment facilities is related to their provision of personally identifiable territories in contrast to the anonymous collectivity of the large hospital and prison. Recently, Russel Barton [2] described the use of room dividers to give each patient his own space, in these terms: "Every patient, no matter how sick he is, needs some privacy and a place he can call his own where he may store his personal possessions. After all, man, like other animals, has territorial instincts."

REFERENCES

1 Ardrey, R. 1966. The Territorial Imperative. Athenaeum, New York.
2 Barton, R. 1966. The patient's personal territory. *Hospital and Community Psychiat.* 17:336.
3 Fisch, R. 1964. Home visits in a private psychiatric practice. *Family Process.* 3:114–119.
4 Friedman, T., A. Becker, and L. Weiner. 1964. Psychiatric home treatment service: Preliminary report of five years of clinical experience. *Am. J. Psychiat.* 120:782–788.

5 Hall, E. 1959. The Silent Language. Doubleday, New York.
6 Horowitz, M., D. Duff, and L. Stratton. 1964. The body buffer zone: An exploration of personal space. *Arch. Gen. Psychiat.* **11**:65-69.
7 Lorenz, K. 1952. King Solomon's Ring. Methuen, London.
8 Lorenz, K. 1966. On Aggression. Harcourt, Brace and World, New York.
9 Morgan, R. 1963. The extended home visit in psychiatric research and treatment. *Psychiat.* **26**:168-175.
10 Nice, M. 1941. The role of territory in bird life. *Amer. Midland Nat.* **26**:441-487.
11 Scott, J. 1958. Animal Behavior. University of Chicago Press.
12 Tinbergen, N. 1958. Curious Naturalists. Basic Books, New York.
13 Tinbergen, N. 1951. The Study of Instincts. Oxford University Press, London.

Reading 5

The Patient and the Family

Victor A. Christopherson

The images that come to mind when we encounter the term patient would make an interesting and possibly profitable study. To what extent, we might ask, would these images reflect uniformities among patients or types of patients? If, indeed, there were pronounced uniformities, to what extent would they be valid, and to what extent convenient but questionable stereotypes?

Individuals who have physical limitations differ markedly, of course, in terms of such variables as pain, the progressive or stabilizing nature of the disease, the residual endurance and mobility, the extent of body involvement, and the length of time afflicted. If there are basic or generic qualities that are shared and that characterize the patient to fit into some sort of subculture, it would seem that first he would have to undergo a certain amount of taxonomic shuffling in terms of the particular condition, the relative severity of his case, and his unique reactions. The symptoms and sequelae arising from each disabling agent are frequently condition-specific, or peculiar to the condition or disease in question.

The condition-specific uniformities, for the most part, are physical. For example, among those suffering from arthritis of particular variety, we could expect to find a considerable amount of pain, progressive deterioration of joints and muscles, a progressive loss of mobility, endurance, and motor function, certain side effects due to prolonged treatment with steroids, and probably a number of other symptoms. Even so, when his specific physical

Reprinted from *Rehabilitation Literature*, vol. 23, no. 2, pp. 34-41, February 1962.

limitation is compared with all others in the same category, when his material resources are considered, and when his own unique adjustment to the limitation is taken into account, the significance of the uniformities gives way to that of the individualized aspects of the patient. "The patient" like "the average" becomes an amorphous image in the mind's eye, a statistical myth that takes on meaning only in terms of his many alter egos.

Understanding of a given patient becomes grounded in the critical, evaluative perception of him as he functions in relation to the particular limitations and as he interacts with those who occupy his social world. In this framework it might be argued that a physical limitation is not so much a determinant of behavior as it is a catalyst that reveals and throws into sharper relief the more basic personality and behavior tendencies already present.[1]

DIMENSIONS OF DISABILITY

Physical limitation then can serve to emphasize the patient's unique qualities rather than submerge them under the general rubric of disability. An emergent need is for a means of perceiving the patient at once as an individual effecting a personal adjustment to a particular limitation and as an interacting member of a number of social groups, in each of which he has a productive level and a productive potential. In order to provide such a means for characterizing the patient the following dimensions[2] of disability are suggested: protensity, intensity, extensity, and autoviability.[3]

Protensity is intended to indicate the length of time from the onset of the limitation to the present. This dimension has somewhat different implications for the different limiting conditions. The implications of time for a progressively deteriorative-type disease are obviously different from those of the disease that stabilizes after a certain time with no foreseeable recurrence likely. Presumably, the medication, therapy, vocational goals, avocational

---

[1] The reactions to physical limitation are typically highly individual and are not infrequently as productive of the disability as the degree of limitation itself. To put it another way, the manner in which the individual takes his physical limitation into account or integrates it into a larger plan of life is often more important in gauging the actual extent of disability than is the actual, objective, or measurable amount of physical limitation present. The distinction suggested here between physical limitation and disability is an operational one—it depends upon the way one uses words and the meanings one intends to convey. The meaning here intended is that disability and physical limitation are not synonymous but that the former derives from the product of the limitation per se and the individual's reaction to it.

[2] The term dimension of disability is suggested in this context because each of the dimensions discussed can be quantified on the basis of objective facts and formulas. Thus all patients having a certain type of physical limitation fall at different points along the particular dimension under consideration in relation to all other individuals having the same type limitation.

[3] The first three terms were introduced and discussed briefly by the author in *Rehab. Lit.*, vol. 21, no. 4, p. 113 (footnote), April 1960. These dimensions are being researched at the University of Arizona through the provisions of a grant by the Office of Vocational Rehabilitation and the Agricultural Experiment Station at the University.

pursuits, and relationships with others would vary accordingly. Time, moreover, is an important variable to be considered in terms of the different stages through which each individual to some extent goes regardless of the specific nature of his limitation. There seems reason to suspect that the quality and nature of the individual's adjustment to physical limitations will vary in terms of the protensity dimension.

Intensity, the second dimension, is more complex. It is an estimate of the relative severity of the disabling agent in relation to that of all other persons who suffer from the same type of limitation. The calculation of intensity is based upon measures of endurance; loss of motion, mobility, and function; medication; active symptoms; and apparent disease or condition-related residuals. The interpretation of the measure of intensity depends to a large extent upon a knowledge of the peculiar characteristics of the specific physical limitation.[4] The pain with which the arthritic lives imparts a somewhat different meaning to this dimension than is found in disease that has stabilized and is largely measured by residuals with few or no active symptoms. For the latter, the problem might be principally that of learning to develop reserve potential and to utilize some sort of mechanical advantage in order to compensate for the loss of function. For the arthritic of comparable intensity in terms of loss of function, there would be the same problem,

---

[4] The measurements referred to are made by an interview instrument designed to reveal the extent of limitation and loss of function at five time intervals ranging from the time of onset to the present. Weights are then assigned and employed in formulas in the calculation of the status of the individual in relation to the particular dimension. For example, the intensity status is determined as follows once the individual's weighted scores have been found:

Derivation of Intensity (I) from Mobility (M), Endurance (En), and Disease Intensity (Ib):

$$\text{Motor Deterioration Factor } (MDF) = \frac{(100\text{-}M) + (100\text{-}En)}{2}$$

This is simply the average of the deterioration of the subject's Mobility and Endurance.

$$\text{Degree of Normal Health } (DNH) + (100\text{-}Ib).$$

This is the amount of good health of the subject as opposed to "bad" health or Disease Intensity. (The sum of DNH and Ib is always 100.)

$$\text{Friction Factor } (FF) + MDF \times DNH.$$

This shows the amount of "drag" effect the accumulated physical deterioration of a subject has on his health.

$$\text{Intensity } (I) = Ib + FF$$

Intensity is, then, the sum of the accumulated physical attrition (FF) of the subject and active attritional process (Ib).

Combining the above, the formula for Intensity is

$$I = Ib + \frac{(100\text{-}Ib)}{100} \left[\frac{(100\text{-}M) + (100\text{-}En)}{2} \right]$$

but also the additional problem of enduring the pain caused by the rotation of inflamed joints. The intensity of a progressive disease will fluctuate over time, whereas the intensity of a stabilized disease will remain relatively level after it once settles down. Of course, the "settling down" might come at a very high level.

Extensity, the third dimension, is one of the most complex of all. It might be most accurately described as the effect the physical limitation has had upon the personality and behavior of the individual. In a sense, extensity reflects the individual's adjustment to the limitation. Those who have considerable experience with the physically limited will readily agree that the severity of the condition does not always enable one to predict with any degree of accuracy the effect of the limitation upon the individual. To put it another way, extensity cannot be predicted accurately from a knowledge of the individual's intensity. As a result, the estimate of extensity must be arrived at by the independent estimates and measures.

It seems quite probable that the hopes of a number of persons with apparent and severe limitations have been dimmed by premature negative prognoses on the part of the diagnosticians and counselors who have made their judgments on the basis of something roughly corresponding to intensity. There is little doubt that such initial orientation can influence the way the person orders his life. When the handicapped person is perceived in relation to both of these dimensions as they inevitably interact, a much more adequate basis for prescription is provided.

There are many dramatic examples of severe intensity combined with low extensity; there are also, however, many less fortunate combinations where relatively mild intensity is combined with high extensity. The fact that extensity and intensity are often found in somewhat independent relation indicates that increased sophistication with these dimensions might well preserve premature discouragement and lack of striving toward constructive goals. The objective of rehabilitation with the physically limited is always to lower extensity, thus maximizing the physical and personality resources of the individual.

Autoviability, the fourth dimension of disability, is obviously a term synthesized from the combining word auto, meaning self, and the word viability, meaning the state of being able to sustain life or live. There are two quite distinct categories of elements implied by this dimension to be considered. The first category contains an inventory of the individual's intrinsic and extrinsic resources. The second includes a careful appraisal based upon all available evidence of the extent to which the individual is utilizing these resources in his present living and in his long-range plans.

Intrinsic resources are such factors as intelligence, motivation, determination, strength, endurance, and mobility, while extrinsic resources include the individual's economic means, his living accommodations, the quality of care available to him, his friends, equipment, education, and occupational training. The thesis that few so-called normal persons achieve at the level at which they are inherently capable is well known. The unknown level of achievement of which the individual is capable in any given direction or endeavor is very likely established by his heredity; however, the extent to which a given individual approaches this level is, in a broad sense, a function of culture. The person with a physical limitation cannot always afford the luxury of a half-hearted attempt to realize his inherent and remaining possibilities. His resources are reduced to the point where, if he is to make his way in our competitive society, he must utilize his resources at a relatively high level of efficiency. A function of the rehabilitation counselor and worker is to help the individual discover and appraise his resources and then to motivate and instruct the individual to the end of the most functionally integrated and productive utilization of his resources in the transactions of daily living.[5]

The dimensions of disability as described above are useful and possibly valuable only to the extent that they enable us to perceive the person with a physical limitation with more insight and more comprehension. One can never lose sight of the fact that a human being, physically limited or normal, is a social or gregarious creature. He operates and functions in a social milieu. It is in this context that ultimately we must view the handicapped person.

THE FAMILY

In the hierarchy of social settings, the family undoubtedly would appear as the most eminent. The primary group for the handicapped individual must be considered very carefully, for, other things being equal, the extent of dependence upon the family very likely varies directly with the extent of disability. This should not be construed as any lack of emphasis upon the significance of secondary or tertiary groups, however. We see about us and read daily evidence of the often-stated importance of the family to all of its members. We see evidence in the personal and social disorganization of those in our society who through fate, or of their own choosing, have been deprived of the stabilizing influence the family can have. We see evidence

---

[5] The matter of welfare provisions for the physically handicapped person might logically be considered a part of his autoviability. However, the generous intent of the welfare state not infrequently acts as an impediment to subsequent rehabilitative efforts. The individual receiving industrial compensation who remains bitter over his accident and who believes, unconsciously or not, that the world (state) owes him a living might be cited as a case in point. There seems to be considerable evidence that this problem is assuming expensive proportions in both financial expenditures and wasted manpower. The reduction of extensity in such instances is undoubtedly one of the important tasks facing the rehabilitation team at the present time.

also in the tenacity with which people cling to family membership even when the particular family in question might be characterized as an unhealthful social environment for those who dwell within it.

The beneficial functions of the family and the wholesome effects upon the individual that derive therefrom are so well known that extended elaboration becomes tautological. The assumption that the family is the most basic unit in society has become a sociological truism. The complexity of its organization and processes, however, is frequently underestimated. Family failure cannot be measured accurately by the very crude indexes of divorce and desertion. Divorce and desertion point up merely the structural failures of the family by means of legal or illegal dissolution of the structure. However, the incidence of functional failure of family life can only be estimated. Estimates that are alarmingly high are not thought to be exaggerated. Attention might be called to the fact that the family has undergone a considerable amount of change in recent years as a result of the general cultural change of our society. No one individual nor one family can be said to contribute much to the total process of social change, yet each one is affected and involved in the change in some way.

Having erected a few cautionary perceptual sets concerning the image of the patient, we might well inquire as to the nature of the image—the picture in the mind's eye—of the family in America today. One might argue that the family, like the patient, is nonexistent. Rather, there are many types or kinds of families in America today. One we might designate as the majority type is the Protestant, Caucasian, urban, middle-class, neolocal, nuclear family. Such a family is, in a sense, like the patient, a statistical myth. Again, it takes on meaning in terms of its hundreds of alter egos—the many representative types of families in our national subcultures. Before specific consideration of the home and family of the patient, it would be worthwhile to catch an over-simplified glimpse of the statistical composite family or the mythical majority-type American family as it exists in our society today.

The contemporary family is characterized as neolocal, which means the family moves frequently to new locations and feels no particular obligation or ties that might hold it in the community where its members were born and reared and where the parents and relatives of its members may still reside. This tendency leads to a general weakening of kinship bonds and results in the apparent prevalence of a type of structure called the nuclear family, meaning father, mother, and offspring. Missing from the scene, in particular, are extended kin and additional members. One of the implications of the nuclear family structure is that there is a general man- or woman-power shortage when one of the regulars is sent to the sidelines by illness or accident or [when he] departs the field by divorce or desertion. Thus it is that, even though one might argue that this family type having burned its bridges is productive of self-reliance and independence of a kind valued in our society, he would have to accept at the same time the probability that the nuclear setting is not one where economic, emotional, and other human resources are always or often sufficient to provide for a chronically ill or disabled member.

In addition to the neolocal tendencies of modern families and their nuclear structure there has been a large-scale transfer of institutional family functions to community agencies. For example, such family functions as the protective function, the religious function, the educational, recreational, and to some extent the economic function have transferred from the family to appropriate community agencies. There is general consensus that the transfer of functions has done little to orient the family toward mobilizing its resources and consolidating its ranks for the long, demanding haul occasioned by chronic illness, mental, emotional, or physical limitation.

Another factor is that our family culture has adopted norms for reciprocal emotional weaning as the child grows toward maturity. When one of the two parties to the process fails to conform to the norms, friction and perhaps tragedy can result. For the parent, the unhappy result may come in the form of disappointment and heartache and, for the child, in the form of emotional suffocation, incompetence, or some other equally unfortunate manifestation. The normal rupture between parents and child that occurs as emotional weaning climaxes is replaced by a new relationship that stresses friendly, benevolent, and even loving but nonentangling prerogatives on the part of both generations.

When a member of the family sustains an injury or suffers a disease that results in a fairly permanent physical limitation, cultural norms can no longer operate except by considerable modification. If the victim is a child, in addition to all other stresses imposed by the limitation, the inclination toward reciprocal weaning is frustrated. The child may remain relatively helpless in the face of mounting years, and the parents' control of the child's destiny from the child's point of view becomes more deeply entrenched. If we could peek into a household wherein the invalid child had progressed chronologically to adulthood, we might find the parents refusing to let the 25-year-old daughter wear lipstick, smoke, read detective stories, watch Westerns, or in fact do anything of which they disapproved. If the individual were a male, we might see a mother or father refusing to let the son shave, or grow a beard, or have girl friends visit him, or again do anything contrary to the parents' values and standards.

The conflict between generations that might arise—particularly between mothers and sons—over some of the finer points of indoctrination into the male subculture is not difficult to visualize. Seriously handicapped males testify that the complete lack of heterosexual association, or even its prospect, is more difficult to bear and more damaging to the self-image than almost any other single item. As one of the more verbal individuals with a physical limitation put it, "When you people put sex back into rehabilitation, the status of rehabilitation will have matured into something worthwhile." As a society, apparently we are not yet ready to face this issue or to deal with it except by ignoring its presence. It would be well to remember that the individual with the physical limitation has needs that are probably more nearly like those of physically normal people than they are different. The differences that do exist very likely are of a quantitative rather than a qualitative nature.

The handicapped person perhaps needs more intensely than most of us to be valued as a person, as an individual with his own tastes, values, interests, and characteristics. He frequently finds, however, that care implies control as well. He finds too frequently that others react more readily to the obvious and apparent characteristics imposed by the disability, or to the obligations of care thrust upon them, than to the more intimate basic qualities of this person.

STAGES OF DISABILITY

We might consider the person with a physical limitation in terms of four stages, recognizing of course that an individual's history will vary with the specific determinants involved. The significance of these stages is not that they are immutable, sacrosanct, or inevitable, but that they do enable us to sharpen our perception of the patient in his important relationships. The first of these stages might be termed the acute stage. This stage is the initial stage, the time when seemingly without rhyme or reason a member of the family is stricken with some sort of disabling condition.

There is frequently some degree of panic in the family as the members first realize what is happening and vaguely begin to contemplate the long-range implications. Well-educated families, otherwise rational, become vulnerable to the suggestions of uninformed advice-givers or folk-medicine[6] specialists, and even of persons who would prey upon and exploit those who would go to any expense to help a newly stricken person. Some families

---

[6] A distinction should be drawn between folk medicine and quackery. Folk medicine typically is concerned with the welfare of the patient, and some of the folk remedies have proved to be effective and of scientific value. For example, digitalis was found in the flower foxglove, which had been used for centuries by primitives for heart disease. Quackery on the other hand is, from the first, an attempt to defraud and exploit. Unfortunately, each of the "cures" has its share of seeming successes. After a given treatment, temporary or permanent remission of symptoms has been noted. Arthritis, for example, is by nature characterized by spontaneous remission—usually temporary. It stands to reason that, if a patient takes enough treatments of any kind, sooner or later there will be a fortuitous circumstance that suggests a cause-and-effect relation. Unwarranted reinforcement occurs in the form of the well-known *post hoc, ergo propter hoc* fallacy, or "after this, therefore because of this."

come close to bankruptcy because of frantic, ill-considered attempts to reverse or modify medical diagnoses or prognoses.

In short, while acknowledging the probable effect, that crisis of this kind might act as a cohesive agent within the family, uniting the members for a task that confronts them, the acute stage of disability is, nevertheless, a time when most families need guidance in order to utilize their economic, emotional, and physical resources in the most productive manner. Frequently, guidance at this time is limited to medical advice only, important as this is. Even at the earliest stage of illness in the hospital or the home, it is highly desirable to establish a constructive and dependable routine. Routines provide a sense of direction and meaning for all concerned. To the extent the physically limited patient is able to avail himself of the services of the rehabilitation team, the acute stage is not too soon for the team to begin to function.

As a rule, the emotional relationships between the patient and his family are good in the acute stage. The patient receives the support of the family in rather complete measure. In the interest of reconstruction, these resources should be employed in intelligent and conservative fashion.

The second stage is termed the reconstruction stage. There is nothing intrinsically valuable or historical in this term nor in the names of the other stages employed in this discussion. They probably do not appear in professional journals concerned with rehabilitation nor in medical texts. The extent of their worth will depend upon the operational concepts they suggest, bearing in mind that each individual will not go through each of the stages necessarily, nor will his experience in the several stages be of the same nature. The reconstruction stage is intended to suggest that period of short or relatively long duration when the individual has passed the acute stage and is now attempting through surgery, physical therapy, exercise, and other types of treatment to regain as much of his former physical status as possible.

From the standpoint of the patient's outlook, it is a very critical time in many respects. He may realize intuitively that his chances of recovery are small. It may be that the evidence indicating a future of confinement, limited physical facility, and social insulation will be overwhelmingly clear. It is common for realistic perception to vary between the patient and his family in either direction. Recently, an almost completely immobilized arthritic patient indicated that his parents fully expected him to walk until two years ago. He had known he would not for seven or eight years. On the other hand, the patient can be unrealistically optimistic against a background of family realism.

It is not at all unusual for the person with a severe physical limitation to feel a kind of peripheral status with regard to his principal reference groups.

In part, status change, felt or real, may derive from alteration in appearance and apparent function, and in part from modification in occupational, social and sex roles.[7] Perhaps at this point the ideal rehabilitative goal is realistic perception. The patient left entirely on his own psychic devices may alter his perception too far toward the periphery of his social-occupational world. On the other hand, he may resist any perceptual adjustment and set or keep unrealistic goals. Rehabilitation counseling at its best can do much to help the patient and family to see the situation in a realistic but, hopefully, flexible light. Meaningful integration can proceed from this point.

In the interest of regaining as much of the loss caused by the disabling agent as possible, whatever its nature, the patient and his family should receive all the guidance necessary to the end of high motivation, intelligently expressed. Obstacles can arise in many forms along the way. The intensity of the patient's limitation obviously has to be considered. The initial extensity may be affected by bitterness the patient feels over the arbitrary way he suddenly has been included in an exceptional population. His world has become painful as the result of the condition itself or corrective measures. His contacts with the world have become dull and largely circumscribed. The resultant emotional involvement may affect the individual's autoviability, which becomes central in terms of the inner resources at the person's command, and the extent and nature of the family's ways and means of providing the necessary assistance. The expense of treatment, medication, and confinement are highly practical matters that are bound to concern all members of the family. At this time, however, even though the expense of treatment and emotional problems the affliction has caused the family are difficult to manage, the fortunate patient receives the physical care and emotional support he needs. It is not at all unusual, however, for patients to prefer the dependable hospital routines and the hospital-ward brand of humor to the less sure and anxious reactions they encounter within their own families.

Presumably the patient begins to perceive each increment of progress as worthwhile, even though it falls short of his original hopes. The fortunate person makes sufficient progress in this state to become largely independent again and to resume many of his former roles and activities.

The majority of patients find themselves at a place where further medical reconstruction rapidly approaches a point of diminishing return. Thus the patient, medically speaking, moves into the plateau stage. This term is meant to imply that all reconstructive measures available to the patient have been taken. He is now concerned with maintaining what gains he has made, in preserving the status quo, and in developing compensatory skills and

---

[7] A study of the role modifications of disabled males is currently in progress at the University of Arizona.

attributes. From the standpoint of family relations, this may be the most difficult stage of all—primarily because hope for improvement has diminished or gone, a long period of considerable or total care and confinement confronts both patient and family, and financial and emotional resources have been worn thin.

Should the limitation be one of sufficient intensity so that the patient is confined, the family faces a difficult and possibly eroding sort of situation. Over a period of time, confinement and the attendant care and services performed by other members of the family can destroy what might once have been good relationships and, on the part of the family members, good mental and physical health. It is of cardinal importance that family members pursue outside interests and that they be able to count upon time of their own outside the home.

Confinement and interaction with those who administer to the needs of the confined person over a protracted period again can easily result in what might be termed a locked relationship. In this kind of relationship the patterns of interaction of the two parties become stereotyped and stylized. Neither seems able to modify his behavior to an extent sufficient to break the tension cycle that is usually a negative concomitant. The intelligent intervention by a third party by way of suggestion, possibly even a suggested change in the timetable of daily care, can sometimes provide for better relationships. Frequently, the parties to a locked relationship are much relieved by imposed change or aid in modifying the situation.

The term plateau, like the other stage designations, is not entirely satisfactory. The implication is not so much a static, passive acceptance as it is the end of medical reconstruction. The time period of the plateau or postreconstruction period is of relatively long duration, and many of the relationship problems derive from the protensity consideration.

Our experience indicates that too many families and patients pin their hopes to the star of reconstruction. When it stops rising in the sky, the hopes—goals—suddenly stop with it. Family rehabilitation counseling might well attempt to place reconstruction, whatever its degree of success, in its proper perspective, as a means of helping the patient more easily and completely achieve his goals. Families and patients frequently need assistance in perceiving compensatory alternatives and in encouraging constructive striving toward realistic objectives. Too frequently growth is stunted by the family's lack of co-operation or interest in the patient's progress.

After reconstruction the family may be tempted to place a television set in the patient's room to keep him entertained and occupied. A more adequate concept of the postreconstruction period would be for the family and patient to plan together for the family to support the patient in his plans, to widen his circle of friends, to develop or adapt vocational and avocational competencies and interests, to find ways to overcome limitations of energy and mobility, and in general to increase productive articulation with society in all its aspects. Medical counseling only, or any other limited approach that does not include the cultural family contact in which the patient resides, will very likely enjoy the limited success characteristic of attempts at psychotherapy with children when the parents are not co-operatively involved.

The fourth and final stage might be called the deteriorative stage. This stage is intended to characterize the time where the patient gives way to a long process of attrition or when he suffers a terminal attack. It should be re-emphasized that these stages are loosely conceived and are not, in any sense, mutually exclusive. On the other hand, they might, like the dimensions of disability, enable us to see more order in the field of rehabilitation as it attempts to meet the needs of the physically limited.

The superordinate-subordinate relational structure between the patient and the other members of the family warrants careful scrutiny. It is probably both easy and tempting for the family to dominate the patient in ways that the patient finds to be keenly humiliating. Occasionally the family may need guidance to prevent the patient from dominating matters through poorly organized routine and requests or by exploiting the "helpless" role. Families may unwittingly encourage the patient to depend too much on the so-called secondary aims of invalidism.

Actually, the patient's role in conserving the family is very nearly as important as the reciprocal role of the family toward him. He must learn, for example, that plenty of advance notice should be given when he requests a service. Spontaneous requests upset schedules and routine. It is imperative for the patient to space and plan his requests. He should try to have a few things done each time someone comes. Otherwise, the assisting members might be overwhelmed by long, complicated requests. The patient must learn to take the schedules of other members of the family into account in planning his requests and activities. He must learn also to utilize and organize his time between the major events of routine care. There is bound to be a certain amount of reciprocal ambivalence between the patient and other family members. Intelligent planning can do much to minimize the antagonism.

In so-called normal families, misunderstandings among siblings are not uncommon. When the patient is a child, other children in the family may misinterpret the care and attention accorded the physically limited child as preferential treatment. They may be sensitive also to the atypical nature of the afflicted child in terms of the reaction of other children. A great deal of patience and understanding on the part of the parents is necessary to avoid reinforcement of these perceptions. When the patient is a parent, there is a delicate balance between imposing unnecessarily heavy burdens on the able-bodied children and denying them the privilege to serve, commensurate with their age and ability, by assuming reasonable responsibilities. Just where the dividing line occurs on the continuum depends on the situation and the individual personalities involved.

In the interest of productive and harmonious relationships, families should be sensitized to the importance of honoring the patient's own unique hierarchy of felt needs. This hierarchy of needs could be expressed as a type of homeostatic adjustment. In determining the needs or constancies that the individual maintains, his own history is basic. If a given patient should express a strong desire for a hospital bed in preference to a new television set, the chances are the request is a valid and meaningful one. The relationship between expressed needs and the extensity should always be kept in mind.

As a case in point, an arthritic with a very high intensity expressed the desire to have a recording machine and a telephone rather than a television set and other expensive means of entertainment. His family denied him this request, and it was only after many months of struggle, conniving, and work that he was able to obtain the equipment he desired. In retrospect, those who know him are convinced that the telephone and tape recorder, which enable him to dictate and express his thoughts, were responsible for the degree to which this individual was able to rise above his physical limitations, or in effect, to lessen the extensity of his physical limitation.

We can perhaps now see more clearly the relationships among the dimensions of the disability and also the significance of these dimensions in terms of the person's relationships. In the example cited above, concerning the phone and dictating machine, this might be described as an increase in the person's autoviability; specifically, his extrinsic resources were increased. This enabled him in turn to overcome aspects of his limitation that he could not overcome without the equipment, it enabled him to function more like a normal person in terms of the end product of his endeavors, and thus the extensity, or the effect of the disability upon the personality and behavior of the person, was lessened. The reduction of extensity is always the ultimate aim of rehabilitation.

Medical progress pointed toward the preservation of life and restoration of limb and function has obviously been remarkable. One of the most eloquent expressions of the higher values of mankind, particularly in Western civilization, has been the relative disregard of eugenic considerations. Having defined and determined life as a birthright, we have directed immense energy and resources to the preservation of life for all persons. We have, in effect, reversed or replaced nature's law of survival of the fittest by a moral and ethical law of survival of all from weakest to strongest and youngest to oldest.

Inherent with this concept of life is the responsibility of restoring people with physical limitation to the optimal function of which they are capable. Function and restoration, however, is but a part of the over-all responsibility of complete rehabilitation. To neglect the interpersonal competency of the individual is in effect to thrust him prematurely into the deteriorative and final stage of his life. Attrition can result as surely from emotional wear and tear as from physical accident or failure.

Realistically, we cannot assume that the families of physically limited individuals will necessarily have the intelligence, the values, the education, the motivation, or even the interest to enable them, as a family unit, to proceed independently toward the goals of rehabilitation. Some families have fewer resources than others that can be mobilized, as well as lower thresholds of tolerance to frustration and crises. In this respect families are like individuals; many families and individuals barely able to keep their heads above water under normal circumstances become quickly submerged by the imposition of a serious physical handicap or the addition of an older relative to the household. It seems obvious that special counsel, special rehabilitation education, needs to have the interpersonal competence of the person and the family as a central goal. Perhaps such a focus will better enable the potentialities inherent in the patient, the family, and the situation to be combined most productively for the good of all.

Section B

Psychological Considerations

One of the many avenues of approach to the rehabilitation of the disabled or handicapped patient is through an understanding and utilization of the concept of role. The major cultural sex role of the male in our society is undoubtedly that of breadwinner or family provider. When the individual is forced to retreat from this role before the onslaught of some form of physical disability, it is highly likely that some degree of role disequilibration ensues. Objective reality may or may not correspond closely to perceptual reality, consequently, the new role alternatives available to the disabled individual may be completely overlooked in his perceptual organization, or they may be seen only dimly. Christopherson discusses various degrees and kinds of role modifications of the disabled male and suggests ways the nurse can utilize the concept of role modifications to bring about gains in the rehabilitation process—including extreme modifications of role, or role reversals, for which the patient without assistance may perceive no acceptable cultural precedent.

Whether professionally credentialed as a psychologist or not, each person who works in a therapeutic relationship with a patient is practicing what at least in a popular sense could be considered a kind of psychology. Not many members of the therapeutic team can afford the luxury of a great deal of formal training in psychology—or learning that body of knowledge that some psychologists teach to other psychologists. At the same time, if one is to bring true professional competence to bear in the sphere of influence in which he is most instrumental in patient recovery, some knowledge of the characteristic modes of patient behavior is essential.

Few of us stop to consider how well adapted our bodily design is with regard to the functions it performs. Indeed so dependent upon the accomplishment of seemingly ordinary skills and functions do we become that we have great difficulty in adapting to any limitation of these functions. Reva Rubin counts this a blessing, however, for it is through this frustration and impatience that the motivation and determination to overcome is born. She suggests that the achievement of integrated functions does not register with the same impact as its loss. When any of the body functions become involuntary or get out of control, we become distressed. One of the manifestations of this distress is shame. Rubin suggests that enabling another to achieve or maintain control has been called the process of "lending ego"—a new description for graciousness—which is certainly a therapeutic capacity well within the province of the rehabilitation nurse.

One of the most neglected areas in rehabilitation, and possibly one of the areas whose importance is most underestimated, is that of sex adjustment. Perhaps, on the other hand, the complexity of the area is well known but the answers are not. At any rate the typical attitude is to ignore sex as a problem area of rehabilitation as if it did not exist, or if problems do exist, the implicit expectation is that they will disappear spontaneously. Frankel offers some examples of the onset and nature of sexual disturbances. One of the problems in rehabilitation is that few professionals have had either training or experience to deal with them. Under such circumstances it becomes extremely important to know the resources for appropriate referral. Frankel also suggests that where there are few opportunities for referral insight can be gained by listening to the patient and discussing with him the relevant aspects of the problem as one would with any other specific area of disturbance in the rehabilitation process.

Smith begins his essay with the assertion that illness is, in addition to all else, a psychological event. To the extent this is true, it would seem essential for the nurse to become as well informed as possible concerning the wide spectrum of patient response to illness. One need not accept the entire Freudian model to acknowledge the benefit of recognizing the existence of an intrapsychic conflict in the patient's behavior. Unless the nurse is sensitive to the possibility of a struggle between the conventional ego on the one hand and the contrary unconscious on the other, her own response may be antithetical to the patient's real needs.

The patient can bring only his own frame of reference to bear on a given situation and frequently illness or disability is a new or confusing experience to him. His subjective appraisal of what is happening and the implications of the events are likely to be distorted. The nurse is in a strategic position to interpret the nature and meaning of the illness to the patient in order to help him resolve his conflicts in a constructive fashion. The nurse must be able to recognize and deal with regression, masochism, dependency, transference, and other inappropriate adjustive mechanisms. Smith also points out some of the potential difficulties that can occur between nurse and patient over the problem of pain. One of the pitfalls is that of projection. The nurse may unwittingly reinforce a response to pain that has as its only justification a minimum of trouble for her. The author provides a number of valuable cues that can be incorporated into the rehabilitation process to very good advantage.

A comprehensive, up-to-date article on human sexuality that deals with both specifics and generalities in unusual circumstances pertaining to health is provided by Isadore Rubin. As an acknowledged authority and author in the area of human sexuality, Rubin covers topics with which the rehabilitation nurse will likely have to deal. Answers are provided to common questions that patients will ask, and in many cases Rubin's discussion indicates that their concern may be exaggerated. Contained in Rubin's paper is the implicit assumption that sexual functioning, particularly for the male, is tied in very intimately with mental health and will to live or recover. Failure to take proper cognizance of this fact may well constitute one of the common sins of the healing professions.

Reading 6
Role Modifications of the Disabled Male
Victor A. Christopherson

It has been estimated that disease and disability cost the United States some 35 billion dollars each year [1]. Rheumatoid arthritis, muscular dystrophy, multiple sclerosis, cardiac and respiratory disorders are some of the leading disease contributors to that toll, with automobile, farm, mining, and construction accidents adding many more names to the roster.

The fact that human beings are not entirely predictable is sometimes as much related to disability as the disease or accident factor per se. Our research with physically handicapped individuals of both sexes indicates a surprising independence between the relative seriousness of the physical condition and the disability of the individual [2,3,4].

Much actual disability occurs as a result of the way an individual takes his condition into account and how he is able to adapt himself and his residual abilities to the new requirements and opportunities imposed or offered by society. After acquiring the disability, he finds much of the structure of his world changed, and he finds, too, that the new structure requires new statuses—some ascribed to him by others and some which he must strive to achieve. The new statuses will yield different privileges, expectations, rewards, and deprivations, and will require his assuming new or modified roles.

Many of the nonproductive disabled persons represent failures in the psychologic and sociologic aspects of rehabilitation rather than in the physical and physiologic aspects. The application of role concepts—particularly role modifications—as a frame of reference within which to consider implications for rehabilitation may help to reduce this deficit.

Role can be defined as a system of related behavior that a person regularly performs in a certain group or social situation as a result of his "notions" of (1) the general and characteristic nature of the situation, (2) the expectations of the group members concerning him, and (3) his own obligations and capabilities. In effect, an individual's role is the behavior that, to him and others, seems indicated in terms of his status in the group or situation. Role is, in a sense, the translation of status into behavior.

Reprinted from *American Journal of Nursing*, vol. 68, no. 2, pp. 290-293, February 1968. The research on which this paper is based was supported by grants from the Agriculture Experiment Station, University of Arizona, and the Vocational Rehabilitation Administration, Department of Health, Education and Welfare.

THE CRIPPLE ROLE

When the visibility of a disability is high—as, for example, when a person has an amputated extremity or deforming rheumatoid arthritis—the individual is keenly aware of one of his ascribed statuses. He is "pegged" by those he encounters as a cripple or a physically handicapped person. His reference groups change, and he finds himself coming to terms with new norms to which he may or may not adjust readily. He is implicitly expected to assume roles in keeping with what the observer deems appropriate for a cripple in the various areas of life.

Interested and seemingly sympathetic persons will register shock, disbelief, and disapproval on receiving reports from a physically handicapped individual that he has been dancing, golfing, hunting, getting married, or has otherwise violated the expectations that the well-bodied have of him.

Occasionally, this happens within the family constellation. One of the persons included in the role research project was a young man in his late twenties who, because of severe arthritis, was no longer able to support his own weight or to get around unless carried. His father promptly placed a television set in his son's bedroom and encouraged him to pass his time watching programs and reading. Instead, the son was determined to keep active and productive. He organized a market research firm, ran a telephone answering service, learned computer programming, and became more active in many respects than most able-bodied individuals. All these activities were disapproved and resisted by his well-meaning parents. This illustrates what might be characterized as the principal developmental task of the disabled individual—as he modifies his roles, he must effect a compromise between his own shifting self-image and the expectations society derives from his apparent physical cues.

When visibility is low, as in cardiac disorders, the problem may be just as acute but of a different nature. The disabled individual attempts to modify his roles in accordance with his real, though not apparent, physical limitation, but he lacks the support and sanction that a visible disorder provides. In order to assume appropriate modification, the individual frequently needs help to utilize, and to keep in balance, legitimate rationalizations for the support of his self-image and for the maintenance of his ego.

THE SEX ROLE

One of the significant categories in which role modification takes place is the cultural sex role. In all societies for which ethnographic data are available, there are divisions of behavior—duties, privileges, and responsibilities—along sex lines. Men and women each have unique sex roles prescribed by the culture of the society to which they belong. When a disability forces a retreat from the sanctioned sex role, the impact can be very serious. Generally, there is a means of modifying the role rather than abandoning it completely. The fact that each sex, in effect, represents a separate subculture in society, warrants giving special attention to each rather than considering both entirely equivalent.

In spite of a certain amount of popular journalism to the contrary, there is relatively little confusion of sex roles in our society. There is some overlapping to be sure, but this condition leaves no one really in doubt as to what the basic sex roles are. The sex-role image of the American male, which serves as a major referent for his self-concept, is that of a fully employed, able-bodied man who assumes all or most of the support of his family. The able-bodied man generally can rationalize quite easily the fact that his wife helps contribute to the family's economic welfare. Often, he sees the condition as temporary and feels no particular threat. Or, if she works by choice, he attributes the situation to his own largess and takes credit accordingly.

This kind of rationale is not always available to the disabled male who cannot maintain his breadwinning role as before. He frequently must be helped to see alternative ways to cope with his sex-role task. He may need help in coping with the image problem on a modified level that is in keeping with his physical and energy characteristics as they are at the time. Too frequently as real limitations are imposed by disability, the tender psyche of the newly disabled male responds with withdrawal and passive role modifications.

The fact that many disabled individuals have made imaginative and constructive sex-role modifications indicates the feasibility of learning to guide and facilitate the process. Our culture has provided only limited precedent for sex-role modification, but there may be generalized solutions that can be successfully applied once role modification configurations are better understood.

The virtual exchange of sex roles between husband and wife has been termed role reversal. Dorothy Canfield dealt with this situation some years ago in her novel *The Homemaker*. She described a disabled father who stayed at home to manage the household and take care of the children while his wife went out to earn the living. When he was physically able to resume his breadwinning role, the couple found to their surprise that they both preferred the modified arrangement and continued with it.

This extreme mode of role modification can be successful only if worth and challenge are perceived in the substitute role. A perfunctory or forced assumption of a reversed or highly modified role has a rather poor prognosis in the long run. Perception—how a man "sees" his condition vis-à-vis his life space and all it contains—is as important a factor, if not more so, than the extent of the physical damage or loss sustained.

The primary, biologic sex role is also a vital part of the integrated ego of the male. Even though the sex problems per se of the disabled male were not a particular focus of the role modification study, they arose with sufficient frequency to warrant serious attention. Three main kinds of difficulties were described: (1) impotency caused by disease, injury or psychological factors; (2) lack of available sex partners for the seriously disabled male who seems destined to remain single; and (3) physical or emotional barriers to the sex act. Barriers included the inability to move or adopt the necessary positions, physical frailty interfering with weight bearing, or difficulty of the able-bodied or disabled partner to accept changes in the so-called normal techniques.

The significance of sexual adequacy with regard to the total adjustment configuration is illustrated by the history of Harold P. who developed arthritis at the age of 10 but managed to finish high school with his class. During the next 10 years he enjoyed several periods of good health interspersed with a number of serious exacerbations of the disease. At the age of 27 he was under steroid therapy and was mobile enough to drive a car and walk short distances with a cane. However, he usually used crutches because of severe knee involvement. His family's economic resources had dwindled markedly, and at the age of 28 he sought aid from the vocational rehabilitation agency. He was sent to business college, and at the end of a year he obtained a clerical job in an insurance office.

Harold had a reputation for constant preoccupation with sex that preceded him wherever he went. He complained to his friends about spending considerable amounts of money on a number of girls, wining and dining them—"setting them up"—but never quite succeeding. He was particularly bitter over one girl whom he had never even kissed, but on whom he had spent over $200.

As he grew more and more blunt and incessant in his determination, his friends and acquaintances grew correspondingly less enthusiastic about him. Finally, upon the suggestion of an acquaintance, he contacted a girl known to come to specified locations on a paying basis. He made a date for her to come to his room one afternoon when his mother was scheduled to be away until evening. The girl arrived. Harold became fearful lest his mother return prematurely and find him in bed with the girl. He was unable to perform and finally the girl left after accepting his money and expressing her sympathy over his failure.

This appeared to be a definite turning point in Harold's life. He stopped working and stopped trying. He withdrew from his friends, had no more dates, and died in his sleep at the age of 30 years, less than a year after the call-girl episode.

THE OCCUPATION ROLE

When an occupational role modification takes place, it is usually from a higher to a lower order or level. There are the occasional upward modifications brought about by specialized vocational training, but these are much less common modifications than the other way around. The change from more rewarding to less rewarding occupational roles involves more than loss of income; it almost always is associated with a lowering of general community status. By and large, a family's status in the community derives from the man's occupation. The disabled man not only has to contend with the primary problems of his own adjustment resulting from the role modification, but also with the status change and all its implications in which the entire family is caught up.

The family that suffers a loss of status and benefits can become a nontherapeutic community in its strict sense. Vocational counselors, nurses, and physicians alike have seen their efforts go up in smoke as the glimpse of hope they have given their patient is extinguished by the skepticism, overprotectiveness, or outright opposition of a nonsympathetic or uninformed family. Possibly the time will come when the release of a patient with a serious disability from the hospital without the careful involvement of the family will be considered in the same light as child therapy without parental conferences.

If a man is single, there are comparable status problems and questions which affect his self-image—whether or not he will be able to attract a mate, marry, support a family, and so forth. The not infrequent despondency and depression of the newly disabled person reflects the sense of loss and futility he experiences. The nurse as one of the most instrumental figures in his life at this point should not underestimate the power at her disposal to affect the patient's outlook and resolve. In effect, she can be very important as a "setter of mood."

The occupational role modification made by a highly trained civil engineer who moved to Arizona because of his son's asthma illustrates the point very well. He developed a severe case of arthritis some time after arriving in the state and was subsequently hospitalized. Faced by his own and his son's hospital bills and by the prospect of increasing disability, he became extremely distressed. His words, taken verbatim from an interview schedule, were as follows:

> . . . At that time I was ready to call it quits. One of the nurses on the floor said something encouraging to me each time she came in, and her visits did as much, or more, for me than any part of the treatment I received. Her encouragement changed me on the inside. She told me I'd be fine, that I had what it takes, and that I was luckier by far than many she sees. The thing I remember in particular was that in a very matter-of-fact way she told me she'd seen others just like me who were doing very well with their families and in their jobs.

Mr. S. completed a course in business training under provisions made by the vocational rehabilitation agency and has now been with the same company for several years in the bookeeping department.

A cursory examination of these words spoken by the nurse suggests very little that could be judged new or profound. Very likely other supportive interaction between the nurse and patient, less clearly recalled by Mr. S., was also significant in the outcome. On the other hand, the few words repeated by Mr. S. might well be a clue to the most strategic role of the nurse at the time when a disabled man's "set" for role modification is at the most impressionable state. They suggest, moreover, the value of moderate, confident optimism expressed by the nurse in the interest of normalizing a new and frightening experience.

THE SOCIAL ROLE

The social world of the disabled male can dwindle very quickly. Sometimes intentionally, and sometimes in spite of good intentions, old friends stop coming by and immediate family members soon constitute the man's social relations matrix. His own children, if he is a father, begin to find other ways to spend their leisure time. His wife may be too physically and emotionally exhausted to provide much in the way of companionship. Soon he may turn to other disabled individuals with whom he has common interests and who can share similar experiences. Social contacts with other disabled persons are all right in themselves, but when they are limited to the disabled, the whole fabric of the social milieu becomes too lean and circumscribed to satisfy most men's gregarious needs. Other disabled persons also provide too narrow a foundation for the expansion and replacement of social contacts necessary for a healthy and ongoing social relations network. This, of course, is more of a composite model than a prescription for, or description of, the case of any given individual. However, in establishing the usual hierarchy of treatment and services necessary for a newly disabled person, the significance of helping him adjust his social life to his new circumstances is sometimes overlooked. It is very easy to assume that someone else on the team will attend to the matter.

In order to avoid conforming to the model above, a disabled man will frequently need a boost from a figure whose authority is accepted and respected. He needs competent assurance that he is still possessed of sufficient bases for establishing meaningful social relations. Sometimes the balance between successful or unsuccessful role modification rests upon a very thin line. A little push of the right kind by the right person at the right time can accomplish disproportionately good results.

Role modifications are in a sense behavioral changes and they are not easily made, nor made without exacting a price. When they do occur, particularly in a constructive and creative fashion, they often have started through some significant contact with a person in an important therapeutic role early in the rehabilitation process. Our respondents have suggested, over and over again, that nurses have marked influence in such situations.

REFERENCES

1 Jones, Boisfeuillet. Organizing medical research to meet the health needs of Americans. *Amer. Acad. Polit. and Soc. Sci. Ann.* **337**(9):20-28, 1961.
2 Christopherson, V. A. Role modification of the handicapped homemaker. *Rehab. Lit.* **21**:110-117, April 1960.
3 ———. Patient and the family. *Rehab. Lit.* **23**:34-41, February 1962.
4 ———. Role Modifications of the Disabled Male with Implications for Counseling. Final report to U.S. Vocational Rehabilitation Administration on Project No. 755. Tucson, Ariz., University of Arizona, 1963.

Reading 7
Body Image and Self-esteem
Reva Rubin

It seems that today we are all zeroing in toward a statement about nursing care that is more precise than just "comfort and safety of the patient." Comfort has a broader, more significant context, it would seem, that has to do with self-esteem, or at least self-acceptance, and this last is decisively a factor of the controlled, functionally operant body image.

Picture a youngster walking along a sidewalk curbing or the top of a fence, deliberately placing one foot in front of the other, balancing for an upright position with his arms and trunk, and concentrating on the challenge of walking within a rigid, limited space without falling off. Or watch another child jump to a rhythmically turned rope; her jumping is restricted to a limited space and coordinated with the appearance of the rope at a specific time and place. These games, like so many of childhood, serve as proving grounds for purposefully coordinated body functioning in direct engagement with one's environment.

Blake, among others, describes these activities of childhood in terms of attaining mastery of body parts and body functioning [1]. Piaget avoids any consideration of motivation and describes these and related activities of

Reprinted from *Nursing Outlook*, vol. 16, no. 6, pp. 20-23, June 1968.

childhood in terms of adaptation [2]. Both viewpoints, one representing internal striving and the other external achievement, seem useful. Freud has suggested that the ego is primarily and essentially a body ego [3]. Erikson bases his theory of psychosocial identity on the activities, modes, and modalities of body organs and functions [4].

The capacity for functioning is dependent on the biological structure or equipment, organic, skeletal, and neuromuscular, available to the individual. The newborn infant cannot chew food, see, or bear his own weight to effect postural change. His limitations are "normal"; that is, his functional limitations or inadequacies coincide with our, and perhaps his own, expectations. Objectively, we know that the infant's incapacity in functioning is relatively temporary, and we expect that, with time, biological structures and equipment will develop to provide the capability for these activities and behaviors. Subjectively and experientially, however, the infant is considerably less future-oriented and less phlegmatic about his own limitations in functioning.

It is doubtful whether at any age we can accept functional limitation or incapacity in ourselves with the same equanimity, tolerance, and realism that, so readily and spontaneously, we can muster for others. Such intolerance of our own functional inadequacies is perhaps one of our greatest strengths. It provides us, somehow, with energy or drive, with purpose or motivation to *do* something, to actively master the functional capability. Acceptance and tolerance of our own functional incapacities and limitations cut off the source of energy for development, for potentiation, for a future condition of anything different or better.

Functional development is an open-ended process. There is a progression in levels of functional achievement and a progressive substitution of goals. The baby clutches, then grasps and holds, then picks up—actions which bring objects into his immediate environment through his own manipulations. After a while, using the same body parts, he writes, constructs, makes, and fixes—actions which enlarge his environmental space and scope of interaction with that space [5]. The same progression is seen in postural development that permits him to turn over, then sit, stand, crawl, and walk, so that his increased capacity brings objects of his environment into his sphere of contact and interaction. A little later, he not only walks, but runs, skips, climbs, cycles, and skis. His contact-environment is enlarged in space. Speech, progressing from sounds, to words, to social communication, follows the same pattern to enlarge interpersonal space. The available environment for stimulation and interaction, socially and physically, is directly dependent on the scope and capacity for functional development.

The element of time is of paramount importance in functioning. In the socialization of the child, both time and place are conditions of adequate functioning. There is an appropriate time and place for each action, whether evacuating the contents of the bowel, running, or shouting. Subjectively and experientially, it becomes even more important to coordinate activities, mentally and physically, in terms of appropriate or available time and space. The timing and placing of a person's actions are dependent for effectiveness on situational time and space. Whether it is the trapeze artist in position to catch his partner, or the person who knows at last what and how he should have said something hours after the situation has passed, it is apparent that functional competence and achievement are inconsequential without coordination of situational time and place.

The ability to function with control for time and place is held in personal, social, and cultural esteem. The ability to use himself in such a way, functionally, as to achieve precisely what he intended—no more, no less, and precisely at the right time and place—gives a person a sense of high accomplishment. We distinguish the skilled worker by these criteria; we evaluate excellence in every sport by these criteria; we elect to admire those performers in the entertainment and cultural arts who have perfect time and placement control of their body movements.

When we consider the high value placed on a person's capacity to use himself in action to accomplish what he wishes to do when and where he intends to do it, we can estimate and understand to some degree what happens personally and experientially when he succeeds or fails. In fact, it is possible to consider a sense of personal success or personal failure in terms of the congruence between intent or expectation of self and the effectiveness of functional control. Certainly, self-respect is measured in these terms.

After an individual has achieved a certain level of control in one dimension of functional activity, there is little pleasure, or even awareness, of its value. Despite years of assiduous effort to achieve a particular level of body functioning and control, once achieved it is assimilated into the total personality or identity. It is no longer an achievement; it is "the way I do." It may have taken two years of a very short lifetime to achieve the kinesthetics of walking; but a 6-year-old child would consider us witless if we complimented him on this ability. It takes considerably longer to produce speech sounds in combinations of social significance; but the adult would be bewildered if he were complimented on his ability to produce selectively and appropriately for time and place an achieved and integrated phrase like "thank you" or "please."

SUCCESS OR FAILURE

These seemingly trivial achievements in functioning have resounding personal importance when they are lost. We are not impressed with our abilities in functional control when we reach for a cup and saucer. But if this ability were lost, through either neurological impairment or psychological preoccupation, we would, at least, experience frustration. If the situation recurred, with the loss of control in action, not the relationship of cup to saucer, anxiety would replace frustration. If the situation persisted, fear would supplant anxiety. To lose or be threatened with the loss of a complex, coordinated, and controlled functional activity which has been achieved and integrated into the personal system is to lose or be threatened with the loss of self. Psychosocially, the loss, or threat of loss, of self is equivalent to loss of life. Emotional responses serve as warning signals of the extent of danger, and we immediately mobilize energies for self-protection and self-preservation.

We have seen the look of dismay when a postpartum patient, unaware of the hemodynamics of delivery, tries to get up after 12 hours of staying in bed and finds that supporting her body in the upright position is a burdensome effort. Ages ago, the simple act of supporting herself in the upright position was worked through. That it should be a problem now simply does not fit with her self-expectations and self-concept. It is not only disconcerting, but even disorienting. The experience is typical postpartally but it is not typical in any sense of the word to her. There is a vast difference between viability and living.

A postoperative patient may expect weakness, but rarely expects to be unable to marshal energy to turn from side to side or to sit up. This is a fearsome regression: if one loses so much functional control, how much more will one lose? With every bit of functional control lost from the available personal resources, a bit of personal life space is lost.

Many of us are familiar with the work of Margaret Bourke-White, an outstanding photographer, who besides her technical competence was able to convey illuminating insights, perspectives, and viewpoints about her subjects. In order to take her pictures, she often had to strap herself into some preposterous position—under the wing of a moving airplane, or from the top of a slightly swaying skyscraper. This actively involved, functionally competent person was stricken with a degenerative disease that immobilized and confined her to the restricted life space of her bed for several years. When she started to recover, she wrote about the experiences in an issue of *Life* with the same insight and capacity for meaningful portrayal that had characterized all her work. One phrase she used to describe her feelings about the situation stands out: "I felt trapped, trapped within the boundaries of my own body."

Can there be a more devastating situation? The woman who, at the end of labor, does not have enough energy to raise her arms to wipe the sweat from her face and neck or to raise her head to drink is helpless and relentlessly victimized by her own body discomforts and discharges. She is

BODY IMAGE AND SELF-ESTEEM

trapped within her own body. The newborn infant, attacked from within his own body by the pains of hunger or by the beginning of a bowel movement, has energy but cannot localize or direct his energy to alter the situation. In his helplessness he, too, is trapped and victimized by his own body. If the situation of helplessness is unaltered, the trapped feeling in both the maternity patient and the newborn results in panic. Panic, unlike fear, cannot be sustained for long; it may be incompatible with life.

Those of us who are grossly uncomfortable when we are restricted, alone, to a small room and quickly identify our dislike of the situation as claustrophobia can understand some element of the subjective experience of being trapped. Prisons are designed for just this punishment. If we are free, we can move out of or bring movement or activity into that box of a room. Being free, however, requires available energy and then control of that energy for direction, purpose, and effectiveness. Neither the patient approaching the end of labor nor the newborn has that control.

In contrast, the same maternity patient a few minutes later, given the changed situation of imminent delivery, musters all her energies for an immense physical effort and is relieved to be able to "do something." If she cannot be effective enough to meet her own expectations, she is frustrated, even angry, but not frightened and certainly not panicked. Despite the fact that pain remains unchanged (though, in truth, the force of contractions increase), the difference between the two situations of marked curtailment of activity in labor and of action potentiation in delivery is remarkable. Also, the newborn, a few months later, can now propel his own body through space, at his own initiative, and through his own resources; here is gleeful contrast to that earlier situation when he was trapped within his own body boundaries.

MOTION ESSENTIAL

We cannot underestimate the indispensability of motion. Each organ has a function, a movement, an action. Motion is essential for physical survival; movement is essential for physical and mental well-being. But movement, action, or function is not enough; one must be able to control it. Our postpartum patients who cannot void spontaneously on their own initiative are distressed and dismayed. It is not enough that the bladder can be emptied with help from another by catheterization. The catheterization is not a welcome procedure to a patient. An enema is more tolerable because it does not eliminate the patient's volitional efforts. A patient may well be pleased or relieved with what she produces as a result of an enema, but she is never pleased or relieved by the removal of urine, no matter how worthwhile the results. It is very nice to survive, to be kept living, to exist. But, in itself, it is not enough.

Vomiting, coughing, and sneezing are functions that maintain and protect the organism. Most of them are acquired after birth, assimilated into the body schema, and taken for granted as endowments [6]. But let any of these functions become involuntary or get out of control and we become sorely distressed. Beyond the infantile stage of neurological development these acts are not just simple reflexes. We can inhibit or delay any discharge, any so-called reflex, at will [7]. We have impulses, but we are not driven or victimized by them. We can select that stimulus, time, and place to which we will respond. If inner stimuli conflict, we select for priority the stimulus we will respond to on a purely situational-value basis.

Some inner stimuli can be very forceful. Who has not had the experience of suddenly and desperately needing to cough during a sermon or a concert? If the coughing persists, we are embarrassed, and restrain those responses until we are safely out of the auditorium. Coughing is embarrassing only when it occurs in the wrong place and at the wrong time. The forcefulness of the stimulus in diarrhea preempts attention and disrupts all other occupations. If a person is in public or far from a toilet he responds with apprehension, then with anxiety, and then with fear bordering on panic. The degree of emotional response is in direct relationship to the intensity of the struggle to maintain control. Once body function, time, and place are appropriately coordinated, that function becomes a pleasurable relief.

Further evidence of the significance of control over body function in relation to time and place is provided in clinical nursing practice. Ostensibly, the hospital is the appropriate place and hospitalization is the appropriate time for priorities of physiological functioning over socially acceptable behavior. But the desperate cries of "I have to go!" or "I have to vomit!" are appeals for help to coordinate time and place more precisely for the body function. Immediate accessibility of a bedpan or emesis basin to a patient at such a time miraculously removes all his anxiety and tension; he is in control. Similarly, a patient moved swiftly and unpredictably through space on a stretcher or in a wheelchair becomes apprehensive and perhaps disoriented because he has no sense of being in control in terms of time or space.

PROBLEM OF SHAME

Loss of control produces shame. There is nothing shameful about any function of the body, per se. It is the inability to control for appropriateness in time and place that produces shame. If we lose our tempers (and we often refer to this as "losing control"), we are ashamed. If a child or a patient inadvertently soils himself, his clothing, or his bedding, he is ashamed. If a maternity patient screams during labor, she is ashamed. If she inadvertently jerks away during a pelvic examination or during a venipuncture, she is ashamed. If a patient cries, he is ashamed.

One is ashamed of one's self [8]. One expects one's self to be in control, especially in the simplest functions. Shame is the personal, private judgment of failure, passed on self by self. And it is a merciless judgment. To have one's shame seen by others only serves to reverberate and amplify awareness of shame. Since this is an ego failure, all defenses are mustered—withdrawal, denial, rationalization, and, fortunately, repression.

Enabling another to achieve control of function appropriately in time and space may well be a succinct description of nursing. Essentially the same concept has been expressed in nursing by the phrase "helping the patient to cope." The advantage of the concept of control over that of coping is that control lends itself to a breakdown into component factors: functional capacities or limitations, the values of the patient, and the situation in time and space.

We might, then, formulate some operationally useful nursing definitions. Frustration results when an individual wishes or intends some action, but coordination with the other factors of time and place is not obtained and the action cannot be carried through. If the individual is able to perform the activity, he will try again until time and place are more closely coordinated. If success is not achieved after repeated trials, he will stop trying, but not without feelings of humiliation or anger. If frustration and anger are viewed as a continuum of the extent and degree of ineffective control over a person's actions in relation to a physical situation, we have still another possible nursing definition of anger. We also can appreciate the intensity of the emotional response as directly dependent on the extent of the subjective experience.

If frustration and anger are outcomes of an experienced failure in coordination or control of functional activity, time, and place, anxiety and fear can be operationally defined as anticipations or expectations of such failure. When a person anticipates some experience with a sense of well-being and competence and there is plenty of time before the experience occurs, he "plans" for it. When he anticipates an experience with some concern about his adequacy, but there is plenty of time before the experience occurs, he "worries." When, however, an individual is concerned about his adequacy and the experience is imminent, he becomes "anxious." If the same experience comes into the immediate present and a person is deeply concerned about his adequacy to control his actions, then he is "frightened." If these definitions are appropriate identifications of behavior, it would be possible to determine which components can be altered by nursing intercession on behalf of the patient's control and which components cannot be altered.

Enabling another to achieve or to maintain controls has been described as a process of "lending ego." This may be a new way to describe what has sometimes been referred to as graciousness.

REFERENCES

1. Blake, Florence. The Child, His Parents and the Nurse. Philadelphia, Pa., J. B. Lippincott Co., 1954.
2. Piaget, Jean. Construction of Reality in the Child, trans. by Margaret Cook. New York, Basic Books, 1954.
3. Rappaport, David. Collected Papers, ed. by Merton M. Gill. New York, Basic Books, 1967.
4. Erikson, E. H. Childhood and Society, rev. ed. New York, W. W. Norton and Co., 1964.
5. Piaget, op. cit.
6. Schilder, Paul. Image and Appearance of the Human Body. New York, International Universities Press, 1951.
7. Harlow, H. F., and Woolsey, C. N., eds. Biological and Biochemical Bases of Behavior. Madison, Wis., University of Wisconsin Press, 1958.
8. Lynd, Helen M. On Shame and the Search for Identity. New York, Science Editions, 1961.

Reading 8
Sexual Problems in Rehabilitation
Alan Frankel

Most people have unconscious conflicts about sex which they keep buried, and continue to live in a relatively satisfying manner. But a devastating injury or disease serves to unearth these conflicts, with their attendant anxiety. An injury which impairs bowel and bladder function brings to the surface an individual's hitherto buried conflicts about his sex role and creates further emotional disabilities.

When anxiety about sex is a significant problem to an individual with a physical disability, how does he cope with it? Most people are not willing to talk directly about sex. However, it is quite common for persons with a physical disability to express concern about their physical status. Sex-related anxiety, therefore, can be displaced to concern about ability to function physically, ability to function in the sexual role—omitting intercourse, and concern about bowel and bladder function.

An in-dwelling catheter may be unconsciously interpreted in a highly sexual manner. For example, a young girl, after a serious automobile accident, was left with a residual quadraparesis, ataxia, and loss of bowel and bladder function. She had an in-dwelling catheter and was almost completely physically helpless. She began to complain about men coming to see

Reprinted from *Journal of Rehabilitation*, vol. 33, no. 5, pp. 19-20, September-October 1967.

her at night, lurking in the shadows, and molesting her. Her reports of being molested diminished dramatically after her catheter was removed.

Rehabilitation personnel who are from time to time confronted by patients' sexual problems may feel uneasy and unqualified to discuss sex with them. Nevertheless, the patients' problems exist and must be handled. The great variation among patients as well as among personnel and agencies precludes any uniform approach. However, it may help to begin with an analysis of some of the reasons patients may talk about sex.

Depression and denial are two of the hallmarks of reaction to physical disability. In this context sexual material may be yet another symptomatic expression of feelings of worthlessness, e.g., "my spouse doesn't want me." Conversely, if denial and reaction-formation are operating within a depression, a person may brag about his premorbid sexual prowess in an attempt at restitution of his former self-image.

These two examples represent the reaction of an individual in the initial stages of his disability and are probably the least anxiety-producing for the rehabilitation worker. However, as a patient progresses through a rehabilitation program and thinks about return to the community, the meaning of sexual material may change.

For most people, the sex relationship serves as "interpersonal currency," i.e., a way of buying and selling in the interpersonal marketplace. Sexual behavior often reflects the characteristic style of participation in interpersonal relationships. For example, I was asked to see a 34-year-old woman who was exhibiting herself. She would frequently lie on her bed completely nude. At other times, she would stand at the wash-basin in her room, drop her skirt and underwear, and wash herself. Two months prior she had had a stroke.

As exhibitionism is frequently an attempt to disprove what is most deeply feared (she was afraid she was not a woman, but exposure of her genitals proved she was), I tried to understand what being a sexual woman meant to her. In essence, it meant insurance about being taken care of. Prior to her stroke, being taken care of was the central theme in her life. She would often offer her body either in gratitude or as prepayment for this.

With her perceived bodily disfigurements subsequent to her stroke, she now feared the loss of nurturance. Her exhibitionism represented a plea for caretaking (from the rehabilitation staff) and in part a testing out of her former mode of adaptation.

Her exhibitionism disappeared with a good deal of mothering from the nursing staff, and, equally as significant, with the beginning of a flirtation with a male patient.

Perhaps not as directly, but to a greater or lesser extent, we all use sex in this way or feel that if we wanted to, we could.

Sexual problems are, of course, usually related to the nature of the disability. Take the individual with a spinal cord lesion, for example. If it is true that sex is so interwoven with our interpersonal life, particularly in our middle-class American culture, then for the person with the spinal cord lesion, his very psychosocial existence is threatened.

RETURNING TO NORMAL

Getting back to normal implies resuming the patient's premorbid role within the family. The impact of a disabled member is considerably different after he returns home from an active rehabilitation program. Any social activity on weekends may have been enjoyable when the patient was in the hospital. However, the same activity may now have a new context. It is now carried out not in isolation from the daily life of the family at home, but as part of the fabric, including the wear and tear, normally encountered in family life.

If a wife with multiple sclerosis is in the hospital all week, but returns home for weekends, husband and wife may eagerly look forward to all the satisfactions, including sexual intercourse, of being together. If the wife is home permanently, weekends may be seen by the husband as a time of rest because he may have two jobs, his regular one plus parttime attendant to his wife. Or weekends may be seen by the husband as a time of family relaxation and an opportunity for the family to enjoy things together.

THE HUSBAND'S PROBLEM

If the wife is home and has a visiting rehabilitation worker during the week, the following situation could occur: The husband stops the worker on the way out and says in an agitated manner, "I don't know what to do. It's very hard for me to talk about it, but maybe you could help me." He then goes on to say that his wife has become sexually demanding. This is not like her and he doesn't know what to do. He may go on to talk about fear of pregnancy, fear of physically hurting her, concern about her catheter, etc.

The most therapeutic approach at this time is to *listen*. The husband and the worker both have very little idea of what the husband is saying except that he is upset about what should be a normal aspect of marriage.

Or, the husband may say that he wants to have sexual relations, but his wife refuses. It would seem profitable that the worker listen and try to answer some of these questions: How is the husband trying to use the worker—in collusion against his wife? In an attempt to coerce the wife? As a sympathetic ally? As a medical expert? As another human being to share his troubles with?

Understanding the communication and the nature of the marital relationship is of primary importance. The resolution of emotional conflicts is not the primary goal of most rehabilitation workers. However, a worker can use his sensitivity, experience, and sophistication to understand the emotional climate within a family.

EMOTIONALLY LOADED TOPIC

What a worker does with his understanding depends on many things. In my experience, rehabilitation personnel not infrequently feel concern, anxiety, fear, and a vague distress when patients talk about sex. The personal feelings of the worker, his inadequate academic preparation, agency restrictions, and the simple fact of an emotionally loaded topic all contribute to his uneasiness.

Sexual problems in a client are generally not expected by rehabilitation workers, who have probably experienced little exposure to this type of material in their training. Didactic course work, or even field work, seldom provides them with adequate guidelines. The policy of the agency may limit the scope of a worker's participation. For example, if the agency is oriented toward vocational placement or training, any significant personality problem may be handled by referral to another treatment person—or by ceasing to work with the client until the emotional problems are resolved.

In view of this, several ways of handling the problem are suggested below.

The organizational nature of the agency can provide a comfortable structure which enables the rehabilitation worker to deal with this type of problem. If he works in a comprehensive medical rehabilitation setting, there are colleagues with whom he can discuss this type of problem and, if indicated, to whom he can refer his client or patient.

It would seem that, in such a setting, the first person to whom the patient should be referred is his physician, especially when the patient has a spinal cord lesion. It is imperative that the patient and doctor work closely together on the physiological as well as the emotional aspects of sexual functioning, so that the patient has, at the very least, an intellectual understanding of his sexual capabilities. Once the patient has this understanding, it in no way insures that he will have an emotional understanding of it.

If, after working with an individual, the physician finds that he has reached the limits of his capability in dealing with the problems, he then may refer the patient to that rehabilitation worker who has established the best relationship with the patient.

Depending upon the policy of the agency, the security of the rehabilitation worker, and the willingness of the patient, there is no inherent reason why any rehabilitation worker cannot help a patient to talk about and work through feelings dealing with sexual problems. The mere title "nurse," "occupational therapist," etc., should not in any way affect whether a given rehabilitation worker handles this type of problem.

It would probably be agreed that sexual problems present much more difficulty where the rehabilitation worker is the only professional person in an agency, or where the worker does not have immediate access to other members of the traditional team.

What might the worker do in a situation where, for example, a person who is in psychotherapy comes to the agency worker and spills out sexual problems that are being worked through with the patient's psychotherapist?

The worker could best help the client by trying to understand the reason why the client is telling this to the worker at this time. Is he using the worker as a friend? Is he using him as an antagonist to the psychotherapist? Is it in the client's best interest to declare this topic off-limits? The latter might be the most productive type of support that the rehabilitation worker can offer. What may be supported is the client's inability to stop talking. To accomplish therapeutic support in this instance would involve, at the very least, talking with the patient's psychotherapist.

Another situation might occur in a sheltered workshop, where the clients are mentally retarded and adolescent and suddenly begin to act out sexually. Parents are disturbed, and it really looks as if a crisis is brewing.

In this situation it would seem best to consider any deviant behavior on an individual basis, i.e., to ask, "Why is *this* person acting out?" rather than to ask, "How can we stop *them* from doing this?" Such consideration, rather than rushing to smooth things over by a quick administrative decision, is often more effective, even though this type of approach is difficult to interpret to nonprofessionals, including parents.

IN SUMMARY

Within the interpersonal context of rehabilitation worker and patient, sexual thoughts and conflicts sometimes distress patient and worker alike. Talking about sex is a symptomatic expression of the current state of the patient and family and should be dealt with as one deals with any expression of psychological symptoms, i.e., by exercising good clinical judgment.

Reading 9
The Psychology of Illness
Sydney Smith

Illness, however else it may be classified, is a psychological event. How the emotional elements of an illness are understood and handled by the nurse may have a great deal to do with the patient's accessibility to treatment and his rate of recovery. Her ability to understand her own emotional reactions to illness may also affect the care she gives the patient and his response to her care.

WHAT ILLNESS MEANS TO THE PATIENT

The reactions patients have to illness, or the expectations they have of it, are of various kinds: those that are related to the symbolic meaning that illness has for them; those that pertain to the threats imposed by the state, or fact, of illness; and those connected with the pain that accompanies illness.

THE SYMBOLIC MEANING OF ILLNESS

Why is a person sick? The patient can often give reasonable justifications for his illness, sometimes in scientific terms, but the unconscious is not so logical, and the patient may entertain many subterranean fantasies about the meaning of his illness.

It is not uncommon to find people looking upon illness as a providential retaliation for their sins or as a punishment for their evil ideas or desires. If, at some deep level of his psychological organization, the patient believes that illness is punishment, what implications would this belief have for his getting well or, for that matter, for his having fallen ill in the first place? [1] Nurses often tell of their exasperation with the patient who gives lip service to his eagerness for recovery, but at the same time "forgets" to take the pills so dutifully laid out for him, subtly undermines the doctor's orders, and somehow manages to pull back from every sign of progress favorably commented on by the staff. It is sometimes difficult to remember that it is the patient's unconscious with which the nurse must do battle, and perhaps, like the good psychotherapist, she must ally herself with the patient's ego, identify with the sources of his inner strength, and thus help shift the balance of energy in the direction of recovery. If a man's guilt becomes aroused, it is possible for him to label himself as "bad" in the same fashion that his parents, earlier in his life, called him a "bad boy" for his misdeeds. Illness may be one way which the badness has of breaking out, so that whatever the nature of the germ or virus lurking in the body, it may be abetted by the patient's deep-seated need to purge himself of the psychic stress.

During illness, it is the fear of loss of the whole or a part of the body that appears to be the focus of psychological concern. While the anxiety is conscious, the idea of loss may not be conscious at all; such an idea may be so grave a threat to the ego that the whole matter is repressed.

That the idea of loss is at the basis of the patient's anxiety is dramatically portrayed in some cases of surgical or accidental amputations. I can remember seeing, in an emergency clinic, a young child whose middle finger had been blown off by a home-made explosive device. While the surgeon was attempting to sedate him and was preparing to repair the damage, the child pleaded with him and the nurses to release him so that he could recover the remainder of his finger.

Although amputations furnish particularly pertinent examples of the relation between anxiety and fear of loss, it seems likely that every illness contains some degree of threat to body integrity. Serious illness especially arouses a fear of loss of function, or loss of capacity for undertaking daily routines, or the sudden awareness of loss of control over one's own activities.

The threatened bodily damage implied in surgical procedures may have profound meaning for the patient. A study by Jessner, Blom, and Waldfogel on the emotional reactions of children undergoing a tonsillectomy or adenoidectomy provides a good illustration of the point [2]. The removal of the tonsils or the adenoids is a simple, usually uncomplicated surgical procedure, and yet the child's fantasy life regarding his fate may be extremely active.

When one leaves the patient in ignorance about what is going to happen to him, one provides a fertile field for the activation of fantasy. All kinds of distortions, many of a fearful nature, may creep into the patient's thinking. Jessner and his colleagues, for example, found that many of the children in their study did not even know where the tonsils and adenoids were located. When, prior to the operation, their fantasies were explored, it was found that many of them feared the mutilating results of the operation, and others felt that the operation would leave them castrated or would literally change them from boys into girls. Some of them associated hospitalization with pregnancy and had vivid fantasies about the birth process; others had identified themselves with another person's illness that was very different from their own, so that their fantasies were strangely deviant from reality. Disturbing fantasies of this kind are not limited to children, but are just as rampant in adult patients.

Unless dealt with at the time of illness, these threats to body integrity can have permanent effects. Janis's study of the implications of illness [3] suggests that exposure to any stress involving the threat of bodily damage—as, for example, in surgery—will facilitate the revival of disturbing childhood memories. It is remarkable how often any surgical procedure will leave an indelible psychic scar which, not infrequently, will be reported in later years as a significant childhood memory.

Psychiatrists and psychologists find these memories diagnostically important and can appreciate their dynamic meaning. If a patient comes to us with a psychiatric disturbance, we systematically explore his fantasies and his childhood memories. On the other hand, if a patient comes to us with a complaint of a physical nature, his fantasies and his early memories are ignored, despite the fact that these psychological realities may contain the key to a complete understanding of his illness.

THE THREAT OF ILLNESS

In addition to the unconscious, and often unrealistic, fears that a patient may have, illness is accompanied by some very real threats to his ego. In the first place, illness, by its very nature, tends to preoccupy its victims. Discomfort or pain in the body results in a withdrawal of whatever psychic investments one has made in the outside world. The patient almost involuntarily finds his concentration focused upon his own misery to the exclusion of whatever is happening around him. Most illness and its accompanying pain are likely to be transitory, but for the period of time an illness dominates its victim's consciousness, there is a shift of psychic energies to the self that results in an enlarged egocentricity.

Illness means not only increased narcissism but also increased regression. It is, in a sense, normal for a patient to withdraw from the world and to concentrate upon his body and his needs. A person often gives the first warning of an impending illness by discontinuing an active, outgoing contact with his environment. The child, especially, often becomes isolated and apathetic, curling up in a corner and remaining unusually quiet. There is good reason to believe that these features of the patient's behavior may be as psychological in origin as they are physiological, and that they may even be a beneficial and necessary part of the patient's adjustment to his own illness.

The need to adjust, however, may constitute another threat. Not uncommonly, a person faces in his illness the trial of unfamiliar states of dependency and passivity which may prove frightening and arouse considerable resistance to the acceptance of help.

The physical weakness and the limited motility which the patient sometimes suffers often given rise to an emotional intolerance for his illness that complicates the processes of recovery. Then, he must renounce ownership of his own body and passively permit it to be handled and manipulated by those who purport to nurse him back to health. He is dressed and undressed, regardless of his preferences; he is washed like an infant; while his bed is made he is pulled and pushed from one side to the other; the processes of urination and defecation are suddenly no longer private affairs; and he is subjected to the final indignity of having his nakedness exposed to the hospital personnel regardless of their sex. As a result, his attitudes, not surprisingly, often turn out to be ones of resentment, although they are frequently looked upon simply as "management problems."

One might think that in the case of the child patient the problem would not be quite so severe, since the child is closer to his own infancy and thus does not have so far to regress. But if the child is at an age when he has only recently come by his independence, his resistance to relinquishing it is even stronger than that of the more sophisticated adult; he does not wish to become a baby again and fights the loss of his ego control. For this reason, the child patient becomes the most difficult nursing problem the hospital faces.

While this typical reaction of children may be a source of despair for the nursing staff, the psychologist, in the safety of his academic distance from the hospital, sees it as psychologically healthy. It is the child who readily and completely surrenders his ego control and slides back into infancy without the least effort to do battle with his nurse for the preservation of his independence who is the one most likely to experience a severe emotional aftermath of his illness. Ego achievement so quickly lost may be a long time in redeveloping. Once it is abandoned for a return to the comfort of an infantile symbiotic relationship, it may not be easy to persuade the child again to tread the path of ego development.

These considerations underscore the necessity, in good nursing practice, of encouraging the independence of the patient whenever such encouragement is medically feasible. And it is feasible far more frequently than psychologically unsophisticated nursing routines would lead one to believe. In most instances, and this is especially true of the child patient, the nurse who is interested in preserving the patient's ego autonomy will get ample support from the patient. Every pediatrician and many mothers can recount cases of seriously ill children who will stand upright in the crib in the face of raging fevers and severe physical discomfort rather than surrender to the regression implied by lying down.

One can see an interesting re-emergence of this pattern of behavior in cases of senility. The older patient may be convinced, often on an unconscious level, that to relinquish ego control is tantamount to relinquishing life; to give up the ownership of his body in illness is to give up his claim to life itself.

THE PROBLEM OF PAIN

The psychological aspects of pain are not yet well understood. Pain is obviously one means the organism has of warning itself against the risk of further injury. However, pain frequently becomes exacerbated when it appears in the context of anxiety: The greater the anxiety in the patient's response to his illness, the more crippling the pain becomes, not only because of the manifest physical reaction, but also because of its unconscious determinants. To put it another way, the more the illness is invested with psychological meaning, the more vulnerable the patient becomes to pain. Pain, in turn, interferes with accessibility to treatment.

The more pain the patient experiences, the more he becomes preoccupied with the avoidance of further pain. His defenses may become phobically organized in that all of his fears may become focused on the needle or the pill or some special treatment procedure. One or another of these factors is perceived as the source of all discomfort; it is therefore regarded as something that must be avoided, regardless of the consequences insofar as the illness itself is concerned.

Pain that is intolerable to one patient is ignored by another with casual abandon, but precisely why such wide variations in the tolerance to pain exist is still something of a mystery. Hospital staffs often have an unfortunate tendency to use labels in describing patients who have variable reactions to pain; the more sensitive the patient is to pain, the more likely he is thought to be cowardly, whereas the patient who tolerates pain easily is referred to as courageous, or heroic. The nursing staff in any hospital will systematically discourage "cowardly" behavior, while encouraging the behavior of the patient who tolerates pain easily. One suspects that this nursing reaction stems more from a self-interest in the avoidance of management problems than from an understanding of the psychological meaning of pain.

Patients vary not only in their tolerance to pain, but also in their emotional reaction to suffering. Some patients become angry when they experience pain, others become filled with rage, still others become fearful; and there are those who, surprisingly, feel guilty in the face of pain. It is sometimes difficult to explain these specific reactions, but it seems likely that they arise from the patient's underlying unconscious fantasies about the personal meaning of his illness. Sometimes these fantasies can be exposed in a psychiatric interview or expressed in certain psychological tests, and in the hands of a skilled person this information can be used to help the patient cope with his anxiety and his pain.

Nurses and physicians have frequently remarked that some patients who, because of the nature of the treatment procedure, have suffered a great deal of pain at their hands form strong emotional attachments to them. It is as if the patient slips into a passive masochistic response to the sadism expected of the physician or the nurse. Although it is not appropriate here to engage in a detailed account of masochism as a defense against pain, it is not out of place to warn nurses that the "love" their patients express for them may be nothing more than a libidinizing of the painful aspects of their treatment.

Patients also differ with respect to their expectations of pain. Janis, in his study [4], found that a good many patients were defending themselves against their disturbing fantasies about surgery by denying the likelihood of suffering. The patients whose denial of pain or the implications of their illness was marked showed little anxiety prior to the operation. However, these patients were the ones most likely to react with anger and resentment in the postoperative crisis period. Janis explains that an intellectual denial of suffering leads to the anticipation of little pain, and that when this illusion is shattered, the patient experiences a reactivation of early childhood disappointment. In a sense, nurses and physicians become, for a time, symbolic parents, and the patient's early disappointment in his parents is rekindled.

THE PREPARATION FOR TREATMENT

If the patient's emotions are properly dealt with—that is, if in preparation for a treatment he is given some understanding of, and help in coping with, his feelings—much can be done to reduce the emotional complications of illness. Recently, I worked with an emotionally troubled boy who, eight weeks before, had entered a hospital to have an inflamed appendix removed. He had been sedated and wheeled into the operating room in a drowsy state, but not asleep. Moments before the anesthetic was to be administered, a hurried conference among the staff resulted in a quick switch of plans. The child was wheeled to one side of the room to make way for another patient, also a child, whose tonsils were to be removed. With mounting panic, the first patient heard and partially observed the entire tonsillectomy.* This child has made a slow recovery, during which he has suffered from repeated nightmares, insomnia, and anorexia.

Although this may be an extreme case, it helps to underscore the fact that adequate emotional preparation of the patient for a treatment procedure is a matter almost entirely neglected in the hospital setting. We all have failed to realize that the fears that accompany illness are often mingled with the fear of death. Our knowledge of the patient must include an understanding of his emotional reactions to illness. Furthermore, dealing with these feelings in a constructive way should become a standard part of any treatment regimen.

The importance of such an approach is demonstrated in a report by Plank and Horwood [5] that describes the detailed and careful preparation of several weeks' duration provided for a four-year-old girl whose leg had to be amputated. Both the parents and the surgeon wished to hide the facts of the illness from this child, but they were overruled by the psychiatric social workers, who realized that, if this were done, the child would feel angry and resentful toward her parents because they had not been strong enough to protect her from such a terrifying fate. The operation was delayed as long as was medically feasible, not only so that the child could be prepared psychologically for the loss of her leg, but also so that she could be helped to accept the idea of wearing an artificial limb.

* Incredible as this event may seem, its details were later verified by the hospital staff.

The authors describe how the idea of amputation was introduced and how the need for the amputation was for a time displaced to the leg of the child's doll. Together, the psychiatric social worker and the child made an artificial leg for the doll and spent several days in fitting it on the doll and disassembling it, until eventually the child understood what the doctor would do, why it was necessary, and what the aftermath of her own operation would be.

The patient's need for understanding can be seen in his tendency to relive the experience of his illness again and again. In the case of the child, such experiences may be acted out, as when a youngster who has suffered pain in the dental chair comes home to re-enact the experience with his younger sibling. In the adult, the reliving of the experience is more likely to take the form of verbal expression. Who has not been socially trapped by a friend's endlessly detailed and fatuous account of his operation?

Illness has unconscious meaning for the nurse as well as for the patient. In spite of the adequacy of her formal training, her application and scholarship, and the wisdom of her teachers, she will inevitably have emotional reactions to illness and, equally inevitably, to patients. When it is possible, it is wise to examine the unconscious motives for entering a given career. Just as the policeman may enter his field of work to protect himself against his own unconscious criminal tendencies, or as the psychologist may be gratifying his unconscious need for voyeurism, so the nurse may have a need to overcome her internal weakness by dominating and infantilizing her patients. A nurse's failure to respond to the psychological wavelengths of the patients is frequently due to the fact that her own emotional needs have interfered with her acceptance of the patient's reality.

Death and incurable illness are two realities that are very difficult for a nurse to accept. Her personal needs often lead her to view illness as something to be conquered. Her need is to deny death and to emphasize eventual recovery, even when these attitudes seem hypocritical. If the patient can be snatched from the jaws of death, she will not only have the feeling of job success but also will have convincing proof that people do not have to die. In saving the patient, the nurse is also saving herself.

When her patient does not get well, or when his impending death stares out starkly from the hospital bed, the nurse may feel that she has been a failure. The feeling of depression that follows upon a patient's death stems in part from the nurse's feelings of hopelessness and despair because she has been unable to protect him from death. In some cases, the nursing staff withdraws from the seriously ill patient or from the patient whose death is imminent. The withdrawal of emotional investment in such a patient is a defensive maneuver on the part of the nurse, who must manage her own feelings of failure and her own emotional reactions to the meaning of illness and death.

Admittedly, it is not easy to view death as a natural phenomenon or see that, in some cases, the nursing function is one of helping the patient to accept his illness. The difficulty of embodying these realities in one's philosophy of life underscores the importance of mental health concepts in the nurse's background. The job of training in such concepts is not simply one for the undergraduate years in a nurse's college or hospital experience. Continuing education is necessary for her to face the mental health issues that inevitably intrude upon her work situation.

A sign of progress in recent years has been the recognition, by many schools of nursing and hospitals, of the need for mental health consultants. However, many promising possibilities have yet to be explored. As one of many examples, take the possible role of the psychiatrist or psychologist attached to a general hospital. Consider the important job such a specialist could do in helping patients to accept the necessity for surgical intervention, or the preventive work that could be accomplished in saving patients from unnecessary postoperative reactions. How many postpartum depressions, how many dysphoric reactions to hospitalization, how many emotional blocks to recovery could have been prevented if the need had been recognized, if the time had been taken, if the care had been provided? In how many cases are the emotional problems of the patient's family and relatives handled perfunctorily, often without compassion, because feelings are no one's special job?

However, it is not just the patient and his family who need help; the entire hospital staff must be brought to a better understanding of the meaning of pain and the symbolism of the patient's reaction, and to an appreciation of their own emotional responses to the patient. The psychology of illness is a psychology of humanity, and in humanity we all have a share.

REFERENCES

1. Stephen, Karin, *The Wish to Fall Ill*, Cambridge University Press, 1933.
2. Jessner, L., G. Blom, and S. Waldfogel, "Emotional Implications of Tonsillectomy and Adenoidectomy in Children," *The Psychoanalytic Study of the Child*, 7:126-168, 1952.
3. Janis, I., *Psychological Stress*, New York: John Wiley & Sons, 1958.
4. Ibid.
5. Plank, Emma, and Carla Horwood, "Leg Amputation in a Four-Year-Old: Reactions of the Child, Her Family and the Staff," *The Psychoanalytic Study of the Child*, 16:405-422, 1961.

Reading 10
Sexual Adjustments in Relation to Pregnancy, Illness, Surgery, Physical Handicaps, and Other Unusual Circumstances
Isadore Rubin

As William F. Sheeley has noted [1],

> Sexual feelings and activities, whether normal or disordered, are the final common pathway of a complex constellation of numerous and various influences and conditions. They certainly have roots in physiological function. But they also have roots deep within the psychological being of the individual and within his interpersonal adjustment with other people.

Being physiologically and psychologically controlled, sexual feelings and activities are inevitably affected both by the anatomic and functional changes resulting from illness, chronic disease, or surgery and by the psychologic and interpersonal reactions to these changes. Particularly in cases of surgery or disease involving genital or reproductive structures, the physician should prepare the patient for possible changes in sexual functioning and should forestall needless damaging anxieties or difficulties caused by his indifference to possible sexual problems. Aging men who are already beginning to have problems with impotence need every encouragement that can realistically be given concerning the likelihood that needed surgery will not diminish their sexual potency [2]. A negative attitude or even silence on the part of the physician will sometimes pronounce a death sentence for a patient's sexual life.

For the couple whose sexual adjustment has been precarious, a prolonged period of abstinence following illness, surgery, or pregnancy may bring about further deterioration in marital relations, and may even serve as a convenient pretext for ending sexual activity permanently. For this reason, Oliven [3] recommends that the physician allow, or even encourage, the greatest possible sexual freedom to a couple at the earliest possible time following a period of abstinence necessitated by the physical condition of the husband or wife. In some cases, of course, special precautions may have to be recommended. Oliven's advice is based not so much on a desire to allevi-

---
Reprinted from Clark E. Vincent (ed.), *Human Sexuality in Medical Education and Practice*, 1968, pp. 532-551. Courtesy of Charles C Thomas, Publisher, Springfield, Ill.

ate the hardship caused by abstention from sexual activity as on the belief that lengthy periods of abstinence may have unpredictable disruptive effects on marriage. Masters and Johnson [4] have pointed out, for example, that the unnecessarily long period of abstinence traditionally prescribed after delivery causes many men to turn to extramarital sexual relations for the first time.

The physician should prepare the patient for the fact that, because of general body weakness, lack of confidence, or other factors, the first attempt at sexual relations following illness or surgery may not be satisfactory. Many men and women, not realizing that a temporary discomfort related to their physical condition may make sexual activity unattractive for a time, jump to the conclusion that their sexual functioning is permanently impaired. For many men, a failure in the first attempt at intercourse may reinforce this erroneous belief, paving the way for future failures.

In a study of men who had had heart attacks one to nine years previously, three cardiologists underscored the importance of providing guidance concerning sexual activity following a serious illness [5]. Most of the men were under fifty, and virtually none of them had received from their physician any detailed and specific advice about sexual activity. Only about a third of these men had resumed their normal pattern of sexual activity, and 10 per cent had become completely impotent. The most significant finding, however, was that the pattern of sexual activity bore no relation to age or to the severity of the heart attack; it depended almost entirely on the patient's attitude.

Unfortunately, traditional attitudes toward sex still constitute in most areas what a distinguished British jurist called "a legacy of the ascetic ideal, persisting in the modern world after the ideal has deceased" [6]. It is difficult for most persons to rid themselves of this legacy even within the normal marital relationship. When this relationship is complicated by unusual physical conditions—or even by a condition as usual as pregnancy—the physician will need to assume an active counseling role in order to help the couple overcome the handicap imposed by these traditional attitudes. Patients find it difficult to ask questions about sexual problems even under ordinary circumstances. In the face of a serious illness involving life or death, anxieties about sexual functioning may be considered by the patient too shameful or trivial to be mentioned and, by the spouse, as showing a selfish lack of consideration. By making questions of this nature a routine part of medical practice, the physician can insure that proper attention will be given to this important aspect of marital interaction.

Golden has emphasized the importance of the physician's attitude in the management of sexual problems [7]:

There is often implied by the doctor's behavior an attitude of rejecting the patient, perhaps conveying to one already embarrassed that his concerns are evil, unacceptable, or otherwise beneath consideration. On the other hand, physicians can bring about successful change in a patient as much by the persuasive effects of the physician's personality as by the information he conveys.

Golden stressed the need for the physician to become aware of the extent to which his own attitudes toward sex affect his relationship with his patients. "If he personally is uncomfortable discussing sexual matters," he warned, "or if his attitudes are too rigidly moralistic or too flagrantly antisocial, he is vulnerable to error." This advice is particularly applicable in cases involving illness, disease, or serious handicaps.

PREGNANCY AND THE POSTPARTUM PERIOD

Medical journals and textbooks have devoted little attention to the question of sexual relations during pregnancy and the postpartum period, although it is clear that this is an important problem for most couples. It is traditional to prohibit coitus during episodes of threatened abortion or unusual bleeding as well as during the last four to six weeks of pregnancy and the first six weeks after delivery. This may add up to the disruption of marital relations for a period of three consecutive months. In spite of the lack of sufficient research evidence, obstetricians are beginning to challenge the traditional blanket prohibition of coitus before and after delivery and to adjust their advice to individual circumstances [8]. Many believe that intercourse should not be prohibited during pregnancy, or in the period following delivery, for the woman who has no significant pain or discomfort and who desires coitus.

Increased attention is also being paid to the emotional problems of the husband during pregnancy and to the need for preventing, so far as possible, any feeling of exclusion on his part. To this end, it is important that the expectant father have ready access to his wife's physician to discuss any problems or questions he may have.

MEDICAL CONDITIONS

Heart Disease and Hypertension

Despite the common belief that normal sexual relations are no longer possible after a coronary attack, there is general agreement among cardiologists that the vast majority of patients are able to resume sexual activity within a few months [2]. There is, of course, no blanket rule to cover all cardiac patients; the physician must base his advice not only on the type of heart condition the individual has, but also on his emotional makeup and the circumstances of coitus. It should be noted that suppressed libido causes considerable tension [9,10].

Although cases of hemiplegia, stroke, or death occurring during intercourse and other sexual activities have been reported, these are, according to the Kinsey group [11], not at all frequent. Sexual excitement and climax have distinct effects on the pulse rate and blood pressure and, consequently, on the heart. Pulse rates of 110 to more than 180 have been recorded during intercourse [11,12]. In addition to the increase in pulse rate from 70 to 80 to as high as 170 or 180, the blood pressure may rise from 120 to more than 250, and the respiratory rate, normally 16 to 18 per minute, may increase to more than 40 per minute. As the Kinsey investigators noted, these rates approach those of an athlete during his maximum effort, or those of a man involved in heavy labor. They return to normal very quickly after intercourse, however. Masters and Johnson [12] reported that higher cardiac rates were found during female masturbation than during intercourse.

It is generally agreed that no patient with any type of acute cardiac disease should engage in intercourse [13]. Patients with angina pectoris have been warned to be very cautious regarding intercourse. In other cases it is generally agreed that sexual activity is permissible as long as it causes no subjective discomfort, shortness of breath, palpitation, or undue fatigue [14].

The precautions to be observed regarding sexual intercourse following a heart attack are the same whether the husband or the wife is the patient [15]. Some men believe that the relatively passive part women play in intercourse does not constitute undue exertion. The physician should explain to the husband of a cardiac patient that emotional rather than physical factors are responsible for raising the blood pressure and heart rate during coitus. Masters and Johnson, as well as other researchers, have shown that these rates are generally similar in males and females.

Special precautions that may be advisable for the patient include the use of nitroglycerine before coitus; having coitus in the morning rather than at the end of the day; selecting a comfortable and relaxed position (side positions may be advantageous); avoiding intercourse after a large meal, while wearing constrictive garments, or under unusual conditions of heat, cold, or humidity [13]. Coitus interruptus is considered unwise, and special caution is needed in cases of delayed ejaculation.

In general, Oliven has advised the need for "moderation" and "relaxation," pointing out that moderation in the amount of intercourse can be defined only in terms of individual need and habit: "Although one may rather arbitrarily set an average figure of one or two times a week, frequencies as high as five times a week probably do not, per se, constitute harmful excess in couples accustomed to, and genuinely and mutually desirous of this rate." He defined "relaxed" or "sedate" coitus as coitus taking place in the presence of a good, affectionate relationship, where the spouse is willing to cooperate in all necessary measures. Coitus is less apt to be relaxed when it takes place in an atmosphere of emotional tension, in nonmarital ventures, and between newlyweds.

Estrogen has been found useful in the treatment of men who have had coronary attacks, but its side effects have made it undesirable for some men. The effect of the therapy on libido is still a matter of controversy. One group of investigators [16] reported that 84 per cent of patients on estrogen therapy experienced either a decrease or a total loss of sexual desire and ability; another [17], that changes in libido were rarely noted in 125 patients treated for as long as twenty-five years.

In discussing the management of high blood pressure, Irvine H. Page, chairman of the Medical Advisory Board of the Council for High Blood Pressure Research of the American Heart Association, declared [14]:

> When intercourse is followed by the normal feeling of relaxation and peace of mind, it is altogether beneficial. On the other hand, a state of sustained though mild sexual excitation, whether following intercourse or not, can only result in a steady tension, which is especially undesirable for the management of hypertension.... There is no rule for the frequency of intercourse for those who have high blood pressure. They may well apply the dictum that should govern all their lives—moderation.

Diabetes in the Male

In recent years it has been discovered that diabetes in men may have important effects on the sexual function, sometimes causing erectile impotence, difficulty in ejaculation, or retrograde ejaculation into the bladder.

The connection between diabetes and impotence was first investigated by Rubin and Babbott [18], who found that a number of women with infertility problems reported that their husbands were impotent. Follow-up investigation showed that the rate of impotence in diabetic males was two to five times higher than the average reported by the Kinsey group.

Schoffling and his colleagues [19] found erectile impotence in 51 per cent of their series of 314 diabetic men. Klebanow and MacLeod [20] found that one-third of the impotent males among their diabetic patients complained, not of weakness of erection, but of difficulty in ejaculation. This difficulty became progressive until complete loss of function resulted. Greene and his colleagues at the Mayo Clinic [21] have described cases of retrograde ejaculation caused by diabetic neuropathy. Severe diabetes apparently damages the nerves which control the closing of the bladder neck during coitus.

The mechanism responsible for sexual disorders in diabetics is still a matter of conjecture [20,21,22]. Impairment of pituitary gonadotropic function may be one factor; another may be calcium deposits in the smooth muscles of the genital tract and the walls of seminal vesicles, which are known to occur earlier in diabetics than in normal persons. Another possible explanation is degeneration of the nerve fibers responsible for sexual functioning; it seems likely that this might occur as part of diabetic neuropathy.

As in other disorders, physicians must not overlook the psychologic factor resulting from anxiety or loss of confidence produced by the physical disability. Learning that one must reorganize his dietary habits and way of life may cause considerable emotional trauma.

Every patient with the complaint of impotence should be checked for possible diabetes. The physician should be careful, however, not to convey to any diabetic patient the impression that impotence is a necessary consequence of this disease. The data are not yet all in. Wershub [23], finding few diabetics among the impotent males he has treated, sent out a questionnaire to selected internists who treated many diabetic patients. The majority indicated that they had found no increase in the incidence of impotence among diabetic men. Schoffling and his colleagues [19] reported that therapy with combined chorionic gonadotropin and testosterone corrected impotence in most of their diabetic patients under forty years of age; patients over forty were treated with testosterone alone, with improvement in sexual potency and general well-being.

SURGICAL CONDITIONS
Prostatic Surgery

A considerable proportion of middle-aged and elderly men have prostate trouble, and many require prostatic surgery. Since these problems are likely to occur at the time of life when most men have some concern about their sexual capacities, prevention of anxieties about sexual functioning should be an essential part of the urologist's treatment. Research in recent years has made it clear that impotence following prostatectomy—regardless of the surgical route employed—is surprisingly rare in men who were sexually active prior to surgery; some men even claimed improved sexual functioning.

Stearns [24] found that 81.4 per cent of a series of patients who had undergone retropubic prostatectomy (at an average age of 76) claimed ability to have sexual relations following the operation. Finkle and his colleagues [25] found that 70 per cent of their series of men who had undergone prostatic surgery of various kinds retained their potency. A study by Holtgrewe and Valk [26] showed that 382 of 840 men who had undergone transurethral prostatectomy at an average age of 69 reported satisfactory sexual performance thereafter. Even after radical perineal prostatectomy, which results in considerable damage to the nerves responsible for sexual functioning, at least 10 per cent of patients retain potency [27].

In cases of prostatic cancer, the surgeon may remove the testes as well as the prostate, or institute treatment with estrogen—sometimes in addition to removal of the testes. Ellis and Grayhack [28] have reported that many men retain some degree of normal sexual functioning following the castration. Even in the group treated by estrogen therapy in addition to orchiectomy, 27 per cent of the patients remained potent. One sixty-two-year-old man in this group had intercourse about fifteen times per week!

Physicians may contribute to impaired functioning following prostatectomy in different ways. Some, by their silence, confirm the patient's belief that sexual activity will no longer be possible. Others, as a measure of protection against lawsuits, contribute to the psychologic causes of impotence by asking men to sign a statement to the effect that they are aware that the surgery may result in impotence. Surgeons who comment that impotence is inevitable after certain types of surgery such as radical perineal prostatectomy help to insure impotence in patients who have this operation.

Finkle and Moyers [25], stressing the importance of psychologic factors in bringing about impotence following prostatic surgery, cited the case of a patient, supposedly made impotent by the surgery, who regained his potency following hypnotic suggestion. They noted the following psychologic factors which can explain impotence after a prostatectomy: (1) For a certain number of men the operation provides a convenient excuse for ending sexual activity which may have been maintained only with difficulty in the face of declining desire, ability, and performance; (2) the patient's fear of impotence may have been reinforced by the attitude of the urologist; (3) many men believe that sexual activity following any operation will weaken the incision or endanger health; (4) certain negative attitudes toward sex that existed before the operation are strengthened after it.

Men should be made aware of one important sequel of most prostatectomies: retrograde ejaculation into the bladder as a result of surgical damage to nerves controlling the muscle that closes the bladder neck. Often neither the patient nor his partner is aware that normal ejaculation of semen has not occurred. In younger men the condition may be discovered only after medical advice is sought because of infertility.

It is quite clear that the retention of sexual function following prostate surgery depends in some measure on the attitudes which the surgeon communicates to the patient. The physician has a responsibility to prevent any postoperative impotence of iatrogenic origin and to make a positive contribution by uncovering and assuaging the anxieties which this type of surgery creates in both the patient and his wife.

Hysterectomy

Adequate care of a patient who must undergo hysterectomy, Shipps has cautioned, "involves more than the mechanics of a properly performed surgical procedure" [29]. It involves consideration of the woman both as an individual and as a member of the family unit. According to Shipps, it is essential that the husband be brought into consultation before surgery. The family physician and the hospital personnel "all have a role to play" in the outcome of the hysterectomy, "to say nothing of the friends and visitors who stop by to play their part for better or for worse."

Aside from the occasional shortening of the vagina which may result, hysterectomy causes little physiologic or anatomic change that should diminish the sexual satisfaction of either the husband or the wife. Hormonal therapy can compensate for the loss of estrogen resulting from removal of the ovaries. It is possible that removal of the cervix deprives some few women of a sensation resulting from movement of the uterus during deep penetration [30]. For the majority of women, however, sexual functioning is unchanged after a hysterectomy [31].

Like any surgery involving the reproductive organs, hysterectomy may have important psychologic repercussions for some men and women, particularly if they are not prepared for the operation. Psychoanalytic studies have revealed that women view hysterectomy as a castration in some degree, and many of them not only fear possible loss of sexual feelings but are also afraid of becoming unattractive, of aging prematurely, and of developing masculine characteristics [32]. It is important to note that these studies all involve patients who have sought psychiatric treatment for emotional disturbance, and that these women are therefore not necessarily typical of all those who have undergone hysterectomy. In a study of persons admitted to a psychiatric institute, Patterson and Craig [33] found that only 15 per cent of the women had been admitted during the first year after hysterectomy; this finding suggested that removal of the womb had not in itself been particularly stressful. Investigating the hypothesis that the uterus is of tremendous psychologic significance to the average woman and that, when it is removed, she feels "mutilated" and "nonfeminine," these researchers found this attitude in only six of one hundred patients who had had a hysterectomy. In some of these cases, too, they found reasons other than the surgery for such feelings. Half of the women considered themselves to be "well and whole, better than before."

A severe depressive reaction, however, follows hysterectomy in a small percentage of women, particularly those in the younger age group. Melody's study of women who had these depressive reactions revealed that all of them had had at least one depressive episode during the five years preceding the hysterectomy. In each case, it seemed clear that the depressive reaction following the surgery was precipitated by some event which the patient interpreted as serious rejection by someone important in her life.

Melody's analysis showed widespread misconceptions about hysterectomy, which should be countered by the physician whenever possible. In a few cases, hysterectomy had a serious effect on the husbands. Two became impotent—one because he felt his wife was now just "a shell of a woman"; and the other, because he feared penile injury from coitus with a "desexed woman." One husband deserted because he was fearful of contracting cancer if he resumed sexual relations with his wife, who had had cancer of the uterus; and two accused their wives of infidelity and adultery "after that operation." Obviously it is essential that a clear understanding of what happens during and after hysterectomy, the vast majority of couples continue a satisfactory sexual life without any complications. In a South African survey conducted by three physicians, 40 per cent of the women replying stated that marital relations were unchanged, and an additional 38 per cent reported that they had improved [35]. These physicians found, however, that at the time of the six-week checkup some of the women asked the physician to advise them to postpone the resumption of intercourse.

Mastectomy

The removal of the female breast is not likely to have any direct physical effect upon sexual functioning. Because the breasts have important sexual connotations for both men and women, however, mastectomy may have a serious effect on the husband-wife relationship. In summarizing the result of research with cancer patients, Waxenberg said [36]:

> The loss of an important part of the body may disrupt a person's total pattern of psychological adaptation. The more critically the organ has been involved in a pattern, the more difficult is readjustment likely to be and the more important is psychological understanding of the patient.

According to Bard and Sutherland [37], the removal of a breast is a terrifying experience that has an enormous impact on any woman from the moment she discovers the first symptoms throughout the course of treatment and convalescence. They have pointed out that the focus of anxiety varies greatly for each patient, and that it is essential for the physician to determine the particular source of anxiety in each case before trying to deal with it.

The prerequisite is the establishment of a warm and supportive relationship with the patient; otherwise, factual discussion may aggravate rather than lessen the patient's problems. Bard and Sutherland also emphasized the importance of including the husband in any discussion of radical mastectomy since the operation may constitute a real threat to the marriage. A good marriage will probably weather the problems imposed by the operation. In a marriage habitually fraught with tension, marital distrust, and sexual incompatibility, mastectomy almost inevitably leads to some deterioration in the relationship; in such cases, referral to a family counseling service may be advisable.

Oophorectomy

Removal of the ovaries, either because of ovarian disease or because of the potential effect upon other organs, does not essentially alter the patient's sexual response and activity [38]. However, removal of a woman's adrenal glands (performed in some cases as part of the treatment for cancer of the breast) has caused a sharp decrease in sexual desire, activity, and responsiveness in the majority of cases [39,40]. This has been attributed to the loss of the androgen produced by the adrenals; the so-called male hormones are now considered to play a critical part in maintaining the patterns of sexual response in the human female as well as in the male [41].

Colostomy and Rectal Surgery

Many factors contribute to the sexual difficulties that often follow this operation [36]. Although women generally retain sexual function, surgical damage to pelvic nerves may lead to erectile and ejaculatory impotence in men. Fear of rejection by others is an important factor in many cases; some patients do not ever allow their spouses to view the colostomy. More than half the patients in one study gave up intercourse altogether following colostomy, for reasons ranging from abhorrence on the part of the partner to impotence on the part of the patient. This situation, of course, poses a serious threat to many marriages. Weigel has urged careful preparation to minimize the panic, despair, or confusion with which a patient may react when informed of the need for this surgery. In cases of impotence following colostomy, according to Weigel [42]:

> Where sexual relationship was good prior to the onset of impotence, the emotional rapport continues to be good between husband and wife. In the case of pleasureless and unstable marriages before the advent of the colostomy, the emotional relationship deteriorates and the colostomy is used as a rationalization for the situation.

Studies of sexual activity following surgery on the rectum [43] have shown varying results, apparently depending upon the extent to which nerves essential for functioning have remained unharmed, as well as upon unknown psychologic factors. In a large number of cases, sexual functioning has not been disturbed.

Vaginal Surgery

Operations performed on or through the vagina may adversely affect the sexual functioning of older women and their husbands. Apareunia and dyspareunia are common after operations for prolapse of the uterus [44]. It has been estimated that, in approximately 20 per cent of the women who have this operation, the resultant vaginal narrowing and scarring are sufficient to cause loss of feeling or pain on intercourse. The narrowing may result partly from senile atrophy and vaginal disuse, but the method of suture is also a factor. It is important for surgeons to take every possible precaution to avoid shortening the vagina. The patient should be re-examined six weeks after surgery and given specific instructions about the resumption of coitus.

DISABLING PHYSICAL HANDICAPS

In most of the problems discussed thus far, the physician's primary role has been that of providing reassurance and encouragement and of dispelling wrong attitudes and anxieties which may interfere with satisfactory marital relations. We cannot overlook the many cases in which serious physical handicaps make it difficult or even impossible for the patient to engage in coitus. Helping a couple to readjust to such a situation often requires the physician to reevaluate his own thinking, especially if he has held rigidly to certain beliefs. As Branson has pointed out [45],

> The consensus in our culture is that the handicapped person is to be cared for and indulged regularly. Yet little consideration is given to the fact that a victim who is married is not disabled alone. His mate suffers a form of disability, too, one that also requires adjustment and rehabilitation.

Faced with a disabling handicap, many couples will find their own solution: sexual gratification by noncoital methods such as mutual hand stimulation of the genitals or oral-genital contacts; the use of positions not usually employed in coitus; sexual relations outside the marriage, with or without the consent of the handicapped partner; or the use of masturbation by the nonhandicapped person.

It is not the function of the physician to propose a particular solution, but rather to help the couple make the wisest choice among alternatives as is possible in the light of their needs and their values. The physician must guard against imposing his own values system upon them, either overtly, or covertly by a biased evaluation of the options open to them.

Paraplegics were formerly believed to be without sexual capacity. It is now recognized, however, that most types of injuries to the spinal cord permit varying degrees of sexual functioning for both the male and the female [46,47,48]. For the male paraplegic, erection will be the reflex type brought about by manual stimulation of the penis or scrotum or inner sides of the thighs. Coitus is generally possible for the female. The paraplegic may have strong libidinal urges, based on mental imagery. Because of cord damage, orgasm or ejaculation produces no sensation; nevertheless, paraplegics often find coitus desirable for its effect on their ego and sense of adequacy, as well as to permit gratification of the partner. Few paraplegics, according to Oliven, need to remain total "sex cripples" [47].

> It is possible to help them to explore what they are capable of and to develop a vita sexualis adapted to the life circumstances, personality, past experience, cultural background and temperament of each one of them. Ideally, this is an integral part of the rehabilitation program for these patients.

In the case of youngsters growing up with serious handicaps from birth or from an early age, most families tend to regard them as nonsexual entities and fail to prepare them in any way to accept a feminine or masculine role. Physicians who deal with these families must help the parents to realize that normal sexuality is as important for handicapped people as for others [49]. Although a few such individuals are forced, by virtue of their handicaps, to suppress their sexual desires, many can be satisfactory wives or husbands. Parents should be encouraged to accept the developing sexuality of these young people and to provide an environment where the child can come to grips with his sexual feelings, realize his limitations, and develop skills that will help as much as possible to compensate for these limitations. Parents should especially be cautioned against overprotecting these youngsters and thus depriving them of the opportunity to mature emotionally.

OTHER UNUSUAL CIRCUMSTANCES

Epilepsy

Children with epilepsy present a special problem. Most parents consider them unmarriageable, and some states have laws against the marriage of epileptics. However, a study by a counselor (herself subject to epileptic seizures) of fifty marriages in which one or both partners were subject to seizures indicated that epilepsy in itself need not interfere with normal sexual union and successful marriage [50]. Naturally these couples face special problems in adjustment, and careful medical management may be required in the period of courtship and the early days of marriage. For those whose condition is hereditary, sterilization or very careful contraceptive measures are advisable.

Mental Retardation and Mental Illness

For understandable reasons, attitudes toward the sexual needs of the mentally retarded and of persons in mental institutions have been most restrictive. Parents—with the approval of society—have concentrated all their energy on repressing or controlling any expression of sexuality in the mentally retarded rather than encouraging expression of the individual's sexual needs in ways which would not be harmful to society. Physicians should begin to help parents adopt this carefully encouraging attitude rather than a completely restrictive one [51]. In mental institutions, the general practice has been to deny libidinous feelings in patients. As Wolff has said, however, "Sexual interest may be present even in psychotic and confused patients," and understanding of libidinous impulses and empathy on the part of the therapist "may make the difference between a cure or a failure in treatment" [53,54]. Although Wolff's statement was made with reference to geriatric patients, it is even more applicable to younger ones.

Institutional Isolation

Many circumstances other than mental illness require institutional isolation and separation from one's regular sexual partner. Among these circumstances are diseases like tuberculosis or leprosy, some geriatric conditions, and imprisonment in penal institutions. Money has commented on this situation as follows [48]:

> Our society has not yet seen fit to formulate a rationale of its policy of depriving people of a sex life who are not able to love out of custody. . . . In an age of effective contraception and liberalized public sentiment on sexual matters, the time seems ripe in our own society for a reformulation of the rules of arbitrarily imposed abstinence on patients and prisoners institutionally segregated from society at large.

DISFIGURING INJURIES AND DISEASES

As a result of heredity, embryonic development, or injuries in later life, there are a number of ugly, maimed, or deformed people whose "index on the popularity parade . . . is at the bottom of the list" [48]. When nothing further remains to be done surgically, the physician can help the patient to build self-confidence and courage. Often the biggest problem is one of simply meeting suitable prospective partners. To accomplish this purpose, Money [48] has suggested, "Lonely Hearts Clubs" and marriage bureaus deserve more serious attention than the snickering they generally receive. Special clubs for the handicapped and disfigured are also useful.

CONCLUSION

In counseling patients concerning sexual adjustments in relation to various normal and abnormal conditions, the physician has a key responsibility. As the person best trained to give advice concerning the physiologic effects of particular conditions upon sexual response, he is accorded an authority in this area possessed by no other individual. This very authority obligates him to become familiar with the psychologic aspects of these conditions so that he can deal adequately with the anxieties which they arouse concerning sexual function.

REFERENCES

1. Sheeley, W. F.: Sex and the practicing physician. *JAMA*, **196**:139-143, April 11, 1966.
2. Rubin, I.: *Sexual Life after Sixty*. New York, Basic Books, 1965, chaps. 11 to 13.
3. Oliven, J. F.: *Sexual Hygiene and Pathology*, 1st ed. Philadelphia, Lippincott, 1955, p. 215.
4. Masters, W. F., and Johnson, V. E.: *Human Sexual Response*. Boston, Little, 1966, chap. 10.
5. Tuttle, W. B., et al.: Sexual Behavior in Post-myocardial Infarction Patients. Abstract of paper presented to the College of Cardiology, February 1964, p. 128 of program.
6. Williams, G.: *The Sanctity of Life and the Criminal Law*. New York, Knopf, 1957, p. 51.
7. Golden, J. S.: Management of sexual problems by the physician. *Obstet. Gynec.*, **23**:471-474, March 1964.
8. Israel, S. L., and Rubin, I.: *Sexual Relations during Pregnancy and the Post-delivery Period*. SIECUS Study Guide No. 6. New York, Sex Information and Education Council of the U.S., 1967.
9. Reichert, P.: Does heart disease end sex activity? *Sexology*, **29**:76-81, September 1962.
10. Klumbies, G., and Kleinsorge, H.: Circulating dangers and prophylaxis during orgasm. *Int. J. Sexology*, **4**:61-66, November 1950.
11. Kinsey, A. C., et al.: *Sexual Behavior in the Human Male*. Philadelphia, Saunders, 1948, pp. 597, 599, 636.
12. Masters, W. F., and Johnson, V. E.: *Human Sexual Response*. Boston, Little, 1966, pp. 34-36, 174-176.
13. Oliven, J. F.: *Sexual Hygiene and Pathology*, 2nd ed., Philadelphia, Lippencott, 1965, pp. 269-271.
14. Quoted in Ellis, A.: *If This Be Heresy*. New York, Lyle Stuart, 1963, chap. 12.
15. Weiss, E.: *Don't Worry about Your Heart*. New York, Random House, 1959, chap. 10.
16. Kaplan, B. M., and Grunes, J.: Emotional aspects of estrogen therapy in men with coronary atherosclerosis. *JAMA*, **183**:734-736, March 2, 1963.

17 Marmorston, J., et al.: Clinical studies of long-term estrogen therapy in men with myocardial infarction. *Proc. Soc. Exp. Biol. Med.,* **110**:400-408, June 1962.
18 Rubin, I., and Babbott, D.: Impotence and diabetes mellitus. *JAMA,* **168**: 498-500, October 4, 1958.
19 Schoffling, K., et al.: Disorders of sexual function in male diabetics. *Diabetes,* **12**:519-527, November-December 1963.
20 Klebanow, D., and MacLeod, J.: Semen quality and certain disturbances of reproduction in diabetic men. *Fertil. Steril.,* **11**:255-261, May-June 1960.
21 Greene, L. F., et al.: Retrograde ejaculation of semen due to diabetic neuropathy. *Fertil. Steril.,* **14**:617-625, November-December 1963.
22 Norris, H. J., and Yunis, E.: Age changes of seminal vesicles and vasa deferentia in diabetics. *Arch. Path.* (Chicago), **77**:126-131, February 1964.
23 Wershub, L. P.: *Sexual Impotence in the Male.* Springfield, Thomas, 1959, pp. 33-34.
24 Stearns, D. B.: Retropubic prostatectomy, 1947-1960: a critical evaluation. *J. Urol.,* **85**:322-328, March 1961.
25 Finkle, A. L., and Moyers, T. G.: Sexual potency in aging males. IV. Status of private patients before and after prostatectomy. *J. Urol.,* **84**:152-157, July 1960.
26 Holtgrewe, H. L., and Valk, W. L.: Late results of transurethral prostatectomy. *J. Urol.,* **92**:51-55, June 1964.
27 Finkle, A. L., and Prian, D. V.: Sexual potency in elderly men before and after prostatectomy. *JAMA,* **196**:125-129, April 11, 1966.
28 Ellis, W. J., and Grayhack, J. T.: Sexual function in aging males after orchiectomy and estrogen therapy. *J. Urol.,* **89**:895-899, June 1963.
29 Shipps, H. P.: Preparation and care of a patient for hysterectomy. *Med. Times,* **91**:20-24, January 1963.
30 Clark, L.: Answer to question 6414. *Sexology,* **30**:621, April 1964.
31 Oliven, J. F.: *Sexual Hygiene and Pathology,* 2nd ed. Philadelphia, Lippincott, 1965, p. 328.
32 Bieber, I., and Drellich, M. G.: The female castration complex. *J. Nerv. Ment. Dis.,* **129**:235-242, September 1959.
33 Patterson, R. M., and Craig, J. B.: Misconceptions concerning the psychological effects of hysterectomy. *Amer. J. Obstet. Gynec.,* **85**:104-111, January 1, 1963.
34 Melody, G. F.: Depressive reactions following hysterectomy. *Amer. J. Obstet. Gynec.,* **83**:410-413, February 1, 1962.
35 Study by Dodds, D. T., et al., cited in Patterson and Craig: Misconceptions concerning the psychological effects of hysterectomy. *Amer. J. Obstet. Gynec.,* **85**:104-111, January 1, 1963.
36 Waxenberg, S. E.: Some biological correlatives of sexual behavior, in G. Winokur (ed.): *Determinants of Human Sexual Behavior.* Springfield, Thomas, 1963, pp. 52-75.
37 Bard, M., and Sutherland, A. M.: Psychological impact of cancer and its treatment. IV. Adaptation to radical mastectomy. *Cancer,* **8**:656-672, July-August 1955.
38 Kinsey, A. C., et al: *Sexual Behavior in the Human Female.* Philadelphia, Saunders, 1953, pp. 734-735.
39 Schon, M., and Sutherland, A. M.: The relationship of pituitary hormones to

sexual behavior in women, in H. G. Beigel (ed.): *Advances in Sex Research.* New York, Harper, 1963, pp. 33-47.
40   Schon, M.: Hypophysectomy as a psychological experience. *Dis. Ner. System,* Monograph Supplement 24 (no. 4), April 1963.
41   Money, J.: Sex hormones in human eroticism, in W. C. Young (ed.): *Sex and Internal Secretions.* Baltimore, Williams & Wilkins, 1961, pp. 1383-1400.
42   Weigel, C. J.: Quoted in *JAMA,* **187**:29, March 14, 1964.
43   Bors, E., and Commar, A. E.: Neurological disturbances of sexual function with special reference to 529 patients with spinal cord injury. *Urol. Survey,* **10**:191-222, December 1960.
44   Francis, W. J. A., and Jeffcoate, T. N. A.: Dyspareunia following vaginal operation. *J. Obstet. Gynec. Brit. Comm.,* **68**:1-10, February 1961. See also *Obstet. Gynec. Survey,* **18**:1006-1008, December 1963; **16**:587, August 1961; and **15**:763, October 1960.
45   Branson, H. K.: When a mate is disabled—what sex solution? *Sexology,* **34**:98-100, September 1967.
46   Williams, J. G.: Sex and the paralyzed. *Sexology,* **31**:453-456, February 1965.
47   Oliven, J. F.: *Sexual Hygiene and Pathology,* 2d ed. Philadelphia, Lippincott, 1965, pp. 424-426.
48   Money, J.: Sexual problems of the chronically ill, in C. W. Wohl (ed.): *Sexual Problems—Diagnosis and Treatment in Medical Practice.* New York, Free Press, 1967, pp. 266-287.
49   Branson, H. K., and Branson, R.: Sex and the handicapped. *Sexology,* **30**:561-563, 1964.
50   Branson, H. K.: Epilepsy in marriage. *Sexology,* **29**:379-381, January 1963.
51   Johnson, W. R.: Sex education of mentally retarded children. *Sexology,* **33**:410-414, January 1967.
52   Stokes, W. R.: Sex life of the retarded. *Sexology,* **33**:170-173, October 1966.
53   Wolff, K.: Definition of the geriatric patient. *Geriatrics,* **12**:102-106, February 1957.
54   Wolff, K.: *The Biological, Sociological, and Psychological Aspects of Aging.* Springfield, Thomas, 1959, p. 45.

Reading 11
The Doctor-Nurse Game
Leonard I. Stein

The relationship between the doctor and the nurse is a very special one. There are few professions where the degree of mutual respect and cooperation between co-workers is as intense as that between the doctor and nurse.

Reprinted from *Archives of General Psychiatry,* vol. 16, pp. 699-703, June 1967. Copyright 1967, American Medical Association.

Superficially, the stereotype of this relationship has been dramatized in many novels and television serials. When, however, it is observed carefully in an interactional framework, the relationship takes on a new dimension and has a special quality which fits a game model. The underlying attitudes which demand that this game be played are unfortunate. These attitudes create serious obstacles in the path of meaningful communications between physicians and nonmedical professional groups.

The physician traditionally and appropriately has total responsibility for making the decisions regarding the management of his patients' treatment. To guide his decisions he considers data gleaned from several sources. He acquires a complete medical history, performs a thorough physical examination, interprets laboratory findings, and at times obtains recommendations from physician-consultants. Another important factor in his decision making are the recommendations he receives from the nurse. The interaction between doctor and nurse through which these recommendations are communicated and received is unique and interesting.

THE GAME

One rarely hears a nurse say, "Doctor, I would recommend that you order a retention enema for Mrs. Brown." A physician, upon hearing a recommendation of that nature, would gape in amazement at the effrontery of the nurse. The nurse, upon hearing the statement, would look over her shoulder to see who said it, hardly believing the words actually came from her own mouth. Nevertheless, if one observes closely, nurses make recommendations of more import every hour and physicians willingly and respectfully consider them. If the nurse is to make a suggestion without appearing insolent and the doctor is to seriously consider that suggestion, their interaction must not violate the rules of the game.

Object of the Game

The object of the game is as follows: The nurse is to be bold, have initiative, and be responsible for making significant recommendations, while at the same time she must appear passive. This must be done in such a manner as to make her recommendations appear to be initiated by the physician.

Both participants must be acutely sensitive to each other's nonverbal and cryptic verbal communications. A slight lowering of the head, a minor shifting of position in the chair, or a seemingly nonrelevant comment concerning an event which occurred eight months ago must be interpreted as a powerful message. The game requires the nimbleness of a high-wire acrobat, and if either participant slips, the game can be shattered; the penalties for frequent failure are apt to be severe.

Rules of the game

The cardinal rule of the game is that open disagreement between the players must be avoided at all costs. Thus the nurse must communicate her recommendations without appearing to be making a recommendation statement. The physician, in requesting a recommendation from a nurse, must do so without appearing to be asking for it. Utilization of this technique keeps both from committing themselves to a position before a sub rosa agreement on that position has already been established. In that way open disagreement is avoided. The greater the significance of the recommendation, the more subtly the game must be played.

To convey a subtle example of the game with all its nuances would require the talents of a literary artist. Lacking these talents, let me give you the following example, which is unsubtle, but happens frequently. The medical resident on hospital call is awakened by telephone at 1 A.M. because a patient on a ward, not his own, has not been able to fall asleep. Dr. Jones answers the telephone, and the dialogue goes like this:

This is Dr. Jones. *(An open and direct communication.)*

Dr. Jones, this is Miss Smith on 2 W—Mrs. Brown, who learned today of her father's death, is unable to fall asleep. *(This message has two levels. Openly, it describes a set of circumstances, a woman who is unable to sleep and who that morning received word of her father's death. Less openly, but just as directly, it is a diagnostic and recommendation statement; that is, Mrs. Brown is unable to sleep because of her grief, and she should be given a sedative. Dr. Jones, accepting the diagnostic statement and replying to the recommendation statement, answers.)*

What sleeping medication has been helpful to Mrs. Brown in the past? *(Dr. Jones, not knowing the patient, is asking for a recommendation from the nurse, who does know the patient, about what sleeping medication should be prescribed. Note, however, his question does not appear to be asking her for a recommendation. Miss Smith replies.)*

Pentobarbital mg 100 was quite effective night before last. *(A disguised recommendation statement. Dr. Jones replies with a note of authority in his voice.)*

Pentobarbital mg 100 before bedtime as needed for sleep, got it? *(Miss Smith ends the conversation with the tone of a grateful supplicant.)*

Yes I have, and thank you very much, doctor.

This is an example of a successfully played doctor-nurse game. The nurse made appropriate recommendations which were accepted by the physician and were helpful to the patient. The game was successful because the cardinal rule was not violated. The nurse was able to make her recommendation without appearing to, and the physician was able to ask for recommendations without conspicuously asking for them.

The Scoring System

Inherent in any game are penalties and rewards for the players. In game theory, the doctor-nurse game fits the nonzero sum game model. It is not like chess, where the players compete with each other and whatever one player loses the other wins. Rather, it is the kind of game in which the rewards and punishments are shared by both players. If they play the game successfully they both win rewards, and if they are unskilled and the game is played badly, they both suffer the penalty.

The most obvious reward from the well-played game is a doctor-nurse team that operates efficiently. The physician is able to utilize the nurse as a valuable consultant, and the nurse gains self-esteem and professional satisfaction from her job. The less obvious rewards are no less important. A successful game creates a doctor-nurse alliance; through this alliance the physician gains the respect and admiration of the nursing service. He can be confident that his nursing staff will smooth the path for getting his work done. His charts will be organized and waiting for him when he arrives, the ruffled feathers of patients and relatives will have been smoothed down, his pet routines will be happily followed, and he will be helped in a thousand and one other ways.

The doctor-nurse alliance sheds its light on the nurse as well. She gains a reputation of being a "damn good nurse." She is respected by everyone and appropriately enjoys her position. When physicians discuss the nursing staff it would not be unusual for her name to be mentioned with respect and admiration. Their esteem for a good nurse is no less than their esteem for a good doctor.

The penalties for a game failure, on the other hand, can be severe. The physician who is an unskilled gamesman and fails to recognize the nurses' subtle recommendation messages is tolerated as a "clod." If, however, he interprets these messages as insolence and strongly indicates he does not wish to tolerate suggestions from nurses, he creates a rocky path for his travels. The old truism "If the nurse is your ally you've got it made, and if she has it in for you, be prepared for misery" takes on life-sized proportions. He receives three times as many phone calls after midnight as his colleagues. Nurses will not accept his telephone orders because "telephone orders are against the rules." Somehow, this rule gets suspended for the skilled players. Soon he becomes like Joe Bfstplk in the "Li'l Abner" comic strip. No matter where he goes, a black cloud constantly hovers over his head.

The unskilled gamesman nurse also pays heavily. The nurse who does not view her role as that of a consultant, and therefore does not attempt to communicate recommendations, is perceived as a dullard and is mercifully allowed to fade into the woodwork.

The nurse who does see herself as a consultant but refuses to follow the rules of the game in making her recommendations has hell to pay. The outspoken nurse is labeled a bitch by the surgeon. The psychiatrist describes her as unconsciously suffering from penis envy and her behavior as the acting out of her hostility toward men. Loosely translated, the psychiatrist is also saying she is a bitch. The employment of the unbright outspoken nurse is soon terminated. The outspoken bright nurse whose recommendations are worthwhile remains employed. She is, however, constantly reminded in a hundred ways that she is not loved.

GENESIS OF THE GAME

To understand how the game evolved, we must comprehend the nature of the doctors' and nurses' training which shaped the attitudes necessary for the game.

Medical Student Training

The medical student in his freshman year studies as if possessed. In the anatomy class he learns every groove and prominence on the bones of the skeleton as if life depended on it. As a matter of fact, he literally believes just that. He not infrequently says, "I've got to learn it exactly, a life may depend on my knowing that." A consequence of this attitude, which is carefully nurtured throughout medical school, is the development of a phobia: the overdetermined fear of making a mistake.

The development of this fear is quite understandable. The burden the physician must carry is at times almost unbearable. He feels responsible in a very personal way for the lives of his patients. When a man dies leaving young children and a widow, the doctor carries some of her grief and despair inside himself; and when a child dies, some of him dies too. He sees himself as a warrior against death and disease. When he loses a battle, through no fault of his own, he nevertheless feels pangs of guilt, and he relentlessly searches himself to see if there might have been a way to alter the outcome. For the physician a mistake leading to a serious consequence is intolerable, and any mistake reminds him of his vulnerability. Little wonder that he becomes phobic.

The classical way in which phobias are managed is to avoid the source of the fear. Since it is impossible to avoid making some mistakes in an active practice of medicine, a substitute defensive maneuver is employed. The physician develops the belief that he is omnipotent and omniscient, and therefore incapable of making mistakes. This belief allows the phobic physician to actively engage in his practice rather than avoid it. The fear of committing an error in a critical field like medicine is unavoidable and appropriately realistic. The physician, however, must learn to live with the fear rather than handle it defensively through a posture of omnipotence. This defense markedly interferes with his interpersonal professional relationships.

Physicians, of course, deny feelings of omnipotence. The evidence, however, renders their denials mere whispers in the wind. The slightest mistake inflicts a large narcissistic wound. Depending on his underlying personality structure the physician may worry for days about it, quickly rationalize it away, or deny it. The guilt produced is usually exaggerated and the incident is handled defensively. The ways in which physicians enhance and support each other's defenses when an error is made could be the topic of another paper. The feelings of omnipotence become generalized to other areas of his life. A report of the Federal Aviation Agency (FAA), as quoted in *Time* magazine (August 5, 1966), states that in 1964 and 1965 physicians had a fatal-accident rate four times as high as the average for all other private pilots. Major causes of the high death rate were risk-taking attitudes and judgments. Almost all of the accidents occurred on pleasure trips and were therefore not necessary risks to get to a patient needing emergency care. The trouble, suggested an FAA official, is that too many doctors fly with "the feeling that they are omnipotent." Thus the extremes to which the physician may go in preserving his self-concept of omnipotence may threaten his own life. This overdetermined preservation of omnipotence is indicative of its brittleness and its underlying foundation of fear of failure.

The physician finds himself trapped in a paradox. He fervently wants to give his patient the best possible medical care, and being open to the nurses' recommendations helps him accomplish this. On the other hand, accepting advice from nonphysicians is highly threatening to his omnipotence. The solution for the paradox is to receive sub rosa recommendations and make them appear to be initiated by himself. In short, he must learn to play the doctor-nurse game.

Some physicians never learn to play the game. Most learn in their internship, and a perceptive few learn during their clerkships in medical school. Medical students frequently complain that the nursing staff treats them as if they had just completed a junior Red Cross first-aid class instead of two years of intensive medical training. Interviewing nurses in a training hospital sheds considerable light on this phenomenon. In their words they said, "A few students just seem to be with it, they are able to understand what you are trying to tell them, and they are a pleasure to work with; most, however, pretend to know everything and refuse to listen to anything we have to say, and I guess we do give them a rough time." In essence, they are saying that those students who quickly learn the game are rewarded, and those who do not are punished.

Most physicians learn to play the game after they have weathered a few experiences like this one. On the first day of his internship, the physician and nurse were making rounds. They stopped at the bed of a 52-year-old woman who, after complimenting the young doctor on his appearance, complained to him of her problem with constipation. After several minutes of listening to her detailed description of peculiar diets, family home remedies, and special exercises that have helped her constipation in the past, the nurse politely interrupted the patient. She told her the doctor would take care of the problem and that he had to move on because there were other patients waiting to see him. The young doctor gave the nurse a stern look, turned toward the patient, and kindly told her he would order an enema for her that very afternoon. As they left the bedside, the nurse told him the patient had had a normal bowel movement every day for the past week and that in the 23 days the patient had been in the hospital she had never once passed up an opportunity to complain of her constipation. She quickly added that if the doctor wanted to order an enema, the patient would certainly receive one. After hearing this report the intern's mouth fell open and the wheels began turning in his head. He remembered the nurse's comment to the patient that "the doctor has to move on," and it occurred to him that perhaps she was really giving him a message. After this experience and a few more like it, the young doctor learns to listen for the subtle recommendations the nurses make.

Nursing Student Training

Unlike the medical student, who usually learns to play the game after he finishes medical school, the nursing student begins to learn it early in her training. Throughout her education she is trained to play the doctor-nurse game.

Student nurses are taught how to relate to physicians. They are told he has infinitely more knowledge than they, and thus he should be shown the utmost respect. In addition, it was not many years ago when nurses were instructed to stand whenever a physician entered a room. When he would come in for a conference the nurse was expected to offer him her chair, and when both entered a room the nurse would open the door for him and allow him to enter first. Although these practices are no longer rigidly adhered to, the premise upon which they were based is still promulgated. One nurse described the premise as, "He's God almighty and your job is to wait on him."

To inculcate subservience and inhibit deviancy, nursing schools are for the most part tightly run, disciplined institutions. Certainly there is great variation among nursing schools, and there is little question that the trend is toward giving students more autonomy. However, in too many schools this trend has not gone far enough, and the climate remains restrictive. The student's schedule is firmly controlled and there is very little free time. Classroom hours, study hours, meal time, and bedtime with lights out are rigidly enforced. In some schools meaningless chores are assigned, such as cleaning bed springs with cotton applicators. The relationship between student and instructor continues this military flavor. Often their relationship is more like that between recruit and drill sergeant than between student and teacher. Open dialogue is inhibited by attitudes of strict black and white, with few if any shades of gray. Straying from the rigidly outlined path is sure to result in disciplinary action.

The inevitable result of these practices is to instill in the student nurse a fear of independent action. This inhibition of independent action is most marked when relating to physicians. One of the students' greatest fears is making a blunder while assisting a physician and being publicly ridiculed by him. This is really more a reflection of the nature of their training than the prevalence of abusive physicians. The fear of being humiliated for a blunder while assisting in a procedure is generalized to the fear of humiliation for making any independent act in relating to a physician, especially the act of making a direct recommendation. Every nurse interviewed felt that making a suggestion to a physician was equivalent to insulting and belittling him. It was tantamount to questioning his medical knowledge and insinuating he did not know his business. In light of her image of the physician as an omniscient and punitive figure, the questioning of his knowledge would be unthinkable.

The student, however, is also given messages quite contrary to the ones described earlier. She is continually told that she is an invaluable aid to the physician in the treatment of the patient. She is told that she must help him in every way possible, and she is imbued with a strong sense of responsibility for the care of her patient. Thus she, like the physician, is caught in a paradox. The first set of messages implies that the physician is omniscient and that any recommendation she might make would be insulting to him and leave her open to ridicule. The second set of messages implies that she is an important asset to him, has much to contribute, and is duty-bound to make those contributions. Thus, when her good sense tells her a recommendation would be helpful to him she is not allowed to communicate it directly, nor is she allowed not to communicate it. The way out of the bind is to use the doctor-nurse game and communicate the recommendation without appearing to do so.

FORCES PRESERVING THE GAME

Upon observing the indirect interactional system which is the heart of the doctor-nurse game, one must ask the question, "Why does this inefficient mode of communication continue to exist?" The forces militating against change are powerful.

Rewards and Punishments

The doctor-nurse game has a powerful, innate self-perpetuating force—its system of rewards and punishments. One potent method of shaping behavior is to reward one set of behavioral patterns and to punish patterns which deviate from it. As described earlier, the rewards given for a well-played game and the punishments meted out to unskilled players are impressive. This system alone would be sufficient to keep the game flourishing. The game, however, has additional forces.

The Strength of the Set

It is well recognized that sets are hard to break. A powerful attitudinal set is the nurse's perception that making a suggestion to a physician is equivalent to insulting and belittling him. An example of where attempts are regularly made to break this set is seen on psychiatric treatment wards operating on a therapeutic community model. This model requires open and direct communication between members of the team. Psychiatrists working in these settings expend a great deal of energy in urging and rewarding openness before direct patterns of communication become established. The rigidity of the resistance to break this set is impressive. If the physician himself is a prisoner of the set and therefore does not actively try to destroy it, change is nearly impossible.

The Need for Leadership

Lack of leadership and structure in any organization produces anxiety in its members. As the importance of the organization's mission increases, the demand by its members for leadership commensurately increases. In our culture human life is near the top of our hierarchy of values, and organizations which deal with human lives, such as law and medicine, are very rigidly structured. Certainly some of this is necessary for the systematic management of the task. The excessive degree of rigidity, however, is demanded by its members for their own psychic comfort rather than for its utility in efficiently carrying out its mission. The game lends support to this thesis. Indirect communication is an inefficient mode of transmitting information. However, it effectively supports and protects a rigid organizational structure with the physician in clear authority. Maintaining an omnipotent leader provides the other members with a great sense of security.

Sexual Roles

Another influence perpetuating the doctor-nurse game is the sexual identity of the players. Doctors are predominantly men and nurses are almost exclusively women. There are elements of the game which reinforce the stereotyped roles of male dominance and female passivity. Some nursing instructors explicitly tell their students that their femininity is an important asset to be used when relating to physicians.

COMMENT

The doctor and nurse have a shared history and thus have been able to work out their game so that it operates more efficiently than one would expect in an indirect system. Major difficulty arises, however, when the physician works closely with other disciplines which are not normally considered part of the medical sphere. With expanding medical horizons encompassing cooperation with sociologists, engineers, anthropologists, computer analysts, etc., continued expectation of a doctor-nurse-like interaction by the physician is disastrous. The sociologist, for example, is not willing to play that kind of game. When his direct communications are rebuffed the relationship breaks down.

The major disadvantage of a doctor-nurse-like game is its inhibitory effect on open dialogue which is stifling and anti-intellectual. The game is basically a transactional neurosis, and both professions would enhance themselves by taking steps to change the attitudes which breed the game.

Part Two

Teaching and Prevention

Section A

The Role of the Nurse as a Teacher

The base of health and medical knowledge in Western society is probably adequate to enable most people to maintain reasonably good health. The problem, as pointed out by Coulter, is not lack of knowledge but lack of application. The problem stated another way is that too few are knowledgeable—and perhaps even among these, a problem of application exists.

It would be difficult to trace with any degree of accuracy all the philosophical traditions or practical exigencies that have influenced patient care on the part of the nurse. It seems probable, however, that perception of nursing responsibility has been limited too frequently to ministering to the patient's immediate needs with too little attention devoted to his future adequacy. In a sense, when we can no longer see the patient our feeling of responsibility toward him ends. Increasingly, however, nursing has become a professional field with equal emphasis on both present and future utility. It is not enough to operate on a crisis resolution basis or to perform repetitive services for the chronically ill. In many situations the understanding the nurse can impart to the patient and the competence she can help him achieve concerning self-care will be the most significant input she can make. The teaching function of the nurse can be the difference between a home- or activity-bound individual and one who has regained autonomous function.

Coulter discusses the teaching function of nursing in a comprehensive fashion. She raises a number of questions to help the nurse discharge this function more effectively, and points out some of the possible advantages of group teaching situations.

Peplau approaches the teaching function from the experiential point of view. In so doing the author is reflecting a teaching trend that extends beyond the field of nursing. There is, in fact, little opposition to the theory of learning by doing. Education at all levels is making a concerted effort to increase the meaningfulness of content by tying theory and practice together. That this approach is given recognition in nursing procedures is a good sign. Both Peplau and Coulter help bring the teaching function of the nurse into focus and they give it the emphasis that in some quarters may be long overdue.

Reading 12

The Role of the Nurse
in the Prevention of Illness and in Health Teaching
Pearl Parvin Coulter

Included in the long history of the human race is an account of persistent effort to alleviate suffering, to treat illness, and to prolong life. These efforts were at first somewhat occult and later became experimental. They were characterized by trial and error, and after years of experience with varying degrees of success or failure, some finally became validated scientific knowledge.

Health practices are derived from scientific theory in this country to put such health components as good nutrition, industrial and highway safety, immunization against communicable diseases, and specific drug therapy within the grasp of the total population. Even with these rich resources society falls far short of attaining the goal of maximum health for all. Since the problem is not lack of knowledge but lack of application, a failure in the delivery of service, it is incumbent upon the vast army of health workers to add teaching to their respective roles.

A preventive modality such as immunization is dependent upon scientific discovery. When the technique is perfected, application to the total population is comparatively simple. Technical skill for preparation and administration of the immunizing agent and sufficient public cooperation for the majority to submit to the procedure is required. This approach has accomplished a great deal toward prolonging life and eliminating human suffering. Prevention of some of the chronic diseases and adding new dimensions to the quality of life are not as simple. Dealing with these problems is probably more difficult because they are more intimately associated with the details of everyday living, the life-styles that have been adopted by individuals, families, communities, and nations. Such habits as eating, rest and exercise, and handling anxieties appear to be transmitted from parent to child and from social group to social group, not as genetic characters, but as a part of the cultural heritage. Though these activities are taught in very subtle ways, they may influence behavior as much as genetic inheritance. While the causal relationship between behavior and health is only dimly appreciated by the general public, it should be crystal clear to the health professionals. To those members of the patient care team who have this knowledge and understanding, negative health behaviors present a vast challenge—namely, (1) to accept health teaching as a legitimate and urgent responsibility, and (2) to recognize health teaching as an effective means of achieving high-level "wellness" for all.

In addition to the well-accepted role of curing, health professionals must include prevention and restoration. Theoretically, if the general public as well as the health workers placed a high priority on the achievement of maximum wellness, a large segment of the population need never be sick or disabled, and few would require therapeutic or restorative services. This health utopia is contingent upon individuals learning about appropriate health achievement and maintenance. They must become involved in controlling the quality of their own health. Much illness and disability must come to be regarded as a teaching and learning failure.

The human tragedy is not that we do not have the means to achieve and maintain high-level health, but that we lack the self-discipline required for success. When the main thrust of health services focuses on prevention of illness and the promotion of health, the resources and effort formerly allocated to therapy can provide a plentitude of well-being and freedom from sickness, disability, and pain. The current trend is for community and national health programs with emphasis on prevention. This trend may indicate that the public will not much longer tolerate sick-oriented health practitioners.

The nurse is an accepted member of the patient care team, and the public appears to rate her high in both her knowledge about health and illness and her technical skills. There seems to be an assumption on the part of both the public and the practitioner that this knowledge and skill will automatically endow the nurse with the interest in and the ability to teach appropriate health behaviors. The range of information which the nurse is expected to impart might vary from facts directed toward the patient's orientation to the hospital environment to health practices requiring extensive changes in a well-entrenched life style. The focus is now shifting to ways of preventing illness and, failing that, to better understanding of a specific pathological process—how to recover from it or how to live as productively as possible in the wake of a devastating disability.

It is difficult to evaluate the quality or quantity of the actual health teaching performed by nurses. Some nurses are nonplussed when asked for examples of their teaching. They are prone to project their teaching failure onto the system in which they work—there is not time, there is no suitable equipment, the administrative climate is not compatible with patient teaching. Some of these statements are well founded. Other nurses appear to equate teaching with telling: "I told him to quit smoking or his cough would get worse" or "I told him to take his medicine three times a day" may be cited as examples of teaching. These statements indicate that the nurse believes she has fulfilled her teaching responsibility when she has remembered to tell the patient, immediately prior to discharge, the things she has decided he should know in order to carry on his activities outside of the hospital.

In addition to her storehouse of scientific knowledge, the nurse committed to her teaching role will be aware that individuals are unique in their response to extrinsic efforts designed to change their behavior. If she is working with a sick patient, the nurse usually has the advantage of a learner who wants to get well. She also has the benefit of extremely relevant and interesting material. She needs an approach appropriate to the learner's capacity. For the purpose of expanding her options in method, she will explore the literature where a variety of ways of attractively and effectively packaging and presenting health information can be found. She will also keep records of her own experience in order to improve teaching. Teaching may range from a chance remark derived from the nurse's perception of desirable behavior on the part of the patient to structurally planned teaching developed from clues regarding patient's needs, selection of methods which seem most likely to succeed and involving the establishment of learner-teacher goals toward which they will work. Without doubt, some nurses are superb teachers. Many patients credit nurses with providing the impetus which started them on the road to restoration and good living.

Teaching performed by patient care personnel can be considered in the following categories:

1   Incidental
2   Planned

INCIDENTAL TEACHING AND LEARNING

There is a great deal of evidence that ill or disabled persons are highly motivated toward regaining health. People tend to take health for granted until they are deprived of it. When ill, if they can overcome their sense of futility and depression, they bend every effort toward recovery though they may have made little or no effort to maintain health when they were comparatively well. Sick or disabled persons are threatened with pain, loss of capability, and death. They may have been deprived of their ability to engage in lucrative and satisfying work, which has resulted in economic dependency added to physical inadequacy. Often hospitalized children believe that they have been abandoned by their parents, and even adults are fearful that their illness and disability will deprive them of the support and affection of those they love. For various reasons they feel depressed and unworthy.

It seems obvious that a large number of patients and their families have implicit faith in the therapeutic value of hospitalization and are ready to assume that all hospital practices should be accepted and perpetuated.

Unfortunately, many hospitals seem to give more consideration to perpetuating a system congenial to the personnel rather than one focused on the patient's needs. Hence, there is danger that the patient care personnel may fail to take advantage of the wonderful motivation generated by the patient's dependency. They may foster dependency or other patient behaviors which are actually detrimental to the restoration and maintenance of health rather than contributing to the enrichment or prolongation of life. It should, of course, be understood that hospital personnel do not willfully try to disadvantage patients or to teach them behavior patterns that are harmful. The patient's negative learning is "fall-out" from the system because there is not conscious planning to involve him positively in his own recovery. Without any effort on the part of patient care personnel, the patient is immersed in the care system and tends to assume that "it must be good for him." Some of the things he learns are by default—the failure to explain that certain treatments and medications are emergency measures required because of enforced inactivity and the pathology involved. In this connection the professional nurse cannot afford to overlook the impact of various types of nurses functioning in her jurisdiction who may need help in their relationship with patients. Because they are not clear about their limitations, these persons sometimes attempt teaching or make suggestions that are detrimental. Such practices as the continued use of sleeping pills, laxatives, and enemas to which the patient has been introduced in the hospital may be perpetuated by the patient long after he should have returned to normal function. A conscious effort to help the patient reestablish a normal regimen can hasten his return home unfettered by artificial devices to stimulate body function.

The personal example of the patient care team can be of great value. These persons are important components of the patient's environment. He regards them as "health experts," and their behavior has tremendous impact on him. This impact may be either positive or negative. The health worker who is not himself a practitioner of high-level wellness may not only be a poor example, but he may find it difficult to present information to the patient which is essential to the patient's recovery but inconsistent with the life-style of the practitioner. For example, it is hard to persuade an emphysemic or cardiac patient that he will be advantaged if he stops smoking when the teacher carries a strong tobacco odor about; it is difficult for the obese worker to present the hazards of overweight to a patient who should be encouraged to lose weight. The patient will reason that the teacher does not really believe what he is teaching. While it is the prerogative of each practitioner in the health field to determine the extent of his own commitment to patient care, he should be aware of his influence on patients who have entrusted their welfare to his keeping. The extremity of need provides strong motivation, and the patient assumes health personnel to be knowledgeable and their behavior exemplary. Patients may be unable to identify the various types of personnel who contribute to their care, hence the tendency to think of all of them as "health experts."

It is also essential for personnel to be aware that patients will learn throughout a hospital experience and that the potential for learning to establish and maintain maximum health can be exploited or it can be left to chance acquisition of health knowledge. The option is whether the learning will be directed and assisted by expert professionals or allowed to follow a haphazard unplanned course with little or no attempt to assess the learning, either in terms of suitability or in terms of changed behavior. While health learning should not be left to chance, it is possible to take advantage of chance opportunities to encourage behavior change.

PLANNED TEACHING AND LEARNING

All teaching is based on the assumption that behavior can be changed. The person who undertakes to teach must be careful that the changes in the behavior of another are initiated thoughtfully and with considerable assurance that, if accomplished, they will help him. The patient must be encouraged to develop a sense of his own value on the therapeutic team—he must decide what he can do for himself and how he can utilize the professional assistance offered to him.

The nurse who aspires to a truly professional role will not be able to abdicate her teaching responsibilities but will expand them to include patients and personnel working with patients. Her success in effecting behavior change may be one of the greatest measures of her professional stature. The would-be teacher must understand pathology while maintaining an orientation toward wellness and the application of basic science principles in the clinical setting. She must become a skilled observer of human behavior and learn how to interpret her observations. To this end she gathers data with a purpose. She selects relevant data and subjects them to analysis which enables her to transform them into action. The results of learning must be evaluated so that both teacher and learner know how nearly the accepted goals have been reached. The dynamics of the situation may require continuous data collection and reevaluation as progress is made. The nurse will know that it is seldom necessary to try to share all her knowledge about pathology and health with the patient. Patient teaching must be geared to the needs and capabilities of the individual concerned, taking into consideration such variables as age, intellectual capacity, level of education, desire for information, and appreciation of the need for his own involvement in the therapeutic process.

Planned teaching may be conducted on either an individual or a group basis. A number of questions should be asked and answered in arriving at a choice between these two options:

1 In which setting will the patient under consideration learn best?
2 Is there a sufficient volume of patients with common needs to form a group?
3 What segment of teacher and learner time can be made available?
4 What space is available for teaching?
5 How can the content to be learned be best presented?

In general, too little use has been made of group teaching. At its best this way of teaching is quite informal, but it can be sufficiently structured to challenge the teacher to make the best preparation of which she is capable. There are a number of advantages in group teaching for both teacher and learner. Patients tend to approach a group session psychologically prepared to learn. The activity has been scheduled and they recognize it as a learning opportunity. It takes place in a designated area which affords protection from distractions and interruptions, which seem inevitable in the patient's room. Most important of all advantages is the support and stimulation which members of the group generate for each other. They gain by participation in a shared experience. They begin to realize that others have the same problem and that together they can work toward solutions. Some content material, such as information about exchange foods, techniques for administering medications or treatments, testing urine, relief of anxiety, lends itself to group teaching. Anxiety of preoperative patients, of patients who have terminal illness, or of the families of disabled or seriously ill patients will often yield to group sessions. They gain strength from each other in the process of considering their concerns in a climate of mutual assistance. The teacher facilitates these developments by organizing the group and setting the stage for their discussion.

From the teacher's point of view, teaching a group is time-saving. It reaches more people for the effort expended. It enables the teacher to make better preparation and it makes possible the use of more elaborate teaching materials. The benefits of group teaching are not necessarily automatic. There is nothing magical in getting a group together. The dynamics of the group must be utilized in such a way that learning goals will be attained. There are obviously many situations in which group teaching is not feasible. They may range from insufficient numbers of patients with common learning needs to problems which are so intimate and individual that the patient will prefer to learn by himself. Individual teaching may eventually progress to group work. For example, the patient who is coping with a colostomy may require individual instruction in the early management of his disability, but may need the support of a group later. The alert nurse-teacher will not discount the value of including members of the family in the group. Family members are invited when their understanding is needed. A male patient whose adjustment is dependent on diet may look to his wife or children to prepare his meals, and a patient who has rest prescribed as part of his treatment should be in a household able to adjust to his limitations. The patient's own motivation to change his way of life is important, but his determination is greatly reinforced when he is surrounded by a supportive family. When members of the family are relied upon to administer medications and treatments, they, as well as the patient, must understand the therapeutic goals.

Whether group or individual teaching has been selected, rehabilitated former patients can be a great resource. They serve as models for the person embarking on a rehabilitation program. They have been through a similar experience. While the nurse may have worked with many patients, her relationship to the problem remains vicarious. The willingness of graduate rehabilitated patients to help others is heart-warming and inspiring. Their effectiveness has been beyond measure. A woman who has suffered a breast amputation may be better motivated by another woman who has survived the same experience and adjusted to a prosthesis which has helped her regain her poise, self-assurance, and attractiveness than she would from the attempts of any professional to present these possibilities to her. The professional service is arranging the encounter. The patient who has just lost a leg may be more stimulated toward recovery by seeing a graduate amputee dance, ski, or just walk unaided into the room than by any amount of encouragement by the health team. It is reassuring to the patient with a recent colostomy to see former patients dressed and going about their normal work or for the laryngectomy patient to hear a person talk who has had similar surgery. A housewife who, because of residual paralysis from a stroke, is confined to a wheelchair can be helped greatly by a visit to another paraplegic patient who is managing her household tasks as she moves about in a wheelchair. These rehabilitated patients not only have a tremendous impact on new patients, but they also receive a great deal of personal satisfaction from this unique opportunity to be of service.

In some respects the plan for teaching and learning is a form of self-fulfilling prophecy. The teacher and learner have made a compact; they have a target to hit, a goal to attain. Their mutual declaration of intent to achieve may be the most important step in its actualization.

In order for both learner and teacher to be assured that learning has progressed to the point of goal achievement, evaluation is necessary. The proof of teaching is in the learning, and the proof of learning is the demonstration of changed behavior. Health teaching is of little value until it extends well beyond verbalization. Health learning should be expressed in health performance. During the learning process, periodic tests may be utilized which let the learner know how much of his goal has been achieved. A weekend at home may satisfy him that he is ready to manage alone, or it may indicate to him that he needs more practice under guidance before he is ready to be independent. If the learner's goal is to learn to walk with the aid of crutches, it is necessary to see that the crutches are of the type prescribed and that they are the correct length for the person who will use them; but this is not enough. He must walk with them on the various types of surfaces he will encounter in daily living, including going up and down steps. He must be encouraged to practice until he can perform without either undue fatigue or anxiety.

The rehabilitation process is referable to the patient—his willingness to capitalize on his remaining assets. One of his greatest resources in changing his behavior to accommodate to his loss or disability is the guidance, support, and encouragement of the various members of the patient care team. Their dedication and creativity in devising strategies that will help him progress is teaching. To satisfy the need, it must be of a high order.

Reading 13
What Is Experiential Teaching?
Hildegard E. Peplau

"Learning by experience" is a phrase that is widely used. It suggests that a person's experience can be used to promote his learning. To understand the phrase, therefore, it is necessary to grasp and use the concept of learning and the concept of experience, and to know the teaching method that can be used to promote learning by experience.

The purpose of this paper is to propose definitions for these two concepts and to describe the form of teaching in a way that clarifies the meaning of the phrase and distinguishes the method from more traditional or didactic forms of instruction. Experiential teaching is an important function performed by nurses in their work with patients. An understanding of this method of teaching should facilitate health teaching in all types of nursing situations.

Reprinted from *The American Journal of Nursing*, vol. 57, no. 7, pp. 884–886, July 1957.

WHAT IS EXPERIENCE?

Experience is anything lived or undergone. It is the inner perception that a person has of events in which he participates. It consists of the "felt relations"—the connections which a person feels concerning an event—or the inferences he draws. It is, for example, the inferences which occur to nurses in a relationship with a patient.

These "felt relations" or inferences can be identified. Descriptions of responses of the separate senses, reports of the total organism, and observations which the nurse makes of others are the major components of the raw data from which nurses formulate what they experience in a work situation. Thus, when experiential teaching is the method used in nursing education, the nurses identify and describe what has been seen, felt, thought, or done in a situation with a patient, and what has been noticed concerning the patient.

Experiential teaching aids students (or staff nurses in an inservice program) to organize the meaning of experiences in clinical situations, and has three principal components: (1) what the nurses or students have *experienced,* as just described; (2) what is *learned,* or the meaning of that experience; (3) the *instructional process,* or the interacting roles of teacher and students in discussion of clinical experiences. The nurses or students bring the content to the classroom with them and the teacher functions as a critical auditor and facilitator in formulating meanings.

In traditional education the content is usually decided upon, prepared in advance, and introduced by the teacher, possibly from a course outline or teaching files, and the students are expected to absorb what is said and later recall and use it in their work. So this is one difference. In experiential situations, reports of events are presented by students, usually verbally, sometimes from notes. In the discussion of these, data are analyzed and the meaning abstracted. A blackboard helps to keep formulations before the students as they are made and revised. These may be statements of problems encountered, as they emerge from discussion. They may be generalizations to explain what went on in the clinical situations. They may be hypotheses or clinical hunches, which serve as guides for future observations. Discussion often reveals biases and misconceptions, particularly those of very young student nurses. In these situations, individuals can learn something useful when they become involved as participants—when what has actually been experienced is organized and its meaning to the observer checked against experiences of others in the peer group.

In undergraduate and graduate training programs, formal and informal events (called "learning experiences") are usually arranged or occur so that students have a series of varied experiences which permit them to see relations between different kinds of experience. In inservice programs, the everyday work situation provides many experiences which ought to be analyzed and organized in their meaning to nurses. This can be crucial to the recovery of patients. What nurses actually experience when patients are anxious, self-derogating, expressing feelings of worthlessness, resentment, hatefulness, and the like, influences these situations.

Knowingly or unknowingly, nurses make inferences—assign meanings to what is experienced—and these are part and parcel of the meaning to which they respond. Some awareness of this is needed and effort at such awareness is the nurse's obligation. Otherwise, the nurse and patient act in juxtaposition, each observing the other's behavior, without seeing her own participation. And, short of mechanical restraints, the nurse cannot really control the behavior of patients. She can only be aware of, and in some degree control, what goes on in her responses.

WHAT IS LEARNING?

Learning is a concept that is often used very loosely in the literature. It is used to indicate formation of automatic or habitual responses, as a result of trial and error, reward and punishment, and the like. Other concepts, such as conditioning, adaptation, integration, and so forth, are often defined as though they were synonymous with learning. It is uncommon to find in the literature the opinion that pathological patterns, such as those in patients diagnosed schizophrenic, are learned. From the standpoint of this paper, these patterns would be called adaptations.

A workable definition of learning, which educators and therapists alike would find useful, ought to help make the use of this concept, especially in the field of education, more precise.

Learning can be defined in terms of the behavior of the person who is in the process of learning. Such behavior can be observed or inferred from behavior that is observed. The process involves a series of operations, each one reached by the learner at a given time. The operations, in the order of their appearance, are as follows:

1 A person who is in the process of learning *observes what goes on* in the course of an experience, event, or situation in which he is participating, actively or passively, overtly or covertly. A person who is reading a book, hearing a lecture, watching a patient, listening to a colleague, is observing. To observe means to use the five senses to notice the details of an event as it is happening. One of the most important interferences with noticing the details of what goes on is anxiety.[1]

---

[1] Sullivan, H. S. *The Interpersonal Theory of Psychiatry*, edited by Helen S. Perry and Mary L. Gawel. New York, W. W. Norton and Co., 1953, p. 26.

2 As the next step in the process of learning, the person *describes what went on and what was noticed* during the experience. Anxiety can also interfere with this step. Perception and attention are selective—to maintain comfort, one might see the familiar rather than the new, or hear only those ideas that are in agreement with one's personal views on a subject. The tendency of all people to avoid anxiety is supported by patterns of selective perception and selective inattention. Severe anxiety, therefore, may automatically rule out description of some facet of experience that was not noticed enough to be described. To describe what was observed means to tell it to somebody else, or to be able to write down a verbatim account of what transpired during an event or after it has occurred. In this way, using observation and then description, the learner *collects the data of an experience* from which something will be learned.

3 A person who is learning then *analyzes the data collected* so that the possible and significant meanings can be determined. Identifying the significance or abstracting the essence from the variety of details in an experience is a principal task of the learner. Here, too, anxiety and parataxic distortion (the tendency to see present events only in terms of past experiences) often operate to hinder learning. Data are analyzed by sorting out the common and the unique elements, by comparing one aspect with another, by applying known concepts to explain the data, and by drawing inferences as to the connections among the various occurrences that were observed and described. Analysis should lead to fresh, new inferences from the data of an experience, or should suggest other data which may be required before conclusions can be drawn.

4 The learner then *formulates the significance* of an experience by making statements which reflect precisely the gist of what went on. These formulations are the learning products; they are the conclusions drawn from data secured while undergoing experience. The most common interference with this step is the tendency in our society to assign clichés to denote the meaning of experience. It is common to have students conclude, "I liked her," "it's terrific," "she didn't cooperate," and to offer other such noncommunicative phrases as the significance of their richly varied observations. In formulating the significance of an experience, various standpoints must be considered—the significance to the learner, to the teacher, to the author of a book, or to its reader, for example.

5 A person in the process of learning *validates* the learning product. Validation, as it is used here, refers to checking the meanings, the inferences drawn, for their correctness in the light of data collected. The nurse who is using experiential teaching with a patient helps the patient to formulate the meaning of his experience and then checks that meaning with him to see whether they both agree on it.

6 Finally, the learner *tests a learning product through usage,* and, with this step, the learning process—with reference to the particular experience—is brought to a close. Through such testing, learning products are evaluated as one step in the development of foresight which will be useful in later experiences.

COMPARING LEARNING AND ADAPTATION

Both learning and adaptation are influenced by the tensions of need, by anxiety, and by conflict in which there are opposing goals. Both learning and adaptation go on during, and as a result of, experiences, but they lead to different products. We have already shown that a learning product is developed by sustaining anxiety, tension, or conflict while collecting and analyzing data in order to determine the meaning of an experience. Adaptation indicates more static patterning.

The steps in adaptation include: (1) observing a difficulty that is felt, or experiencing vague discomfort, or feeling an unexplained and immediate need for comfort or relief in the form of approval or disapproval (as relief from indifference, for instance); and (2) using familiar patterns which in earlier situations reduced tension automatically—that is, without critical examination of the meaning of what is experienced. It would clarify thinking in the field of education if the formation of patterns that work automatically merely to relieve tension were classified as adaptations, or as products of conditioning. The term "learning" could then be used in a more precise way, indicating use of critical faculties, such as the capacity for conceptualizing experience, for generalizing, for abstracting the meaning of events in original patterns—that is, responses that are new, spontaneous, and significantly specific to a current situation.

The operating difference, then, in these two concepts lies in the recognition and handling of anxiety, and the use of available skill in sustaining doubt, delay, and uncertainty until an experience has been understood. In this concept of learning, anxiety would be recognized as an aspect of the data collected, would be analyzed as a relevant part of the experience, and would provide the energy for use during a stage of inquiry. Anxiety-relieving phenomena offer security by restricting awareness; the relief is a sort of payoff for not noticing, not profiting from experience, not grasping the meaning of what has been observed. Everyone has seen phenomena such as transferring blame from the nurse-as-observer to patients or other personnel, operating on the basis of wishes rather than what is experienced or observed, shifting a discussion from the point of focus, or being otherwise distracted from a task at hand. These are examples of automatic actions used to relieve tension.

In this sense, then, "learning by experience" (which the psychiatry textbooks say "psychopaths" do not do) implies generalizing from what is felt, thought, or done as a participant in an event. It implies development and refinement of the human capacities—to conceptualize, to comprehend, to formulate significant relations as they are experienced in a situation, and to use and refine this ability in personal and work situations. This, then, is one component of preventive psychiatry in education. Experiential teaching in nursing education offers nurses a way of using and refining their capacities as persons and as nurses.

THE TEACHER'S ROLE

When experiential teaching is used as a method, the role of the teacher is rich and varied and is limited only by the boundaries of endowment, training, and the policies of an educational institution. The teacher has two principal functions—as a *critical auditor* and as *facilitator*. She listens intelligently to students' descriptions of experiences and uses her own capacities and skills to encourage learning, that is, the recognition of what can be generalized from these descriptions.

She might act in the following ways: ask for further description of the situation in which a student participated; frame simple but provocative questions which challenge the student to clarify an experience or to notice other possible meanings; suggest gaps in data which require delay in making inferences; pose likely alternatives to generalizations made by students; call attention to sources for further exploration of relevant information; restate what has been presented to suggest a new relation, theme, or variation; and the like. These actions stimulate constructive use of capacities to clarify what has been experienced in a clinical situation.

The teacher must be sensitive to latent, or partially recognized, creative capacities in others and be able to observe and to relate herself to these constructive aspects. An optimistic bias—an expectation that the student can and will learn—is particularly helpful when coupled with sensitive observations of the interaction of teacher and students.

The intention of the student to learn becomes a central feature of the kind of educational situations described. Knowledge that is useful and practical, relevant to the work situation, is an inevitable outcome. Helping students to find out what they know intuitively, or what they know more fully, of their experience and participation with patients is at first the aim of the teacher, but the students soon recognize this and make it their aim, too.

Nurses want to be as helpful as possible, to intervene constructively in the nursing problems of patients. To function in this way, expertness of a particular kind is required of them. The kind of expertness needed is determined by the nature of problems, and by the kind of intervention likely to reduce the strength of, or solve, those problems with patients. I think this kind of expertness can, in some degree, be described, and that there is a relationship between it and the outcomes of experiential teaching situations.

USING EXPERIENTIAL TEACHING

Health teaching is a part of the work role of the staff nurse in all situations. In psychiatric nursing, however, experiential teaching may, at this time, have wider applicability.

Technical or mechanical expertness is not the major requirement of psychiatric nurses. The problems of patients in psychiatric situations are problems of living—unawareness, disorders of feelings, thinking disorders—problems which have to do with communication, symbolization, perception, and the like. Professional nurses, who get into more or less immediate touch with the patient undergoing stress in the ward situation, need particularly to observe, conceptualize, and comprehend how the situation looks to the patient. They ought to be able to observe changes in situations and the concomitant shifts in the behavior of participants. This requires rather expert use of their conceptualizing capacities. It requires development and continuing refinement of the abilities to observe, to recall vividly, to describe and record significant details, to analyze situations and determine the nursing problems, to generalize and infer meaning from observational data, to formulate and state problems and generalizations, and to validate with other nurses and patients the meanings inferred. These abilities are needed by nurses in their everyday work role, and for improving the collaborative relations with other professional workers, particularly in hospital situations. Research which involves nurses can hardly proceed without these important abilities and opportunities for refining them.

OBSERVATION, PARTICIPATION, AND INTERVENTION

To summarize another way, the predominant features of the work role of nurses in psychiatry are observation, participation, and intervention in social interactions within the hospital ward or the professional work situation. In this work situation, day in and day out, both nurses and patients experience something. There is, therefore, always the possibility of learning something useful to living, here and later, through the nurse-patient relationship. If nurses focus on the learning possibilities and view psychiatric hospitals as special educational institutions in which neglected learnings—gaps in learning by experience in the past—can be rectified, this can be an important element in the patient's recovery.

Instead of this view of psychiatric hospitals (where patients learn about living by learning from experience in the ward situation), there are various current views and misconceptions. One particularly important here is the idea that if you work in psychiatric hospitals long enough, you will become "crazy" too. Perhaps under present conditions, and in some situations, there may be a kernel of truth in this. Given a ward situation in which the pathology of perhaps 30 patients operates all day, every day, and the nurse is more or less unaware of the possible meanings of that pathology and of her own participation in relation to it, she may be affected by it.

There is a vast difference, however, between that kind of situation with its long-range effects on patients and personnel, and a nursing situation in which the nurse is competent. And by competent I mean that she has become fairly adept and is interested, in a continuing way, in identifying and using what she experiences. This kind of participation—conceptualizing that "inner component" of ward events and situations while participating with patients—is guided by awareness, intention, purpose, and foresight as well as some inferences concerning the consequences of her actions.

Nurses can only communicate and interact in terms of what they actually know, or are aware of—by way of their feelings, thoughts, and immediate actions. Experiential teaching offers a way of both clarifying and expanding that awareness and self-knowledge.

In the nursing profession, and particularly among psychiatric nurses, there are many who are expecting fruitful outcomes of the research projects now being conducted. What is available in textbooks gives us some plausible explanations of what is observed in nurse-patient situations in psychiatry, and there are some useful guides to action. But there are carefully selected and able nurses, participating in research activities, whose observations should prove valuable in enlarging and clarifying the principles of psychiatric nursing practice. To get these observations formulated for review, and to give these nurses full opportunity for refining their skills, I suggest inservice educational programs, using experiential teaching as a method for finding out what does go on in nursing situations. This would seem more useful than relying on textbooks, which can only tell us about what others believe does, or should, go on.

The informal review of day-to-day experiences may well provide a fresh view of psychiatric nursing practices. It may indicate the points at which nurses tend to reinforce or go along with the pathology of patients, instead of helping them to learn something new about living among people. It may clarify this method of "learning by experience" as a preventive-psychiatry aspect of education, as a way of identifying roles and activities of nurses which are most useful to patients, and as an aid to nurses themselves in learning healthy ways of living with people.

Section B

The Role of the Nurse in Disability Prevention

There is so much evidence that a very large percentage of illness and disability can be prevented that mention of it seems redundant. However, there is almost an equal amount of evidence that health personnel as well as the general public tend to be strongly oriented toward pathology and, therefore, do not exploit the vast potential for the prevention of illness and disability and the promotion of health. Much of the progress that has been made to date can be attributed to public health workers who for many years focused primarily on the prevention of communicable diseases through immunization programs and the sanitation of the environment. This has resulted in the virtual disappearance of such scourges of childhood as diphtheria and pertussis. Poliomyelitis with its subsequent deformity has also become a rarity. It is largely to this effort that lower mortality and disability among infants and children are attributed. It has resulted also in greatly extended life expectancy.

Emphasis on prevention has more recently turned to accidents and chronic diseases. Theoretically all accidents are preventable. This is an important fact, since vehicular and other accidents are now listed among the five most common causes of death. Though death takes a high toll, accidents also leave in their wake a residue of suffering and disability.

Preventive aspects of chronic illness have been neglected. Recent studies have illuminated the role of nutrition, exercise, and the intelligent utilization of medical care in heart disease. Habits of daily living are difficult to correct because they are so intimately integrated into the life-style of people. Ideally, positive health habits acquired in early childhood could be firmly entrenched by the time the individual reaches maturity. The young adult who did not acquire good living habits during childhood has a twofold problem—he must live with the increment of already acquired problems, such as a diet high in saturated fats, while attempting to replace established practices with new ones.

Reorientation of the general public toward better health practices is largely educational, and every member of the health team has a responsibility for it. Not as much is known about prevention of cancer, but it is very clear that the best hope for preventing death from cancer is early detection with subsequent surgical intervention or other inhibitive treatment. It is simpler, cheaper, and infinitely more desirable to teach a woman to engage in periodic self-examination of the breasts to detect abnormal growths than it is to teach her to adjust to a radical breast amputation with all its accompanying mutilation and anxiety. It is not unusual for discharged hospital patients such as those with leg amputations or colostomies to find themselves unable to cope with their problems of self-care even when the hospital personnel attempted to teach them. Some of these inadequacies are related to psychological blocking or lack of family support, but others may be related to limited skill, inability to improvise equipment, or lack of realistic arrangements for the privacy which the patient requires.

Since immobility is itself a cause of disability and thus a complicating factor with regard to patient recovery, controlled exercises would seem to be the logical preventive and therapeutic measure to be employed. In her article on "Exercises for Bedfast Patients" Kelly is explicit in placing the burden of prevention on the nurse, and she is very explicit in outlining this responsibility in terms of nurse-initiated exercise regimens for the bedfast patient.

Even patients who are able to independently exercise their joints and muscles will require encouragement to persist in the repetition of monotonous movements. One way to relieve the monotony is to permit the patient to get exercise through some of the activities of daily living. However, the nurse will have to observe carefully to find out whether or not the patient taking his own bath or brushing his teeth is getting the full range of wrist motion. If he is not, the bath or brushing activity will have to be supplemented with further exercise. Patients require a great deal of supervision and encouragement if they are to maintain a consistent, restorative exercise program. It is essential that the nurse assume her preventive role early in the acute stage of disability; almost immediately after the patient has been admitted. She must continuously guard against allowing the demands of the acute condition to obliterate her equally valuable preventive and restorative role. If she fails to give suitable emphasis to her responsibilities for prevention, she risks greatly prolonging the patient's hospitalization. It is of little value to keep a patient with multiple hospital-acquired disabilities alive if he will never be able to resume normal living activities.

Of the many hazards in life, many are objectified in the external environment; others appear as infectious diseases. Olson and her collaborators[1] also discuss the effects of immobility. Their particular concern is in regard to: the cardiovascular function, respiratory function, gastrointestinal function, motor function, urinary function, metabolic equilibrium, and psychosocial equilibrium. The basic assumption underlying these articles is that a very substantial reduction in disability can be brought about through intelligent rehabilitative nursing care. Inasmuch as the patient is perceived as having the right to maximum utilization of his potential resources in each of the areas discussed, the procedures covered by the authors should not be considered optional in the nursing care, but as necessary guidelines for optimal results.

---

[1] Bonnie Jean Johnson, Joyce A. McCarthy, Lida F. Thompson, Ruth E. Edmonds, Lois M. Schroeder, and Mildred Wade.

Reading 14
Exercises for Bedfast Patients
Mary M. Kelly

Nursing is a preventive science as well as a healing science. The nurse's responsibility for protecting her patients from complications due to inadequate skin or mouth care is universally accepted. The nurse's responsibility for protecting her patients from complications due to inadequate exercise is, unfortunately, not as widely accepted. Far too frequently a patient, following a period of complete bed rest, complains of stiffness and pain in muscles and joints which were strong and healthy before he became bedfast. Far too frequently, complications which might have been prevented through an effective exercise program prolong an individual's stay in bed and increase his financial burden.

Studies of bedfast patients have shown repeatedly that confinement to bed can predispose an individual to constipation; urinary retention and infection; nephrolithiasis, metabolic disturbances, circulatory disturbances including thrombosis and embolus, dizziness and fainting, hypostatic pneumonia, stiffness and pain in joints and muscle groups, muscle atrophy, loss of strength, contracture of muscle groups, bone demineralization, skin breakdown, loss of appetite and of weight, and, needless to say, discouragement. The same studies have shown that planned exercise programs can markedly reduce the frequency and severity of these complications. Exercise, essential to the well-being of the normal, healthy person, is essential for the bedfast individual as well.

Range-of-motion exercises are those in which each joint in the body is moved through the complete range of all the movements which that joint is capable of performing normally. The muscle groups which move each of these joints are the real focus of the exercises. Contraction of a muscle group as it moves a joint is essential in preventing stasis of venous blood and fluids in the body tissues and in maintaining muscle tone.

Range-of-motion exercises are not used in corrective therapy in a "rehabilitative" sense. Their purpose is to maintain the normal functioning of healthy muscle groups in individuals who are not able to obtain sufficient exercise through normal activity. For this reason, the exercises are carried out by a nurse in most patient-care situations, without a physician's order. The physician indicates the amount of activity in which he wishes the patient to engage (for example, bed rest or bathroom privileges), but, beyond this, it is the nurse's responsibility to plan a program of exercises appropriate for her patient's capabilities. For the few patients for whom range-of-motion exercises might be contraindicated, either in several joints (for example, a patient with arthritis in both hips) or in all joints (for example, a patient with congestive heart failure), the nurse would need more specific directions for exercise from the physician.

Figure 14-1 [pp. 120-121] shows the range-of-motion exercises suggested for a bedfast individual.

All inactive muscles lose tone and strength. A decrease of muscle contraction and relaxation is an important factor contributing to systemic complications associated with bed rest. The muscles which lose tone and become weak most rapidly are those of the ankles, knees, hips, and abdomen that normally maintain and balance the person in the upright posture.

In addition to exercising muscle groups by moving the joints through a full range of motion, setting exercises are of value. Setting exercises are accomplished by alternately tightening and relaxing the muscles without joint movement. Setting exercises are particularly useful for maintaining the tone of postural muscles of the buttocks, abdomen, and thighs. The patient can set the quadriceps, gluteal, and abdominal muscles separately, or he may set all of them simultaneously by lying supine with legs extended and hands at his sides, then lifting his buttocks off the bed, bearing his weight on shoulders and heels. Deep breathing and coughing exercises are of value not only for maintaining respiratory efficiency but also for concomitant exercise of the abdominal muscles.

Since actual contraction of a muscle group is essential, the bedfast patient must be encouraged to perform the exercises himself. Passive exercise in which the muscle does not do the work itself, but is moved through the various exercises by the nurse, is of less value. For the patient who is unable to perform the exercises himself, passive movement is, obviously, of more value in preventing the complications of bed rest than no exercise. For these patients the nurse must move each healthy joint through the exercises using as wide a range of motion as possible without discomfort to the patient. Normal, healthy joints should not be painful on movement as would diseased or injured joints or muscle groups. Discomfort, particularly the day or so following strenuous activity, is more probable, but the bedfast patient is unlikely to exercise to this extent. Footblocks, sandbags, pillows, and other artificial measures to insure proper alignment are essential for the patient who is unable to exercise actively. For the patient who is able to move his extremities, these devices may inhibit movement and prevent him from exercising freely and continuously. Any artificial measures to help him maintain proper alignment should be used judiciously. These artificial measures are not a substitute for exercise.

EXERCISES FOR BEDFAST PATIENTS

The bedfast patient who is encouraged to carry out as many of his daily activities as possible will be using many of the range-of-motion exercises of his upper extremities as he combs his hair, takes his bath, or rearranges the articles in the drawer of his bedside table. Because the lower extremities are not used for their normal daily functions of standing and walking, when the patient is able he can be shown how to use his feet and legs to push himself up toward the head of the bed, to turn, and to position himself comfortably. Footboards and footblocks are useful for the patient to push his feet against as he moves himself. Linen over the foot of the bed should be kept loose so that movement of the lower extremities will not be restricted.

The nurse needs to make careful observations of the various movements her patient is using in his daily activities. It is possible, for example, for a patient to bathe himself without completely flexing, hyperextending or laterally flexing his wrist. Those movements which the patient is not using regularly or is using through an incomplete range in his daily activities are those upon which the nurse needs to focus attention.

Since full range of motion of all joints will not occur spontaneously in the normal activities of the bedfast patient, planning an exercise regimen is essential. A patient should be started on a program of exercises as soon as possible after he becomes bedfast. Since most patients do not realize how rapidly their muscles can become weak and stiff, the nurse needs to help them understand the effects of inactivity and that exercise will help to maintain their strength.

Although the type and amount of exercise will depend upon the patient's capabilities, he should start gradually, exercising frequently during the day for short periods of time. In time, the patient who is able should be encouraged to perform the exercises for each joint at least five times, and to repeat the entire series of exercises at spaced intervals four or five times a day. No effective program of exercises can remain static but must change as the patient's capabilities for exercise change. As his physical status improves, the nurse may find that some of the exercises may be omitted entirely, while others may need more emphasis. Most wheelchair patients and many ambulatory patients will benefit from an exercise program until they can return to their normal activities at home.

The patient who is able to participate in planning his exercise program and can take responsibility for carrying out the exercises becomes less dependent on the nurse and more dependent upon his own ability in helping himself to return to normal activity. The nurse should assist him to set up a schedule for his exercises at times convenient for him. He may, for example, wish to start his exercise program each day by doing his exercises along with his morning hygienic care. His schedule for exercises should be planned so that they won't conflict with regularly scheduled treatments, appointments, and visiting hours. The bedfast patient needs to understand that having a

All exercises can be performed from the supine position in bed except hyperextension of the spine, hips, and shoulders, and flexion of the knees for which the person must lie prone or on his side.

Spine:

Cervical

lateral flexion — rotation — flexion extension hyperextension

Trunk

lateral flexion — rotation — flexion extension hyperextension

Shoulder

abduction
adduction

rotation: outward inward

flexion extension hyperextension

Hip

rotation: outward inward

abduction
adduction

flexion extension hyperextension

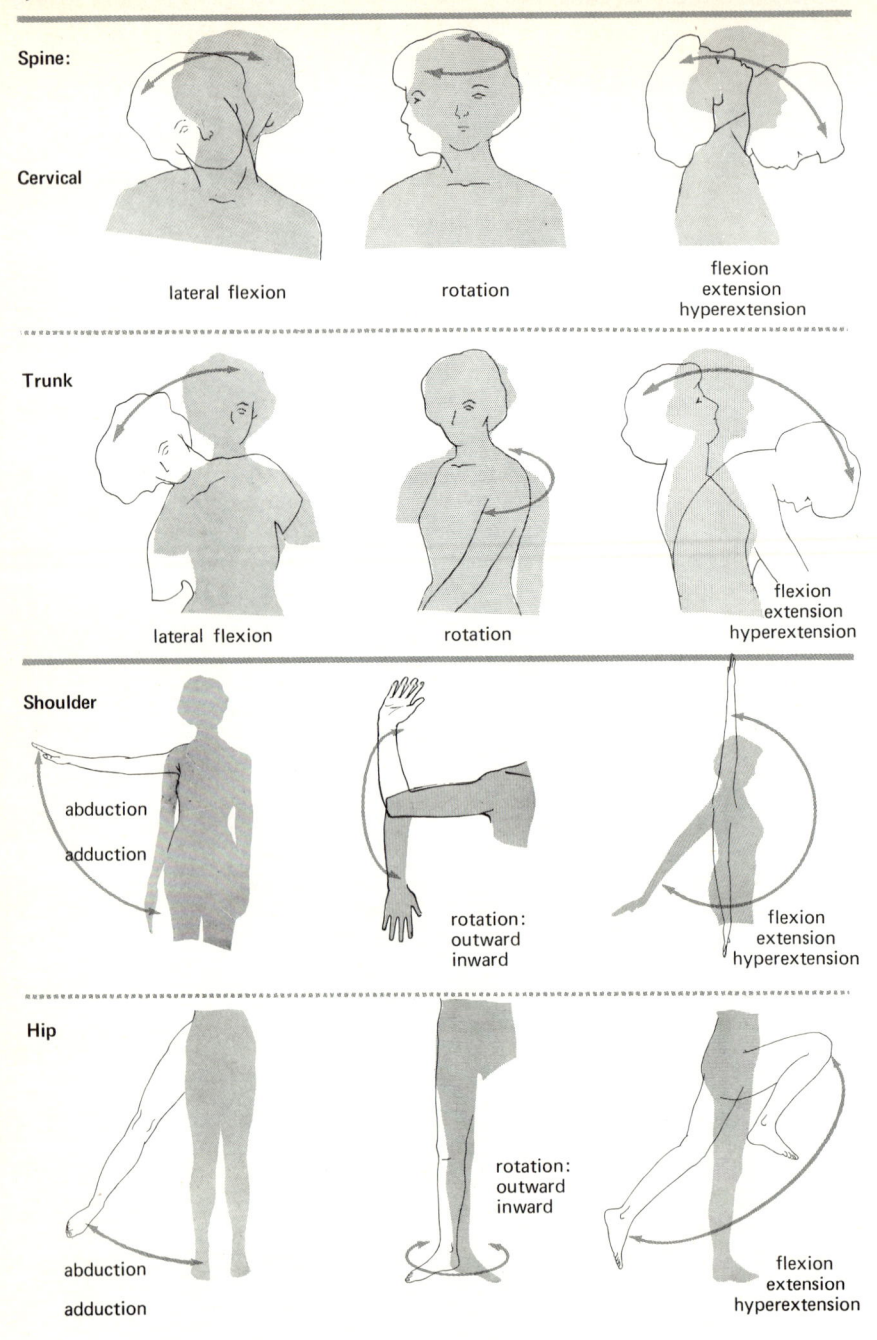

Figure 14-1 *Ranges of Motion.* All exercises can be performed from the supine position in bed except hyperextension of the spine, hips, and shoulders, and flexion of the knees for which the person must lie prone or on his side.

120

Elbow

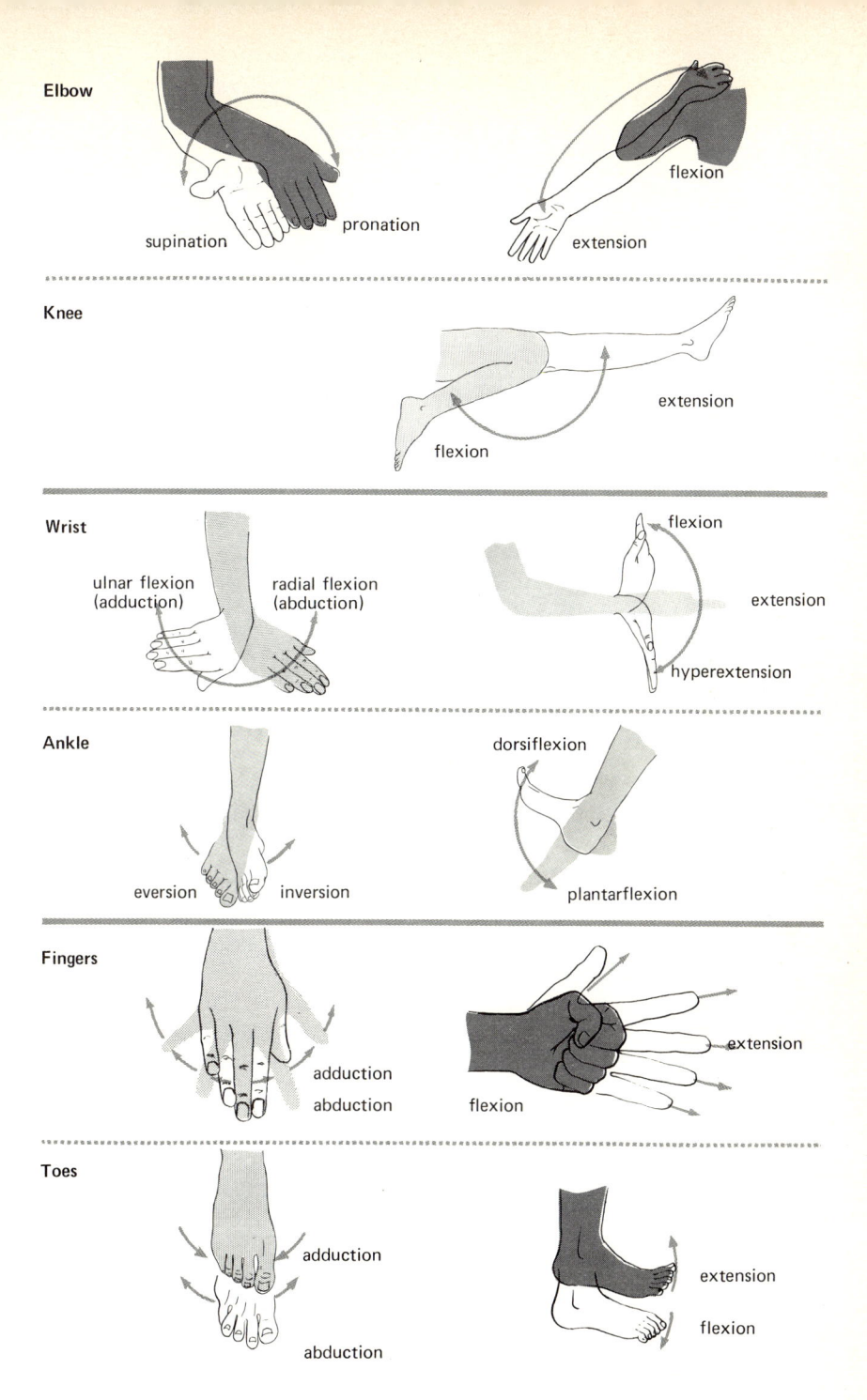

supination — pronation | flexion — extension

Knee

flexion — extension

Wrist

ulnar flexion (adduction) — radial flexion (abduction) | flexion — extension — hyperextension

Ankle

eversion — inversion | dorsiflexion — plantarflexion

Fingers

adduction — abduction | flexion — extension

Toes

adduction — abduction | extension — flexion

121

schedule does not mean that he is to remain immobile between periods of planned exercise, for the more exercise he can obtain, the less likely he is to develop complications. Once they have learned to do the exercises, many patients can carry them out independently with only periodic observation and guidance by the nurse.

The patient's exercise program should be outlined in a written plan of care available to all nursing personnel, physicians, and physical therapists. Progress the patient is making should be shared by members of these groups and changes made accordingly in the patient's program of exercises.

Only through a well-planned program of range-of-motion exercises for all bedfast patients capable of activity can nurses hope to prevent the physical complications and discouragement which patients can experience as a result of confinement to bed.

Reading 15
Effects on Cardiovascular Function
Edith V. Olson
with
Bonnie Jean Johnson

The cardiovascular system, including the heart, the arteries, the venous channels, and the lymph vessels, is designed to deliver blood to and from the capillaries where the exchange of the vital respiratory gases and other metabolic substances occurs. Three major changes in cardiovascular system function have been identified as resulting from immobility: orthostatic hypotension, increased work load of the heart, and thrombus formation.

ORTHOSTATIC HYPOTENSION

Perhaps the most dramatic of these changes is the deterioration of the ability of the autonomic nervous system to equalize the blood supply when a person who has been recumbent for a long period attempts to stand up. All nurses are aware that when patients first get up after several days in bed, they may suffer from weakness, dizziness, or giddiness. They may even faint.

Taylor found that when healthy young men were put to bed for 21 days, the ability of the cardiovascular system to respond to the upright posture was not regained for more than five weeks after activity was resumed [1]. This was due to two factors: loss of general muscle tone and decrease of

Reprinted by permission from the *American Journal of Nursing*, vol. 67, no. 4, pp. 781–783, April 1967.

efficiency of the orthostatic neurovascular reflexes. The loss of muscle tone resulting from complete disuse is estimated to be 10-15 percent of strength per week. One potent factor assisting venous return is the so-called venopressor mechanism in which the contraction of muscles causes pressure on veins. The venous valves which prevent the backflow of blood close, hence muscle action assists venous return of blood to the heart. In the absence of this type of assistance, the venous blood tends to pool in the lower parts of the body.

The second factor, decreased efficiency of the orthostatic neurovascular reflex control of the vessels themselves, is a puzzling complication. At the very time that there is an inability to maintain blood pressure when erect, patients show signs of strong activity of the sympathetic nervous system such as palmar sweating, pallor, and restlessness, which proves that the nerves are intact and central function is normal. Birkhead, who also demonstrated that persons show decreased tolerance to the erect posture after 42 days at bed rest, found a normal autonomic response to exercise in the supine position which confirmed positively that the problem is a peripheral rather than a central nervous system one [2]. Browse reported that this local failure of the nervous system may result simply from its habituation to the lower pressure, higher flow, and increased diameter of vessels in the supine position [3]. In such a situation the blood vessels cannot react to the nervous stimuli and the increased intramural pressure suddenly thrust upon them.

INCREASED WORK LOAD

The second change in cardiovascular system function resulting from immobility is that the heart itself works harder in the resting supine position than in resting erect position. The physiologic effect on the heart of bed rest as a method of treatment for myocardial infarction has received much attention in recent literature. Coe demonstrated that the heart works 30 percent harder when a person is in the recumbent position than when he is in a sitting position [4]. Several physiologic factors are involved in this phenomenon.

Changes in the vascular resistance and the hydrostatic pressure associated with lying down alter the distribution of blood within the body. With the release of gravity pressure, part of the total blood volume leaves the legs to be redistributed in other parts of the body, thus increasing the volume of the circulating blood which must be handled by the heart. The cardiac output and the stroke volume increase with lying down. Studies by Chapman found a 24 percent increase in the cardiac output and a 41 percent increase in the stroke volume when healthy men were put on enforced bed rest [5]. Also the heart rate itself increases progressively as the patient remains bedfast. Taylor found that, even in healthy young men who were confined to bed, the cardiac rate at rest increased approximately 0.5 beat per minute per day [1]. After three weeks of bed rest, these men showed an increased heart rate of 40 beats per minute during moderate work. They required 5 to 10 weeks of reconditioning before their heart rates during work matched those prior to the prolonged bed rest. This progressive increase of the resting heart rate and greater tachycardia during work indicates progressive decrease of ability in cardiovascular function. During tachycardia the recovery time for the heart muscle is decreased and the heart muscle fatigues more quickly. Taylor demonstrated that the ability of healthy young men to walk 3.5 miles an hour on a 10 percent incline was decreased by 75 percent after only three weeks in bed due to decreased cardiac reserve [1].

Another factor affecting the work load of the heart during bed rest is concerned with the Valsalva maneuver. When a person uses his arms and upper trunk muscles to expedite moving about in bed, he fixes his thorax and usually holds his breath. In so doing the breath is pressed forcibly against the closed glottis—the Valsalva maneuver. The same basic action occurs with straining at the stool. During this period of thoracic fixation without expiration, the intrathoracic pressure is elevated and interferes with entry of venous blood into the large veins. With release of the breath, there is a consequent fall in intrathoracic pressure and a large surge of blood is delivered to the heart at one time. This can result in tachycardia which, in turn, can result in cardiac arrest if the heart is not functioning optimally. Estimates on the frequency with which this maneuver is used by bedfast patients range from 10 to 20 times per hour.

THROMBUS FORMATION

The third major hazard to cardiovascular function resulting from immobility is thrombus formation. It is believed that immobility predisposes to thrombus by contributing to venous stasis, hypercoagulability of the blood, and external pressure against the veins. Venous stasis in the legs results from the lack of muscular contraction which ordinarily promotes venous return. Evidence that bed rest actually contributes to hypercoagulability of the blood is difficult to document, but several theories have been presented. Some physiologists believe that bed rest results in an increased concentration of the formed elements in the blood which by increasing viscosity would predispose to clotting. Dehydration which often accompanies immobility also is considered a factor leading to hypercoagulability of the blood. One familiar hypothesis of blood coagulation states that prothrombin is activated by material from the platelets and calcium to form thrombin, which, in turn, becomes the activating enzyme for the conversion of fibrinogen to fibrin. It is believed that the vital role of calcium in this process of coagulation supports the theory that the increased blood level of calcium resulting from immobility may result in hypercoagulability of the blood.

Another factor predisposing to thrombus formation, external pressure on the blood vessels, is well known to nurses. The danger of restricting circulation by allowing pressure from the bent-knee gatch or pillows under the knees is often voiced. However, the lateral recumbent position so often used in positioning patients may also result in both circulatory stasis and damage to the intima of the blood vessels. The upper leg will rest heavily on the lower leg unless care is taken to prevent it. When the intima is damaged a layer of platelets is laid down over the damaged area, and this plaque may be the basis for a clot.

While studies related to predisposition to thrombus formation because of immobility are contradictory, a report by Sevitt and Gallagher showed that on autopsy the number of thrombi found was in direct proportion to the length of time patients were at bed rest [6]. Their findings support the contention that venous stasis and the other effects of immobility play a major etiological role in venous thrombus formation.

NURSING IMPLICATIONS

These effects of immobility on the cardiovascular system dictate that no patient should be allowed to remain immobile any longer than absolutely necessary. Even when bed rest must be imposed, nursing measures, implied from the physiologic changes discussed, can prevent the hazards of immobility.

Exercises to prevent loss of muscle tone and to promote muscular pressure on veins to assist the return flow of blood to the heart should be included in any nursing care plan for the immobilized patient. These might include passive and active range-of-joint motion, isometric exercises, and self-care to the maximum permitted.

Seeing that the patient's position is changed frequently will alter the intravascular pressure and provide stimulus to the neural reflexes of the vessels and help prevent hypotension. Probably the most effective measure is changing the patient's position from horizontal to vertical. This can be achieved by elevating the head of the bed, or, when permissible, sitting the patient in a chair.

Patients need to be taught how to move and change position in bed without building up intrathoracic pressure. An overbed frame and trapeze can be provided if necessary and the patient taught to use it properly. To prevent the dangers inherent in repeated Valsalva maneuvers, he should be told to exhale rather than hold his breath while moving in bed.

The normal person changes position every few minutes, so that to plan position changes only every two hours is to condemn the person to discomfort or to the use of his own means of shifting weight or position.

Preventing constipation and positioning the patient for defecation in a well-supported sitting or squatting position also will reduce the work load on his heart. And, finally, as activity is permitted, it must be graduated carefully to avoid fatigue.

REFERENCES

1. Taylor, H. L., and others. Effects of bedrest on cardiovascular function and work performance. *J. Appl. Psychol.,* **2**:223-239, November 1949.
2. Birkhead, N. C., and others. Circulatory and metabolic effects of prolonged bedrest in healthy subjects (abstract). *Fed. Proc.,* **22**:520, March-April 1963.
3. Browse, N. S. *Physiology and Pathology of Bedrest.* Springfield, Ill., Charles C Thomas, Publisher, 1965.
4. Coe, S. W. Cardiac work and the chair treatment of acute coronary thrombosis. *Ann. Intern. Med.,* **40**:42-47, January 1954.
5. Chapman, C. B., and others. Behavior of stroke volume at rest and during exercise in human beings. *J. Clin. Invest.,* **39**:1208-1213, August 1960.
6. Sevitt, Simon, and Gallagher, Niall. Venous thrombosis and pulmonary embolism. *Brit. J. Surg.,* **48**:475-489, March 1961.
7. Dietrick, J. E., and others. Effects of immobilization upon various metabolic and physiologic functions of normal men. *Amer. J. Med.,* **4**:3-32, January 1948.
8. Beland, Irene L. *Clinical Nursing: Pathophysiological and Psychosocial Approaches.* New York, Macmillan Co., 1965.
9. Leithauser, D. J. *Early Ambulation and Related Procedures in Surgical Management.* Springfield, Ill., Charles C Thomas, Publisher, 1946.
10. Bockus, H. L., and others. *Gastroenterology,* 2d ed., vol. II. Philadelphia, Pa., W. B. Saunders Co., 1964.
11. Asher, Richard A. J. Dangers of going to bed. *Brit. Med. J.,* **2**:967-968, Dec. 13, 1947.

Reading 16
Effects on Gastrointestinal Function
Edith V. Olson
with
Joyce A. McCarthy

Immobility markedly reduces the energy requirements of cells and their metabolic processes. It sets in motion the complex physiologic phenomena associated with disuse which lead to psychologic and mechanical effects on gastrointestinal function.

Reprinted by permission from the *American Journal of Nursing,* vol. 67, no. 4, pp. 785-788, April 1967.

Bed rest and immobility may be considered as affecting the three main functions of the gastrointestinal system: ingestion, digestion, and elimination. The effects described here, however, deal primarily with ingestion and elimination.

INGESTION

An experimental study by Deitrick, Whedon, and Shorr demonstrated the effects of immobility upon metabolic and physiologic functions of healthy male subjects [7]. Clinical findings revealed that within 6 to 10 days following immobilization of these men, their nitrogen balance had reversed to a negative state. When anabolic and catabolic activities are equal, an individual is in a dynamic state of nitrogen equilibrium. The accelerated catabolic activity during immobility produces a rapid breakdown of cellular materials, leading to a protein deficiency and consequently to changes in the normal tissues.

Frequently, patients in a prolonged state of negative nitrogen balance suffer from anorexia. Failure to eat further contributes to their existing malnutrition. The disease process is then significantly prolonged since the cells of the body do not receive the nutrients necessary for the building and the maintenance of cellular processes. According to Beland, almost all sick persons have some disturbance in their capacity to ingest, digest, absorb, or utilize food [8]. The factors influencing food intake are difficult to study because of the interrelationship of psychologic, pathologic, and physiologic components.

In spite of decreased energy requirements, the immobilized individual needs appropriate and sufficient nutrients to maintain his basal metabolic needs and compensate for losses due to immobility-induced catabolism. In most instances, the immobilized patient does not feel like eating. His likes and dislikes must be determined and every effort made to provide him with a satisfying and adequate diet. Small, frequent feedings are usually more appealing to the anorexic patient than large meals. Nutrients necessary for cell metabolism should include an increased intake of protein and adequate carbohydrate and fat. A deficit of protein may be overcome by supplying the patient with increased amounts of complete protein foods. Eggs, meat, and milk provide some of the essential amino acids necessary for tissue synthesis and for the regulation of certain body functions.

During immobility, each individual is confronted by stress. If this stress is excessive, beyond the individual's ability to cope with it, the continued stimulation of the parasympathetic nerves will produce such symptoms as dyspepsia, gastric stasis, distention, anorexia, diarrhea, or constipation. Nursing intervention must be directed toward tension-reducing mechanisms for the individual which may help to alleviate these distressing problems and prevent their return.

ELIMINATION

Elimination is the other major gastrointestinal function affected by immobility. Normally, this process depends upon the integration of smooth and skeletal muscle activity and complicated visceral reflex patterns. Immobility may interfere with these mechanisms and, because of diminished expulsive power or the loss of the defecation reflex, or both, may cause constipation.

The primary muscles involved in the elimination process are the abdominals, the diaphragm, and the levator ani. These are necessary to increase the intra-abdominal pressure preliminary to the act of defecation and for the expulsion of the fecal mass. Muscular atrophy and loss of tone occur in the immobilized, the debilitated, or the malnourished patient. Too, lack of exercise brings about a generalized weakening of the muscles which may interfere with the mechanical expulsive mechanism. Thus, the patient is unable to assist with the elimination process and retention or incomplete evacuation of fecal material results.

SUPPRESSION OF DEFECATION

In many instances, one effect of immobility on bowel activity is the failure of the individual to heed the defecation reflex. Deterring factors for the individual may be his strange environment, the disruption of his familiar patterns of daily living, and the unnatural position he is often forced to assume. The act of defecation is initiated by a mass peristalsis which forces the fecal contents from the sigmoid colon into the rectum. The distended rectum stimulates the nerve impulses that create the reflex activity of emptying the rectum. If one fails to allow defecation to occur when the reflexes are excited they will become progressively less and less strong over a period of time. Habitual neglect in responding to these impulses may lead to the complete absence of the defecation sensation. Postponing this act when the stimulus is present may also produce an inhibition of the colonic motility and a weakening of the gastrocolic reflex.

The physiologic posture for defecating is the squatting position. Sitting changes the position and the tone of the muscles of the pelvic floor. The patient who must use a bedpan is placed in an abnormal position at best with his hips flexed to about a 90-degree angle and his knees extended. As a result, most of the normal mechanisms and reflexes are not stimulated. Furthermore, in our culture, the defecation act is performed in the privacy of one's bathroom. Psychologically as well as physiologically, it is very difficult for a person to defecate while sitting on a bedpan and screened only minimally from others. The unavoidable odor, the expulsive noises, and embarrassment cause most people to ignore or suppress this act until more suitable conditions prevail. Over a period of time, suppression of the act may lead to the development of constipation. Without proper treatment, fecal impactions and a mechanical bowel obstruction may develop.

Constipation is such a common problem of immobilized individuals that nursing personnel should anticipate and prevent it rather than accept it as inevitable. Although pharmacologic agents, dietary modifications, environmental changes, and decrease in physical activity may be individual predisposing factors, constipation is usually the result of a combination of these and other factors. Whatever the cause, the patterns of colonic motility are altered and manifestations associated with constipation—headache, anorexia, distention, malaise, vertigo, pain in the buttocks and sacrum—are seen. It is believed that these symptoms are of reflex origin.

Fecal impactions and fecalomas result from prolonged retention of feces in the rectum or the colon. When the fecal material remains in the bowel, water is continually withdrawn from it, and the material becomes increasingly more dry and hard. Excessive hardening of the stool can also be caused by medications or diet. The bulk of the stool may become so great that the person has a continuous desire to defecate. The rectal muscles contract but, due to the hardened consistency of the stool, it cannot be molded for expulsion. Such pathologic conditions as cerebral vascular accidents, hemorrhoids, fissures, ulcers, and rectal prolapse and heart block may be accompaniments of excessive straining at the stool.

The older person may have a relaxation of the rectal musculature. When the rectum is distended with stool he will have no desire to defecate due to the blunting or the loss of the defecation reflex.

The earliest symptom of an impaction is the frequent passage of liquid material around the impacted stool. Often this situation is erroneously treated as diarrhea, thus increasing the magnitude of the patient's problem. A slight degree of cramping abdominal pain and distention may be present when an impaction is present in the rectum. However, when the impacted material is located higher in the colon these symptoms increase in severity.

Mechanical bowel obstructions, partially or completely occluding the intestinal lumen, may result from fecal impactions. With this blockage there is an immediate interruption of the normal pathways of intestinal propulsions and absorption of liquid and gas. Stasis of fluid within the intestine produces distention and an increase in the intraluminal pressure. With the expansion of the intestinal wall the mesenteric vessels are stretched to the point of occlusion and impaired circulation to the area occurs. Intestinal function becomes depressed, dehydration occurs, and absorption ceases with a resultant fluid and electrolyte imbalance. The distention produces pain and discomfort for the patient. His respirations may become difficult as the intra-abdominal pressure interferes with the expansion of the diaphragm.

According to Leithauser, the increased pressure on the large veins of the abdomen may retard venous return from the legs and contribute to the formation of thrombi in the veins of the lower extremities [9].

PREVENTING CONSTIPATION

Since constipation is a problem that confronts all immobilized individuals, intelligent management to maintain the individual's state of homeostatic equilibrium must be initiated before serious complications develop. Prevention must be the primary focus of nursing action. Bowel hygiene management should be a program planned jointly by the patient and the nurse, and should involve three essential steps: obtaining a history of the patient's elimination habits, educating him about the physiology of elimination, and planning a course of action to maintain and promote normal colonic function.

Each person has a different pattern of elimination. It is learned and usually it is established early in childhood. Therefore, the patient's habits prior to his immobility should be determined and incorporated into the nursing care plan. The patient's regular pattern should be supported and when this is disrupted it should be re-established. Mass peristalsis occurs most often following meals and is believed to be the strongest following breakfast. To establish regularity the patient should be taught to eat breakfast, to respond to the signal for defecation, and to allow at least 10 to 15 minutes for this process. If feasible, the patient should be permitted to use the lavatory, or for the immobilized individual the environment can be modified to provide privacy and make it possible for him to assume a position that best promotes evacuation. Gentle, digital stimulation to the anal sphincter may be helpful in activating evacuation for some patients.

An explanation of the process of defecation aids the patient in overcoming the misconception that a daily bowel movement is necessary. It is generally accepted that evacuation twice a week in sufficient amounts and consistency is compatible with healthy body function.

The dietary regimen, also an important aspect of the bowel hygiene program, needs to be individualized. Because foods have a varying effect on each person it is imperative to learn what foods have a natural laxative effect for the patient and to supply these in the necessary amounts. Prune juice is universally considered the most effective laxative. Adequate fluids and fruit juices are encouraged to stimulate reflex activity and to assure enough water in the feces. The diet must contain sufficient amounts of bulk and cellulose material. This poses a problem for the edentulous patient and the nurse and dietitian who plan his diet.

To maintain normal bowel habits, such patients often must use stool softeners. Stool softeners or mineral oil are also advocated for the hypertensive patient to decrease the likelihood of straining at stool. The use of laxatives and enemas should be discouraged. The abuse and misuse of these agents may lead to an interruption of normal colonic motility patterns and to cathartic habituation.

Bockus recommends the following two exercises for individuals with weak abdominal muscles [10]:

1 Instruct the patient to recline on the bed with his arms folded across his chest and to rise to a sitting position without allowing the heels to be raised.

2 Instruct the patient to assume a supine position with shoulders flat on the bed and to raise both legs without bending the knees. These exercises should be performed twice daily until the patient's abdominal musculature is strengthened.

Many persons who have been ill or immobilized for a prolonged period, and most elderly persons, should begin with more simple, less strenuous modifications of these exercises. For example, lying with his knees bent, the patient can raise his head and shoulders from the bed, or from the same position contract his abdominal muscles, letting his pelvis roll and his back flatten. It may be necessary for some individuals to wear abdominal binders or corsets for visceral and postural support until the strength of their abdominal walls has been increased through a systematic program of exercises.

Astute observations regarding the frequency, color, amount, and consistency of the stool can provide the nurse with guidelines for action. She should also be alert for any signs or symptoms of discomfort associated with the process of elimination.

Even with a well-planned bowel hygiene program, fecal impactions may develop, especially in the aged or in patients with neurologic diseases. An impaction should be dislodged and removed by gentle digital action. Some authorities recommend that this be followed by an oil retention enema and three saline or soap-suds enemas. It may be necessary to repeat this treatment for several days until the patient is free from ensuing problems. Suppositories and digital stimulation (and perhaps enemas) may be required for several weeks until normal patterns are re-established. In every case, however, daily enemas are contraindicated.

Prevention of the physiologic effects of immobility on the gastrointestinal system is contingent upon knowledgeable nursing intervention to maintain the patient's homeostatic equilibrium.

REFERENCES

1 Taylor, H. L., and others. Effects of bedrest on cardiovascular function and work performance. *J. Appl. Psychol.,* **2**:223-239, November 1949.
2 Birkhead, N. C., and others. Circulatory and metabolic effects of prolonged bedrest in healthy subjects (abstract). *Fed. Proc.,* **22**:520, March-April 1963.
3 Browse, N. L. *Physiology and Pathology of Bedrest.* Springfield, Ill., Charles C Thomas, Publisher, 1965.
4 Coe, S. W. Cardiac work and the chair treatment of acute coronary thrombosis. *Ann. Intern. Med.,* **40**:42-47, January 1954.
5 Chapman, C. B., and others. Behavior of stroke volume at rest and during exercise in human beings. *J. Clin. Invest.,* **39**:1208-1213, August 1960.
6 Sevitt, Simon, and Gallagher, Niall. Venous thrombosis and pulmonary embolism. *Brit. J. Surg.,* **48**:475-489, March 1961.
7 Dietrick, J. E., and others. Effects of immobilization upon various metabolic and physiologic functions of normal men. *Amer. J. Med.,* **4**:3-32, January 1948.
8 Beland, Irene L. *Clinical Nursing; Pathophysiological and Psychosocial Approaches.* New York, Macmillan Co., 1965.
9 Leithauser, D. J. *Early Ambulation and Related Procedures in Surgical Management.* Springfield, Ill., Charles C Thomas, Publisher, 1946.
10 Bockus, H. L., and others. *Gastroenterology,* 2d ed., vol. II. Philadelphia, Pa., W. B. Saunders Co., 1964.
11 Asher, Richard A. J. Dangers of going to bed. *Brit. Med. J.,* **2**:967-968, Dec. 13, 1947.

Reading 17

Effects on Respiratory Function

Edith V. Olson
with
Lida F. Thompson

Full utilization of his available pulmonary energy for the activities important to him is the patient's right—his right to breathe. Respiration as a physiologic process is the gaseous exchange between an organism and its environment. Oxygen is absorbed and carbon dioxide is eliminated. The purpose of the respiratory movements is to renew the air in the alveoli, to ventilate, to move air in and out. The lungs lie within the thorax and communicate with the environment via the bronchioles, bronchi, and trachea. As the thoracic cavity changes in size through the contraction and relaxation of the muscles of respiration (abdominals, external and internal intercostals,

Reprinted by permission from the *American Journal of Nursing,* vol. 67, no. 4, pp. 783-785, April 1967.

and the diaphragm), the lungs also change in size because of shifts from negative to positive air pressure. The lungs expand on inspiration (compliance) and relax on expiration (elastic recoil). These movements are normally so rhythmic and easy that the individual is not aware of his breathing.

Gaseous exchange can only occur when the air is in the alveoli, in close contact with the circulating blood, and when the air is constantly being changed, providing a fresh supply of oxygen and removing the carbon dioxide as it accumulates. Physiologists have found that in order for the exchange of gases to occur there must be a large, thin, moist, permeable membrane and a difference in the concentrations of molecules of the gas on either side of that membrane. There is a tendency for such a difference in concentration to be equalized through the movement of molecules from a higher concentration to the lower concentration. The alveoli and capillaries provide the large, thin, moist membrane. The differences in the pressure of the gas in the capillaries and in the alveoli provide the differences in molecular concentrations. The pressure of oxygen in the alveoli is higher than the pressure of oxygen in the capillaries. The reverse is true of carbon dioxide. Thus, oxygen is absorbed into the blood and carbon dioxide is eliminated.

Changes in the normal physiologic functions of the respiratory system during short periods of immobility may at first be compensatory or adaptive as the body strives to preserve homeostasis. During immobility the basal metabolism is decreased, and the cells require less oxygen for use in the synthesis of proteins. As a consequence, less carbon dioxide as a byproduct of cell metabolism is produced. Respirations become slower and less deep in order to compensate for the lessened demand and maintain the needed and constant concentrations of these two elements, oxygen and carbon dioxide, in the blood and extracellular fluids.

Three physiologic effects on the respiratory system may occur as a result of immobility—decreased respiratory movement, decreased movement of secretions, and disturbed oxygen-carbon dioxide balance.

DECREASED RESPIRATORY MOVEMENT

Respiratory movement may be limited by the counterresistance of the bed or chair to chest expansion when the patient is allowed to sit too long or lie too long on his back or side, or in a prone position. Chest-cage expansion may also be limited by sitting or lying postures, which compress the thorax, by abdominal distention (secondary to an accumulation of feces, gas, or fluid), and by the use of tight abdominal or chest binders. Anything that creates intra-abdominal pressure will prevent the normal descent of the diaphragm and limit inspiration. Movement of the chest may also be hindered by a diminution of muscle power and coordination, as a result of muscle disuse or decreased innervation. Further, the administration of anesthetics, narcotics, sedatives, and other pharmacologic agents acting on the central nervous system may limit the rate and depth of respiratory movement by depressing the respiratory center in the medulla, the sensory and motor areas of the cerebral cortex, and the cells of the spinal cord.

These limitations to chest-cage expansion necessarily result in a limitation of lung expansion and, eventually, in a substantial decrease in the compliance and elastic recoil of lung tissue. Thus, decreased lung expansion hinders the normally efficient and effective ventilation or the movement of air in and out of the lung tissue.

STASIS OF SECRETIONS

The normal movement of secretions out of the tracheobronchial tree is decreased whenever one of the normal cleansing mechanisms, such as coughing and changes in posture or position, is made ineffective. Prolonged immobility causes stasis and pooling of secretions. The maintenance of a patent airway may be threatened or disrupted as the secretions collect. Poor fluid intake, dehydration, or anticholinergic drugs may render secretions thick and tenacious and further interfere with their movement.

With the stasis of secretions, it is no surprise that the immobilized patient frequently contracts a tracheitis, bronchitis, or that old enemy, hypostatic pneumonia. Moreover, the collection of unmoving secretions provides an ideal medium for bacterial growth within the body, especially for pneumococcic, pseudomonal, staphylococcic, and streptococcic organisms.

Anesthetics, narcotics, and sedatives may also contribute to respiratory complications by decreasing the rate and depth of lung expansion and ventilation, by depressing the cough center, and by slowing the reflex action of the epiglottis and thus permitting aspiration of secretions from the nasopharynx. The bulk of the unmoving secretions or the inflammatory edema may eventually obstruct the airway. The combination of the necessity to overcome resistance to chest and lung expansion, diminished muscle power, and an obstructed airway will require more subjective effort for the act of breathing. Increased oxygen will be used and more carbon dioxide will be produced, in turn demanding that the immobilized patient try even harder to breathe at a greater rate and depth in order to counteract this deficient ventilation.

OXYGEN-CARBON DIOXIDE IMBALANCE

A decrease in respiratory movement and a decrease in the movement of secretions, therefore, result primarily in deficient ventilation and in turn, limited diffusion of oxygen and carbon dioxide via the alveolar and capillary membranes. The exchange of oxygen and carbon dioxide may be further diminished by functional disabilities on the capillary "side" (as compared with changes on the lung "side" of the membrane) because of the cardiovascular changes during immobility. The disturbance in the exchange will alter the normal oxygen-carbon dioxide balance in a cumulative manner, with a continuing build-up of carbon dioxide in the blood because it cannot be adequately expired and a developing hypoxemia, creating tissue hypoxia, because adequate oxygen cannot be inspired.

At first, the increased concentration of carbon dioxide in arterial and venous blood acts as a respiratory stimulus, but continued strong stimulation of the respiratory centers in the medulla and pons will eventually depress them, and carbon dioxide narcosis will occur. A lowered oxygen concentration in the blood may provide respiratory stimulation via the aortic and carotid bodies for an interval, but, again, continued stimulation will lead to depression and this mechanism will also become ineffective.

Increasing arterial and venous concentrations of carbon dioxide, as carbonic acid and hydrogen ions, will create a respiratory acidosis, or narcosis will lead to respiratory failure or cardiac failure and death. Thus, a fourth possible physiologic effect of immobility on the respiratory system is death!

NURSING IMPLICATIONS

Preventing respiratory physiologic changes from becoming functional disabilities is of primary importance in the preservation of the patient's right to breathe. Many of the activities the nurse performs daily pertain to respiration. One of the most important of these is observation of respiratory function. While observing a patient's respiratory rate, she should also note the quality of the respirations. Are they deep or shallow? Wet or dry? Easy or labored? Is the patient using his neck muscles or abdominal muscles in breathing? Does he present any neurologic signs, such as restlessness or forgetfulness, which often are early indications of a deficiency of oxygen supply to the tissues? Does he have the late signs of hypoxia, cyanosis, and dyspnea? An anxious patient, perhaps using his neck muscles to facilitate breathing that is shallow, wet, or labored, needs the nurse's immediate care—and means that the nurse was late in recognizing his need to breathe efficiently.

Another nursing activity is to help the patient routinely turn, cough, and breathe deeply. Patients as well as nurses must understand how beneficial it is to chest and lung expansion for the patient to turn off his back or side, stretch out, and sit up straight at regular and frequent intervals. Also, how coughing secretions up and out facilitates adequate oxygen-carbon dioxide exchange. If the patient is unable to cough effectively, it may be necessary to suggest and use chest tapping to help loosen secretions, and postural drainage to remove them from the tracheobronchial tree.

The nurse must be able to teach a patient how to breathe deeply using his abdominal muscles, diaphragm, and intercostals in facilitating deep inhalation and prolonged expiration, and to encourage him to do breathing exercises regularly.

The use of these common nursing measures and the promotion of physical mobility through self-care activities will contribute to the prevention of the functional respiratory disabilities which may result from the physiologic effects of immobility. They will help preserve the patient's ability to breathe and to use his available cardiopulmonary energy for the activities which are important to him.

REFERENCES

1. Taylor, H. L., and others. Effects of bedrest on cardiovascular function and work performance. *J. Appl. Psychol.,* **2**:223-239, November 1949.
2. Birkhead, N. C., and others. Circulatory and metabolic effects of prolonged bedrest in healthy subjects (abstract). *Fed. Proc.,* **22**:520, March-April 1963.
3. Browse, N. L. *Physiology and Pathology of Bedrest.* Springfield, Ill., Charles C Thomas, Publisher, 1965.
4. Coe, S. W. Cardiac work and the chair treatment of acute coronary thrombosis. *Ann. Intern. Med.,* **40**:42-47, January 1954.
5. Chapman, C. B., and others. Behavior of stroke volume at rest and during exercise in human beings. *J. Clin. Invest.,* **39**:1208-1213, August 1960.
6. Sevitt, Simon, and Gallagher, Niall. Venous thrombosis and pulmonary embolism *Brit. J. Surg.,* **48**:475-489, March 1961.
7. Dietrick, J. E., and others. Effects of immobilization upon various metabolic and physiologic functions of normal men. *Amer. J. Med.,* **4**:3-32, January 1948.
8. Beland, Irene L. *Clinical Nursing; Pathophysiological and Psychosocial Approaches.* New York, Macmillan Co., 1965.
9. Leithauser, D. J. *Early Ambulation and Related Procedures in Surgical Management.* Springfield, Ill., Charles C Thomas, Publisher, 1946.
10. Bockus, H. L., and others. *Gastroenterology,* 2d ed., vol. II. Philadelphia, Pa., W. B. Saunders Co., 1964.
11. Asher, Richard A. J. Dangers of going to bed. *Brit. Med. J.,* **2**:967-968, Dec. 13, 1947.

Reading 18
Effects on Motor Function
Edith V. Olson
with
Ruth E. Edmonds

Motion is a fundamental property of most animal life. It is necessary for the maintenance of the structural stability and the metabolism of the musculoskeletal system, and requires both basic tonicity and intermittent work loads

Reprinted by permission from the *American Journal of Nursing,* vol. 67, no. 4, pp. 788-791, April 1967.

of the skeletal muscles. The daily mechanical stresses of normal activity promote strength, endurance, and coordination of the muscles; permit a balance of activities within bone to maintain its solidity and its capability to support the weight of the body; and contribute to cell nutrition by maintaining the muscle pump activity upon the blood circulation.

Motor function is a highly complex process of interaction of man and his environment, of integration of learned and reflex patterns, and of coordination of muscles, bones, skin, and the senses through the nervous system. Musculoskeletal deterioration from immobility is manifested in three major complications: osteoporosis, contractures, and decubitus ulcers.

OSTEOPOROSIS

Osteoporosis affects the osseous structure of the body. Bone is a living structure. The vital matrix is fundamental to its growth and development and carries the calcium which gives the bone its solidity. Throughout life, the matrix and its calcium are continuously being built up and broken down by opposing cell forces in a dynamic state of equilibrium. Osteoblastic cells form the osseous matrix, while osteoclastic cells are continuously destroying the matrix through their opposing function of absorbing and removing osseous tissue from the bone. Since osteoblasts depend upon stresses and strains of mobility and weight bearing for proper functioning, normal motor activity is necessary to their function of building up the bone matrix. If there is no activity, as with complete immobility, there is an absence of these daily stresses and strains.

As a consequence, the process of building up the bone stops, but the osteoclasts continue their destroying function, disrupting the state of equilibrium and causing structural changes until the supply of bone calcium becomes severely depleted. At the same time there is increased excretion of bone phosphorus and nitrogen, and the bone becomes demineralized. This change in bone composition results in the condition known as osteoporosis, or porous bone. As the decalcification process continues, the bones become spongy or porous and may gradually compress and deform. Because of the lack of structural firmness, the bone may be easily fractured.

A healthy, active person is not aware of the weight of his body straining against his bones for there is no sensation from these stresses. However, the person with osteoporosis may experience very intense pain when the bones must bear weight. Advanced osteoporosis causes more pain than many other chronic diseases, and yet it is often unrecognized and undiagnosed because at least 30 percent of the calcium must be lost from the bone before decalcification is revealed on an x-ray film.

Nurses must be aware that decalcification takes place during immobility regardless of the quantity of calcium intake. Increasing calcium in the diet is not recommended for it will not be used by the bone of the osteoporotic patient or the immobile patient. Unneeded calcium will only be added to the very large amount of calcium being excreted, often precipitating from the urine as renal calculi. Or it may be deposited in the muscles, resulting in myositis ossificans, or in the joints, causing osteoarthropathy.

Osteoporosis can be largely prevented or decreased by the maintenance of weight bearing and muscle movement and the avoidance of complete immobility. The "normal" stress on the bones can be promoted through placing the patient in a weight-bearing position on a tilt table or an oscillating bed, or by having him stand or walk between parallel bars if he is able. A daily program of muscle activities against resistance should be planned. Not to be underestimated is the value of encouraging the patient to participate in his care to his maximum ability, and thus contribute to his mobility.

CONTRACTURES

Contractures involving the muscles and other soft tissues surrounding a joint are the second major complication from decreased mobility. Muscle makes up 40 percent of the body. It is very important to the individual because it provides the power for movement and interaction with his environment. All tissues subjected to prolonged immobility undergo atrophy and functional incompetence from disuse. Atrophy, or the wasting away of muscle tissue, leads not only to a decrease in the muscle size but also to a decrease in functional movement, strength, endurance, and coordination.

Contractures occur when muscles do not have the activity necessary to maintain the integrity of their function—that is, the full range of shortening and lengthening of their fibers. Contractures may occur with muscle imbalance in which one muscle is weak and its antagonist is stronger, or spastic, or both. Mild muscle spasm is one of nature's means of preventing further disability from osteoporosis and of splinting a part to prevent pain. Edema may mechanically splint a part and prevent muscle activity. Probably the main cause of contracture of which the nurse must be ever cognizant is that of prolonged immobilization of a joint in one position. This may occur as a therapeutic measure or when emphasis has been on the establishment and maintenance of proper body alignment rather than on mobility and maintenance of function.

Whatever the predisposing cause of the contracture, the fibers of the involved muscle shorten and atrophy, resulting in a limited range of motion of the joint. Such a process may initially produce a reversible contracture that can be overcome by exercise and stretching, but eventually it will involve tendons, ligaments, and the joint capsule and become irreversible, requiring surgical intervention or prolonged mechanical stretching for its release.

Because the prevention of contractures is much easier than the treatment, nursing measures are of great value. The first objective is to maintain body joints in their most functional anatomical position. Special care must be taken to prevent hip and knee flexion contractures which may result from prolonged, faulty positioning with improper placement of pillows, or from gatched beds that keep the hips and knees continuously flexed. A bed board and a firm mattress are helpful in maintaining correct body positioning. A footboard can be beneficial in preventing foot drop, but only if it is used properly. It should be placed firmly against the bottom of the patient's feet to hold them at a right angle with the legs. It should not be placed at a distance where stretching to reach it will inadvertently create the plantar flexion position of foot drop. In such a position the board is only useful for keeping the bedclothes from resting on the toes.

Nursing activities should include frequent and scheduled change of patient positioning and range of motion of all the joints. These should be combined with the use of appropriate devices for temporary maintenance of the functional position of such parts as the wrist, hand, and fingers. Whenever possible, the patient should assume some of the responsibility for checking his position and for performing range of motion exercises. Health teaching which encourages the participation of the patient and his family can be vital in the prevention of contractures.

The skin may also be seriously affected by immobility. A normal, active individual with unimpaired sensory and motor function will change his position every few moments during waking hours and quite frequently during sleep. The patient who is paralyzed or debilitated may be unable to move himself. The patient who is without sensation to a part will not automatically move, for the stimuli of discomfort that usually lead to automatic shifting of position are not felt.

DECUBITUS ULCERS

Decubitus ulcers occur under many different circumstances. Since proper circulation of the arterial and venous blood flow is partially dependent upon normal muscle action, muscle disuse during immobility often decreases the circulatory exchange in the soft tissues. Prolonged pressure on an area causes disturbances in the nerve impulses to and from this area and also decreases the blood supply, which in turn diminishes the nutrition of that part. In addition, constant pressure, particularly over bony prominences such as the sacrum, trochanters, ischial tuberosities, and heels, compresses and obstructs the blood flow, causing ischemia or local anemia of a tissue. Ultimately, ischemia leads to necrosis and ulceration. The ulcerative areas can become so massive that it may take many months or years of treatment and cost thousands of dollars to repair them, during which time the patient's mobility will be further limited. Although decubitus ulcers may occur in healthy persons from pressure against a part, with resultant ischemia and progressive tissue deterioration, they are more likely to appear in malnourished persons who are in negative nitrogen balance. Once the patient regains a positive nitrogen balance, and there is more nitrogen intake than output, there will usually be improvement in regeneration and growth of the tissues.

When a patient has a decubitus ulcer the prevention of infection is a prime nursing concern. Infection not only retards healing of the ulcer, but also may lead to systemic infection. This in turn may cause osteomyelitis, for example, or even death.

Osteomyelitis seriously affects motor function. The infection destroys the blood supply to the bone. The bone deprived of nutrition acts as a foreign object, and a haven for organisms. In order to promote healing, the necrotic bone is surgically removed and the part is immobilized until the bone regenerates.

Nursing precautions to prevent such occurrences are paramount. The development of a decubitus ulcer in any person who has sensation is completely unwarranted with the present knowledge that is available. Even in persons who have experienced a loss of sensation, the development of a bedsore is to be considered an unnecessary complication. The immobilized patient should be turned frequently. Definite patterns of helping the patient to shift body weight off the bony prominences are necessary or pressure areas will develop and tissue will break down. Such aids as turning frames, oscillating beds, or air-filled or water-filled alternating pressure mattresses are useful but do not obviate the need for constant care to vulnerable areas.

During each position change, the skin should be inspected for areas of tenderness, edema, coldness, or redness. Meticulous skin care should be given and a dry and wrinkle-free bed provided. A regular toilet schedule on a 24-hour basis, time-tailored for each individual patient, will reduce the incontinence that contributes to skin breakdown. Two long-standing techniques of routine hospital care should be abolished. One is the use of rubber rings and doughnuts, which do not prevent decubitus ulcers, but actually compress a larger area around the pressure point, decrease circulation to it, and contribute to the formation and enlargement of the ulcer. The other is the use of alcohol for skin massage, since this dries the oils of the skin and creates cracks and subsequent broken-down areas.

If a pressure area should develop, prompt measures should be taken to promote healing, to close this portal of entry for infection, and to reduce the loss of serum proteins. The diet should provide enough protein to compensate for these losses should they occur, and enough carbohydrates and fats so that maximum utilization of the proteins is possible.

NURSING GOALS

In summary, prevention is the common thread weaving through nursing care plans for coping with musculoskeletal deterioration in the immobilized patient. The main objectives of such nursing care should be: to avoid complete immobility through a planned program of exercises and activities geared to the capability of the patient; to give close visual observation to the body positioning and alignment, as well as to skin condition; to see that the patient has a well-balanced diet, supplemented as necessary to meet special needs; and to instruct the patient and family so they can assist in such prevention.

REFERENCES

1. Taylor, H. L., and others. Effects of bedrest on cardiovascular function and work performance. *J. Appl. Psychol.,* **2**:223-239, November 1949.
2. Birkhead, N. C., and others. Circulatory and metabolic effects of prolonged bedrest in healthy subjects (abstract). *Fed. Proc.,* **22**:520, March-April 1963.
3. Browse, N. L. *Physiology and Pathology of Bedrest.* Springfield, Ill., Charles C Thomas, Publisher, 1965.
4. Coe, S. W. Cardiac work and the chair treatment of acute coronary thrombosis. *Ann. Intern. Med.,* **40**:42-47, January 1954.
5. Chapman, C. B., and others. Behavior of stroke volume at rest and during exercise in human beings. *J. Clin. Invest.,* **39**:1208-1213, August 1960.
6. Sevitt, Simon, and Gallagher, Niall. Venous thrombosis and pulmonary embolism. *Brit. J. Surg.,* **48**:475-489, March 1961.
7. Dietrick, J. E., and others. Effects of immobilization upon various metabolic and physiologic functions of normal men. *Amer. J. Med.,* **4**:3-32, January 1948.
8. Beland, Irene L. *Clinical Nursing; Pathophysiological and Psychosocial Approaches.* New York, Macmillan Co., 1965.
9. Leithauser, D. J. *Early Ambulation and Related Procedures in Surgical Management.* Springfield, Ill., Charles C Thomas, Publisher, 1946.
10. Bockus, H. L., and others. *Gastroenterology,* 2d ed., vol. II. Philadelphia, Pa., W. B. Saunders Co., 1964.
11. Asher, Richard A. J. Dangers of going to bed. *Brit. Med. J.,* **2**:967-968, Dec. 13, 1947.

Reading 19

Effects on Urinary Function

Edith V. Olson
with
Lois M. Schroeder

Man's renal and urinary excretory system is designed to function optimally when he is in the erect position. What happens to this function when he is ill, supine, and allowed to remain immobile?

Reprinted by permission from the *American Journal of Nursing,* vol. 67, no. 4, pp. 791-793, April 1967.

The anatomy of the kidney is such that in the erect position the hilus of the kidney emerges from the medial aspect. When man is in the erect position, the urine flows out of the renal pelvis and into the ureter in accordance with the laws of gravity. There is only a small portion of the renal pelvis where stasis of urine might occur. But when a man is in the supine position, the hilus of the kidney is uppermost, and all urine formed must be expressed into the ureter against gravity. Because peristaltic contractions are not of sufficient and continuous strength to overcome this resistance, the renal pelvis may fill completely before the urine is expressed into the ureter. If the supine position is maintained for even a few days, urinary stasis occurs. Any particle contained in the urine may settle into the calyces and become the nucleus for formation of a renal calculus or the focus for infection.

Once urine is formed and propelled into the bladder, it must be excreted. Normal micturition is dependent upon the integrated action of the external sphincter, internal sphincter, and the detrusor muscle of the bladder wall. Man can consciously relax the perineal muscles and the external sphincter. This initiates an autonomic reflex causing contraction of the detrusor muscle. In turn, this contraction increases intrabladder pressure and forces the internal sphincter to relax so that micturition occurs.

When man remains in the supine position, he often has difficulty relaxing the perineal muscles and external sphincter, so that the reflex action is not initiated and micturition does not occur. However, the normal sensation to void is felt and intra-abdominal pressure can be increased to normal levels. But if the sensation to void is not heeded, the bladder distends and, with extensive stretching of the detrusor muscle, the sensation is no longer felt. Subsequently, with bladder distension, overflow incontinence occurs. This becomes a source of shame and embarrassment to the patient, undermining his morale and often precipitating depression. The presence of urine on the skin also makes the skin more prone to breakdown and decubitus ulcer formation.

In time, bladder distention may lead to back pressure and damage to the functioning unit of the kidney, the nephron. Infection may also occur, especially if the individual is catheterized to relieve the distention. Studies have shown that, except with extremely good technique and a closed drainage system, infection is likely when an indwelling catheter is used for any length of time.

URINARY TRACT STONES

In preceding articles of this series, disuse atrophy, protein breakdown, and decalcification of bone were noted as effects of immobility. Prolonged bed rest has little effect on the physiologic function of the kidney nephron. To maintain the homeostasis of body fluids and electrolytes, it continues its selective excretion of the constituents in excess in the blood plasma and its preservation of those in deficit. The changes in the composition and volume of urine are a result of hemodynamics and metabolic changes. Thus, the kidney excretes larger amounts of the minerals and salts released into the blood plasma as a result of the effects of immobility on other body organs.

Dietrick et al. found that with prolonged bed rest and the resultant protein breakdown the excretion of nitrogen, sulfur, phosphorus, sodium, potassium, and calcium was increased [7]. Calcium excretion began within two days after confinement to bed, reached a maximum level after the fifth week, and remained at this high level as long as bed rest continued. A study by Birkhead et al. showed similar results [2].

The majority of the "stones of recumbency" are composed of calcium salts. Factors favoring the precipitation of excess calcium salts are stasis, infection, alkalinity, increased concentration of phosphates, decreased volume of urine, and insufficient citric acid. The urine becomes more alkaline because without muscular activity there are fewer acid end products to excrete.

Two theories about the mechanism by which stone-forming salts may be held in solution have been advanced: (1) adsorption to the colloids suspended in the supersaturated urine, and (2) combination with the citric acid present. When the colloids are dispersed in the urine they present a large surface area for holding salts in suspension, but, with stasis and decreased volume of urine, the colloid particles tend to coalesce, decreasing the total surface area and allowing precipitation of the stone-forming salts. Urinary citrates assist in forming undissociated calcium complexes for excretion of ionized calcium.

The factors which promote calcium precipitation may cause many chronically ill and inactive individuals who are allowed to remain inactive to develop "stones of recumbency." The presence of these calculi may be manifested by hematuria, dull flank pain or backache, or severe bouts of colic-like pain with nausea and vomiting. If man is maintained in the supine position, stones are most likely to form in the renal pelvis and bladder, while the renal stones that are passed into the ureter are more likely to lodge in the ureteropelvic junction. All calculi may injure the mucosal lining of the urinary tract and make the tract more susceptible to infection.

A patient has the right to remain free of urinary tract complications when simple and conscientious nursing care with mobilization will prevent them. Thoughtful consideration of the reasons for the complications of stasis, infection, overflow incontinence, and calculi make preventive nursing measures evident.

Schedule Activity around the Clock

Active and passive exercises, frequent turning of the patient, ambulation, positioning in a chair or on a tilt table—these activities will help to prevent stasis.

Periodic Check for Distention of Bladder

This is especially necessary if incontinence occurs. To facilitate normal urination, male patients should stand whenever possible or be helped to a sitting position to allow relaxation of the perineal muscles and to initiate the micturition reflex. Manual pressure on the lower abdomen may be of value. Women should be in a sitting position to void.

Adequate Fluid Intake around the Clock

Measure intake and output. If the urine is kept dilute, calcium particles are less likely to precipitate, and stasis with resultant infection is less likely to occur.

Acid-ash Diet

The amount of calcium in the diet may be limited, depending upon the need for bone formation. An acid-ash diet will lower the urine pH.

Foods that have an acid residue include cereals, meat, poultry, and fish.

Prevention of Urinary Tract and Systemic Infections

Catheterization should be initiated only after other measures to empty the bladder have failed. Scrupulous aseptic technique for indwelling catheter care must be followed.

Physicians may order physical therapy and medications to prevent or treat urinary tract infections. However, additional measures should not be necessary if nurses conscientiously apply the above measures and promote patient mobility.

REFERENCES

1. Taylor, H. L., and others. Effects of bedrest on cardiovascular function and work performance. *J. Appl. Psychol.*, **2**:223-239, November 1949.
2. Birkhead, N. C., and others. Circulatory and metabolic effects of prolonged bedrest in healthy subjects (abstract). *Fed. Proc.*, **22**:520, March-April 1963.
3. Browse, N. L. *Physiology and Pathology of Bedrest.* Springfield, Ill., Charles C Thomas, Publisher, 1965.

4 Coe, S. W. Cardiac work and the chair treatment of acute coronary thrombosis. *Ann. Intern. Med.,* **40**:42-47, January 1954.
5 Chapman, C. B., and others. Behavior of stroke volume at rest and during exercise in human beings. *J. Clin. Invest.,* **39**:1208-1213, August 1960.
6 Sevitt, Simon, and Gallagher, Niall. Venous thrombosis and pulmonary embolism. *Brit. J. Surg.,* **48**:475-489, March 1961.
7 Dietrick, J. E., and others. Effects of immobilization upon various metabolic and physiologic functions of normal men. *Amer. J. Med.,* **4**:3-32, January 1948.
8 Beland, Irene L. *Clinical Nursing; Pathophysiological and Psychosocial Approaches.* New York, Macmillan Co., 1965.
9 Leithauser, D. J. *Early Ambulation and Related Procedures in Surgical Management.* Springfield, Ill., Charles C Thomas, Publisher, 1946.
10 Bockus, H. L., and others. *Gastroenterology,* 2d ed., vol. II. Philadelphia, Pa., W. B. Saunders Co., 1964.
11 Asher, Richard A. J. Dangers of going to bed. *Brit. Med. J.,* **2**:967-968, Dec. 13, 1947.

Reading 20

Effects on Metabolic Equilibrium

Edith V. Olson
with
Mildred Wade

The effects of immobility on the metabolic processes cannot be discussed without some reference to closely related endocrine functions or some explanation of how interference with metabolic homeostasis profoundly influences the efficiency of all physiologic processes and other homeostatic mechanisms.

Functional changes resulting from immobility include reduced metabolic rate, tissue atrophy and protein catabolism, bone demineralization, alterations in the exchange of nutrients and other substances between the extracellular and intracellular fluids, fluid and electrolyte imbalance, and gastrointestinal hyper- or hypomotility.

When a person is consigned to bed rest and inactivity, his metabolic rate falls in response to the decreased energy requirements of the cells and the disequilibrium of metabolic processes. Anabolic processes are retarded

Reprinted by permission from the *American Journal of Nursing,* vol. 67, no. 4, pp. 793-794, April 1967.

and catabolic activities are accelerated. Many of these have already been discussed in relation to the dysfunction of various other body systems: the process of protein breakdown leading to protein deficiency and negative nitrogen balance; the formation of decubitus ulcers; the excretion of electrolytes when catabolic processes are accelerated; the demineralization of bone as a consequence of reduced muscle tension and absence of weight-bearing stress on the skeleton; and the formation of urinary tract stones. And there are still other factors associated with bed rest that affect metabolism and fluid and electrolyte balance and have important implications for nursing. One of these is body temperature.

Bedclothing prevents the loss of heat by conduction and radiation. The supine position dilates blood vessels, and, in order to throw off accumulating heat, the patient will sweat wherever skin surfaces touch. In the creases in the neck, under the breasts, the abdominal folds, the surfaces where the arms rest against the chest and in the axillary and perineal regions, sweating increases. All of this fluid loss carries with it essential electrolytes—sodium, potassium, and chloride.

It is known that the supine position reduces the production of adrenocortical hormones, although the exact mechanism whereby this occurs is not known. There are two groups of adrenal-cortical hormones that influence metabolism. One is the glucocorticoids which affect the metabolism of carbohydrate, protein, and fat; the other is the mineralocorticoids which are concerned with electrolyte balance (especially of sodium, potassium, and chloride).

Authorities currently are examining the influence of immobilization on other hormones produced in the body, but definitive information is not available at this time. Recently, a second hormone (thyrocalcitonin) has been isolated from the thyroid gland. Its function seems to be an adaptive one wherein it attempts to lower an elevated serum calcium.

Increased urinary excretion sometimes occurs when the patient is placed at bed rest, especially during the first few days of immobilization. This is due to the fact that the circulation to the kidneys is increased in the recumbent position.

Stress reactions, both psychologic and physiologic, are commonly associated with immobilization and illness. The effect of stress on fluid and electrolyte balance, and on other physiologic functions and psychologic behavior, should be kept in mind.

Diurnal patterns are the variations which occur in the physiologic operation of the body during the periods of day and night. While an individual is awake, his metabolic rate, body temperature, hormonal levels, and renal functions are active. During sleep the demands on these homeostatic mechanisms are reduced to a minimum. Whether the individual is asleep or not, the supine position in itself will result in the same minimal functional output. It is important for the nurse to consider these factors as they may affect the patient who is not allowed to sleep for any length of time, as in intensive care units; the individual who sleeps most of the time; and the patient who is awake all night and sleeps during the day. Each of these patients will have altered nutritional and fluid requirements.

The nursing measures which can help prevent some of the foregoing problems are not complex.

The patient should remain up until the need for bed rest is strongly apparent. Allowing the patient to be "up and about," while dressed in daytime clothing, would produce a more natural metabolic state. If the patient is unable to ambulate, sitting in the chair would tend to prevent fluid and electrolyte loss from perspiration and prevent the basal metabolic rate and hormonal level changes that occur in the supine position.

For the patient who must be on bed rest, elevation of the head and upper torso on a schedule similar to turning schedules would alleviate many of the problems previously discussed. Minimal but sufficient bedclothing which is not tight enhances loss of heat by conduction and radiation, thus reducing the patient's fluid and electrolyte loss.

Increased fluid intake and high-protein nutrition are essential to the patient regardless of the stage of his mobility if healing is to be hastened and electrolyte balance maintained.

The prevention of atrophy and of elevated serum calcium levels can be partially attained by range of motion, passive or active exercises, and weight bearing within the limits of the individual patient's capability.

Since metabolic homeostasis provides the framework for the composite of human function, any person when immobilized is confronted with aspects of the stress cycle. Reducing the effects of this process is contingent upon the nurse's ability to perceive, to interpret, and to intervene in the physiologic and psychologic pressure mechanisms.

REFERENCES

1. Taylor, H. L., and others. Effects of bedrest on cardiovascular function and work performance. *J. Appl. Psychol.*, **2**:223-239, November 1949.
2. Birkhead, N. C., and others. Circulatory and metabolic effects of prolonged bedrest in healthy subjects (abstract). *Fed. Proc.*, **22**:520, March-April 1963.
3. Browse, N. L. *Physiology and Pathology of Bedrest.* Springfield, Ill., Charles C Thomas, Publisher, 1965.
4. Coe, S. W. Cardiac work and the chair treatment of acute coronary thrombosis. *Ann. Intern. Med.*, **40**:42-47, January 1954.
5. Chapman, C. B., and others. Behavior of stroke volume at rest and during exercise in human beings. *J. Clin. Invest.*, **39**:1208-1213, August 1960.

6 Sevitt, Simon, and Gallagher, Niall. Venous thrombosis and pulmonary embolism. *Brit. J. Surg.,* **48**:475-489, March 1961.
7 Dietrick, J. E., and others. Effects of immobilization upon various metabolic and physiologic functions of normal men. *Amer. J. Med.,* **4**:3-32, January 1948.
8 Beland, Irene L. *Clinical Nursing; Pathophysiological and Psychosocial Approaches.* New York, Macmillan Co., 1965.
9 Leithauser, D. J. *Early Ambulation and Related Procedures in Surgical Management.* Springfield, Ill., Charles C Thomas, Publisher, 1946.
10 Bockus, H. L., and others. *Gastroenterology,* 2d ed., vol. II. Philadelphia, Pa. W. B. Saunders Co., 1964.
11 Asher, Richard A. J. Dangers of going to bed. *Brit. Med. J.,* **2**:967-968, Dec. 13, 1947.

Reading 21
Effects on Psychosocial Equilibrium
Edith V. Olson

Professional nurses concerned with comprehensive patient care must be aware that immobility can cause disturbances in the ego identity of man as an individual and as a social being, as well as in his homeostatic processes.

Human behavior is defined as an integrated developmental process of action and interaction of the physiology, personality, society, and culture of the individual. All human beings grow through a series of interrelated and interdependent age-related life-stages.

The individual begins life as an entity produced out of biologic functions and prepared to act in a socialized world through an intricately balanced and highly organized biologic mechanism. A personality forms and becomes organized through the socialization process of sensory and motor interactions with the environment and by cerebral integration of these interactions. Each life-stage calls into play new understandings, new definitions, new social groups, and new tests of one's psychologic organization. The human responds to each situation in terms of his own judgment of the nature, meaning, and significance of that situation. His motivation and learning, his body image, the expression of his drives, expectancies, and emotions, his sensory and perceptual interaction with his environment, his adequacy and flexibility in fulfilling his societal role, and his participation in free choice—all of these and more form the aggregate called ego identity. Immobility tends to fracture this personality.

Reprinted by permission from the *American Journal of Nursing*, vol. 67, no. 4, pp. 794-797, April 1967.

In the fields of learning and motivation, studies of immobilized or isolated individuals have demonstrated the subjects' decreased learning of original material, their decreased retention, and their decreased learning in transfer and generalization. In the area of problem-solving there were also lessened motivation, a loss in the ability to receive necessary content for problem-solving because of decreased sensory stimulation, and a decrease in the ability to discriminate.

Such evidence should cause us to question whether or not our expectations that patients should participate in problem-solving are realistic when directed toward patients who are immobilized for a prolonged period of time. Are we expecting too much of the immobilized person when we expect him to be highly motivated to fulfill his particular social roles?

Drives, expectancies, and emotions are influenced by immobility. Drives are such physiologic constructs as hunger, sex, and motor activity that represent internal events of the organism leading to behaviors that may satiate states of physical deprivation or arousal. Expectancies are defined as general responsiveness and anticipation, while emotions are internal events of the organism demonstrated by bodily changes and by behavioral changes. Studies have indicated that drives and expectancies were greatly diminished by immobility, while emotions were expressed in various ways. Examples of emotional expression included apathy, withdrawal, frustrated anger, aggression, or regression.

One of the fascinating paradoxes of the human condition is that the human body, which unites and identifies man as a biologic species, gives rise, in each of us, on a psychologic level, to a body image that is one of the subtly unique features of the individual personality. A person's conception of his own body as a whole and of different parts of the body contributes greatly to his conception of his own personality and of his relations with other people. To a certain extent, the body image is culturally determined in America by our emphasis on youth, vigor, strength, physique, wholeness, and constant activity. However, the intimate association of body image with a person's sense of his own worth and his place among other people goes even deeper than this. To the original self-concept of the child are added the body image changes and emotions from sequential life experiences. Although the emotional components develop into mature and rational associations, irrational and symbolic representations may linger in the unconscious.

Immobility often sets the stage for the expression of either exaggerated or inappropriate emotional reactions, for example, expressions of loss of personal worth, fear, wounded pride, guilt, disgust, or anger. The psychologic reactions to therapeutically realistic and necessary immobility may be related to changes in body image influenced by immobility-induced sensory deprivation as well as to modifications of body image secondary to illness or injury.

PERCEPTUAL BEHAVIOR

Two types of functional changes in behavior can be caused by immobility: perceptual and motor. The motor changes—skeletal, muscular, and systemic—which alter the capacity of the individual to manipulate his environment have been discussed in the preceding pages, therefore emphasis here is on changes in perception.

Immobility reduces the quantity and quality of sensory information available to the organism and reduces the ability of the individual to interact with his environment. We maintain contact with the environment through the senses and seek to control behavior in various aspects of the environment by responding to the perceived sensory stimuli. The process of perception requires the interpretation of complex stimuli. Immobilization reduces the efficiency of the sensory processes, and the individual suffers sensory deprivation.

Numerous clinical studies indicate that sensory deprivation causes a decrease in the perceptions of pattern and form, weight discrimination, pressure, and temperature sensitivity. It also tends to decrease the speed of perception.

In the world of time there may be distortions of time metric, time order, and time direction. Time metric refers to one's ability to estimate time intervals and is an attitudinal state relative to one's physical and/or emotional states. For example, we often say that "time hangs heavy" or "time flies." Time order refers to the relationships of past, present, and future. Time direction designates the sequence of events and the distortion of reality and fantasy in them. In our social world there is a strong relationship between time, space, and energy expenditure since we plan to expend our energy in a specified social role to fill a given time.

Activities like work, sleep, eating, visiting, vacationing, and even sex are largely regulated by culturally conditioned conceptions and interpretations of time. The world of immobility is often nearly devoid of sensory stimulation and filled with behavior aberrations (both physiologic and psychologic) traceable to sensory deprivation. The world of immobility either excludes or turns topsy-turvy the routines ordered by time.

SOCIAL ROLES AND MOBILITY

Our American culture also reflects its value orientation and its social attitudes and norms through its prescriptions for or prohibitions against attitudes, beliefs, or behavior. These determinants are declared essential to orderly human social intercourse and role behavior and center on wellness, work, individual independence, social justice, and social responsibility. Since these determinants tend to cluster together around social functions, they become social institutions in which the individual has a social role. The most important of these social institutions are the family, education, work, religion, and leisure. Throughout his life-stages the individual plays a series of roles set out for him by society. The American ideal of the well-rounded personality, or the development of "ego differentiation," is likely to result in role flexibility and need satisfaction.

Immobility changes role activities through decreased physical activity, decreased occupational activity, and decreased sensory and motor interaction for social responsibility and cultural participation. At the same time there is increased leisure time for the recreational role, but diminished physical ability and energy to expend in recreation. The roles of spouse, parent, sexual partner, employee, club member, and leader may be altered, reversed, or eliminated.

The American culture also encourages mobility to a higher social class via such achievements as greater monetary affluence, increased education, or professional stature. Immobility with its consequent psychologic and sociocultural deprivation often forces downward social mobility. In a society which stresses youth, physique, and energy expenditure, the person disabled because of immobility has diminished personal worth. In a society which places prime value on the worker role, the non-worker role is generally to be interpreted as a movement to a lesser position, with consequent lowering of status in the societal hierarchy.

Our culture, which increasingly includes leisure in its life but which is still work-minded and rurally oriented, has not yet developed an attitude toward leisure as end time, capable of its own interest values. In leisure the world comes to the individual, in work the individual goes to the world. How much stress is created by these moves? And to what extent or under what circumstances do they involve a cumulative tendency to deviance?

NURSING MEASURES

Since the physiologic and psychosocial effects of immobility on the ego identity of man as an individual and as a social being are interrelated and interdependent, the professional nurse, with a philosophy of promoting mobility through her nursing, helps patients move from the dependency role of immobility to maximum mobility.

In the illness setting, the patient may be separated from his family and the ordinary sensory stimuli of his familiar environment. He may be fearful of the unknown as he learns the new role of being immobilized. His body image may be torn asunder. His orientation to the passage and content of time may be distorted. His sociocultural and economic status may be altered.

The nurse, cognizant of the ill person's individual needs and resources, can facilitate the patient's adjustment to his illness environment and sick role by a careful nursing assessment and plan of action with ongoing evaluation. Placement of a clock and calendar in his room, as well as frequent reminders about reality, will help him maintain his orientation. Planning and participation in his own care will promote physical and psychological mobility toward independence. Extending the patient's environment beyond his room will provide him with the opportunity to experience more sensory stimulation, to be physically (at least spatially) mobile, and to reconstruct his body image, his ego identity, and his social roles. A compassionate approach by the nurse that promotes independence rather than dependence will stimulate physiologic and psychologic mobility.

REFERENCES

1. Taylor, H. L., and others. Effects of bedrest on cardiovascular function and work performance. *J. Appl. Psychol.*, **2**:223-239, November 1949.
2. Birkhead, N. C., and others. Circulatory and metabolic effects of prolonged bedrest in healthy subjects (abstract). *Fed. Proc.*, **22**:520, March-April 1963.
3. Browse, N. L. *Physiology and Pathology of Bedrest.* Springfield, Ill., Charles C Thomas, Publisher, 1965.
4. Coe, S. W. Cardiac work and the chair treatment of acute coronary thrombosis. *Ann. Intern. Med.*, **40**:42-47, January 1954.
5. Chapman, C. B., and others. Behavior of stroke volume at rest and during exercise in human beings. *J. Clin. Invest.*, **39**:1208-1213, August 1960.
6. Sevitt, Simon, and Gallagher, Niall. Venous thrombosis and pulmonary embolism. *Brit. J. Surg.*, **48**:475-489, March 1961.
7. Dietrick, J. E., and others. Effects of immobilization upon various metabolic and physiologic functions of normal men. *Amer. J. Med.*, **4**:3-32, January 1948.
8. Beland, Irene L. *Clinical Nursing; Pathophysiological and Psychosocial Approaches.* New York, Macmillan Co., 1965.
9. Leithauser, D. J. *Early Ambulation and Related Procedures in Surgical Management.* Springfield, Ill., Charles C Thomas, Publisher, 1946.
10. Bockus, H. L., and others. *Gastroenterology,* 2d ed., vol. II. Philadelphia, Pa., W. B. Saunders Co., 1964.
11. Asher, Richard A. J. Dangers of going to bed. *Brit. Med. J.*, **2**:967-968, Dec. 13, 1947.

Part Three

Rehabilitation Nursing Care in Non-Life-threatening Conditions

Section A

Neurological Deficits

This section on rehabilitative care of the patient with neurological deficit focuses on the problem of the stroke patient in particular. This is not to deny that other brain-damaged patients have problems, but the nursing problems with loss of function from brain damage have many commonalities, and the stroke patient is used as an example. One contrast does occur. The stroke patient is usually from the older age group, while brain damage occurs from birth to death. It is estimated that 50 percent of car accidents are accompanied by head injury. Motivation may be a function of age, with the older age group having a tendency to feel a greater degree of hopelessness.

No one part of an individual can be affected without affecting the whole. It is never possible, moreover, to consider the pathology apart from the context of the person and his life situation. Loss of function will be widespread—extending into remote parts and activities of the body and personality. Man as a whole is affected, never only a part of man. To carry this one step further, one might suggest that the family and community to which man belongs are also affected.

As one example of the totality, perceptual disturbances are found. Studies of hemiplegic adults who have suffered strokes reveal that half showed signs of perceptual difficulty which was not related to the location or extent of brain damage. It may correlate in disturbances and fluctuations in consciousness and life rhythms such as sleep, eating, and toilet habits. Those with perceptual difficulties tend to be less motivated than other patients. Since the perceptual problem can be located within the sensing-integrating-motor system, it is easier to understand the picture of great emotional distress which is frequently presented.

Diller believes that the distress presents a problem which could be termed an identity crisis. The patient should be challenged by the idea that he is more than a lost leg; ability must be stressed over disability. "I know you feel bad because you can't use your hand or talk, but who are you as a person—a hand, an arm, a voice, a leg?"[1]

Application of the newer theories of perceptual problems can be made by the nurse who assists the patient with brain damage. Spatial disturbances have been noted. Seated in a dark room, hemiplegics had a problem determining the shift of a luminous line in space, particularly from horizontal to vertical. In a lighted room there was no difficulty. Implications are that patients must be taught in a well-lighted room, since the orientation to vertical and horizontal are essential to ambulation. This may involve the nature of the sensory deficit in hemiplegia, the effect of one sensory deficit on another and the interaction of sensory and motor factors. Right-handed persons with damage on the left or dominant hemisphere tend to show verbal deficits, while patients with right hemisphere damage tend to show visumotor deficits. Where this is true, the patient with a left-sided hemiplegia should receive more help from verbal assistance, while the patient with right-sided hemiplegia would receive most help from demonstration. Transferring from a bed to a wheelchair, which is a simple motor act, is accomplished much more easily by the right hemiplegiac than the left. Learning tends to be related to the extent of the deficit in visumotor or verbal skills. Analysis of task demands must be related to the pattern of skills.

Rehabilitation of any patient with neurological deficit starts with the first day of illness. Prevention of disability is the nurse's responsibility during the acute phase. The simple measures of positioning, turning, relieving pressure, range of motion, and the careful handling of extremities to prevent contractures or trauma are important. The physiological measures of adequate fluid intake, nutrition, and elimination fall into the realm of nursing responsibility. The simple undramatic nursing measures which take place

[1] Diller, Leonard, "Some Insights into the Psychological Problem," *Journal of Rehabilitation*, November-December 1963.

during the acute illness may save the patient hours or days of rehabilitation later. Decubitus and contractures may prevent early restorative measures.

Schultz has given a blueprint for the nursing care of the patient with stroke, but it is applicable to any patient with neurological deficits or to long-term patients. Not usually listed among the physical measures is a section on prevention of intellectual regression. The fact that an aphasic individual still recognizes inflections of the voice and looks of displeasure may be forgotten when verbal communication becomes difficult.

An article by Hodgins, who suffered a stroke and speech impairment, expresses just what having a stroke means to the patient, and he begs "Listen! Listen to the patient." He reminds us that no doctor whose propioceptive sense has been knocked out on one side is still in active practice. Therefore he finds it amazing that physicians can understand a condition that the patient cannot even describe. However, Hodgins's description helps to give some insight into the condition which probably can be generalized into all neurological disabilities.

Steele has given case studies of three children with meningomyelocele. From the three it is possible to generalize. One of the grave problems is that of urinary incontinence. A person is socially acceptable only if his bowels and bladder are under voluntary control. This problem alone demands nursing perseverance, especially in reaching these children early. Few if any children born with meningomyelocele have escaped constant and early medical surveillance. This early contact must be utilized in bringing these problems under control.

Buck, who suffered both a stroke and aphasia, and is now a speech pathologist, speaks with the authority of a specialist in the field of speech. He has much to tell nurses who care for the brain-damaged person. As in Hodgins's article, the insights gained through hearing the story from the patient himself furnish a new dimension in planning nursing care. It is a story that is especially well told since the two men are able to picture their interaction with others so vividly. Buck reminds us that the patient is not unconscious and that he has a long memory. He pinpoints areas which can be used to encourage the aphasia patient, and he highlights those interactions which lead to withdrawal and apathy. The experience with homonymous hemianopsia leads to recommendations which may save the personality of the patient from total disintegration. In his experience, Buck seems to sum up the writers in all the preceding articles and place their ideas in a more meaningful mold.

The last article by Wolanin was prepared especially for this volume. The conceptual taxonomy suggested by the author and the final note of realism provide a valuable orientation.

Reading 22
Nursing Care of the Patient with a Stroke
Lucie C. M. Schultz

PROLOGUE

The catastrophic impact of cerebrovascular accident on the patient and his family presents tremendous physiological, psychological, and sociological problems. Once the diagnosis has been made, the multiplicity of these problems necessitates immediate, intelligent nursing intervention if complications are to be kept at a minimum.

The nursing needs of the patient with a stroke vary according to the severity of the trauma. The many life-saving drugs and treatments that may be utilized must be prescribed by the physician, and thus are dependent functions of the nurse. Even though the physician orders these drugs and treatments, the nurse is responsible for knowing about the drugs, the proper dosage, and possible side effects, also how to perform competently the various treatments that the physician may prescribe.

PREVENTIVE NURSING MEASURES

Immediately upon admission of the patient with a stroke, nursing measures should be instituted to prevent contractures, pressure sores, and intellectual regression resulting from sensory deprivation. It is axiomatic that the nurse should be a thinking individual, knowledgeable in her special field, and have the ability to assess the needs of the patient and to plan the nursing care to meet them. Consequently, the nurse needs intellectually and emotionally to accept the fact that merely passive functioning is not sufficient. In addition to carrying out the orders of the physician, she must be capable of utilizing initiative and judgment in making a nursing diagnosis, in planning and implementing the patient's care, and in evaluating and modifying the plan of care as the patient's needs change. Competent nursing of the patient with a stroke makes it mandatory that the nurse be fully informed regarding the cause of the stroke and complications which must be considered in planning the nursing care. It is equally important that the nurse communicate her plan of care to the physician and other members of the health team. All nursing personnel, professional and auxiliary, must fully understand the projected plan and why it is necessary that the specific measures be implemented throughout the 24 hours of each day. Although institution of special

Selected paper from The Clinical Nursing Conference, Nov. 14–15, 1969, Council on Cardiovascular Nursing, American Heart Association, Dallas, Texas.

post-traumatic preventive measures is often referred to as rehabilitation nursing, it is obvious that such procedures also constitute good, comprehensive nursing *per se*. Unless appropriate preventive measures are initiated at the onset of the trauma, the patient with a stroke may suffer severe and irreversible complications. If complications are not ameliorated, the patient's return to society may be permanently impeded. In some cases, unfortunately, ineffective or incomplete nursing care may cause the patient to become totally dependent on others for his care [4].

Too frequently, the patient with a stroke is left merely to lie in bed. This do-nothing nursing approach allows development of pressure sores and contractures, loss of self-respect and dignity, intellectual deterioration, and unrelieved incontinence of bowel and bladder. This need not occur if the nursing personnel concentrate their activities on the patient's abilities rather than his disabilities. Preventive measures must be directed toward the paralyzed muscles as well as the non-affected muscles to prevent atrophy in the uninvolved areas. It should be remembered that the danger of "what the patient does not use he will lose" is a constant risk [4].

BASIC PRINCIPLES OF POSITIONING

The typical position assumed by the patient with a stroke tends to be one in which the affected arm is held close to his body with the elbow and wrist in a flexed position and the fingers and thumb flexed to form a claw-like hand. The affected lower extremity is rotated outwardly at the hip, the knee is flexed, and the foot is in the plantar flexion. Many complications can occur if the patient is permitted to remain in this position. Therefore, it is imperative that nursing efforts be directed toward maintaining the patient in correct body alignment through positioning and frequent change of position [4].

To minimize contractures, development of pressure sores, and respiratory embarrassment, and to provide safety, comfort, and relaxation for the patient, the following basic principles should be utilized:

1 Provide a firm bed to assist in maintaining the patient in correct body alignment;
2 Stabilize the bed to insure safety;
3 Use a footboard that provides a 4 inch space between the mattress and the board;
4 Control the use of the back and knee rest on the Gatch bed to minimize flexion contractures;
5 Minimize development of pressure areas by changing the patient's position every two hours or more frequently, if needed;
6 Check and massage the bony prominences each time the patient's position is changed;

7 Use side-lying and prone position, if the patient can tolerate prone, and avoid using the supine position while the patient is unconscious;
8 Turn the patient toward, rather than away from the nurse; and
9 Use the side-lying prone and the supine positions to assist in drainage of secretions from the lungs [4].

When placing the patient in a side-lying position, the following techniques should be utilized:

1 Use a small pillow under the head to prevent lateral flexion of the neck;
2 Pull the buttocks back and the shoulders slightly forward to keep the spine straight;
3 Use two pillows or more, if needed, under the uppermost leg to keep this leg in a neutral position to prevent adduction or abduction of the hip joint;
4 Support the affected foot to prevent plantar flexion by using pillows or boxes containing sand bags between the foot and footboard; and
5 Change the position of the upper arm frequently to insure comfort and relaxation. The arm is supported on a pillow placed in front of the abdomen, or placed at the patient's back. Alternate using the hand roll and having the fingers extended. Keep the wrist in an extended or hyperextended position to prevent flexion of the wrist [4].

The hand is especially vulnerable to deformity. If the hand tends to deform despite all that can be done, then it is better to allow deformity to develop with the hand in a functional position. The claw-like hand is useless and extremely hard to keep clean. The hand roll can be used to maintain the hand in a functional position. Another device is a partially rolled bath towel, with the patient's thumb tucked under the roll in opposition to the forefinger, and the tail of the towel tightly pinned at the wrist [1].

When the patient has regained consciousness, the supine position can be utilized. Individual needs are determined by the nurse, and the patient is positioned accordingly, keeping the following points in mind:

1 Use a small pillow under the head just to the shoulders, to prevent flexion of the neck and rounding of the shoulders, thus insuring efficient respiration;
2 Keep the forearm elevated at least one hour of the 2 hour period to minimize the development of edema in the affected hand;
3 Alternate positions of the arm so that the elbow is flexed and extended at intervals during the 2 hour period;
4 Use a hand roll to maintain the hand in a functional position, with the thumb in opposition to the forefinger. Alternate this position by extending the fingers and thumb to minimize flexion contracture;

5 Keep the hips flat on the bed;
6 Minimize outward rotation of the affected hip by using a trochanter roll from the waist to the knee;
7 Use a small roll under the knees to provide 5-10 degree flexion to prevent genu recurvatum, or back knee deformity;
8 Keep the affected foot flat against the footboard at a 90 degree angle to the leg to prevent plantar flexion and encourage movement of the non-affected leg. The covers are placed over the footboard to keep the pressure of the bedclothes off the feet, as weight of the bedclothes tends to push the feet into plantar flexion; and
9 Keep the heel of the affected foot off the mattress by letting it hang free between the footboard and mattress to prevent pressure areas. If there is no space between the footboard and mattress, then a small roll should be used under the ankle [4].

The prone position is an excellent one because it provides for full extension of hips; places the shoulders in full external rotation; and aids in moving secretions from the lungs. The following are a few precautions that should be observed:

1 Move patient down in bed to permit toes to hang free of the mattress;
2 Support shoulders with small pads or pillow under chest;
3 Place roll under ankles to provide slight flexion of knees to minimize danger of back knee deformity; and
4 Alternate position of lower extremities by using pillow.

RANGE-OF-MOTION EXERCISES

Immediately upon admission, unless contraindicated, the nurse should initiate range-of-motion exercises to maintain joint motion in the affected extremities. If the patient is unconscious, these activities should be done for all extremities. These procedures can be carried out while the patient is being bathed. Once the patient has regained consciousness, the nurse should continue to put the paralyzed extremities through range-of-motion exercises and encourage the patient to move the non-affected extremities through the same range. In addition, have the patient do things for himself, i.e., reaching for things and assisting in moving about in bed [4].

The patient, the family, and all nursing personnel must understand why range-of-motion exercises are used. The purposes are to increase circulation, maintain joint motion, and to minimize contractures [4].

There are other exercises that the nurse can teach the patient to do which will prepare him for transfer and ambulation. These include biceps and triceps setting exercises, gluteal setting exercises, abdominal retraction exercises, straight leg raising, and gastrocnemius setting exercises [4].

PREVENTION OF INTELLECTUAL REGRESSION

External stimulation or sensory input from the environment is essential to prevent intellectual regression. Some of the factors contributing to sensory deprivation include:

1 *The room arrangement:* The room may be far removed from the nurses' station and the bed so placed that the patient, due to field cut in vision, can only see the ceiling or the one wall.

2 *Attitude of personnel:* Tend to speak to the patient in the third person; assume that if the patient is aphasic and cannot speak he also does not comprehend; no effort is made to communicate with the patient. The nurse must remember that, even though the patient cannot comprehend verbal communication, there is a great deal of non-verbal communication he can recognize and understand.

3 *The patient is left in bed too long:* As soon as the patient's condition is stabilized, he should be placed in a sitting position at least to eat meals.

If the intellectual deterioration occurs, the patient becomes depressed and increasingly dependent. The presence of depression and dependency is manifested by apathy, resentment, and loss of appetite. The patient can become so hostile that urinary incontinence persists or develops. Should this process continue long enough, physical deterioration occurs, e.g., the infrequent turning on the part of the patient plus incontinence leads to the development of pressure sores; or, the passive, depressed, apathetic patient leads to muscular atrophy and contractures. The contractures cause the joints to be painful, which increases the spasticity. The presence of spasticity increases the development of contractures; thus, a vicious cycle occurs.

"Just as a child cannot learn to crawl, walk, or talk without relating to his environment, the patient with a stroke cannot hope to regain speech, judgment, or orientation and motor skills without interacting with his environment" [2].

SUPPORTIVE MEASURES

The nurse coordinates the activities of the nursing team and supplements the activities of the members of other disciplines; therefore, the nurse must understand the functions of each discipline. She actively participates as a member of the health team which includes the patient, and she knows the long- and short-term goals that have been set for the patient. What good does it do for the patient to go to physical therapy once or twice a day if he is not positioned correctly when he returns to the unit? Every opportunity for range-of-motion activity, such as letting the patient carry out his self-care measures, should be utilized. What good does it do for the patient to go to occupational therapy and make a wallet for finger dexterity if the nurses do not encourage the patient to use his hands and arms while on the nursing unit?

Endeavoring to develop a comfortable relationship with the patient and family provides a unique opportunity and responsibility for the nurse to educate them. She should recognize that there may be emotional problems; that the patient has suffered brain damage to a certain extent; and that he may demonstrate various reactions, such as fear, anxiety, anger, loss of inhibitions and susceptibility to over-stimulation. Therefore, she must be aware of these potential difficulties and anticipate them. The nurse should provide an environment wherein the patient and family feel free to express their feelings and concerns without being reproached. Reproving the patient should be avoided, as reproof may precipitate guilt feelings between the patient and his family. The nurse must first analyze her own reactions to the patient with a stroke, for self-understanding enables her to better understand and accept the behavior of the patient. The nurse must realize that sometimes the goals of the patient and his family may be unrealistic. The patient's goal may be to sit for the rest of his life in a wheelchair. If he is capable of doing more than this, then the nurse must find ways to stimulate him so that he is motivated to try to achieve more [4].

RESTORATIVE NURSING MEASURES

Frequently, when the patient with a stroke is brought into the hospital, he finds himself in a completely dependent state, and this adds further insult to his body image. The nursing personnel are with the patient 24 hours a day; thus, they must be alert to clues that will indicate when restorative measures can be utilized to assist the patient.

The nurse, by her facial expression, tone of voice, and approach to the patient, can convey to him that, although he is incontinent and dependent in many of his self-care activities, she still considers him as an individual who expects to be regarded with dignity and respect.

SELF-CARE ACTIVITIES

Self-care activities can be used to strengthen muscles and minimize complications. Handing the patient a wash cloth to wash his face and hands and encouraging him to feed himself, brush his teeth, and comb his hair can do much toward helping him to regain his self-respect and dignity. Teaching the patient how to move about in bed enables him to assist in changing his position, makes it possible for him to reach items on his bedside table, and facilitates ease in giving nursing care. The patient must be taught sitting balance if he is again to dress himself, transfer from bed to wheelchair, use the commode, and take a bath in the tub.

The hemiplegic patient with aphasia presents many challenging problems and particularly if a speech therapist is not available. In order to communicate with the aphasic patient, the nurse needs to know if he understands what is being said to him. The nurse should be alert for clues that will indicate whether the patient (1) responds to his surroundings and the hospital routine, (2) follows commands, (3) gestures, (4) expresses interest in newspaper, get-well cards, or magazines, (5) watches TV, (6) tries to write, and (7) tries to vocalize. The nurse should also determine if his "yes" and "no" responses are reliable. This can be done by placing five or six objects in front of the patient and asking him to point or pick up the specific objects named. Validation of what the nurse has observed can be obtained through sharing these observations with the members of the nursing team and other disciplines to determine if they have made the same observations.

With this kind of information, a communication plan can be developed so that all persons coming in contact with the patient use the same symbols. *Please* do not shout at the patient with aphasia.

Bowel and bladder retraining should be started even if the patient is unconscious. The nurse must first assess the patient's needs, then plan and implement a program to fulfill them. In order for a program to be successful, the nurse must institute the usual bowel and bladder retraining program which includes the following:

1. Determine prior bowel and bladder habits;
2. Develop a program of offering the bedpan at regular intervals;
3. Discuss the plan with the patient, family, and members of the nursing team;
4. Develop a schedule for forcing fluids;
5. Determine if the patient has a fecal impaction;
6. Maintain an accurate record of the intake and output;
7. Keep the patient dry;
8. Encourage activity;
9. Insure privacy; and
10. Consult with the dietitian.

After the first 24 hours, the nursing team should carefully study the patient's intake and output record to determine what his pattern for voiding and bowel elimination has been. After this careful evaluation, modifications in the plan should be made to meet the indicated needs.

As soon as possible, the patient should be placed in a sitting position, either in bed, on the side of the bed, or on the bedside commode, as this is the natural position of elimination. The use of harsh laxatives or enemas should be avoided, as they tend to destroy the natural tone of the colon [4].

EARLY STANDING AND TRANSFER ACTIVITIES

In many instances a physical therapist is not available, and thus the nurse must assume the responsibility of standing the patient and teaching him how to transfer from the bed to the wheelchair. In these circumstances, the nurse must recognize when the patient is ready for these activities and must assume the responsibility of conferring with the physician and obtaining written orders for these procedures [4].

Early standing is an important measure utilized to minimize the deteriorating effects of immobilization. Research indicates that weight bearing or stress on the long bones plays a role in decreasing the rate of demineralization which results from inactivity [3]. In addition, the standing position increases circulation and respiration, aids in emptying the bladder, and assists in minimizing contractures, particularly hip joint flexion. With increased circulation, there is greater exchange of oxygen and carbon dioxide in the lungs, the tissues receive better nourishment, and the digestive process is enhanced. Standing in an upright position also has a tremendous psychological effect upon the patient. He now feels he can look at the nurse rather than having to look up at her as he did when lying in bed [4].

If the patient has been in bed for a long period of time, precautions should be taken to prevent orthostatic hypotension. I will not elaborate on these precautions, because they are good nursing techniques all of you know. Some of the techniques that can be utilized in standing the patient are to place two chairs beside the bed, secure the affected hand to one chair with an elastic bandage, and place the strong hand on the other chair. Another method is to place the wheelchair facing the foot of the bed, lock the chair, and instruct the patient to pull himself up to a standing position. If the affected arm is frail, a sling may be helpful in minimizing subluxation of the shoulder while the patient is standing. The sling should be removed when the patient sits down or goes back to bed.

The following are important points that the nurse should keep in mind when transferring the patient from bed to wheelchair:

1   Use a bed that is low enough to permit the patient to place his feet flat on the floor;
2   Stabilize the wheelchair and bed to insure a safe transfer;
3   Minimize the distance between bed and chair by placing the chair facing the foot of the bed at a 45 degree angle;
4   Place the wheelchair on the non-paralyzed side to enable the patient to pivot with his unaffected foot;

5 Use your knee to block the patient's unaffected knee if the strength of the leg is not known. If the unaffected knee does not buckle, then block the affected knee;

6 Use a web or leather belt, or grasp at the waist to assist the patient rather than pulling on his arm or under the axilla;

7 Instruct the patient to "stand tall" and get his balance before pivoting on the strong leg;

8 Teach the patient to bend at the waist with the head forward when sitting down or coming to a standing position;

9 Use a lapboard, while in the wheelchair, to support the arms and permit the patient to do things with his hand(s);

10 Use a 3 inch cushion in the wheelchair and teach the patient the importance of changing his position frequently to minimize pressure on the ischial tuberosities; and [4]

11 Use a sliding board if the patient is unable to do a standing transfer.

CONTINUITY OF CARE THROUGH REFERRAL

Providing assistance after discharge from the hospital or the rehabilitation center aids the patient in maintaining what he has gained through his rehabilitative program. Discharge planning starts the day of admission to the hospital; therefore, the patient and the family are taught from the beginning how to perform all procedures and the reasons for doing them. Active participation by the patient and family usually can be achieved provided they understand why the procedure should be done. The patient and the family are encouraged to discuss and evaluate the home environment. The patient and family make the final decisions regarding modifications of the home; however, the nurse may assist in the plans, if needed. She anticipates the patient's need for further teaching or supervision, and secures permission from the physician and the family to refer the patient to appropriate agencies, such as the Public Health Department or the Visiting Nurse Association. In some institutions, the medical social worker initiates the referral; however, many hospitals do not provide this service. Therefore, it is the nurse's responsibility to provide continuity of care for the patient when he leaves the hospital [4].

As the leader of the nursing team, the nurse initiates preventive, restorative, and supportive measures, and insures continuity of care after discharge for the patient with a stroke. This total-care program minimizes the dangers of deterioration from immobility and helps to return the patient to his community as a contributing and useful member of society. As Dr. Spencer has so aptly stated, rehabilitation is a concept, an attitude, and a process in which preventive, supportive, and restorative measures are utilized to rehabilitate the patient with a stroke [4].

REFERENCES

1 A Handbook of Rehabilitative Nursing Techniques in Hemiplegia. Kenny Rehabilitation, Minneapolis, 1964.
2 Schoening, Herbert A., and Kottke, Frederic J., "Rehabilitation of the Patient with Hemiplegia," *Current Therapy,* Philadelphia: W. B. Saunders, 1966, p. 561.
3 Abramson, A. S., and Delagi, E. F., "Influence of Weight-Bearing and Muscle Contraction on Disuse Osteoporosis," *Archives of Physical Medicine and Rehabilitation,* **46**:147-151, March 1965.
4 Schultz, Lucie C. M. "The Nursing Care of the Patient with a Stroke," *The Alabama Journal of Medical Sciences,* vol. 5, pp. 27-33, January 1968.

Reading 23
Listen: The Patient
Eric Hodgins

...These are procedures and conventions for the convenience and protection of doctors; their effect and perhaps their intent is to diminish the patient. Doubtless, many patients must be diminished to be made manageable or even tolerable, but diminishing the stroke patient is risky business, for he has already been diminished by act of God, and in addition to his neurologic symptoms, he is full of fear—raw, elemental fear—not necessarily of death but of incapacity or destitution. From whom is he going to draw the courage without which he will not truly recover? Not from a silent practitioner, whether doctor, therapist or nurse, who is aloof. He will draw courage as he perceives human understanding underlying the professional technics of those into whose care he has been given. . . .

. . . I think the stroke patient (I limit myself to him because that is my topic) is entitled to the same understanding compassion as the person who has survived a hard airplane crash. I think he is less likely to get it. The drama of his plight is mostly internal: little meets the eye—no gross injury, no compound fracture, no massive blood loss. But both patients are shocked. Into the bargain, the stroke patient is also deeply enigmatic: in the beginning there is much doubt about what he is going to "do." If he is not going to die he will soon get a lot of examination and neurologic testing. Indeed, it is possible that everyone is going to look so hard at his eyegrounds, watch his reflexes so carefully, and test his gnostic sensibilities so often that he

Reprinted from *The New England Journal of Medicine,* vol. 274, no. 12, pp. 657-661, March 24, 1966. The article is based upon remarks presented at the Maricopa County Medical Society Health Forum, Phoenix, Ariz., Oct. 19, 1965.

himself—the person, the personality, the individual—may become neglected.

Yet there he remains, existing and pleading. The communication difficulties between him and those who want to help him may be considerable. If he is conscious but aphasic the difficulties become tremendous, and much more frustrating to everybody than if he were in a coma. Even if he is not aphasic but has lost his proprioceptive sense on the affected side, he will be at a loss for words with which to describe this. (I have been trying for five and a half years and have not yet come up with anything that satisfied even myself.) Plenty of physicians in practice have broken a bone, come down with a hot appendix, passed a kidney stone, endured a hangover or experienced anginal pain, but the physician whose proprioceptive sense has been knocked out on one side is probably not still in active medical practice. Thus, I think it amazing that doctors can understand a condition that no patient can adequately describe—that is painless but quite disturbing, and into which they themselves cannot enter. It is not surprising, however, that with the best of intentions the doctor-to-patient quotient of understanding, when the patient has had a stroke, is considerably less than 100 per cent—or that the doctor who has just given a remarkable demonstration of his hard-bought second-hand knowledge will then make a remark or issue an order showing that he has instantaneously forgotten it. The patient, however, does not forget. The occupational therapist is much less likely to forget, for this is one of the specific areas of her training; she lives with this sort of thing every day. Not every doctor does. . . .

. . .In stroke there are two basic sets of assumptions which could govern treatment. One set proceeds from what the patient perceives, or thinks he perceives; the other comes from what the doctor knows, or thinks he knows. These are two very different sets of things. Before the doctors among you tell me that this is so with every illness, let me say only that there is something in what the patient says, no matter what it is, so "Listen! Listen to the patient!" A rigid doctor intensifies a rigid patient. And almost everyone who has been in a hospital has seen examples—perhaps not in his own case—where the relations between patient and health personnel have become adversary proceedings. . . .

. . . Meanwhile, I have my own private doubts about the degree to which some physicians, those not themselves engaged in physical medicine and rehabilitation, are aware of the subtleties that separate functioning from nonfunctioning. For example, I go for an annual physical checkup to the medical department of the corporation that used to employ me, and the doctor, having banged a few of my tendons with his hammer, says, "That left side seems pretty good. Squeeze my two fingers as hard as you can with your left hand."

Over the recent years this has come to be an invitation I accept with constantly mounting enthusiasm; I can squeeze quite hard with my "weak" left hand. So I mash his fingers good and proper, whereupon he returns good for evil by saying, "Fine. You can use your typewriter again?" When I say, "No," he looks puzzled as well as hurt. But my ability to crush his fingers in my left fist has nothing to do with my ability to type, which has vanished. Many subtle things are involved here, which the squeeze-and-ouch test tells no one anything about. Let me list a few:

The loss of proprioceptive sense on the left side means that the eye must watch, and help control, what the left hand is doing; it has no time to watch anything else. That upsets one applecart.

Loss of normal tactile sensation in the left hand's finger robs the hand of its knowledge of accomplishment. There goes another applecart.

Although the hand has good power and almost complete freedom of motion, the small muscles of its fingers are disobedient; thus, it cannot perform skilled acts (applecart no. 3).

These are the primary applecarts. There are secondaries. For example, when the left hand stumbles the right hand becomes confused—much as one actor can become confused when another actor forgets his lines, although the first actor knows his part without flaw.

A residual of a cerebrovascular accident occurring in the brain's "dominant" hemisphere (with me the right, since I was born a southpaw) is a certain amount of speech and spelling difficulty. My spelling troubles mysteriously involve the letters *r* and *n,* and words with doubled letters, more than any others. When such words flash across the mind screen, a fuse is likely to blow somewhere in the motor circuits. The mind involved in writing something must then abandon its thought processes (if that's what they were) and give up its selection systems for clothing thoughts in words. Now you must open the syntax switch, unplug the grammar jacks and go fussing around with a flashlight to find out what went wrong in the brain-to-fingertips diagram.

I am using figurative language here because I don't know enough to use the literal. A process like using the typewriter takes place at a sort of fluid gallop. When the fluid flow is disturbed or when something breaks the rhythm of the gallop *everything* goes to pieces. A moment ago things were clear, or reasonably so. Now they are confused. And in confusion I will leave this very deep subject, saying only that an equation between the muscular ability to squeeze and the psychoneuromuscular ability to get a set of words down on paper by pecking at keys with symbols on them simply doesn't exist, even if the words convey no thought deeper than "Now is the time for all good men to come to the aid of the party."

Yet, all in all, the possibilities that today lie in rehabilitation are tremendous: in the prevention of deformity; in improving range of motion; and in coming to hard grips with the activities of daily living. I know that some stroke patients cannot be rehabilitated. But on the other hand, some can be when to the outward eye very little seems left to rehabilitate. When you have rehabilitated a wage-earner you have helped save a family. When you have rehabilitated a housewife you have helped save a family. And when you have saved a family you have helped protect your community, wherever it is.

For *all* illness is communicable; not just the infectious or contagious diseases that are "reportable" to boards of health. All illness is communicable; today we stand only on the verge of recognizing this, and laymen must help the health professions in spreading these tidings. . . .

. . . There always arises, for the recovering stroke patient, the business of the tremendous trifle. I should have used a cane as soon as I was up and about again after my own stroke. I didn't have the brains to. Nor did any doctor ever advise it. (I had no foot drop, but I was tottery.) So I had to fall and crack my hip, thus bringing me into immediate contact with an orthopedic surgeon. After the accident *he* told me to use a cane, and the crack in my greater trochanter has thus been my individual contribution toward the multidisciplinary approach to stroke.

But there are even lesser things. When one hand is adrift and disobedient to your will, and its palm is insensate, making change and handling coins becomes a difficult act. This detail is too small for a physician's attention. But, in our capitalist society, one must go on making change or perish. And where is one most likely to be called on to make change in a hurry? In a taxicab, of course, where even the act of breathing has now been rendered uncomfortable by the implacable designers in Detroit. It was a devoted nurse who solved this change-making problem for me: "Every night before you go to bed empty out your pockets and put all the pennies into that beer mug." She gestured toward a sentimental stein that has never held an ounce of brew. "Then," she explained, "you'll have fewer coins in your pocket and no confusion next day between dimes and pennies." Yes, of course I could have thought of that myself; so could a lot of other people. The point is, they didn't.

I did as I was told—I'm the ideal patient, really—and lo and behold another problem was reduced to manageable size. Moreover, there was a payoff. In my life, and in the present Great Society, the beer mug accumulates $5 worth of pennies every three months. My daughter takes these to the bank, at regular intervals, to relieve the coin shortage—and, of course, keeps the change. Everyone profits, just as Adam Smith said they would.

But there are some things a hemiparetic must learn for himself. Why do I never, in the privacy of my own apartment, go about barefoot or in my stockinged feet? Is it because I am afraid I may step on a tack? No! I have never stepped on a tack in my life, and I am convinced I never shall. The danger comes from above. When your muscular responses are laterally uneven, you are constantly fumbling things and dropping them—particularly things so light and impalpable that you get no neurogenic feedback from their weight on your affected side. Have you ever dropped a light, impalpable letter-opener, point down, on your unprotected big toe? It is a dagger through the heart—all the more so because you get no sensory warning that Brutus is about to lunge. You did not feel the dagger slip; thus, the toe took no evasive action. . . .

Reading 24

Infancy to Adolescence: Habilitation of Children with Meningomyelocele

Shirley Steele

The incidence of meningomyelocele, as well as other handicapping conditions of childhood, is not easy to estimate. Surely a condition as evident as this one is readily identified if the pregnancy continues to term. However, the aborted pregnancies may well be due to such a defect and not be as readily distinguishable. Despite inaccuracies in reporting, the condition has been considered as a "common defect of childhood" and estimated to occur as often as 1 to 3 times in every 1,000 births [Sugar and Ames, p. 362].

In addition, attention has been focused on reports of "epidemics" of spina bifida which occurred in 1962, in two American cities. In each of these areas, Georgia and Vermont, there was an increased incidence in babies born with the condition (Georgia 4.4/1000 and Vermont 2.3/1000) [Ingalls and Klingberg, p. 68]. Investigators are interested in such statistics, as they may eventually lead to information regarding causation. To date, the anomaly seems to be more prevalent in the lower socioeconomic groups, and the incidence is higher in second siblings in the same family, 8 percent [Schulman, p. 855]. As yet, no specific prenatal causes have been found directly related to the development of a meningomyelocele.

There are three classifications of spinal defects which commonly occur together in the literature. They are briefly discussed here to focus attention on the specific condition of meningomyelocele (spina bifida cystica) and how it differs from the other two conditions. *Spina bifida occulta* is the least complicated condition and may easily go undetected. Basically, it is a lack of fusion of the vertebral arches with or without changes in the skin surface, neurological signs, or any pathological changes. Frequently, the only external sign is a "dimple" over the defect. *Meningocele* has the same unfused condition of the vertebral arches, but it also has cystic distention of the meninges without myelodysplasia of the spinal cord; neurological signs are absent. If parts of the cord or nerve roots are in the sac of meninges, they still manage to conduct impulses normally. Meningomyelocele (myelomeningocele) is the most severe form; it has the unfused arches and the cystic distention of the meninges and is associated with myelodysplasia of the spinal cord and neurological symptoms [Smith, p. 5]. Obviously, meningomyelocele will be the most handicapping of the three states, so choosing it as my focus will also provide for transfer of ideas to the lesser-involved types [see Figure 24-1].

To fully appreciate the ramifications of this condition let us focus on Figure 24-1 for a few minutes. The nursing assessment using only observation techniques provides this information:

1 A large sac protrudes from the back.
2 The skin covering is lacking over the sac.
3 There is seepage of spinal fluid from the sac.
4 The neck muscles seem strained by the positioning of the head.
5 The positioning of the feet and legs does not seem normal.
6 The infant sucks his fist.
7 The baby does not seem to be having pain, as evidenced by relaxation during sleep.

Nursing intervention can now be planned to meet the needs of this baby. With an open, draining lesion, it is imperative to minimize infection. The location of the meningomyelocele makes it particularly susceptible to contamination from urine and feces. A shield placed below the external lesion will provide this necessary protection if it is changed frequently. Such a shield can be made from a plastic bag or plastic wrap and attached to the healthier skin surface below the lesion using a mild antiallergic adhesive tape. This application will allow the meningomyelocele to be exposed to air and drying. Another method is to use sterile dressings directly over the sac which act as a protection. The dressings will become wet with the spinal fluid and must be changed to prevent infection.

Although there is not consensus of opinion by the medical experts, many centers are now attempting closure of the sac as early as the first day of life. This early surgical intervention is made possible through advances in pediatric anesthesiology, pediatric surgical techniques, and antibiotics, as well as advanced thinking on the part of medical personnel. The increase in survival rate of these children due to control of infection has made medical

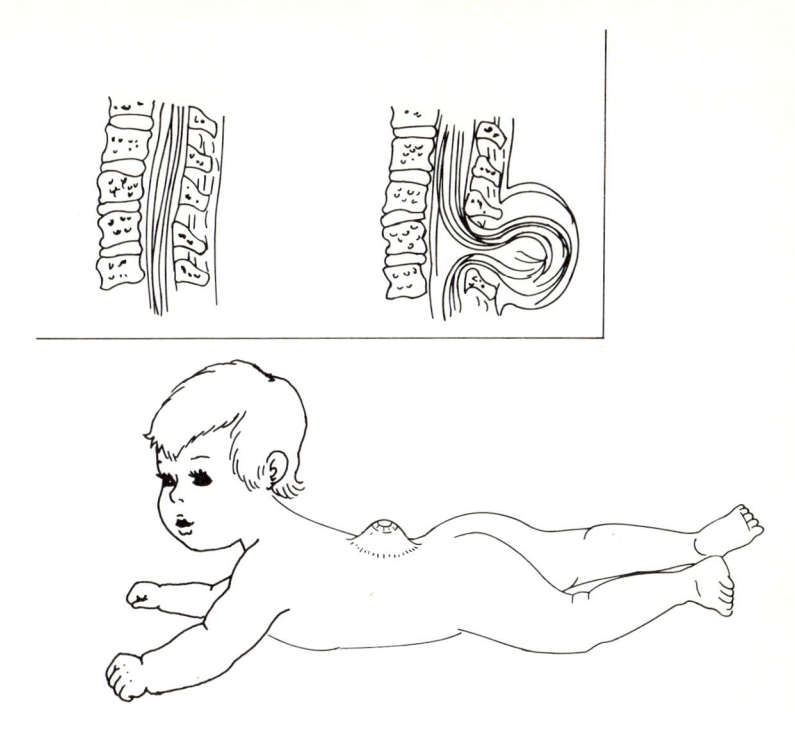

Figure 24-1

personnel more cognizant of the need for making the children as comfortable as possible so they can participate in a habilitation program.

Other nursing intervention in relation to the sac centers on correct positioning of the child. Pressure should be kept off the area, therefore the child will be placed in a prone position. Support may be needed for the sac, depending on its location and size. This support may be provided by the use of rolled receiving blankets or diapers, or the use of padded sand bags. Any restraint or support must be removed frequently to check the baby's circulation to the area. Due to decreased neural functioning the blood supply is also decreased, and the skin condition will not be optimal. Additionally, there may be paralysis present which interferes with frequent ordinary movements of the baby; this may cause complications such as pneumonia if positioning is not changed on a periodic basis.

With the spinal defect, the baby has a decreased capacity to maintain body temperature. This factor usually contributes to the decision to place the child in an isolette for warmth. If this is not done, the baby's lower extremities need protection by wrapping or application of cotton stockings. There is often an accompanying defect to the lower extremities such as a congenital dislocated hip, or clubfeet. If either of these conditions is present, casting may be done, and the casts will provide the additional warmth needed.

Intervention with regard to the strained neck muscles will also take the form of correct positioning. An accompanying hydrocephalus before or after surgical correction of the sac is quite common.[1] The head circumference is measured and recorded at least daily. The fontanelles are observed for fullness. Both these indices will be used by the physician to determine the need for a shunting procedure to control the hydrocephalus. In addition, the nursing observations such as irritability, poor feeding, and inability to sleep will be used in making the decision whether a shunt is indicated. You may ask, "Why irritability?" Irritability is one indication that the infant may have increasing intracranial pressure. This symptom along with increased fullness of the fontanelles or increasing head size is an indication that hydrocephalus is advancing.

The positioning of the feet and legs is most important. Depending on the location of the lesion, they may be completely flaccid due to paralysis, or they may be abnormal due to the conditions described above. Generally, passive exercises are indicated, and a care plan should be designed by the physical therapist. Every attempt should be made to limit contractures or fractures from improper handling or positioning.

The observations regarding sucking and lack of pain relate directly to comfort measures. If at all possible, the baby's arms should be free so he can receive gratification from sucking, and the present positioning should allow enough comfort for the baby to get his much-needed rest. Other positions may be tried, but already one is known that offers comfort.

BLADDER TRAINING

Contingent on the location of the lesion, bladder and bowel incontinence will probably be sources of frustration to the patient and family as well as challenging aspects for the medical personnel responsible for his care. Urinary complications are now known to cause increased concern as children live past the earlier crises. During infancy the flaccid bladder will dribble urine. This will tend toward excoriation of the skin if not given meticulous attention. In addition, the bladder will tend to have residual urine after dribbling. Credé expression of urine is usually begun in infancy. (The physician will give his consent for this technique after a complete urological evaluation, if the bladder is not spastic. In children with meningomyelocele

---

[1] Surgical correction is not used to denote restoration of normal function, as this is seldom possible. I use the term in its broadest sense to denote a surgical procedure done with the intent of providing increased comfort or handling rather than correction.

it frequently is flaccid, and Credé is indicated.) The nurse demonstrates the technique to the parents or guardian who will assume responsibility for the task at home. First the ureters are "milked," using the fingertips, and then pressure is placed over the pubic arch using the palms of the hands to express the urine. With infants care must be taken not to apply undue pressure. If the sac is not repaired, it must also be protected from undue pressure during the procedure.

As the child matures, Credé is adjusted to meet his newly emerging needs. It can be done on the toilet, and the child can be taught to apply the pressure himself. Tudor [1970] describes trigger points which can be stimulated to help in voiding or defecation, such as applying pressure on the vulva, rubbing the internal thigh, stroking the anus, and plunging the hands into water. These techniques are used primarily with children with *spastic* bladders. Additional techniques which can help produce pressure on the lower abdomen are puckering up the cheeks and slowly expelling air through closed lips, blowing up balloons, and blowing on various types of whistle toys (particularly those that offer resistance).

The fluid intake of the child is also important. The child, depending on age, needs enough fluid intake to guarantee adequate urinary excretion. The intake is divided into appropriate quantities and given during the daytime hours and limited after the evening meal. (Note that I have not recommended rigidly stopping fluids at a certain hour, as is sometimes suggested or practiced.) The adequate fluid intake should include the child's favorite fluids as well as emphasizing decreasing calculi formation and limiting infections. Therefore, cranberry juice may be prescribed, or milk limited, but basically the less structured the fluid intake is the better the chance the child will readily accept the needed quantities. A key concept in bladder training is timing of toileting. A consistent plan will help to yield positive results. While some authorities specify a two-hour period, or three-, or four-, depending on the child's age, pattern of wetness, and degree of disability, I prefer to keep this schedule highly individualized. The child's pattern should be planned around the family's schedule and schooling if it is a part of the daily life-style of the child. Many of these children will have braces and use wheelchairs, and therefore toileting is a time-consuming activity. It is not nearly as easy to help the child become self-sufficient in toileting under these conditions. Helpful adjuncts to toileting are rails applied in strategic locations next to the toilet and sink and a box to use as a footstool to support the child's feet and lessen the weight from bracing (see Figure 24-2). Some children find bending forward helps to increase intra-abdominal pressure and aids in voiding. This may be facilitated by using a table in front of the child to protect him as he leans forward.

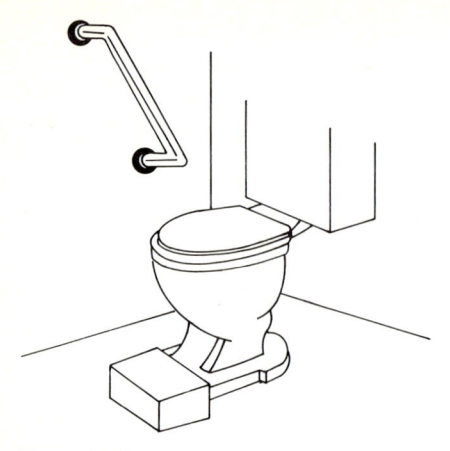

Figure 24-2

Bladder training is not an easy task, and there are many times when success will not be achieved. In these cases, urinary appliances can be used with boys to provide them with dryness, while girls will not be as fortunate and will have to be diapered and wear an incontinence panty. Both of these alternatives demand increased attention to personal hygiene and especially care of the skin which comes in contact with the urine. Cleansing, drying, and use of deodorants are all needed. Special care must be taken for creased areas where skin edges meet. A *light* application of talcum is sometimes helpful during warm weather to decrease irritation. (Emphasis is on light application, as talcum too heavily applied will cake and cause additional irritation.)

During the months or years when the child is being carried on the above routine, a close watch will be kept on his urinary and kidney status. Authorities differ in their opinions regarding diversion techniques, but a general rule of thumb is to do the urinary diversion (ileal conduit) before there is extensive renal damage. The urinary diversion may be done as early as infancy or delayed until symptoms of infection do not adequately respond to medical therapy.

If a diversion is done, additional nursing tasks will include care of the stoma and applicances as well as teaching the parent and child and school personnel about the condition and needs of the child. The teaching will need to include the changes in body image caused by the reconstructive surgery and the implications to the family and child. Let me introduce a specific child to emphasize this point.

Mary was fourteen years old when the physicians decided she was a candidate for a urinary diversion. Mary was an only child and lived with her mother and father in a mobile home. She attended a special school for handicapped children and was an excellent student. Physically she had matured, and menses had begun at 13½. Prior to her menstrual flow, Mary's incontinence somehow did not present any unusual distress. She wore diapering as described above and carried a supply to school. She was able to change her diapering and cleanse herself competently.

Suddenly, with the onset of her menses Mary became very upset about her incontinence, and this roused her parents' anxiety. After much consideration, a urinary diversion was planned for psychological reasons. In the preoperative period it was necessary to introduce the family to the urinary drainage bags which Mary would wear postoperatively. Immediately after the operation a light latex bag was to be applied to the abdomen over the stoma and connected to a urinary drainage tubing and leg bag. This procedure distressed the family, as they did not approve of the visible bag. The necessity for the use of this appliance for an interim period was explained on the basis of (1) the need to limit pressure on the stoma and (2) the gradual change in pressure tolerated by the surrounding skin surface. After the skin had acclimated itself to the lighter appliance, the heavier rubber one which independently collected the urine would be substituted, eliminating the leg bag. In addition, Mary needed help in understanding how her urine would be diverted (illustrations were utilized for this). Despite the fact that she never had achieved continence, she was aware that this procedure would make her very different from her peers. She was introduced to another adolescent who had made a successful adjustment to her ileal conduit, and together they talked over the advantages and disadvantages of the surgical procedure.

One of the major concerns of the parents was the cost of the equipment. The initial output was explained and the decrease in expense over a period of time emphasized. The decrease in expense results because it is no longer necessary to buy diapers and plastic pants. The urinary drainage bags are washed, aired, and reused, and with appropriate care they last long periods of time. Cost varies according to the type of appliance utilized, but it may average as much as $25.00 for the pouch and additional costs for deodorants, belts, cement, etc.

The case of another child with an ileal conduit will be used as an example where helpful intervention was rendered to school personnel. Nancy was ten years old when her family moved from another state. Her mother was a nurse but had not practiced her profession since Nancy's birth. Nancy's father held an executive position, and his advancement necessitated their move. Nancy had a private tutor two days a week in her home, as this was the routine adhered to in her former location. (The possibility of attending public school was rejected on the basis of her physical condition and urinary incontinence.)[2]

Soon after their move Nancy was evaluated, and her renal status was considered serious. Plans were completed and an ileal conduit performed. Nancy responded well and had a quick recovery from surgery. Her parents were delighted with the results and especially pleased that Nancy could now go in swimming.

After a period of time, I approached the idea of seeking to enroll Nancy in school, as she lacked peer associations. Her mother was reluctant, as she remembered her disappointments in their former home state when she made a similar request; but after a few conferences she agreed to contact her local school principal. Following a successful conference with him, she met the teacher whom Nancy would have in class. Despite the teacher's initial hesitation, she agreed to meet Nancy. Nancy won over the teacher, but there was still a degree of concern for assuming total responsibility for her. It was decided that the mother would go to school each day at noon and assist Nancy with emptying and cleaning the bag. I contacted the school nurse, who visited the school only two days per week. It was agreed that she would work with the teacher to offer support and help to ease Nancy's mother of the responsibility to attend school daily. After several weeks this was achieved, and the mother then needed reassurance that she was not neglecting her responsibilities to Nancy. To help fill her free time (which she had very little of since Nancy's birth), she started volunteering service to the local hospital.

BOWEL TRAINING

Bowel training is somewhat easier to accomplish than bladder training. The key factor is to plan a convenient time for the daily routine and try to adhere to it. The child is usually given a glycerin suppository and then placed on the toilet for evacuation. School-age and older children can insert the suppository themselves. The child attempts to retain the suppository for fifteen to twenty minutes before evacuating. This time can be spent doing quiet activities which will help to decrease the chances of early expulsion. After the child is placed on the toilet, he should concentrate solely on moving his bowels, therefore distractions are kept to a minimum. Adjuncts to suppositories, such as stool softeners, fruit juices, food roughage, and pursing the lips to increase intra-abdominal pressure, are sometimes included in the bowel routine.

---

[2] It is realistic to expect that architectural barriers may necessitate rejection from school, but physical handicaps alone should not be cause for rejection.

If the child is hospitalized for any reason, the nurse must find out the child's routine and make every effort to continue it in the hospital. Bowel and bladder training take a long time to establish, and it is unfortunate to disrupt the process unnecessarily during hospitalizations.

LOCOMOTION POTENTIAL

According to the neurological level of the defect of the spinal cord, the child will have differing possibilities for rehabilitation, or, more accurately, habilitation. The following is excerpted from Schulman [p. 858]:

Level T6–T12	Function will vary from being dependent on a wheelchair to gait consisting of a swing to or drag to; elevation limited to low steps.
Level L1–L5	Function varies from wheelchair dependency to a four-point and swing-through gait; elevation using a hand rail.
Level S1–S5	Four-point gait to independent walking and elevation.

The general categories above will give an indication of the child's potential. Other factors which also need to be considered are the accompanying congenital deformities and their state of repair, as well as the general well-being of the child.

I am reminded of a child whose lower extremities are approximately the diameter of a silver dollar. Although she had the potential for ambulation, her small legs would not support the weight of the braces.[3] If she had been fitted for braces, the extremities might easily fracture and her poor circulation was not readily conducive to healing.

When bracing is used, it is imperative to keep the braces in optimal condition and to have them adjusted as the child grows. Improper functioning or fitting of braces will impair the child's ability to reach his maximum potential. The slide locks on the braces should be kept free of dust so they can be moved easily by the child. The braces are attached to shoes which must also be kept in good repair. The child's heel must fit in the shoe properly. Newer shoeing for braces has clear hard plastic heels which allow for checking this fit more accurately and easily. Ill-fitted shoes may cause decubitus to form on the child's feet. Decubitus are difficult to heal, and prevention is vital. To be most effective, bracing must be used consistently, and the parents' cooperation is paramount for this task. The willingness of

---

[3] It is gratifying to know that federal monies are now being utilized to advance bracing designs, as little progress has been made in this area.

parents to commit the time and energy to properly apply bracing cannot be underestimated. To appreciate the time needed to do this one should try doing this task himself. A technique I have found effective in applying long leg braces is to place the child on his side on a firm surface. Move the braces in alignment with the child (the brace is also on its side), and then gently roll the child into the brace. Check to see that the leather waistband is situated correctly; be sure that the legs are in proper alignment and that the feet are correctly positioned in the shoes (the shoes can be detached from the braces and put on first), then buckle all the straps, making them snug but not tight. Check again for constrictions, as the child is unable to feel discomfort. If the child is going to walk, the slide locks are kept locked. If he is going to sit, the locks are opened so that the legs can bend.

Locomotion is also aided by wheelchairs and crutches. Both of these must be properly fitted to the child. A wheelchair should be specifically prescribed for the individual child. Oversized or undersized chairs do not provide comfort and may contribute to deformities acquired in the future. Crutches, too, are fitted directly to the child and must be used properly to prevent paralysis or accidents. Rubber tips and arm cushions must be checked for wear and replaced when indicated. Crutches must be adjusted to provide for increments in growth. (Growth is slower in children with this defect, but this does not excuse professionals from making adequate growth assessments.)

To facilitate ambulation, the child's body, trunk, and upper extremities will have to be kept in maximal condition. This conditioning is provided by the use of games such as table tennis, basketball, catch ball, etc. The games are stimulating and fun as well as effective exercises for appropriate muscle groupings.

In the long process toward locomotion, the child is oftentimes faced with surgical management for correction of orthopedic deformities or procedures for stabilization. Each of these hospitalizations provides the potential for a new crisis situation for the child and his family. Whether to have surgical therapy performed is a difficult decision when the outcomes cannot be guaranteed to result in improvement in function. The parents need time and support to resolve their feelings and proceed with the correct plan of action.

CONCLUSION

From the foregoing discussion, it is evident that the care of the child with meningomyelocele will entail the clinical expertise of specialists in many fields working in close cooperation with the child and his family. I have focused on only a portion of the nurse's role, including some of the most commonly associated problems. Space does not permit an extensive coverage of working with the family, body image, and other possible accompanying handicaps such as mental retardation and hydrocephalus. As with all programs of habilitation or rehabilitation, the focus of care must be on using the child's assets to help him achieve his maximum functioning in the mainstream of society.

REFERENCES

Ingalls, T., and Klingberg, M. Congenital Malformations: Clinical and Community Considerations, in Wolf, J., and Anderson, R. *The Multiply Handicapped Child.* Springfield, Ill., Charles C Thomas, 1969.

Schulman, K. Defects of the Closure of the Neural Plate, in Barnett, H. (ed.) *Pediatrics,* 14th ed. New York, Appleton-Century-Crofts, 1968.

Smith, E. D. *Spina Bifida and the Total Care of Spinal Myelomeningocele.* Springfield, Ill., Charles C Thomas, 1965.

Sugar, M., and Ames, M. "The Child with Spinal Bifida Cystica." *Rehabilitation Literature,* **26**:362-365, December 1965.

Steele, S. Nursing Care of the Child with Congenital Anomalies and Minimal Cerebral Dysfunction, in Steele, S. (ed.) *Nursing Care of the Child with Long-term Illness.* New York, Appleton-Century-Crofts, 1971.

Steele, S. "The Nurse's Role in the Rehabilitation of Children with Meningomyelocele." *Nursing Forum,* **6**:104-117, 1967.

Tudor, L. "Bladder and Bowel Retraining." *American Journal of Nursing,* **70**:2391-2392, November 1970.

Waechter, E. "The Birth of an Exceptional Child." *Nursing Forum,* **9**:202-216, 1970.

Reading 25
Dysphasia: The Patient, His Family, and the Nurse
McKenzie Buck

Cortically traumatized persons are outstandingly dependent on the immediate society in which they must survive, and each individual is an entity unto his family. Unfortunately, this constellation is far too often neglected by all professions, despite the fact that interpersonal family relationships are of vital importance in determining whether the dysphasic patient will remain unchanged or become improved. Thus, our first therapeutic target must be

Reprinted from *Cardio-Vascular Nursing,* vol. 6, no. 5, pp. 51-56, September-October 1970, by permission of the American Heart Association, Inc.

to assist the familial group in detecting the person behind his chaotic screen of overall reductions. There is little we can do to stimulate communicative improvement until relative stability, insight, and appropriate affection are initiated among the members of the familial constellation.

But before going into the effects of the family upon the dysphasic patient, it is important to point out some of the major shortcomings in the hospital environment. These concern bed placement, staff examination discussions, and all too casual consultation with the family. These shortcomings often result from false assumptions about the patient's ability to interpret the language he hears among the staff and family. Much of what follows is based on personal experience as a dysphasic patient myself.

BED PLACEMENT

Awareness of possible disruptions in visual and auditory acuity is essential to emotional security and resultant improvement of communication and maintenance of remaining language. When a patient has a right body paralysis, he may also have a disturbance in the right visual fields of both eyes, or he may be experiencing a collapse of the right eustachian tube, creating a middle ear hearing impairment. On the other hand, some individuals suffer damage to the hearing center in the left hemisphere. Patients with either right or left body paralysis may demonstrate severe startle responses when they suddenly detect persons approaching them on the damaged side. Even slight auditory reductions can stimulate mammoth fear reactions in one who has also little conception of what has happened, who he is, or where he has been. This anxiety is sharply increased among patients placed in the "deaf-blind corners" of the hospital wards. I was one of those unfortunates whose unimpaired left side visual-auditory fields were focused on a blank wall. Personnel rarely squeezed themselves between the bed and the wall to administer medications, meals, or other "disturbances." My wife was the only person to consistently speak to me as she approached to visit on the left side of my bed. Members of the staff contacted me on the left side only when they were after blood samples and pressure measurements.

In an attempt to increase feelings of security, I turned my head to the right, with no resulting security. It seemed as though everyone was compelled to grasp my chin and straighten my head as he passed my bed. Even the patient in the bed to my right was unseen. It was frightening to feel isolated in a room full of patients who, due to blatant circumstances, also ignored my attempts to socialize. Even the most casual language stimulation was absent while I was in that "dead" corner except during the visitations made by my wife.

The preceding complaint is far too common among the patients with whom I've had contact in hospitals, nursing homes, and even in their own homes. Therefore it is highly recommended that the patient's bed be placed so that his paralyzed side and the side of reduced vision face the "blind" corners of the wards. This will facilitate his seeing and hearing others in the environment, help him to retain a need to socialize, and reduce his immediate need for suicide.

The family should also understand the importance of avoiding "blind" corners when they take the patient home, and they should be helped to appraise the furniture placement in their living rooms and bedrooms. They should also understand that the patient is disturbed enough in the most secure environments, and there will be no drive for acceptable language if he is unable to see other persons approaching.

MORNING ROUNDS

Personnel in every profession concerned should be particularly careful to avoid evaluative discussions in the presence of these patients. We must remember that they already have more than they can tolerate without also hearing morbid discussions behind a bland sea of poker faces.

As the staff surrounds the bed, there is always present a tendency to forget that these patients have ears and minds, although the latter may appear to be markedly diminished. Even though our utterances may possibly be beyond the understanding of most patients, we can never be certain when momentary alertness arises. Also, as time progresses, such patients may develop an accurate recall of early events and negative conversations. When this occurs, they can lose all motivation for self-improvement and social recovery.

Even now, thirteen years after my accident, one of the most detrimental of such memories concerns the following statement made by a student during staff rounds: "I predict termination within three months." Eighteen months later I asked my physician what he predicted and mentioned my recall of the statement. He immediately explained that it must have been made in reference to a medication to "reduce vessel blockage" and did not mean expiration of life. I still wonder if that is what the resident really had in mind.

A vast number of patients have revealed a recall of similar comments uttered during routine rounds of the hospital staff. Diagnostic and evaluative discussions should be confined to the staff room; poker-faced countenances should be replaced with expressions of encouraging pleasantness; and an atmosphere of congeniality should be maintained. Most of all, we should remember the totality of the patient's intellect, emotions, and body. These are not separate entities.

FAMILY CONSULTATIONS

When a clinical impression of the brain-damaged patient is based solely on a casual observation of familial stability, unforgivable blunders can ensue. There can be little hope for such a patient if the family group is not given some specific guidance and understanding. Familial understanding cannot be determined by hearsay, nor can it be based on casual or brief consultations.

Ideally, the basic information regarding multiple aspects of neurophysiological disruptions should be provided by the hospital staff prior to the patient's dismissal from the hospital. In this manner, the patient's relatives will be given some cautious anticipation and be more apt to recognize a necessity for regulated contact with medical personnel. No one likes to feel isolated, and no one should be.

With a sudden invasion of the patient's dysphasia, even the well members of the family can experience a disturbance in their use of language. Some, in their state of confused misery, talk excessively and at times frantically. Much of their chatter sounds like nonsense. They seem unable to be quiet. Others retain static facial expressions of sadness, a continuous but inappropriate smile, or even an undefinable blankness of a mask. Many persons are fearful that they are in part to blame for the patient's illness, and they are sick with unwarranted guilt. Their demoralization is terribly contagious, and the patient already has more than he can bear. The family is in profound need of factual support, information, and guidance. They are reacting as would most of us should we be faced with a similar trauma in our own environment.

All members of the various professions must be cautious to avoid false conclusions or snap judgments about the exaggerated behavior of the family groups. Instead, we should stimulate them to discuss personal anxieties, cordially listening to help them gain some understanding. Without such clinical attentiveness familial attitudes may become worse and further devastate the patient's attempts at communication.

In addition to assessing the attitudes of the family, we must be sure that they have a clear conception of the dangers of detrimental depression, which is not a fleeting or even casual state of emotional deterioration and retards all aspects of recovery. It takes considerable time to lessen depression and demoralization in these patients, and there is little if any chance for improvement in behavior until the patient is able to perceive some positive aspects of reality.

It also takes considerable time for the patient to recognize any positive aspects of his situation, since he is organically confused as well as functionally distraught for a long time after his accident. Suicide is a constant threat, particularly if the patient's weakened emotionality and family stability are threatened. The family must be reminded to keep destructive medications, firearms, and dangerous utensils out of sight and out of reach. Medications should be as well guarded in the home as they are in hospital wards. Above all, formal language training is obviously detrimental until the patient has made some recovery of reasonable emotional stability.

It should not be assumed that because the patient is congenial and smiles easily, he is not experiencing suicidal depression. I have had individuals behave in such a positive manner that even I felt there was no need for concern. I have been shocked to learn that they have been hospitalized after consuming a full bottle of medication or have cut their wrists. One individual attempted to drown herself in the bathtub. Severely depressed patients most assuredly do not benefit from any formal stress for improvements in abstract communication, let alone improvement in muscle controls.

SEXUAL RELATIONSHIPS

Nearly all situations of personality deviation produce symptoms of sexual instability and often interfere with one's willingness to discuss them. The extreme limitation in memory and the overabundance of complete depressive withdrawal can result in the patient's total lack of interest in any activity but immediate survival. Therefore in due time there is apt to be some anxiety regarding sexual relationships.

Unfortunately, the literature dealing with the dysphasic patient reveals almost no references to the frustrations experienced by the well members of these marital partnerships. But a large percentage of the patients' wives or husbands will discuss sexual concerns about both their stricken mates and themselves if given an opportunity. With an understanding of the stricken mate's deficit in emotional concentration and the extreme limitations in memory span, the well mate can see that lack of sexual drive does not mean personal rejection.

Most patients eventually regain their drive, but initially they may also lack concern for the satisfaction of their partner. This too can repel and produce conflicts, and the dysphasic may lose motivation for any social recovery or even lack any desire for language recovery. There is little that we can do to help the patient increase verbal confidence if underlying tensions of the marriage are not maximally reduced. If we have any doubts, we should refer the well mate to a properly trained clinician in medicine, psychology, or marital counseling.

THE MATE'S ROLE

The wife of the dysphasic patient does not have an easy role. All sorts of anxieties arise. She too needs an equal amount of attention from all clinical personnel. Should she have symptoms of health disturbances such as weight loss, chronic fatigue, or persistent repetitions of respiratory infections, she should be encouraged to acquire medical assistance. It would do no harm to contact the physician and report observations. He may have had but little contact with her because the majority of his time has necessarily been devoted to her husband. But it should be assumed that the physician is interested and will appreciate our attentiveness. He too knows that the state of the patient's mental health depends on others within the immediate environment. Above all, the effectiveness of all clinical procedures depends upon the mate's ability to make necessary adjustments, and if he or she is physically despondent, emotional or intellectual alertness can hardly be expected. Negative behavior is contagious, and the patient already has more than he can handle in isolation.

The preceding discussion is not meant to imply that the husband of a stricken wife is free from anxieties and sincere concern. He is often more traumatized with feelings of guilt because he must unavoidably neglect his wife. He has to keep working, and very few can afford to take time off for consultations. When he is home, he may be completely lost, since up to the point of his wife's attack, he may have been almost solely concerned with his job. Therefore, the hospital staff must help a husband arrange time to understand his wife's situation more fully. Hospitals and nursing homes have social welfare workers available, and they can be of great assistance in contacting people who may care for the wife during the day while the husband is working. I have found that the majority of these attendants are very helpful in providing assistance in language recovery and are most willing to participate in the clinical procedures of the professional environment. Most assuredly these persons also need guidance from the patient's physicians, nurses, and related clinical staff.

LANGUAGE TRAINING

Too much stimulation and too much disorder can inhibit positive progress and can defeat recovery, despite prolonged training. The brain-damaged adult does not receive or evaluate the messages of sensation in a normal way. Responses to any stimuli are exaggeratedly different from those in pretraumatic existence. The brain-damaged adults cannot consistently perceive the whole of anything. They are unable to sort out substance from shadow and figure from ground. Patterning is most difficult, and things are comprehended distortedly. Most patients recognize this but are unable to understand their misconstructions of reality. Worst of all, neither do some of their clinicians. The patient sees the whole, but it is fogged with numerous details. Often only one minute aspect is comprehended, thus resulting in an endless sequence of misconceptions.

The ability to pattern meaningfully requires continuing but nonthreatening stimulation—not drill books. Human activity is structured by repeated stimulation in the realm of reality. Spurts of progress often occur when a restoration of self-confidence begins to appear.

The word language has a number of implications. Very few professionals are truly aware of what is meant by language. These patients are starting over again, and even their most basic expressions are not wholly dependent upon specific combinations of speech sounds. For example, profoundly deaf persons express language through body movements, and infants communicate with basic body postures and vocal wailing. Even some of our American Indians communicate predominantly via gestures and grunts that are abstract and symbolic. All of the preceding are means of communication.

Fortunately, there are very few damaged adults totally deficient in language usage. Initially at least, as long as they can communicate with gestures and understand some of the verbal body expressions of others, there is reason to hope for some degree of progress in reacquiring symbolic communication. Unfortunately, there is no consistent way to predict the eventual level of verbal recovery other than the response to daily stimulations or careful day-by-day observations. If the patient babbles, at least he is trying to communicate, and even this is good, particularly during the initial stages of recovery. As long as he keeps trying, eventual success may be forthcoming if his damaged brain and his clinical social environment will permit it.

ECHOIC RESPONSES

All of us, particularly the family group, should know that echoic responses are often the first sign of progress. Primitive verbalisms are not strongly structured at first, because perceptions are not highly differentiated. This may appear to be infantile behavior, and far too often we let it imply mental deficiency. In some instances there is a lasting mental weakness, but such should not be assumed prior to extensive communicative assistance and careful familial guidance. Even though the patient is communicating only with himself and not to others, this may be his initial means of holding current perceptions combined with attempts to pattern and stabilize them. Distorted self-talk may be his way of fixing percepts from one experience to the next and may eventually reestablish an orderly arrangement of understanding. But the patient must have a reward for any efforts, and often an objective ear is all the help he needs for several months. This is hard for clinical personnel, and negative attitudes are highly contagious and devastating to the basic morale of the patient. Therefore we must even revise our conception of the patient's behavioral age, which often varies from day to day and even moment to moment. At times the patient may appear to be reduced to a ten-year-old level or less. This often vacillates because there are always instances when he makes sense out of expected nonsense.

AUTOMATICISMS

All of us use slang, have pet phrases, or perhaps express "cuss-words" during our daily conversations. Most of the time we don't hear them, and most of our friends ignore them. Following damage to the cortex, inappropriate automaticisms and expressions will be apt to punctuate speech attempts. The patient's phrases flow without conscious planning, and they are unheard as his words are uttered. As with everyone, the patient does not see a word that he is going to utter and rarely hears an expression that is planned because the planning is instantaneous. However, when the patient observes the facial expressions of his listeners, it may become evident that once again he has failed to communicate thoughts or has said something wrong or shocking. He may immediately try again and become aware of some of the things that he is saying. If he does recognize inappropriate expressions it shocks him, but if his listeners are calm, he may try again. He may or may not improve immediately, but at the very least his own curiosity concerning his listeners' responses is more likely to be satisfied. The important thing is that positive self-awareness, even of his mistakes, is less detrimental to the patient's morale than shocked and mysterious rejection or withdrawal.

Again it must be stressed that the blatant swearing expressed by many patients is quite likely unplanned and unheard by the patient. The swearing can be uttered with a cordial tone of voice, a sad one, or a tone of irritability. Many patients who have never emitted such expressions prior to their accidents demonstrate a profound vocabulary of swear words. On the other hand, patients who have never demonstrated inhibitions regarding swearing cease swearing following their cortical accidents.

Other verbal automaticisms may also dominate expressions. Brief but repetitive phrases, meaningless words, or even portions learned during childhood may appear again and again. Such utterances may last for months in combination with an expansion of meaningful phrases. Gradually the automaticisms may disappear except during periods of extreme fatigue, at which time an occasional automatic utterance will be mingled with meaningful conversation.

COMPREHENSION

Grammatical rules are best learned as babies learn them—indirectly. Rules help but little because the irregularities of our language create an additional handicap. Many words sound alike but refer to different things. Grammatical relationships vary and create further confusion for the patient. When the language deficiency interferes with the patient's accurate assessment of the words of others, they should be restated clearly after a pause or again with a different sequence of words. Much of the time this helps, but we should always keep in mind that it can also fail, particularly in the shadows of needless pressure. Since the patients are not totally insensitive to their lack of comprehension, even though it may not always be apparent, stimulations are as effective as the tone and intensity of the speaker's voice. Sharp impatience only increases the patient's sense of failure. Remember too that the original process of language comprehension and development among infants depends largely on accompanying body movements. Gestures often assist in clarifying the meaning of oral expressions, and such is true of both the patient and the persons with whom he is communicating. There is no one formula for all constellations of dysphasia. Each patient presents a unique problem, and no one patient or family remains static. Variations in responses and understanding will occur, and those around the patient should be alert to use them to facilitate recovery.

ASSUMPTIVE CLASSIFICATIONS

I have seriously questioned the classification of dysphasia ever since my own vascular accident. There is no possible means of accurately measuring how well the patient can understand the words he hears. I had moments and even hours of good reception, but I also had days of severe problems in understanding the words I heard. It was presumed by my own colleagues that my understanding was intact because most of the questions and comments they made required a positive or "yes" response. Many times I nodded my head to get rid of them. I didn't know what they said, and this, combined with much of their ridiculous behavior, insulted me. I also recognized they were assuming too much with the kinds of expressive drills they put me through. The following phrase from a drill book points out a particular trauma to avoid. "I drive a car." I had no use for such a statement! I was still in a wheelchair and couldn't even guide that vehicle without scraping a wall or tearing the bedspread. My right visual field was absent in both eyes, and this thoroughly convinced me that my driving days might be finished. Therefore, I made no effort to repeat the statement, and there were times when I wept as a result of the pressures to say such "stupid things." My greatest desire was to gain a means of communication to let my nurses and later my family know that urinary pressures were almost beyond control. No one made any attempt to give me the word "toilet" or "bedpan," and those were the words I would have practiced and possibly retained. Consequently once I was able to return to professional endeavors with my patients, such drill books were cast aside.

READING

We should also be very cautious with reading activities. It is extremely important to wait for the patient's indication of a need for reading. Usually this does not occur until after the patient is mobile and able to leave the home sanctuary. If, by this time, there has been some evident recovery of reading street signs, labels on grocery containers, and even newspaper headlines, then inquiry into the patient's desire for improvements can be made. Remember, a vast number of our clients have had little need for recreational reading once they departed from the public school. If there is no assurance that the patient has a desire to recover this ability, we may only increase the black crust of demoralization on which he feeds when alone. Reading too soon can even halt conversational progress. But again, there is no generalized program that is applicable to all patients. Each one needs his own therapy design.

WRITING

Even the slightest degree of paralysis in the dominant hand can markedly reduce or eliminate the ability to use the pen. If the patient is unable to organize verbal expressions orally, it seems somewhat ridiculous to have him make attempts to express himself via the written word. Many patients temporarily lose their ability to spell along with their ability to interpret what they read. Most of them have no need to write, so it is senseless to traumatize them with the failures of left-handed script combined with reductions in spelling and interpretations of written words. This should be one of the very last therapeutic procedures to be introduced. The best way to gain insight is to make attempts at left-handed writing and multiply the resulting frustrations by ten to estimate the overall demoralization that occurs among these patients. When the patient recovers enough to have a need for writing, he will make his own attempts and express himself well enough to let his clinician know it's time. Again, the threat of suicidal depression must always be kept in mind.

SUMMARY

We, in each profession, are obligated to keep the family aware of the vital importance of medical care. It is easy to forget the physician when the patient is free from negative health episodes. These patients and their families have to be helped to live within neurological limitations, seizures, hypertension, or arteriosclerotic disease. Mind and body are not separate entities and we must arrange all clinical appointments accordingly.

In many instances, the recovery of language proceeds no faster than the language acquired during infancy. The more successful we are with familial education, counseling, and guidance, the more apt is the patient to reacquire enough communication for satisfactory existence in the home.

We must also bear in mind that none of us is capable of judging chaotic spells of intellectual disorganization or internal emotionality that occur at times. These patients are in vital need of personal support even during the later stages of recovery, because it is at these times that they are most often ignored. Even the most positive degree of self-confidence will have a shadow of negativism for years to come. We must make sure they know that we will be available should they feel a need for supportive counsel. A few moments of our time can save months of recuperative progress if we are willing to be their trusted friend.

Professionally we have come a long way, but our massive literature on dysphasia still rests on a tiny knoll of factual information. We must always be alert to new literature and to the reports of our patients and their families. They must guide us as we also guide them.

Reading 26

Rehabilitation Nursing in Non-Life-threatening Problems

Mary Opal Wolanin

Disability is a disturbance in man's ability to relate to his environment in an appropriate manner. It may be caused by an impairment of his ability to sense the environment, an impairment in his ability to respond to his environment through the motor system, or by an impairment in the integrative mechanism. In the latter the sensory and motor systems may be intact, but the relay pathways in the brain are impaired and do not allow integration of information leading to synthesis and function.

According to Tristan:[1]

> The central nervous system contains mechanisms for the recognition and classification of patterns of outgoing command messages. There is a division of labor; the more complex sensory recognition and processes of correlation between patterns appears to be the specific province of the cerebral cortex. Much

[1] Tristan, D. W. Robert, *Neurology of Postural Mechanisms.* London: Butterworth, 1967, p. 322.

of the routine business concerned with equilibrium and locomotion . . . is carried on in the lower parts of the brainstem. This part of the brain can continue to function even if connections to the higher parts are severed. The reticular formation of the cerebellum and vestibular nuclei together form a close-knit functional group primarily concerned with the routine maintenance of equilibrium and with locomotion.

Disability can take place through interference at any point of this system; problems may affect the sensory system, the integrative system, or the motor system. A smooth functioning whole is necessary for the seemingly effortless adjustment and adaptation which the human constantly makes to his environment. Interruption results in a distortion of reality or inappropriate behavior in response to a situation. Rehabilitation is based on the idea that restoration of function or substitution of another function is possible.

Since the sensory world is apparently learned through experience, it would follow that new experiences would result in new learnings. The nurse must be aware of the learning process and what is involved. The person who is blind from birth learns to sense his environment through sound and pressure. If sight were suddenly given light and color, shape and form, it would have no meaning, for his trustworthy world is sensed through sound and touch. He must learn as the infant learns, although presumably his experience will take less time since he has a knowledge of the world through other modalities.

On the other hand, the person who loses his sight after learning to interpret his world on the basis of vision must learn to use his other senses in a totally new orientation. He is gravely disabled and must learn and unlearn. The smoothly operating system of sensing light and form is suddenly a vacant nonoperative system. It is expressed by Peter Davison:[2]

Capacity, I understand,
Is limited to fixed perfection,
Being a measure of displacement;
The void exists as the bulk defined it,
The cat subsiding down a basement
Leaves a catlessness behind it.

This idea must be central to a nurse's understanding of her patient and his disability. The visionlessness, leglessness, soundlessness of disability becomes just as much a part of disability as the new state. The integrative actions lack the coordinated efforts of each learned act which must be unlearned and relearned in a totally new orientation without the input and output previously known.

[2] Davison, Peter, "The Miracles of Muriel Spark," *The Atlantic,* p. 39, October 1968.

It might be assumed that all disabilities have a neurological component inasmuch as they involve sensing, integrating, or motor problems in adapting to the environment. To illustrate this point the following scheme is presented.

Problems of Input to the Nervous System

Loss of sight	Partial blindness, blindness, hemianopsia, astigmatism, myopia
Loss of hearing	Partial or total deafness
Loss of touch	Temperature or pressure
Loss of proprioceptive sense	Inability to maintain posture (equilibrium and balance)
	Inability to take antigravity measures
	Inability to coordinate locomotion or motion
Loss of ability to sense bladder or rectal content	Spinal cord injury, colostomy, ileostomy, little strokes

Problems of Output of the Nervous System

Loss of innervation to muscle groups	Brain damage—stroke, tumor, trauma, encephalitis, birth injuries, myasthenia gravis, spinal cord injuries
Loss of sphincter control	Bowel, bladder, lips and eyelids
Loss of muscle and bone tissue	Amputations, arthritis, myocardial infarction
Loss of respiratory function	Chronic obstructive lung disease

Problems of Integrating the Sensing of the Environment with Appropriate Motor Action

Sensing apparatus apparently adequate, and the motor system intact but physical response inadequate	Asthma, brain injury or disease
Sensory apparatus and motor apparatus adequate, but emotional response inappropriate	Emotional illness, depression, anxiety, addictions

If one tries to fit each entity into only one niche, he is confronted with the problem of the wholeness of the human body—the inability of one part to act in isolation. The problems of disability must be seen as the total involvement of the nervous system and its related parts—the whole of man. Finally, since each disability involves the interruption of a learned pattern of dealing with one's environment, the human elements of frustration and failure enter in. A simple loss of function may be accompanied by a severe and prolonged depression and inability to adjust. Disability can only be seen in its totality if it is understood as the loss of an integral part of a highly coordinated system.

The problem occurs with a break at any point in the system. Conscious awareness is brought into focus and automaticity is lost. An example is the problem of walking with a blistered heel when every effort is made to protect the damaged tissue from friction and pressure. The loss of smooth transition from one foot to another interferes with the learned act of walking. The person experiences difficulty in using his unaffected areas when there is a break in the system, since loss of a part is not simply a loss of function but of a total integrated system. Without the feedback from the affected part, the unaffected parts must be used in a new orientation. Any loss creates the need for new learning and unlearning. The man who always used his right hand to shave complained when his left hand was paralyzed, "I can't shave myself."

The nurse can use this knowledge effectively when she realizes that the right-handed person who has lost the use of his left hand must be taught to use the right hand without the assistance of the left one. This involves demonstration and suggestion. The nurse may feel this is so obvious that it would offend the patient to call it to his attention. Only by understanding all movement as a highly complex and coordinated activity can she appreciate that the patient has lost a total process, not a part.

Most patients can face their disability if they know what they are facing. All too often, the patient may be the last to be informed. Families may feel the need to protect their disabled member from unpleasant news, but adults must participate in their own decision making. Facing an unpleasant future may hurt, but realistic effort will not be made in the face of deception. It is not fair to build false hopes which can only result in bitterness and depression later.

Section B

Arthritic Conditions

Rehabilitation nursing for the person with arthritis requires a positive approach. It must offer a bridge from despair to hope. It requires maximum prevention of further loss of function reinforced with as much restoration as possible. The patient usually regards pain as a precursor of deterioration and loss of function. Thus, he experiences simultaneously a sense of loss and almost unbearable pain. The great majority of victims develop arthritis during their years of gainful employment, a period when they have responsibilities for themselves and others. The person whose self-concept is associated with his work feels threatened by the necessity of adjustment to less demanding, less prestigious, and less well-paid work. Physical limitations are likely to pose identity as well as economic problems.

The initial steps in the assessment and realization of the patient's full rehabilitative potential are often taken in the hospital in order that the support, guidance, and skills of the hospital staff can be made fully available to the patient. In planning care the nurse will be challenged to help him deal with depression, loss of self-esteem, acute illness, and pain. She defines her task as helping the patient cope with a disease characterized by some remissions but little hope for cure. The patient must be helped to a new way of life requiring the establishment of realistic goals commensurate with his capability for attainment.

THE EXERCISE PROGRAM

In this day of miracle drugs and impressive technology the arthritic patient still faces a regimen which is tedious and unexciting. He must learn, with professional help, during the period of hospitalization that the course of rehabilitation is closely related to his own efforts and perseverance. Frequently, just maintaining the status quo is painful and wearisome.

Throughout hospitalization the nurse must be continuously aware of her teaching role. She can teach the lesson about joint support effectively only if she supports each joint during rest, and if she slowly and carefully assists the patient to engage in the prescribed activity. Even checking the weight of the covers over the patient's toes must be accompanied by an explanation, because slowly but surely the patient is learning to assume responsibility for his own care.

Careful observation and experimentation are needed to determine the amount of exercise the patient can tolerate. Exercises are graded, and it is important to check the pain level after each exercise is performed. In order to take advantage of the most favorable situation possible, the nurse will selectively utilize the environment. Knowledge that joints are most responsive to warmth may suggest that exercises be performed under warm water. Exercises can be facilitated by the use of analgesic to reduce pain. The amount required to reach a level at which the pain can be tolerated can only be determined through experimentation. The patient's involvement in the experimentation is of great importance. Severe pain may prompt him to economize on motion. He may resist any motion in excess of the requirement for minimum activities for daily living and thus fail to make progress. Professional interpretation is needed to help him avoid confusion between random activity and controlled exercises. The patient must learn that exercise should be discontinued at the point of undue pain or excessive fatigue. A suitable balance between rest and exercise should be sought. Full joint activity is the goal of the maintenance exercise program because the joints are needed for all movement. Rest and exercise complement each other, and about fifteen minutes is often as long as an arthritic should remain seated in one position. A patient who becomes discouraged because he is stiff after rest must learn that this stiffness will gradually diminish. It may be necessary to resort to intermittent splinting during rest. The joints are placed in an anatomically neutral position, which reduces the strain on the ligaments surrounding them.

ARTHRITIC CONDITIONS

REDUCTION OF PAIN

The treatment of arthritis involves relieving the joints of pain. This is usually understood and well implemented for the large weight-bearing joints, but the small ones are often neglected. For example, fingers are precision instruments capable of the most intricate movements. Activities of daily living may impose undue strain on them. The fingers can be relieved of the weight of a purse by carrying it on the arm near the elbow; a heavy pan can be lifted with the whole hand from the wrist and elbow; a can opener which does not require twisting with the fingers can be used. The strongest joint available should be utilized for each task, and less strain is imposed upon the joints if they push rather than pull objects.

Heavy bed clothing can distort the position of feet and toes. An electric blanket may be used to ensure a light source of warmth. When joints are swollen, affected tendons may not self-correct in a neutral position, and bracing may be indicated to keep rotating limbs in an anatomically neutral position. Careful support to joints is essential to prevent pull on affected areas. In lifting a limb, the principle of supporting the joint is reversed. Support is applied by grasping the limb near but not at the joint. Joints of the resting patient should be supported in positions of function with splints or rest casts designed for each specific situation. These devices are especially useful at night, when there is danger of overlooking joint strain while the patient is sleeping.

The patient "frozen" in the wheelchair position is an example of what can happen when hip and knee joints have not been allowed to extend through their entire range of motion. Accommodation has been made to the angles of the wheelchair for long periods without relief. Flexion is a position of strain over a period of time. It may be continued in the side-lying position in which the patient assumes the contours of the wheelchair. In the chair the pressure is equal for each arm and leg. While in bed, one shoulder, one hip, and one knee will be uppermost. The pull of gravity results in unsupported positions for these extremities. The arm and leg should be supported to prevent adduction deformities and pull on the shoulder and hip ligaments.

For many patients the wheelchair offers the best means of achieving mobility. The joints of the human organism in the chair still require attention, even though the goal of mobility has been attained. Any position maintained over a period of time impedes circulation because pressure is extended on one side of the joint only. The position in the chair should be changed frequently to prevent further deformity. Slow, coordinated movements should be planned for the patient whose motion is restricted. Such devices as a built-up chair or toilet seat are useful. Good body alignment should be maintained at all times. For the bed patient a firm mattress is desirable, but, lacking that, a board may be placed under the mattress to achieve stability. A wheelchair should have a solid seat. A number of small pillows rather than one or two large ones help in aligning the body because they can be combined in a variety of ways to produce the desired results. Long pillows give good support when placed parallel to a limb, but they should not be used at right angles to the knee. The supine patient may need a foot board. It should be placed at the level of the sole of the foot, and it requires a minimum of padding. The foot board tucked under the mattress is useful as a cradle to keep the bed covers from pressing on the foot, but it should not be confused with the board positioned to prevent foot drop.

Like most other people, arthritics tend to rest in a side-lying position. To help maintain this position they develop knee and hip flexions. If the knee is flexed and pulled forward on the bed, the upper hip joint and the tibial muscles are strained, unless the foot is brought into a position of ankle flexion. In order to prevent hip flexion the patient may have to lie in a prone position. This puts the hip at rest, but the ankle and toe joints are strained unless supported.

Because the ligaments are in tension, the weight of the arms may pull the shoulder down into a strained position. The shoulder socket is shallow, and it depends upon ligaments to maintain the proper shoulder position. If the patient cannot independently assume and maintain correct alignment, he should be helped by straightening the hips and supporting the upper arms with pillows. Reduction of strain during exercise may be made possible by use of an overhead spring, which will help support part of the weight while taking the joint through its full range of motion. Water buoyancy can serve the same purpose.

USE OF ASSISTIVE DEVICES TO REDUCE STRAIN

Assistive devices can reduce both physical and mental strain. Walking appliances lead to support and redistribution of weight and achieve:

Stability through providing a wider base of support and altered center of gravity
Relief of pain
Decreased fear of instability or pain on weight bearing
Prolongation of ambulation in spite of progressive disease

The patient may react positively or negatively to these devices. He may feel that the device labels him a crippled or handicapped person, and he may resist its use. However, when he understands that the more he can be up and about, the less the deformity and the better the circulation, he can usually accept cane, crutch, or walker.

Bed rest produces quadriceps weakness. "Wobbly knees" may develop in as little as twenty-four hours. Walking requires fixation of the knees and a solid base of support while the body is moving through space. To protect the weight-bearing joints of the hip and knee, crutches are advisable. Crutch walking requires good shoulder and arm muscles. Unless the musculature is strong, the patient will tend to lean on the shoulder bar, which can lead to radial nerve compression. When this problem occurs, sensation through the extensors and the triceps is affected, and wrist extensors become weak. Wrist drop may be the earliest sign of nerve compression. It is very important that the crutch fit the person using it. The hand bar must be far enough from the shoulder to prevent the elbow from locking when supporting the body weight. Crutches allow the patient to move at a faster pace. Their use can be adapted to stairs or uneven ground, and they offer greater stability than a cane. Reciprocal action between arms and legs can usually be developed. Sequences required for coordination may be too complicated for some patients. Older patients tend to be apprehensive and may not have the balancing power required for crutch walking. Debilitated patients who attempt to use crutches must be carefully supervised. They may experience weakness in the extremities and are subject to crutch paralysis. A glove attached to the hand support may help the person with poor hand grip.

When 50 percent or more of weight bearing must be relieved, the crutch is the device of choice. To relieve 20 to 25 percent of weight bearing on an arthritic hip or knee, a cane is useful. It widens the base of support and eliminates lurch in the patient's gait. When jerky movements produce pain, a cane can be very helpful in developing a smooth gait. It partially relieves the pull of hip-stabilizing muscles. The patient concerned about appearances may find the cane more acceptable than crutches. It is the least stable of walking appliances, because there is only one point of contact with the upper extremity. It supports the weaker side when used on the opposite side.

The regimen for use of an assistive device should be outlined carefully by a physician and a physical therapist. The musculature must be evaluated in order to make the best use of the strong muscles. Rubber tips are essential for walking appliances, and they should be kept free from dust in order to reduce the possibility of slipping. The large size is usually more effective in maintaining floor contact. A decision regarding padding of the shoulder bar should be made, taking into consideration its value in preventing underarm slippage as well as the danger of damage to the radial nerve. When the device has been prescribed and fitted, the nurse becomes invaluable in assisting the patient to gain independence in walking with the help of the device.

REDUCTION OF EMOTIONAL STRAIN

Scott's article gives an account of the arthritic's proneness to emotional strain. Effective therapy requires that both physical and emotional strain be minimized as much as possible. Such components as acceptance of functional loss derived from chronic illness, socioeconomic factors crucial to the life-style of the person concerned, and the small irritations of daily living present very real problems to the patient. Though to some extent the "system" controls the hospital milieu, the skillful nurse can mitigate a great many of its negative effects on patients.

Swartz also writes from the patient's perspective. His points should be required learning for all nurses from the beginning of their training. Swartz provides free insight to others—insight that he has labored painfully to acquire. Moreover, he does it with a light touch. The message is substantial.

Carroll writes from the physician's view of the management process. His article is basic information that belongs in every nurse's rehabilitation repertoire. In identifying the ADL score at first observation as an important indicator of how much the patient is likely to improve under treatment, he has suggested a potentially valuable tool in designing therapeutic regimens.

Reading 27
Arthritis: A Patient's View
Franklin E. Scott

I have severe rheumatoid arthritis. The disease has had a considerable effect on the pattern of my life, and has given me experiences which I could never have imagined. Even though I had known several people who had suffered from arthritis and was aware of the disease most of my life, I am ashamed that I had to experience it for myself before I really understood their situation. My friends have encouraged me to write about the effect rheumatoid arthritis has had on me, in the belief that it might help others, whether patient or practitioner, to understand it better. This is, therefore, a very personal account of arthritis from the inside looking out.

Eight years ago I had my first attack. Although originally only my right shoulder was involved and the problem was thought to be bursitis, various other joints gradually became painfully swollen and the diagnosis of rheumatoid arthritis was established. During this initial period, I continued to have incidents of swollen painful joints which the doctor called flares. The pain accompanying a flare was usually limited to a single joint, but it also could be generalized and involve the entire body. The isolated joint pain resembled that of an acute sprain or bursitis. It was different from that of the generalized involvement, which could best be described as similar to the aches of severe influenza.

A painful joint is not moved and gradually becomes stiffer and stiffer. This loss of mobility and the accompanying loss of muscle strength left me in a constant state of fatigue. I was so exhausted by the end of each week that I found it necessary to spend the entire weekend in bed in order to be rested enough to face Monday morning.

My general condition gradually deteriorated for the first fourteen months until finally I had to be hospitalized. At this time I was first introduced to the regimen of medication, rest, and exercise which would become part of my daily routine for the rest of my life. The doctor explained the facts and gave me some idea of what to expect in the future. He indicated that episodes of increased joint pain and swelling might continue, that restriction of movement would probably increase, and even that some deformity might develop.

On the other hand, the doctor told me I would have relatively pain-free periods termed "remissions" and finally said that no one could predict either the course of arthritis or the extent to which it would affect any particular individual. His very honest and straightforward explanation made a great impression on me. *For the first time I realized that this arthritis was not temporary, and that I would not be able to overcome it and return to the state of good health I had enjoyed all my life.* It was not a happy outlook, but I remember feeling relieved to learn the facts and to see the possibility of controlling the situation.

As I look back over this initial period, I realize that it was a critical time with respect to my future. Although I was too busy to realize it then, it was a time of considerable stress. My job was very demanding, and trying to reach its goals was extremely frustrating work. I was also completing a spare-time program of study and had several other projects to accomplish. All these obligations kept me in an anxious state, and I gave little thought to my general well-being.

I should have "cooled it," in order to have adequate rest and better follow an organized program of exercise, so necessary at this early stage to maintain joint motion and muscle strength.

Today I cannot help but feel that the effect of rheumatoid arthritis on a particular individual is partly the result of his general physical condition. If I had not allowed myself to become so run down eight years ago, my initial involvement might not have been so severe. This is so important a point that I think every patient should be started on an effective physical conditioning program as soon as his condition is diagnosed. And, because no two cases are alike, each patient's exercise program should be designed by a doctor and a physical therapist.

I left the hospital with a better appreciation of the nature of rheumatoid arthritis but with an incomplete understanding of my medical programs. The need for medication and rest was, by this time, very apparent. Any neglect of either had an immediate effect on my physical well-being. I also understood the need for continuing the exercises, but due to the insidious nature of my ailment, I did not truly appreciate the need for a *formal exercise program.* I felt that my daily activities were sufficient to maintain the necessary muscle strength and joint motion. I continued on my job and completed all my spare-time projects, believing all the time that I was doing everything my doctor had prescribed.

FATIGUE

During the next four years, however, my ability to perform certain activities gradually diminished until I became quite dependent on others. Walking, climbing stairs, rising from a chair, opening doors, and turning on the ignition key of my car (activities we all take for granted) became extremely difficult.

As my general physical condition gradually deteriorated, fatigue once again became a constant companion. The next rest period soon became the most important event of my day, and I could hardly endure the wait from one rest period to the next. The vicious cycle of weakness and fatigue was difficult to recognize, due to its slow progressive nature. Only now, in retrospect, do I truly understand its effects.

In reviewing this second period objectively, one thing becomes very apparent: the need for a combination of a regular medical *and* functional re-evaluation or follow-up. At first glance this may appear to be an artificial separation, but I believe it is very important to all arthritic patients. When conducting his medical evaluation, the doctor is primarily concerned with the control of arthritis through an effective program of medication and rest. The physical therapist, however, is interested in determining the patient's functional capabilities and in establishing an exercise program designed to maintain or improve those capabilities.

Although I received an excellent routine of medical evaluation and supervision, my physical therapy program for the first four to five years was directed more toward the relief of pain (through treatment such as paraffin baths and hot packs) than toward the re-establishment of functional losses. The reduction of pain is an important consideration, but both patient and therapist must realize that it is only a means to an end: greater function through exercise.

One day I fell and had to have help to get back on my feet. Because of this incident, I developed a tremendous fear of repeating the mishap and having no one available to help me. The incident provided critical evidence of my level of dependence, and the image of myself sitting in a wheelchair became more and more troublesome. *I was running scared.*

I mentioned my fears to the therapist on my next visit to the clinic, and he asked me to demonstrate just what had kept me from getting up. I struggled on a large mat as the therapist tried to determine what part of my disability was the result of either pain, joint stiffness, or weakness. *This was the beginning of my functional exercise program.* After several months of rolling, sit-ups, and other exercises, I was able to rise from the floor assisted only by the use of my cane. The vision of the wheelchair became dimmer as the therapist and I began to tackle other functional disabilities through a specific exercise program.

My particular program begins before I get out of bed in the morning. I go through a five- to ten-minute series of loosening-up exercises designed to help me start the day. Later, I take a fifteen- or twenty-minute walk, depending on the degree of discomfort in my feet and legs. To further combat the weakness and stiffness in my legs, I also practice getting up from and down to a low chair (now only twelve inches from the floor), stepping on and off an eight-inch cinder block, and riding a stationary bicycle that I set up in my garage. To maintain the strength and motion in my arms and shoulders, I push and pull against small sections of rubber tubing which are attached to the wall of my garage.

The complete home program requires about an hour a day. Rather than do the entire program in one session, I prefer to break it up into several ten- to fifteen-minute periods. *The exercises are not arduous, and they are valuable because of their daily application.* This day-in, day-out program requires a high degree of motivation. At present my level of motivation is great because I know what will happen if I quit.

Biweekly sessions in an indoor heated pool further supplement my home program. These sessions not only add variety to my exercise program but also allow increased activity because of the heat and buoyancy of the water. *It is the best environment I have found in which to exercise.* The physical therapist in charge of this therapeutic pool periodically reviews my program and modifies it when I am ready to advance.

I have also found it helpful in my daily struggle against arthritis to keep a combined record of performance and progress. Each day I check off the exercises as I do them and note whether there has been any progress. This record not only serves as a constant reminder that my exercises must be completed but also allows me to compare today's accomplishments against those of previous months. It is encouraging to see in this written testimony that some of my previous failures have been eliminated through daily exercise.

I take this chart with me each time I return to the therapist. It serves to familiarize him with my specific exercise program and provides a springboard for his evaluation. If, for example, my joint-motion test indicates that my elbows are not moving as well as they did the previous month, the therapist checks the chart and modifies my program to increase the emphasis on elbow exercises.

This chart usually speaks for itself. If I perform my exercises regularly, both the therapist and I are pleased with the results of the functional evaluation.

The chronic and dynamic qualities of arthritis require constant regulation of medicines. Only through such a careful program can the process of joint involvement be retarded, thereby relieving the pain and allowing rest and exercise sessions to be more beneficial.

In the early period of my involvement I must have tried every home remedy that I heard or read about. As far as I can determine, none of them has had the slightest effect on my condition. I am more convinced than ever that the only way to combat this condition is under the direction of a competent, well-trained physician.

Surgery on involved joints has been performed more often in recent years. Its major goals are the relief of pain and the improvement of function.

I have had four operations on my hands. The specific considerations for surgery can only be resolved by the patient, his physician, and the surgeon. The patient must have confidence that the results of the surgery will be beneficial. But, equally important, he must understand that complete restoration of function is not always possible.

I mentioned earlier the problem of fatigue. My rest must be adjusted as my condition requires. While there have been periods when a good night's rest was sufficient, most of the time I also must take an afternoon nap. At other times, this rest is more effective if broken into fifteen-minute sessions spread out over the day. This program must be well monitored, however, for the tendency to stay in bed is always present and extremely appealing.

Looking back over the past eight years, I think one of the most interesting facets of my condition was the close connection between periods of increased emotional stress and those of increased physical involvement. I can recall many times when particular stressful events preceded a decline in my general physical condition. This was an important discovery, for it helped me to recognize these underlying tensions and to seek the assistance of my doctor in situations beyond my control. My greatest problem in this area was learning to overcome my natural tendency to worry. I finally realized that worry in itself is very tiring and generally accomplishes nothing. My religion has helped a great deal to resolve this problem. My favorite lines are from St. Augustine:

> Live in the present moment, and refuse to worry about that over which you have no control. Leave the past to the mercy of God, the present to His love, and the future to His providence.

Reading 28

The Rehabilitation Process—As Viewed from the Inside

Frank M. Swartz

It is something of a responsibility for me as a patient to tell what I think of the allied health professions. Although I've been in contact with people in these professions much of my life, I've not often been asked for my opinions. I've been led to believe that the only good patient is, if not a dead one, at least a silent one. And I've been a good patient—up to now.

Reprinted from *Rehabilitation Literature*, vol. 31, no. 7, pp. 203-204, 209, July 1970.

First, I must say that I don't like to be thought of as a patient or as an arthritic. Those terms don't describe me to my satisfaction. To be referred to as an "arthritic patient" makes me doubly damned! But don't misunderstand me. I'm not hung up on words, I don't mind these terms; it's the attitude or feeling tone that often goes with them, seeming to deny my humanity. I don't object to being called a patient when it is appropriate; it's a valid term, and to avoid its use would require awkward, cumbersome language. I'll use the term frequently myself. I would remind you, however, that when you call me a *patient,* or an *arthritic,* or a *client,* or a *case,* you are identifying me by negative characteristics, by the flaws in my health or fortune. It certainly isn't as nice to hear as the descriptions "charming," "brilliant," or "good-looking." My mother uses these terms.

Although my name is associated with a rehabilitation center, I have never been a patient there. I work there in an editorial capacity and this gives me no special expertise. I speak only for myself. My qualifications for these comments lie in the fact that I have had arthritis for 32 years. I've been a patient for 32 years—and survived.

I've been told that the allied health professions make up a "team." I confess that the term makes me a little uneasy. I suspect that "team" is a glib way of making the simple acts of consultation and communication sound like revolutionary new techniques. They are essential acts, but I doubt that they are new. I like words and since I knew the term mainly in a sports context, I looked up "team" in my 1947 Webster's. The first definition was obsolete and I passed it by. The second was, "A brood of young, especially of pigs and ducks"; the third was, "Two or more horses or other beasts attached to the same vehicle, the same plow, or the like." I got a mental picture of a patient being dragged along by some health professionals. I doubt that you like that image any better than I. The last definition was more familiar, "A number of persons associated together, as those on one side of a match, or game."

I'm a sports fan and I think that a basketball team that plays well together is a very pretty thing to watch. Of course, that's what they're supposed to do: play well together, blending their talents toward a single goal. I thought of the Los Angeles Lakers; they have three of the superstars of pro basketball, but they don't seem able to put it all together. They have intramural jealousies, they bicker a lot, they have disagreements among themselves and with their coach, and they generally seem to play for their own glory, not for the good of the team. I wonder if some of these problems don't interfere with the efficiency of your team.

And, if there is a team, I wonder if you consider the patient a member of it. I'm not sure what you would say if I asked that question. I think you might say yes, but I don't see much evidence that the patient is regarded as a part of the team. I don't think he is kept well informed. I don't think he is allowed to participate in team discussions and decisions about his own programs, and I don't think his contributions are very well recognized or acknowledged. Obviously, he cannot sit in on all the staffings and consultations that concern him, but I believe he could play an important part on a team.

I address these remarks not only to the paramedical professions but also to the various social and rehabilitation professions. I believe what I say is applicable to all of these: the failure of the allied health professions to help us, the patients, achieve or maintain our self-esteem. I think you, all too often, put us down, belittle us, patronize us, humiliate us; you, all too often, fail to treat us with the dignity and respect that we deserve as human beings. You convey the idea that our feelings are not worth consideration; your manner suggests that we are unable to act constructively, even in our own behalf. I think many of you treat us as inferiors; I'm afraid that many of you honestly believe we are your inferiors because we are ill, crippled, out of work, poorly adjusted to the catastrophes that have befallen us.

This is an attitude to be found in our society-at-large toward the poor, disabled, and culturally deprived. I think it is shameful that the attitude can be found in supposedly enlightened professionals who are trying to help us.

I am unhappy at the way some of you allow personal feelings to interfere with the faithful discharge of your duties. I've seen instances where patients received inferior care or were refused care because they had unattractive personalities or offended the professional in some other way. This may not have been done consciously, but it was easy to rationalize by saying that the patient was uncooperative, or could not be helped, or that someone else needed the care more.

People in many fields, not just the health professions, have an unfortunate tendency to think that advanced technical knowledge in one specialized area makes their preferences more important, increases the validity of their moral judgments, and automatically provides a fuller understanding of politics, economics, religion, and social reform. *This is frequently not true.*

Because you work so closely with people who need help, you have an especial responsibility not to allow your tastes, prejudices, or philosophical views to influence the service you render. Whether your patient is a Republican or an atheist, an advocate of sexual freedom or Medicare or some radical belief, is not very important to your relationship with him. If it doesn't interfere with your work, it should not affect the quality of your work.

Now I don't pretend to believe you can love all your patients. Some of us are undoubtedly exasperating, rude, thoughtless, ungracious, and ungrateful. But that is true of almost any group of people (perhaps even the allied health professions). I know that you can't love all your patients, but you can recognize your antagonisms and prejudices when they arise and you can see that they don't diminish the quality of your work.

I think there is reason enough for me to ask that you give your patients dignity and respect on strictly moral grounds: They are your equals in the sight of God—if not of man. But on a practical basis, you need to help your patients to value themselves enough to believe that their recovery or rehabilitation is worth their strenuous efforts, and yours.

I'm convinced that services that deny the value of the individual do more harm than good. They tend to increase the very dependency they are designed to relieve. They reinforce the person's doubts about his usefulness and give him an easy excuse for not trying very hard. What's the use, after all, of doing tedious exercises, submitting to painful operations, training for a new job, or looking for work, if you think you're not worth very much and the authorities—the professionals—seem to confirm that idea?

I've been lucky that the help I've received has always been on an individualized basis. At every stage I've been given help that acknowledged my role and encouraged my participation and commitment. You cannot build this kind of commitment with superficial, depersonalized service and, without such commitment, I'm not sure your services are worth a damn.

Over the years, I've been disturbed by the lack of communication that seems almost a characteristic of the allied health professions. The professionals seem to be as tight-lipped with each other as gold prospectors sitting on a mother lode. Beyond that, I find them hesitant or unwilling to tell the patient what is happening in any specific and concrete terms. What's the big secret? I think you may be unaware of the agony you can cause us by not letting us know what the hell we're doing. It may not occur to you that circumstances so familiar to you can be frightening, confusing, or embarrassing for your patients.

I've already suggested another side to the communication barrier—the professional's unwillingness to listen to the patient. Perhaps the subject of pain is an example of this, and it may be where the greatest gulf lies between us: We can't *tell* you what our pain is like, and you can't *know* what it is like. You have a certain comprehension of pain on the basis of broken arms and toothaches and childhood accidents, but that can give you only a dim idea of what it is like to have pain every day, perhaps every minute, for many years of your life. As a friend of mine put it one time, arthritis is so damned daily!

The fact that I have pain is just that—a fact. It is not a matter that requires your tears, sympathy, or judgment. It is just one of the many facts that make up my situation. It *is* a matter that calls for the respect and communication that are my themes here. You must give me the respect of accepting the idea that I have the pain I say I have. You cannot judge whether it is as bad as I say, but either it is that bad or there is some reason for my saying or thinking it is that bad. And that may be a call for help, too.

Some professionals who work with people with arthritis seem to pay lip service to the idea that this is a painful disease. They say, "Yes, it is a painful disease," and believe they have done their duty and go ahead and mangle us. Others are so afraid of hurting us that they back away or approach us so gingerly they don't provide the proper care or service. And they don't help us to understand that some pain must be incurred by the patient in any recovery program.

I'd like to end these observations on some happy notes. I'd like to point out that I have not been critical of the *quality* of services you deliver: I have been critical of the *quality* of their *delivery,* and that is something that should be *amenable* to change. I'd also like to say that knowledgeable friends have told me that it is possible to learn how to develop what they call facilitative relationships with the people who are your patients. It is possible, my friends say, to develop the ability to give empathy and respect and to communicate more effectively with your patients and your fellow team members. I am enough of an optimist to believe that, especially if you will remember that your patients are, first of all, people, as I have been insisting.

And if you think I've been pretty hard on you, I want you to know that I could give a stinging address to patients, especially those with arthritis, about what I believe their responsibility to be in this mutual battle against our disease.

Reading 29

Rehabilitation of Patients with Rheumatoid Arthritis
Douglas G. Carroll

Rehabilitation of the patient with rheumatoid arthritis requires a comprehensive and long-term approach, preferably by a single physician. Many badly crippled patients can be helped by rehabilitation techniques, but rarely dramatically. The study of late cases suggests that many deformities could be prevented or significantly ameliorated if treatment and preventive measures had been started and continued at an earlier stage in the disease. Motivation plays a major role in the final outcome.

Reprinted from the *Maryland State Medical Journal,* vol. 18, pp. 71-75, March 1969.

DEFINITION

Rheumatoid arthritis is a chronic inflammatory disease of unknown origin which is systemic in nature and characterized by the manner in which it involves joints [1-5]. It runs a prolonged intermittent course, resulting in severe disability in approximately 30% of the patients. The principal cause of disability is the painful joint and the contracture and atrophy of contiguous muscles. Less frequently there is severe osteoporosis with lysis of the involved joints.

PSYCHIATRIC ASPECTS

Patients with rheumatoid arthritis who come to a municipal hospital are a highly selected group of older people with severe deformities and few social resources. The largest number of acute initial cases of rheumatoid arthritis occur in young females. At this time of life they are either self-supporting or supported by parents or husband. Consequently, they are seen by private doctors in private hospitals as long as they, or their relatives, can pay for private medical care.

The older patients with deforming rheumatoid arthritis are almost always victims of a prolonged, painful, gradually-limiting disease. Consequently, nearly all of them are deeply depressed, have given up hope, and are frequently attached to hospital life. They are often fearful and confused. They receive information about arthritis from friends, from advertisements in magazines, and from popular medical articles. They may shift from one doctor to another, try new remedies, or move to a new part of the country in an attempt to obtain relief.

EVALUATION AND TREATMENT

Since this disease is frequently intermittent and of long duration, treatment must be carried on for long periods of time, possibly the patient's entire life. It is, therefore, important to evaluate the patient carefully when the initial diagnosis is made. Investigation of the activity and extent of the arthritis, evaluation of functional capacity by the use of muscle tests, joint range of motion, and the activities of daily living (ADL) are essential. In addition, a knowledge of the patient's psychological background and outlook, his family and social situation, and his vocational potentialities is necessary in planning management. For these reasons it is helpful to hospitalize the patient for a period of one month to six weeks early in the disease in order to perform the evaluation and determine the mode of management, as well as to educate the patient about his disease.

As for treatment, a number of drugs have proved to be of help in relieving pain in rheumatoid arthritis. Their use will not be discussed here, but any drug or modality which relieves pain promotes the maintenance of range of motion and muscle strength.

REHABILITATION

The purpose of rehabilitation in rheumatoid arthritis is (1) to relieve pain, (2) to maintain muscle strength and range of motion, and (3) to compensate for loss of range of motion and muscle strength late in the disease if severe deformities have occurred.

Relief of Pain

In addition to the use of drugs, there are several methods which are helpful in the alleviation of pain during the acute stage of rheumatoid arthritis.

Immobilization: During the acute stage, bed rest is most helpful in relieving pain. Individual joints may be immobilized by the use of splints.

Heat: Almost any type of heat will give temporary relief of pain in involved joints. When the pain is in the hands or feet the use of paraffin baths once or twice daily is often of significant value. Moist-air cabinets, Hubbard tanks, or hot baths are helpful where many joints are painful.

Maintenance of Range of Motion and Muscular Strength

Positioning in bed: The bed should have a moderately hard mattress. A bed board is usually indicated. A soft mattress results in adduction and internal rotation of the shoulders in the supine position. Ulnar deviation of the wrists and fingers is favored when the patient's body sinks into the mattress. Pillows under the head increase the dorsal kyphosis. Pillows under the knees promote hip and knee flexion contractures. The feet should be protected from the weight of the sheets by a foot board.

Poor positioning in bed can cause irreparable damage in as little as two weeks time in some patients. Lying on the stomach several hours daily helps to prevent hip and knee flexion contractures.

Range of motion: The patient must be taught to treat himself. Interest in this program wanes several months after the patient leaves the hospital unless rapport is established and maintained. A complete explanation of the common deformities and how they may be prevented is essential. Directions to the patient must be simple, and only the most important joints should be worked with. If a joint can be taken through the full range of motion twice daily, range of motion can be maintained.

Selective muscle strengthening: The muscle atrophy which is part of the disease is made worse by disuse. Efforts, therefore, should be made to maintain muscular strength in muscles crossing the most important joints. The patient should understand why he is performing the specific exercises, how often they should be performed, and exactly how to do them. The program should be performed by the patient under the direction of the physical therapist until carried out correctly. A written program should be made out individually for each patient.

Particular care should be taken to maintain motion and strength in the following joints:

Knees—flexion and extension: These are probably the most important joints in the body from the point of view of function in the patient with rheumatoid arthritis. Knee flexion contracture is the most common reason for forcing the patient to bed. Once patients are forced into bed, contractures of the upper extremities follow rapidly.

Hips—flexion and extension
Shoulders—full elevation and abduction of the arm
Forearms—supination
Wrists—dorsiflexion, radial abduction
Thumbs—abduction (abductor policies brevis) and extension
Fingers—index finger abduction (first dorsal interosseus)
Flexion and extension at metacarpal-phalangeal joints [7].

Use of splints: Splints may be used to give complete immobilization of an acutely inflamed joint. This is an effective way to relieve the swelling and pain. The fear that complete immobilization would inevitably lead to contracture has been definitely disproved [8-10]. Acutely inflamed joints may be completely immobilized in casts for as long as a month with the expectation that the joint will regain its function if appropriately treated with physical therapeutic methods on removal from the cast.

In subacute joint activity, splints which are removable several times daily or worn only at night may be effective in promoting immobilization.

Splints may also be used to prevent the gradual drifting of joints into poor position. For this purpose splints may be worn at night.

For complete immobilization, an unlined plaster cast is believed to give the maximum degree of immobilization. New plastic splints have greatly increased the strength and decreased the weight of splints so that they may be worn for months without wearing out [11].

Serial knee splints increase range of motion in the knees, but the knees will contract into flexion again unless the patient uses the legs for walking. Dynamic or lively hand splints are effective in increasing range of motion in the fingers—if used before ankylosis or joint destruction has occurred.

Surgery in Arthritis

A large number of surgeons have become interested in rheumatoid arthritis and are rapidly gaining experience under a wide variety of circumstances in many areas of the body [12-13]. Before undertaking reconstructive surgery in rheumatoid arthritis, it is necessary not only to know the condition of the bones, joints and muscles, but also the motivation, emotional make-up, and vocation of the patient. Even under the best conditions, recurrences of the disease may make well-performed surgical procedures useless.

The general indications for surgery are deformities which produce discomfort, loss of function, or a bad cosmetic appearance, and which cannot be corrected by non-surgical means.

Self-Help Devices

In patients with severe contractures of the back, arms or legs, a number of devices may be used which allow performance of the tasks of daily living when physical or surgical methods are not appropriate or have failed. Patients with severely contracted hips may be helped by a wheelchair. For patients who are unable to bend forward to reach the foot, gadgets to help with putting on stockings and shoes may be helpful. Patients with hip contractures may be helped by a raised toilet seat and by chairs with a slanting seat [14].

RESULTS OF TREATMENT IN PATIENTS TREATED AT BALTIMORE CITY HOSPITALS
Diagnostic Group 1

Twenty-seven patients who had rheumatoid arthritis without associated diseases were treated for six months or more. At the end of the treatment, these patients were arranged in rank order dependent on the degree of improvement they had shown in activities of daily living.

The final ranking was then compared with the ranking of a number of measurements made at initial evaluation. The Spearman Rank Correlation Coefficient (r_s) of final ranking with age when first seen was .46; the r_s of duration of illness with final ranking was .32; the r_s for initial MSCL score with final ranking was $-.16$; the r_s for initial ADL score with final ranking was .68; the r_s for duration of treatment with final rank was .13.

This analysis suggests that the ADL score at initial observation is the most important measurement in predicting how much a patient will improve under treatment. The higher the initial ADL score, the more likely the patient will be to show improvement in the ADL score while under treatment. The patient's age, the duration of the disease, the duration of treatment and the initial MSCL score were of decreasing importance in predicting the outcome of treatment.

Diagnostic Groups 1 and 2—Combined (see Table 1, p. 214–215)

Of the 29 patients in this combined group, one had high blood pressure and the other mild diabetes. Table 1 shows that five reached full independence, two reached an ADL score of 90 to 99, and five improved slightly. Nine did

Table 1 Results of Treatment (29 Patients with Rheumatoid Arthritis in Diagnostic Groups 1 and 2—Treated More than 6 Months)

Column		1	2	3	4	5	6
Finding at initial visit	Categories	Total	Reached full independence: ADL score 100	Reached ADL score 90-99	Reached ADL score less than 90	Unchanged ADL score	Deteriorated in ADL score or died
Cases		29	5	2	5	9	8
Age:	59 or less	20	3	2	4	6	5
	60-69	5	2		1		2
	70-79	2				2	
	80 +	2				1	1
Male		12	2	1	3	4	2
Female		17	3	1	2	5	6
Duration at initial visit	Less than 1 year	3	1			1	1
	1 to 5 years	10	2	2		5	1
	6 to 10 years	5			1	1	4
	11 to 20 years	5	2		3	2	
	21 + years	4			1		1
	unknown	2					1

Table 1 Continued

Finding at Initial visit	Column Categories	1 Total	2 Reached full Independence: ADL score 100	3 Reached ADL score 90-99	4 Reached ADL score less than 90	5 Unchanged ADL score	6 Deteriorated in ADL score or died
Initial MSCL score	0-10	1					
	11-20	9					
	21-30	5					
	31-40	10	2		2	1	1
	41-50	11	1	1	2	3	2
						3	5
MSCL not performed		6					
Initial ADL score	0-20	1					1
	21-40	9	1		4	3	1
	41-60	5	1	1		2	1
	61-80	3	1	1			1
	81-95	7	2		1	3	1
	96-100	4				1	3
Diagnostic group	1	27	5		5	8	8
	2	2		1		1	
Duration of treatment	6 mos to 1 yr	7	2		3	2	
	1 to 2 years	1					1(d*)
	2 to 3 years	7		1		3	3(1d*)
	3 to 4 years	6	2		1	2	1
	4 to 5 years	4		1	1	1	1(d*)
	5 to 6 years	3	1				2(1d*)
	6 years +	1				1	

*d = died

215

not improve, and eight deteriorated or died. The numbers are small but agree with the findings of the Spearman Rank Correlation Coefficient analysis that there is no initial finding of outstanding help in predicting whether the patient will or will not improve significantly in ADL score.

Diagnostic Group 3

The 16 patients in this group had associated manifested disease other than rheumatoid arthritis. Five had heart disease, five had lung disease, eleven had neurological or psychiatric problems. One had osteomyelitis of the spine. This group is in no way comparable to Groups 1 and 2, since rheumatoid arthritis was often only an incidental finding. (The importance of separating patients with multiple diseases from those with only one disease has been emphasized.) Of these 16 patients, two reached full independence, two reached an ADL score of 90 to 99, one improved slightly, nine did not improve, and two deteriorated or died.

REFERENCES

1. National Foundation Conference on Rheumatoid Arthritis. *J. Chronic Dis.,* **10**:365, November 1959.
2. Lowman, Edward W.: *Arthritis, General Principles, Physical Medicine and Rehabilitation.* Little, Brown and Co., Boston, 1959.
3. Short, C. L., Bauer, W., and Reynolds, W. E. *Rheumatoid Arthritis.* Harvard University Press, Cambridge, 1957.
4. Talbott, J. H., and Lockie, L. M. *Progress in Arthritis.* Grune and Stratton, New York, 1958.
5. Rheumatism and Arthritis. Review of American and English Literature of Recent Years, Fifteenth Rheumatism Review, *Ann. Int. Med.,* **59**:Suppl. 4, November 1963.
6. Kelly, M. How to Prevent Crippling in Rheumatoid Arthritis. *Lancet,* **1**:1158, June 5, 1954.
7. Rose, D. L., and Kendell, H. W. Rehabilitation of Hand Function in Rheumatoid Arthritis. *JAMA* **148**:1408, 1952.
8. Partridge, R. E. H., and Duthie, J. J. R. Controlled Trial of the Effect of Complete Immobilization of the Joints in Rheumatoid Arthritis. *Ann. Rheum. Dis.,* **22**:91, 1963.
9. Swanson, N. The Prevention and Correction of Deformity in Rheumatoid Arthritis. *Canad. M.A.J.,* **75**:257, 1956.
10. Kelly, M. The Correction and Prevention of Deformity in Rheumatoid Arthritis. *Canad. M.A.J.,* **81**:827, 1959.
11. Rotstein, J. *Simple Splinting.* W. B. Saunders Co., Phila., 1965.
12. Milch, R., Jr. *Surgery of Arthritis.* Williams and Wilkins Co., 1964.
13. Flatt, A. E. *Care of the Rheumatoid Hand.* C. B. Mosby Co., St. Louis, 1963.
14. Lowman, E. W. *Rehabilitation Monograph VI. Self-Help Devices for the Arthritic Institute of Physical Medicine and Rehabilitation.* New York University-Bellevue Medical Center.

Section C

Bowel and Bladder Disorders

The tiny infant is excused in its incontinent state because it is an infant. But society tends to be less tolerant of deviance from the state of full control over the bladder after the stage of infancy is past. Social acceptance is based on control of elimination among other factors—and, even when all other factors are favorable, the loss of bladder or bowel control seems to dictate the response by others. The paraplegic who has achieved good control works in an office and is valued for his intellectual skills which place him on a par with anyone else in the work situation. However, when an accident occurs and he cannot control his urine, the immediate response is shame and withdrawal on his part and embarrassment by his colleagues. He may never return to the office again, having lost the self-esteem which he needs so desperately. For the cord bladder or neurogenic bladder, Delehanty and Stravino describe the state of the art at this moment. For the bladder problems of the aged, perhaps one of the principal forms of training starts with remotivating the patient—helping him to become more alert as described in the section on nursing the geriatric patient. The hypovigilant patient must be assisted to return to reacting with his environment in a meaningful manner before he can cooperate with any retraining program. The problems of lack of self-esteem may be crucial to involving the patient in regaining his control. Rewards must be given for successful performance and understanding given to failures in order to keep the patient motivated toward return of function.

The principal reward is personal. The discomfort of the wet padding or bed should be a sufficient deterrent to resisting any program for control. However, the reward of social acceptance is quite as important. The control, when achieved, leads to other achievements—participation in group activities or return to one's family. The most tolerant of families tires of the constant battle with odor, skin breakdown, and other problems. The nurse who helps such a family and patient to attain successful management derives immense amounts of satisfaction from her work.

Delehanty and Stravino divide their problems into upper motor neuron and lower motor neuron. Roughly all incontinence seems to fall in these two categories. The aging may have a lesion which is less clearly differentiated—a cortical problem which is linked to the general state of awareness. Total person rehabilitation is sought in these instances before bladder retraining is attempted.

In order to plan an individual program, the nurse must be aware of the physiology of voiding. Delehanty and Stravino have stressed these concepts and their implications for planning.

The problem of the retention catheter is one which deserves a great deal of consideration. Under many circumstances it is essential. In the care of the burn patient, the patient in cardiogenic shock, or the patient in diabetic coma, constant monitoring of the renal function must be done by means of a retention catheter. Following surgery, it is frequently placed as a temporary measure. However, its use is questionable for many other situations in which it is now used. The possibility of introducing infection into the urinary tract justifies critical assessment of the real need. At one time, such a device seemed to solve the problems of urinary incontinence, but it has proved a mixed blessing. Today the tendency is to avoid the introduction of any tubes into the bladder for any reason. Once infection has been introduced into the bladder, it must be eradicated before effective retraining programs can be instituted.

The philosophy of this text is that rehabilitation begins with prevention. This includes the necessity of making critical judgments concerning catheterization of the urinary bladder. It is suggested that the use of sensory stimulation techniques be tried as a means of control both in emptying the bladder and in controlling the incontinent flow of urine.

Hill, Shurtleff, Chapman, and Ansell discuss a special variety of incontinence, i.e., that associated with meningomyelocele lesions. They point out realistic and hopeful alternatives to a life swaddled in diapers. They present a clear picture of the condition and a step-by-step presentation of management considerations.

Katona discusses one of the most difficult self-care management problems in the entire spectrum of rehabilitation problems—the management of the colostomate. Almost all the secondary or residual effects of the colostomy procedure are disagreeable. They may, without skillful nursing example and interpretation, intimidate the patient to the point where his disability is maximized and his capacity for normal behavior is minimized. The author describes the problems and patient trauma in detail, and she emphasizes beneficial nursing procedures and patient orientation.

Reading 30
Achieving Bladder Control
Lorraine Delehanty
and
Vincent Stravino

Establishing a voiding pattern despite complete or incomplete central nervous system injury is as much a challenge for the nursing staff as it is for the patient and his physician. An understanding of the underlying physiologic difficulty and the emotionally disruptive effects of incontinence is basic to the nurse's participation in a bladder training program. This knowledge enables her to recognize potential in patients she may have previously considered hopeless, and she will be willing to accept incontinence as an inevitable aspect of nursing care.

Micturition may be an involuntary or a voluntary act. It is an involuntary act when only the spinal reflex mechanism operates, which occurs in everyone who is not toilet trained. It is voluntary when the sensation of the need to void is carried to the brain, and the person is able to relax the muscles of the perineum and contract the abdominal muscles to help initiate voiding. The normal course of events in urination is as follows:

1 The bladder wall expands with increasing urine volume, usually until a volume of 150 to 250 ml. of urine is reached. Stretch receptors in the detrusor muscle (the three-layered, smooth muscular wall of the bladder) then send impulses to the voiding reflex center in the spinal cord via the visceral afferent pelvic nerves. This reflex for voiding is located in the spinal cord at the level of the second to the fourth sacral segments.

2 The sensation of the desire to urinate is then carried to centers in the midbrain and pons which are under voluntary cortical control.

3 If the time for voiding is appropriate, the brain will send impulses to motoneurons in the sacral area of the spinal cord causing the parasympathetic efferent fibers of the pelvic nerve to stimulate the bladder muscle to contract. Urine is released from the bladder to the external urinary sphincter.

4 Relaxation of the external sphincter, necessary to the act of voiding, takes place through inhibition of the pudendal nerve by the impulses from the spinal micturition center. Normally, the external sphincter is kept closed except during the act of voiding. This spinal center is also controlled by the

Reprinted from *American Journal of Nursing*, vol. 70, no. 2, pp. 312–316, February 1970. The authors wish to express their appreciation to Theodore Cole, M.D., and Thomas Lutz, medical illustrator, for their assistance in preparation of this article.

higher centers in the brain. The pudendal nerve originates in the sacral spinal cord and innervates both the external urinary and rectal sphincters [1].

To summarize, normal voiding is a reflex act under voluntary cortical control. Voiding may be voluntarily inhibited by constriction of the external urinary sphincter. It is through teaching and constant conditioning of this sphincter that the child learns to inhibit the voiding reflex at inappropriate times and, thus, becomes toilet trained.

INCONTINENCE WITH CORD BLADDERS

The term "cord bladder" or "neurogenic bladder" is used to describe bladder dysfunctions which result from lesions of the central nervous system. Incontinence resulting from spinal cord injury is basically of two types and corresponds to the level of the damage to the nervous system. The essential difference between these two types of cord bladder is the presence or absence of injury to the reflex center in the spinal cord. In the bladder with an upper motor neuron lesion, the sacral reflex center is saved; however, it is damaged in the bladder with a lower motor neuron lesion. Other terms used to describe upper motor neuron bladders are reflex, automatic, spastic, and central. The terms nonreflex, autonomous, flaccid, and peripheral are used to describe the lower motor neuron bladder.

In the upper motor neuron bladder, nerve damage occurs above the sacral spinal cord and frees the voiding reflex from voluntary control. This damage produces a bladder which acts independently of the patient's wishes. It is a reflex bladder because it will abruptly empty when the stretch receptors in the bladder muscle wall reach their threshold. The patient has no sensation of bladder filling, and voiding is involuntary. One of the difficulties with this type of bladder is that the external sphincter as well as the detrusor muscle may be spastic, thereby preventing adequate emptying of the bladder.

A lower motor neuron lesion, one in which the innervation to the bladder muscle and the external sphincter is damaged, occurs with such conditions as tumor, infections, or trauma in the sacral cord. There is no interruption of cerebral control, but, rather, no way to effect this control.

In this state of total denervation, the bladder muscle loses its normal tone, and the patient is unable to void by reflex emptying. With continual distension, the bladder wall becomes thin, flabby, and without sensation, retaining as much as 1,000 cc. of urine. In the normal bladder, the sensation of fullness occurs when the bladder contains approximately 150 cc. of urine, and discomfort is noted when the urine in the bladder exceeds 350 cc. The patient with a lower motor neuron bladder frequently voids in small amounts, but this is overflow incontinence. This is especially common during movement such as transferring from a wheelchair to a bed. The patient is not able to sense bladder fullness, stimulate detrusor contraction, or inhibit the leakage of urine which results from overflow dribbling.

Neurogenic bladders do not always exist as pure types. Patients often have a mixed type of cord bladder with either partial sensation or partial voluntary control. This type of "mixed" bladder is seen in the patient with damage to the cerebral cortex, such as cerebrovascular lesion, tumor, or multiple sclerosis. It would be classified an incomplete upper motor neuron bladder. These patients may be bladder-trained more easily than the patient with a complete upper motor neuron lesion because of their remaining partial sensation and control. They must be given a carefully supervised trial period without the catheter in order to determine their voiding abilities. Generally, they have urgency to void but damaged ability to inhibit voiding at inopportune times [2].

The state of a damaged bladder can change with time. For example, in spinal cord injury above the sacral spinal cord, the bladder undergoes a period of areflexia, in which all reflexes are absent, similar to the period of spinal shock in the skeletal muscles. The period of spinal shock with flaccid muscles is followed by the gradual return of spinal reflexes and spasticity in both the skeletal and bladder muscles.

TRAINING CORD BLADDERS

As might be expected, the training for each type of bladder is different—but goals in all cases of urinary incontinence are similar: (1) adequate bladder emptying with low residual urine to eliminate infection; (2) a predictable voiding pattern, that is, one that is socially acceptable.

To determine if a patient with a neurogenic bladder is able to void without the catheter, a trial of voiding is attempted. A trial of voiding requires that any severe bladder infection be eradicated. An adequate fluid intake of between 3,000 and 4,000 cc. a day is encouraged, and urinary antiseptics such as methenamine mandelate, usually with acidifiers such as ascorbic acid, are given to minimize bacterial growth in the urine, which must be expected when the catheter is in the bladder. It is valuable to have a recent cystogram showing no reflux of urine from the bladder proximally into the ureters, and a recent cystometrogram measuring bladder pressures will provide information as to the type of bladder present.

There is some doubt concerning the value of intermittent clamping and unclamping of the catheter as a part of bladder reeducation. On the assumption that clamping may produce acute urinary infections, it is not used at the University of Minnesota Rehabilitation Center.

The patient must be informed of the details of a trial of voiding. He must be told that initial failure or success is not necessarily indicative of permanent failure or success.

UPPER MOTOR NEURON BLADDERS

The patient with the complete upper motor neuron bladder usually does not receive the message of his need to void, but there may be sensations associated with a full bladder such as sweating, restlessness, and abdominal discomfort which warn him of the need to empty his bladder. The nurse can help this patient find "trigger areas" which initiate the voiding reflex when stimulated. Common trigger areas may be found on the thigh, abdomen, or genitalia. Digital stimulation of the anus and rectum is the most effective stimulus, but tapping the abdomen or doing push-ups on the commode chair may also be effective in precipitating voiding.

The trial-of-voiding procedure followed at University Hospitals for patients with an upper motor neuron bladder is as follows: (1) The catheter is removed at 6:00 A.M., and the patient is given 200 cc. of liquid each half hour until 8:00 A.M. (2) Using one of the trigger areas, the patient is stimulated to void. (3) If he is able to void, the amount of residual urine in the bladder is checked immediately. This amount determines whether the trial may safely continue. If the residual is over 100 cc., the patient's catheter is replaced, and the trial is considered unsuccessful. If the residual is under 100 cc., however, the procedure continues and the patient receives 200 cc. of liquid every hour and is stimulated to void every two to three hours. Residual urines are checked at three-hour intervals, depending on the patient's ability to void throughout the day.

The nurse must know exactly what the intake and output are in order to prevent overdistension of the bladder. Overdistension could damage the bladder muscle, could cause ureterovesical reflux, and could predispose the patient to infection. If the patient is voiding in adequate amounts, he is left catheter-free for the night, but stops drinking fluids in the early evening. He is, however, stimulated to void at 8:00 P.M. and 11:00 P.M. The program then resumes at 6:00 A.M. with a glass of liquid each hour.

If the patient is a male quadriplegic and he continues to be successful with the catheter removed, a condom catheter or other external drainage appliance may be used to simplify his self-care and avoid socially embarrassing "accidents."

During the hospital stay, when it becomes apparent that the patient is voiding in good amounts on a regular basis, he is taught to plan a daily home schedule. He learns to space his intake of 3,000 to 4,000 cc. of fluid throughout his waking hours and plans to attempt to void every four hours. In patients with complete upper motor neuron lesions, for example, quadriplegic patients, it is often difficult to achieve success because of the spasticity of the urinary sphincter, which prevents adequate bladder emptying. However, when success is achieved, it is important for the patient to have regular posthospitalization checkups in order to continue determining the amount of residual urine in the bladder after voiding and the condition of the bladder and kidneys.

LOWER MOTOR NEURON BLADDERS

To determine if a patient with a lower motor neuron lesion is able to void without the catheter, a trial of voiding is also attempted, but a somewhat different technique is used. A lower motor neuron bladder shows no spontaneous activity since the reflex arc is broken; therefore, emptying is assisted by external pressure suprapubically on the abdomen as with Credé's method. Straining as in Valsalva's maneuver or contraction of the abdominal muscles, if possible, may also be effective, and these procedures are taught as part of the patient's self-care.

The trial of voiding in the lower motor neuron bladders consists of the following: (1) The catheter is removed at 6:00 A.M., and the fluid intake is restricted to 200 cc. every hour. (2) The patient attempts to void within two hours. (3) The residual is checked after the patient voids. If the residual is under 50 cc., the trial of voiding continues. A residual lower than 50 cc. in patients with lower motor neuron lesions is expected because the external sphincter in this bladder is flaccid, and urine can often be adequately expressed with sufficient external pressure.

Drugs may also be used in the treatment of incontinence. Propantheline bromide (Pro-Banthine) inhibits the action of the parasympathetic nervous system and may be used to decrease the activity of a hypertonic detrusor, such as in a spastic upper motor neuron bladder. In a hypotonic detrusor muscle, muscular contractions may be increased by bethanechol chloride (Urecholine), which mimics the activity of the parasympathetic nervous system.

Diazepam (Valium) shows promise for the treatment of incontinence in spastic bladders. This drug is effective in reducing skeletal muscle spasticity, including spasticity of the external urinary sphincter. Diazepam often allays the patient's anxiety, which sometimes contributes to urinary urgency and incontinence.

The patient with an incomplete lesion, such as the hemiplegic patient, has a good chance for bladder training because his reflex arc is intact, and he also has partial sensation and partial voluntary control of his bladder. The procedure for his trial of voiding is similar to the one for the patient with an upper motor neuron lesion.

Because of impaired sensation in the bladder, the patient must be taught to respond to his diminished sensations. The nursing staff can promote this awareness by encouraging the patient to regulate his intake and to maintain a regular voiding schedule during the day. Any success should be praised. It may also help to have the patient dress in his own clothing to encourage him to remain continent. Since the supine position is inadequate for voiding, the patient should sit on a commode or, if male, stand well supported.

There may be a tendency to have accidents at night; in males, a condom catheter or night urinal within easy reach may be recommended until the patient's awareness has increased. Increased social stimulation may help increase the elderly patient's alertness and self-awareness in cooperating with a bladder training program.

All of the trial-of-voiding procedures require close nursing observations and accurate recording of intake and output, the frequency of voiding, the force of the stream, the patient's subjective sensations, and his behavior during his trial.

DEVELOPING A BLADDER PROGRAM

Unfortunately, bladder training is not a simple procedure. It must be highly individualized, depending on the pathology of the injury and the personality of the patient. The knowledge and interest of the staff is also a determining factor of success.

The image that a person has of himself after loss of bladder function affects his feelings about himself as a whole. There are rather firm ideas established at a young age concerning control of one's excretions. Once a child has mastered control at 16 to 18 months, it is of little concern unless control is somehow lost. One patient made the relationship between incontinence and infancy by stating, "My wife changes the kids all day, and now I'm added to her list."

It is usually advisable to wait until the patient has resolved some of the shock of the disability before approaching him with a bladder training program. Timing, as well as technique, are very important. During these first few months, the patient may tend to ignore his bladder disability and refuse to take part in the necessary procedures. Resistance and denial must be understood as part of a natural process in which the patient is limiting his view of the total disability in order to cope with a few facts at a time [3]. As he asks to participate in his care or shows interest in what the nurse is doing, there is fairly good indication that he is ready to hear more.

The importance of proper timing and sensitivity to the patient's feelings were made evident in the case of Mike S., a 21-year-old college student who sustained a T10 fracture in a skiing accident. His first admission lasted three months, and during this time he was apathetic and easily discouraged. He preferred to stay in bed as much as possible, covering himself from head to toe with a sheet. A common statement heard in reference to Mike was, "He certainly has potential, but just won't use it."

A trial of voiding was attempted even though Mike indicated he didn't care if it worked or not. Needless to say, the trial was unsuccessful.

It was true that Mike did have potential for rehabilitation, but he was unable to mobilize this potential because he did not yet have the strength to accept his disabled body. Not only was his bladder in shock, but also his mind and spirit. Mike was discharged to his home to return in three months. He left as an angry, depressed young man, unable to see much future in his life as a paraplegic.

On readmission, there was a noticeable change in Mike's attitude toward himself. He had obviously used his three-month "vacation" from the hospital in a constructive way. He had developed many plans and ideas to improve his self-care. He was also interested in getting rid of the catheter. Cystometric studies indicated some reflex activity, so another trial of voiding was performed. At 8:00 A.M. on the day of the trial of voiding, the catheter was removed. He had 85 cc. residual. This was high, but within the acceptable limit of 100 cc. He continued on the trial for three days with very close observation. On the third day his residual ranged from 15 to 20 cc., which indicated a successful trial.

Mike was able to reenter college and was most happy to be free of the indwelling catheter. He found the condom catheter to be of much greater convenience for him since he no longer needed to irrigate his bladder and did not need to sterilize equipment, as with the indwelling catheter. It was also pointed out to Mike that success at this time was not necessarily permanent and that close observation of his intake and output was very important.

As with many patients, Mike's time to initiate a trial of voiding was when he was ready for it, when it assumed value for him and his future plans. He had needed to take time to reflect on his total condition and to try to work through some of the body-image difficulties; he was able to become a more efficient problem-solver and, consequently, made significant advances in his self-care.

CONCLUSION

The treatment of incontinence depends on the location of the lesion which is causing the incontinence, whether it is an upper motor neuron lesion or a lower motor neuron lesion. The nurse who assists the patient in bladder training must have a clear idea of the type of lesion and its implications for the training program. An understanding of the emotionally disruptive effects of the loss of bladder function on the patient's total body image is crucial in the treatment of this condition. The individual response to a loss of body function is highly variable, but the sensitive nurse will recognize what meaning this has for the patient and will more accurately determine the correct timing for the introduction of this procedure. This knowledge and sensitive judgment can reduce the needless use of the indwelling catheter in patients who have the potential for bladder training. "Healing," Hippocrates wrote in *Precepts I,* "is a matter of time, but it is sometimes also a matter of opportunity."

REFERENCES

1 Best, C. H., and Taylor, N. B. (eds.). *Physiological Basis of Medical Practice: A Text in Applied Physiology,* 8th ed. Baltimore, Md., Williams and Wilkins Co., 1966.
2 Schutt, A. H., and others. Problems of the bladder and bowel in patients with myelopathies. *J. Lancet,* **87**:187-189, June 1967.
3 Shontz, F. C., and others. Chronic physical illness as a threat. *Arch. Phys. Med.,* **41**:143-147, April 1960.

Reading 31
The Myelodysplastic Child—Bowel and Bladder Control

Margaret L. Hill
David B. Shurtleff
Warren H. Chapman
and
Julian S. Ansell

For the normal child, achievement of toilet control is an integral part of achieving self-identity and self-conceptualization. The child with meningomyelocele, however, rarely achieves this control because of the resultant neurogenic bowel and bladder.

Of all the problems to which handicapped children are subject, urinary and stool incontinence is perhaps the most frustrating and socially unaccept-

Reprinted from *The American Journal of Nursing,* vol. 69, no. 3, pp. 545-550, March 1969.

able. Therefore, at the Birth Defects Center associated with the University of Washington School of Medicine, interdisciplinary efforts have been focused for some years now on the medical and nursing management of the myelodysplastic child. As part of the overall care, we have initiated a program of practical management of incontinence, the goal being to assist the myelodysplastic child to attain the highest possible degree of independence in his daily living.

NATURE OF THE PROBLEM

The lower bowel, bladder, and their sphincters depend upon intact innervation from the lumbosacral nerve roots to precipitate the normal reflex of micturition. This reflex act, however, is subject to voluntary control. The forces of expulsion and retention are reciprocally balanced at all times, and the higher brain centers can facilitate or inhibit these forces at will.

Since most meningomyelocele lesions are lumbosacral, the cauda equina or bilateral roots of the pelvic nerves which carry both motor and sensory fibers controlling micturition are affected in varying degrees. The reflexes essential for micturition are thus interrupted, and the bladder is isolated from the higher brain center. The result is a hypotonic bladder with uncoordinated, arrhythmic contractions, a purely flaccid, or a spastic bladder.

The patient can neither inhibit nor initiate micturition. Clinically, such incontinence is most commonly manifested by two patterns: (1) constant dribbling due to overflow, and (2) intermittent dribbling with one- to two-hour periods of dryness.

The mechanisms involved are, on the one hand, intact autonomous reflexes distal to the spinal lesion which allow uninhibited sphincter and urethral muscular contractions. On the other hand, a weak detrusor muscle with uncoordinated and arrhythmic contractions decompensates while trying to express urine through the tight sphincter and urethra. This muscle imbalance inhibits complete emptying of the bladder; varying amounts of residual urine are retained, and infection follows. Bladder dilation progresses to the point of allowing ureterovesical reflux with progressive hydronephrosis.

A meningomyelocele usually affects the bowel, too, since the levator ani and external anal sphincter musculature are supplied by the sacral nerve outflow. It has been suggested that the functional status of the sphincter ani externum parallels that of the sphincter urogenitalis (urethrae), so that paralysis of both anal and bladder sphincters often occurs at the same time.

The resulting disturbances of bowel function consist of constipation, lack of voluntary anal sphincter control, weakly spastic (stretch reflex) anal sphincter, and, occasionally, rectal prolapse. There is usually a lack of normal contractile tone in the lower bowel and rectum.

Because of sensory loss, there is usually no indication of discomfort or urge to defecate. Poor bowel musculature and the lack of force that results from the absent Valsalva maneuver fail to expel feces past the spastic sphincter. Obstinate constipation will often result; sometimes a false diarrhea of liquid feces around a gross impaction occurs. Chronic, unregulated constipation causes a secondary gut dilatation. However, keeping feces slightly firmer than normal proves advantageous, since involuntary defecation is less likely to occur under these circumstances than with soft or liquid stool.

Of the many defects associated with meningomyelocele, urinary and fecal incontinence is perhaps the most distressing for the child and his family. Certainly, these organic problems create both physical and psychosocial difficulties.

During the first two to three years of life, the incontinence can be managed by the "normal" methods used for that age group: diapers. Beyond that point, however, diapers become socially unacceptable; so do accidents of elimination. The full impact of the situation may not be realized until the child reaches school age and finds himself deprived of school attendance, solely because of the incontinence.

In addition, the child with meningomyelocele often becomes over-dependent upon his parents to provide him with perineal hygiene. In turn, parents become overindulgent and overprotective, thus suffocating the child's individuality and independence. Yet, if it is important for the normal child to have opportunities to develop into an independent individual, how much more so for the child with meningomyelocele.

The progress he makes in this direction is influenced not only by his social environment, but also by his intellectual capacity, educational opportunities, motivation, and the variations in the pattern of complications secondary to the myelodysplasia. In addition, learning must be carefully timed to insure maximum benefit.

Keeping all these things in mind, we have tried to develop a hygiene program that is practical and flexible enough to fit any social environment. Our children progress to as full and nearly independent a life as possible. The program begins in infancy and stresses the early establishment of a socially acceptable method of urine and feces control; special emphasis is put on skin care, fluid and dietary regulation, and awareness of the importance of urinary tract infection. The full understanding and cooperation of the child and his family are necessary and we do everything possible to inform and motivate them.

UROLOGIC MANAGEMENT

Fecal incontinence, unpleasant though it may be, is no threat to the patient's life. However, a malfunctioning urinary tract can result in renal failure. Therefore, a primary consideration in the medical management of these patients is the prevention of renal destruction.

When patients with meningomyelocele or any of the forms of spina bifida cystica are first seen at our center, a complete biologic assessment is made of all systems. This is followed by a conference to ascertain whether the patient needs care for any of the problems associated with meningomyelocele. We will discuss here only bowel and urinary tract management.

During the first two years of life, the chief focus is on detecting any changes that indicate progressive obstruction and recurrent infection in the urinary tract. In our series of myelodysplastic children followed from birth, all manifested some abnormality ranging from infection to massive hydronephrosis by the time they had reached their second birthday. The cinecystogram has been the most valuable diagnostic procedure, since it permits visualization of reflux and detects early deterioration of the upper urinary tract.

During the first few years of life, radiographic studies of the urinary tract are undertaken routinely at six-month intervals and more often if indicated. Urinalysis is done once or twice a month to detect infection during the intervals between roentgenographic studies.

If reflux is present, procedures aimed at lowering residual urine are indicated. These vary from simple internal urethrotomy and/or sphincterotomy to a plastic procedure on the bladder neck (Y.V.-plasty) to open it more widely and allow the urine easier egress. Reimplantation of the ureters has been tried but is usually successful only when combined with a procedure devised to reduce the intravesical pressure. The majority of our ureteral reimplantations have been failures.

An indwelling catheter, draining off urine either through the urethra or directly through the abdominal wall as a cystotomy, has been used with some success by us and by others. However, the catheter acts as a foreign body and is undesirable, with its accompanying infection, stone formation, plugging, urethral inflammation, diverticuli, and fistula formation.

After the age of two, the patient's urinary tracts are reevaluated annually unless signs suggestive of decompensation are detected in the interval. The male bladder is kept intact since the boy has a "spigot," permitting the use of urine collection devices. In the female, however, no adequate collection device has been devised, and a catheter or diversion technique is more often used.

The best known of the urinary diversions is the uretero-ileal cutaneous ureterostomy (ileal loop), in which the ureters are implanted in an isolated segment of the small bowel which is brought out to the side of the abdomen. A watertight collection device is worn on the skin around this opening.

A second method of diversion is the cutaneous vesicostomy of Lapides. In this procedure, a flap of bladder and a flap of skin are joined together to form the circumference of a tube that opens directly from the bladder onto the skin. A collection device similar to the ileostomy collector must be worn over this opening to collect the urine.

These procedures must be coordinated with any necessary orthopedic measures, since either a body cast or a brace might interfere with the placement of collection devices. Besides, spillage of uncollectable urine can destroy a plaster cast very rapidly.

Whatever corrective measure is used, all those associated with the child's care, including his parents, must be alerted to the ever-present possibility of urinary tract infection. Odoriferous urine or the development of chills or fever are suggestive symptoms that should be reported promptly. Children rarely complain of frequency, dysuria, or urgency.

Good urine flow and complete bladder emptying reduce the opportunity for bacteria to multiply in residual urine. Therefore, adequate fluid intake—125 cc. per kilogram of body weight, or 2 ounces per pound—is a daily must. Good drinking habits need to be formed early.

If there is no reflux of urine, parents may be instructed to do a Credé maneuver (application of suprapubic pressure over the bladder) with each diaper change to express residual urine. They need careful instruction and close supervision at first, to be sure that they do it properly. The whole hand should be placed on or above the dome of the bladder to give gentle pressure downward. However, if the procedure requires too much pressure it should be discontinued, as there is danger of producing reflux into the ureters.

As soon as possible, the child should be taught to do the Credé himself. He can do this best in the sitting position, pushing his hand into the suprapubic area and applying pressure downward.

We have devised special urine-collecting equipment (described later) for both boys and girls to use as they grow older and advance beyond the diaper stage. Before these can be used, however, bowel control must be established. From infancy on, special attention must be given to the buttocks and perineal skin, not only because of the incontinence but also because of the usually impaired sensation in these areas.

An adequate bowel program consists of (1) keeping the fecal mass of normal consistency or slightly firmer to insure easy evacuation and (2) a timed, consistent evacuation. The bowel program should be established as early as possible, since the bacterial action of the feces complicates skin care. In addition, impacted feces in the rectum press forward on the urethra to favor retention of urine by preventing proper drainage.

BOWEL CONTROL

We initiate our bowel program when the child is approximately one year old. One-quarter or half of a bisacodyl (Dulcolax) suppository is inserted as high as possible into the rectum every morning before breakfast. The amount of suppository used depends upon the age and size of the child; too much causes abdominal pain, and too little, no action.

The bisacodyl's stimulating action with the gastric-colic reflex following a meal produces evacuation in 20 to 40 minutes. Hence, following breakfast, the child is placed on a pottie chair or toilet with his feet on the floor so that the hips are flexed to the "squat" position. Abdominal pressure is important, so he should lean forward to compress the abdomen against the thighs and/or massage the abdominal muscles. Depending on his age, he can do this himself.

He is encouraged to strain at the same time. For the young child who does not understand the concept of straining, blowing up a toy balloon will serve the same purpose. It is the effort exerted, not just the sitting, that insures success.

As soon as possible, the child is encouraged to take care of the duty of bowel control on his own.

Because the infant will be wet most of the time, the diapers should be changed at frequent and regular intervals during the day. The buttocks and perineum should be cleansed with an antibacterial soap and water and thoroughly dried at least twice a day and every time feces are present at diaper change.

BUTTOCKS AND PERINEAL CARE

Exposing the perineum to the air most of the day and/or to a heat lamp 15 to 20 minutes twice a day aids in preventing or eliminating diaper rashes. Diapers should be soaked in vinegar water or one of several commercially available solutions in an effort to prevent the formation of ammonia salts, which predispose to rashes and decubiti.

Frequent change of position as the child learns to sit will prevent pressure on the atrophied gluteal muscles and ischial tuberosities. If the child is semiambulatory or not able to be up, he can (1) be placed in the prone position on the bed or floor; (2) stand a few hours each day on a tilt table or in a standing box; or (3) when he is old enough, be encouraged to push up from his sitting position every 15 to 30 minutes to raise his buttocks. Such positions allow for circulation of air over and blood through tissues of the buttocks.

A silicone pad placed under the buttocks is beneficial not only in preventing but also in healing decubiti. These pads are available commercially; so is a greaseless silicone cream (Covecon) that can be used to prevent incontinence scald and rashes. The cream puts a protective coating between healthy skin and urine or stool. For best results it should be applied twice a day, after careful cleansing of the soiled areas, during the first one to two weeks of treatment. Less frequent applications are often sufficient thereafter. The ointment should not be used over raw, weeping areas.

URINARY CONTROL

A pediatric collection device for boys and special panties for girls help in the management of urinary incontinence once the child is beyond the diaper stage and "social acceptability" becomes increasingly important.[1]

Boys

The boys, especially if they are ambulatory, are fitted with the collection device at about the age of three. Since the appliance will not function adequately under diapers, bowel control must already have been established. We also recommend prior circumcision for cleanliness and prevention of penile ulceration.

Parents and child are instructed in the special skin and apparatus care necessary to insure proper functioning and to prevent penile ulcerations. These instructions include:

1 Wash the penis and perineal area with soap and water and dry thoroughly before applying and after removing the drainage device.
2 Have two collection devices and use them alternately.
3 Wash the appliance and urine-collecting bag with mild soap and water, dry, and powder with cornstarch. Soak the device in vinegar water 15 to 30 minutes if urine odor persists.
4 Do not use ointments or powder on penis or perineum (unless specifically ordered to do so), as they predispose the area to decubiti by localizing bacteria.
5 If penile ulcerations occur, discontinue appliance until skin clears.
6 Unless contraindicated, use the Credé maneuver to reduce residual urine each time the collection bag is drained.

---

[1] The boys' collection device is manufactured commercially as the Hill Pediatric Urinal and is available from the Davol Rubber Co., Providence, R.I. The girls' panties are not available commercially, but a pattern for making them will be sent on request by the author. Write Mrs. Margaret Hill, Department of Pediatrics, School of Medicine, University of Washington, Seattle, Washington.

Boys wear long pants which fit over the apparatus. A zipper opening in the inner leg seam of the trouser allows for emptying the collection bag.

The appliance should not be worn at night. Instead, pads or heavy training pants can be used to protect patient and bed. A heavy bath towel placed within a specially folded latex drawsheet is helpful. But no diapers, please.

Girls

Management of urinary incontinence in girls is somewhat more complicated because of their anatomy. Many of them, however, are on catheter drainage and they, or their parents, are instructed about skin care, bladder irrigation (if ordered), and care of the catheter and collection bag.

1 Wash the perineum, urethral meatus, and the catheter near site of insertion with a hexachlorophene soap and water daily, to remove accumulated secretions which provide a nidus for infection or concretions.

2 Flush the catheter daily with 15 to 30 cc. of an acidifying and antibacterial solution as ordered by the physician (we use Renacidin). A clean irrigation technique is used unless otherwise ordered. Written instructions for the procedure are provided, which emphasize squeezing the bulb several times to be sure that the solution reaches all bladder areas and leaving the solution in the bladder to be flushed out by the normal urine flow. Attach catheter to collection device at conclusion of irrigation. Soak syringe in soapy water for 10 minutes, rinse, and store in clean towel.

3 At night, attach catheter to night drainage bag that either sits on floor or hangs on side of bed.

4 Have two collection bags and alternate their use daily. After use, wash the bag with mild soap and water. Do not use detergents, as they cause deterioration of rubber.

5 Ointments or powders on perineal area are contraindicated unless specifically ordered.

Catheters are usually changed every four weeks or as necessary. If there is urine leakage around a functioning catheter, a larger size may be indicated. Injection of 8 to 10 cc. of water into the Foley bulb helps prevent leakage. If the patient lives in the area, she comes to the clinic for catheter change; otherwise, the community public health nurse changes it. Occasionally, parents are instructed in changing the catheter.

Patients with catheters are encouraged to drink large amounts of fluid (100 to 150 cc. per kg. body weight every 24 hours). This helps maintain a free flow of urine, prevents crystallization of salts and stone formation, and reduces the hazard of infection. Among the fluids should be cranberry juice to maintain an acid pH (ascorbic or mandelic acid may also be prescribed) and to prevent stone formation, certain types of bacterial infection, and mucus formation (a frequent cause of catheter obstruction).

Girls who are not on catheter drainage or who have an ileostomy are encouraged to discard the diapers at the appropriate age level, substitute the special panties, and follow the routine below:

1   Change inserts frequently (every two to three hours). Inserts can be made from diaper material, or commercial sanitary pads are used.
2   Wash perineum and buttocks area twice a day with mild soap containing hexachlorophene, and dry thoroughly. (We encourage the use of silicone cream on the buttocks area.)
3   If rash develops, expose the area to air or sun lamp for 15 to 20 minutes.
4   Soak inserts and panties in vinegar water before washing. Drip dry following routine wash; spin dry when possible.
5   Don't wear panties at night, but use specially folded drawsheet with towel insert.

Skin and appliance care is equally important for the child who has an ileal loop with collecting bag. We demonstrate the application of the device to the parents and child before she leaves the hospital. Their written instructions include:

1   Wash around the appliance daily with mild soap and water.
2   If bag comes off, wash skin around stoma with mild soap and water and dry thoroughly. Remove any cement left on skin.
3   Do not apply ointment to skin. If the skin is irritated, apply karaya gum powder (we use Healskin). If irritation persists, the physician should be consulted.
4   To prevent odors, put two tablespoons of vinegar in the collection bag each day. (A special deodorizing tablet is available, but vinegar works just as well.)
5   Soak appliance after removal in warm soapy water (nondetergent, please!) and alternate the use of two appliances.

The length of time between appliance changes is individual and may vary from 1 to 10 days; a 3- to 4-day interval is recommended. Parents and child are taught to dilate the stoma by inserting the index finger into the stoma opening and gently rotating it down through the muscle fascia. This prevents contractions at the level of the abdominal wall. The frequency of the dilatations are determined by the physician.

CONTINUED EDUCATION

Continued education and reinforcement of learned processes are essential for insuring the child's progress in achieving self-care skills. We review care with both the parent and child at least every six months, in the hospital or clinic. In addition, a detailed referral containing information about the patient's condition and home care recommendations is sent to the public health nurse and to the family physician.

Intensive home visits by the community public health nurse are crucial when the care program is being learned. However, as families become more independent, less frequent visits are necessary. Frequency of home visitation is determined by the nurse's assessment of the needs of the patient and his family. To insure continuity, she sends us a nursing assessment of the patient's and family's progress prior to each clinic appointment or whenever there is an identifiable problem that needs further follow-up by our group.

PROGRAM EFFECTIVENESS

To determine the effectiveness of our program, a prospective study of 46 children with meningomyelocele was made. The group includes all children seen regularly at the Birth Defects Center from January 1, 1966 to April 1, 1967. Thirty-one of the children were in the preschool (0-4) age group, and 15 were of school age (5-10 years). Each child was categorized at the beginning of the study according to the type of bowel and bladder management program. If he was not on a program, then one appropriate for his condition, age, and sex was initiated. Each child's progress was assessed at three-month intervals.

At the end of one year 76 percent of the study group had adequate bowel management (3 or fewer non-scheduled evacuations per week) as compared to only 13 percent with such control when the program started. In relation to urinary control, approximately 26 percent of the children were using either the male collecting device or the female panties at the end of this study period, whereas none had been previously. An additional 23 percent (all girls) had ileal loops or catheters, in contrast to 11 percent, to begin with. The group on diapers alone had dropped from 54 percent to 2 percent; 48 percent were on diapers and Credé at the end of the study, but under better control.

In other words, those patients with urine collection by ileal loop, penile collector, or panty (almost 35 percent of the group) are currently socially acceptable without odor, skin rash, or decubiti. All girls on catheter drainage in the study are doing well after an initial period of learning to care for and replace the catheter at appropriate intervals. Two of them, however, showed progressive urinary tract dilatation despite adequate symptomatic control by Foley catheter drainage; both have had ileal loop procedures and are now well controlled.

As with catheter drainage, we have observed only partial success with Credé. This maneuver is not prescribed for any child with reflux, since it may increase the reflux tendency. All patients on Credé or catheter management programs should be observed regularly and carefully for signs of urinary tract anatomic deterioration and/or bacterial infection.

This study, plus 10 years of working with these children, has convinced us that:

1 What self-care skills the myelodysplastic child learns depend on his social environment, intellectual capacity, motivation, and disorder.
2 Management of bowel and bladder incontinence depends upon a compulsive, rigorous, and consistent medical and nursing program and upon repeated reinforcement of the learning for parents and child.
3 Regardless of the state of continence, reflux and infection must be treated by appropriate medical and surgical intervention in order to prevent renal failure.
4 Continuous parental education, anticipatory guidance, and treatment with a multidisciplinary approach, including the public health nurse in the community, permit achievement of realistic goals.
5 Early institution of hygienic control insures appropriate timing for learning and a much higher percentage of success in establishing a healthy and socially acceptable method of stool and urine control.

As for satisfactions, hearing a child say proudly, "I don't have to wear diapers any more," or seeing him now able to attend school and engage in social activities, are rewards in themselves.

Reading 32
Learning Colostomy Control
Elizabeth A. Katona

Colostomy control is achieved when fecal material is expelled from the colostomy only during irrigation; at other times, the colostomy is free of spillage. This control is necessary so the colostomate can see himself as a whole person again, an adult in control of his own body.

To achieve this goal, the patient needs to learn the anatomy and physiology of the bowel, how to use the equipment, and how regulating his diet, irrigation routine, and other habits can help him obtain and maintain control.

The nurse needs to decide how much information each individual should have, and in how much detail, since too much at one time will

Reprinted from *The American Journal of Nursing*, vol. 67, no. 3, pp. 534-539, March 1967.

increase his anxiety rather than relieve it. He is taught in a simple and direct manner in the amount and degree he can assimilate and understand. He is told he will be taught one step at a time, and "first things first" are emphasized. And, especially in the early stages, frequent repetition may be necessary.

We first teach the patient what a colostomy is and point out the various locations of colostomies on a schematic drawing of the bowel. Then we show him which type of colostomy he has and discuss its significance in relation to the bowel's absorbing and storing functions [1]. We emphasize not what he has lost but what he has left. This is important because people wonder how they can live without a bowel. They understand better when they can see that what is lost is a part of a reservoir, not essential to life. So we point out that the entire colon can be removed without interference with life processes; that removal of a portion of the bowel is also safe, and a rather common procedure; and that individuals in all walks of life have colostomies and continue to carry on normal daily activities.

Thus the patient learns that the colostomy is an opening into the large bowel, that stool will be evacuated from this opening thereafter, since the rectum will have been removed, and that the protrusion of the bowel through the abdomen forms a round, bud-like structure called a stoma. We tell him there will be a perineal wound where the rectum has been removed and an abdominal wound where the obstruction has been relieved, and that these areas will be covered with a dressing until they are sufficiently healed. After the bowel begins to function (in approximately two to four days) the abdominal dressing will be removed and the stoma covered with a temporary "ostomy" bag. To remove the mystery and fear of what the stoma will look like, and thus help the patient look at it in the early postoperative period, we tell him it is the same type of tissue as that inside the mouth (pointing out that the mouth is the beginning of the alimentary canal) and that it may be pink to reddish in color. We explain that it will later shrink in size and that it changes size with change in body position, so he will not be alarmed when this occurs.

It is my experience that the patient's postoperative ability to accept his colostomy readily is affected by his understanding of it, and whether he gains this through planned teaching or through the interpretation of his fellow patients, friends, or relatives. When the doctor and nurse explain, discuss, listen, and re-explain, many of the patient's anxieties are minimized. However, when relatives or friends tell the uninformed patient about acquaintances who went through this horrible experience, his fears are increased a hundredfold.

His postoperative adjustment also depends on the manner in which he has been cared for during the diagnostic workup. When adequate explanations and direct answers are given, then the threats in his hospital experience are minimized. Trust in the staff is established, he knows he will have help in coping with the situations he faces, and he is more willing to accept the end results.

POSTSURGICAL PROBLEMS

Physiologic problems of the new colostomate are: a changed body by creation of an artifical anus on the abdominal wall; fecal incontinence due to his now-limited reservoir for waste storage; perineal drainage in the early postoperative days; interruption of perineal nerves causing temporary loss of bladder control; and temporary impotence. Occasionally, there may be permanent interference with these latter two functions, depending on the amount of pathology the surgeon finds and whether it can be dissected. Also, there may be development of fistulous tracts between the small and large bowel, or between the bowel and the urinary bladder. A superficial sinus tract may develop which may become infected. Finally, there may be heavy scar tissue formation which will result in a feeling of discomfort and pain in the perineal area. This may be temporary, lasting for weeks, sometimes for months, and, in some patients I have known, it has persisted for several years. Also, I have known several persons who had very persistent intractable itching. Sitz baths, x-ray, antipruritic drugs such as trimeprazine tartrate (Temaril), or local applications (calamine, dibucaine) have been employed but with little benefit.

Care of the perineal wound will depend on the individual surgeon's choice of management. If the closure is a primary one, a drain may be left in place and then removed in a day or two depending upon the amount of drainage. Healing is rapid, and postoperative complaints are few. Occasionally, there may be a slight collection of fluid in the wound which requires incision and drainage or cauterization at a later date. But if the wound is left to granulate and a packing inserted, the patient is much more uncomfortable, and daily wound irrigations and dressing changes are required. In addition, his hospitalization is usually prolonged, as the healing is slow, perhaps taking several months, and he will often complain of pain and discomfort as scar tissue forms.

Patients often ask questions about this perineal wound, and we tell them that sitz baths taken several times a day help to promote healing and keep the area clean; that persistence in drainage should be attended to by the physician; that, occasionally, a healed wound will become infected and drain; and that this, too, should be brought to the physician's attention.

There are two periods when the patient is helped by a fellow colostomate who is adjusting satisfactorily: early preoperatively, when he is preoccupied with the question of survival, and then later, when he starts learning self-care and needs to see that life is possible with a colostomy and that former activities can be resumed. This later contact also gives him an opportunity to prove to himself that he will look like anyone else (the colostomy does not show).

Since the patient's early feelings are primarily related to the need to keep clean, bowel control must be reestablished early. With the gaining of this control the psychologic effect is minimized. The immediate control of fecal drainage by use of temporary ostomy bags rather than bulky dressings eliminates the initial problems of fecal odor and the patient's disgust at being soiled and having to handle feces. The doctor can apply a temporary bag when he opens the double-barreled colostomy, or during the first or second dressing change.

Because fecal odor lingers long after the cause has been eliminated, it should be meticulously avoided as much as possible. When the nurse changes the bag, she should be sure to do it adroitly, aware that the patient will observe her reaction to this task and will believe her attitude to be that of the world at large [1].

If the nurse discusses goals with the patient—what is expected to happen and what is expected of him—she will help reduce the normal anxiety he is experiencing. He should be encouraged and praised for each step he takes toward a goal. Full acceptance of his colostomy will come much later—perhaps months later—but early control and knowledgeable, skillful assistance by an interested staff reduces this time. Both patient and nurse learn that time is a great healer, and that most persons, especially with satisfactory preparation, can accept and adjust to the colostomy. Individuals have far more courage and strength in meeting crises than they are given credit for.

APPLYING THE BAG

The patient should learn as soon as possible how to change the temporary ostomy bag, so that his dependency state—which many patients consider childlike—is not reinforced.

First, the stoma is wiped with paper tissue to remove any mucus or fecal discharge present. Then the skin around the stoma is washed with warm, soapy water and patted dry. If necessary, a coating of tincture of benzoin is applied to that skin area which will come in contact with the adhesive facing or the temporary bag. This coating of benzoin will protect the skin and will also increase the adhesiveness of the bag. The skin should be sticky before the bag is applied. (Karaya gum powder, a karaya gum ring, or surgical appliance cement may also be used.)

If the patient has already learned about the stoma's changes in size according to his position, he will understand the need to allow for this size change by enlarging the ostomy bag opening to about ⅛ inch greater than the actual stoma size. (On the other hand, too large an opening will create skin problems if the stool is liquid or semisolid.)

When the patient has mastered the technique of applying and removing the ostomy bag, his entire manner changes. He becomes less fearful and much more cheerful, very proud of his accomplishment. He should be praised, for he has indeed reached an important goal in rehabilitation. He no longer is dependent on others to keep clean. At home, after he has emptied the soiled ostomy bag into the toilet, it may be placed in a paper bag or wrapped in newspaper and discarded in the incinerator or covered trash can.

Many types of ostomy bags are available. Some are applied with adhesive facing; others have a karaya gum ring facing which is also adherent and valuable to those who are sensitive to adhesive. Still another type is attached with a belt and does not adhere to the skin. These bags may be open at the end or sealed as the individual prefers. The nurse helps the patient select the equipment most suited to his needs, considering his physical abilities and limitations. Rarely, it may be necessary to resort to a more permanent appliance. Several of these have disposable parts which facilitate ease in use and care.

In recent years a wide variety of ostomy equipment has become available. Information about it can be obtained from professional journals, surgical supply houses, or from the United Ostomy Association.

SKIN AND STOMA CARE

To prevent or correct skin irritation around the stoma, we advise the patient to keep the surrounding skin clean by washing with lukewarm, soapy water, rinsing, and patting it dry. Ostomy creams or any protective cream (such as Desitin) will prevent further excoriation. A paste made of boiled Gelusil reduces redness, and a paste made of karaya gum powder and water will protect and heal excoriated skin. Karaya gum powder or karaya gum rings are valuable for very sensitive skins. Both can be applied directly to the skin and a temporary ostomy bag fixed over them.

Patients often ask us whether the colostomy stoma should be dilated. Usually it is not necessary. The physician indicates whether it is necessary to dilate or not. When dilation is recommended, the patient uses a finger covered with a well-lubricated finger cot. A tight stoma may be dilated daily or several times a week. The prescribed method and frequency of dilation should be adhered to.

Sometimes, patients notice blood spots and stains from the stoma.

Such bleeding may result from irritation of the intestinal membrane and should not be cause for alarm; it may be due to the method of catheter insertion. Continuous bleeding should be attended to by the physician.

A person with a colostomy can go swimming. We advise patients to cover the stoma with a large waterproof Band-Aid or a temporary ostomy bag, but to try this first while taking a bath, to see that this covering is effective.

THE IRRIGATION

It is essential that the patient learn to do the irrigation procedure as soon as possible. The doctor should irrigate the colostomy first, in order to determine the patency of the bowel and the need for any special instructions for catheter insertion or for the irrigation.

The second irrigation is done by the nurse, with the patient assisting, and soon by the patient, with the nurse guiding and directing. Before he is ready for discharge, the patient must be able to do the irrigation, bag change, and skin care without any assistance. The only exception to this is when the patient has physical limitations, and then a member of the family is taught to assist as needed. But we believe that the patient can do the procedure more easily and effectively by himself, as he does his other routine daily personal habits such as shaving or brushing his teeth.

The proper irrigation equipment is obtained for the patient while he is in the hospital, and his irrigations are demonstrated with his own equipment. Then when he takes over the irrigations, he does so with this same equipment, and when he goes home, he takes it with him secure in his own skill.

Evacuation from an ascending colostomy will be liquid or semiliquid and therefore more difficult to control. If a patient continues to have frequent liquid or semiliquid fecal discharges throughout the 24-hour period despite attention to diet and irrigations, he should be taught how to select and use an open-ended temporary-type ostomy bag, which permits frequent emptying without removing the entire bag, thus preventing skin problems. It is also more economical to use. However, the ascending colostomy, which I once believed to be uncontrollable, can be controlled with daily irrigations. In fact, one patient has achieved complete control for 24 hours at a time with daily irrigation, and is so confident that he wears only a gauze dressing over the stoma between irrigations.

The evacuation from a transverse colostomy can be controlled more easily, since the drainage is about the consistency of toothpaste. After control is obtained with daily irrigations, it is frequently possible to maintain it with irrigation every two days. However, these persons are troubled with excessive amounts of flatus, and, if this does occur, they should return to a daily irrigation schedule to keep them free of embarrassment.

The sigmoid colostomy, where the drainage is quite solid and dry (similar to feces evacuated from the rectum), is the easiest one in which to achieve control. After control is achieved by a daily irrigation, the patient may be able to irrigate every two or three days. A few persons may even irrigate every four days, but, in general, we caution the patient about delaying irrigation for longer than three days, since severe constipation and excessive gas formation may result from this delay.

Only a few persons have attempted to control the colostomy by using suppositories. Because complete control was not achieved for the entire 24-hour period, the patients I knew discontinued their use, although the frequency of movements did gradually decrease after seven days, and continued to decrease with time. Therefore, we plan to investigate further the use and potential benefits of suppositories, especially for those persons who are unable to use the irrigation method successfully.

TIMING

The time to do the irrigation is an individual matter based on the patient's previous bowel habits, the time of spillage postoperatively, his daily living pattern at home, and his occupation. Many patients find that irrigation is most effective when done about one hour after their largest meal, since this is when the bowel is full and ready to be emptied. Another factor in choosing the time of irrigation is that the average person needs approximately one hour of uninterrupted use of toilet facilities. Later, many are able to complete the irrigation in less than an hour. The hour that the patient selects as the one for his home irrigations is also the one that the nurse selects while he is hospitalized. In this way, by continuing the irrigation at the established hour, the patient is less likely to have spillage or interruption of control when he goes home, if control has already been achieved. A concerted effort to establish this regular time has been essential in gaining control, we have found.

When the bowel is irrigated at the same time each day, control usually is achieved in from three to ten days. Daily irrigation is continued until there is no spillage after the irrigation for 24 hours. Once control is established for one day, the schedule is adjusted to irrigation every 48 hours, again maintaining the same hour for irrigation. By observing the returns, the day to skip irrigation will become self-evident. One day the spillage will be copious; the next day, slight. Finally, there will be little or no fecal drainage with the return of fluid, and that will be the day to skip irrigation. There may be a slight movement on the first day the irrigation is omitted; however, frequently there is only a slight mucous discharge, which is to be expected. The use of a temporary ostomy bag will help to allay fear of a fecal accident.

Initially, adherence to a set time is important in establishing control. Once control is achieved, the time may vary occasionally from one to three hours without disrupting the schedule. Most colostomates find that, if they plan a social activity at their usual irrigation time, an earlier irrigation will provide freedom from worry about spillage and gas expulsion. If one has to forgo the irrigation completely, he should be prepared for spillage, and should wear a protective covering which can be changed easily and quickly. In such a situation, some patients find they can apply gentle pressure to the abdomen to express stool which has collected near the stoma.

IRRIGATION PROBLEMS

The patient may be quite skillful in doing the irrigation and he may have participated in many detailed discussions of the irrigation procedure, stoma and skin care, and dietary regimens. Nevertheless, as soon as he encounters a new difficulty or a new problem with his colostomy he becomes terribly anxious. He wants help and he needs it right away. For this reason, I give each discharged patient a telephone number they can call for help at any time, day or night, and I conduct a weekly nursing care clinic where instructions and assistance are given to patients who are both in and out of the hospital. The following discussion incorporates answers to the questions that are most frequently asked about the irrigation. (A description of the procedure itself can be found in any medical-surgical nursing text.)

Water

Approximately two quarts of water should be used for the irrigation. A general rule is to use enough water to clean out the large intestine, so that toward the end of the irrigation the water is running clear. Many persons have been able to gradually cut down on this amount afterward as they establish their routine. There have been no harmful effects from the use of three or even four quarts of water, which has been necessary in a few instances. But the new colostomate is cautioned to use only an additional pint or quart of fluid if the initial two quarts are not sufficient, lest he keep on irrigating indefinitely and become overtired or retain the extra fluid. When only a pint of water is used, the patient has frequent spillage and control is delayed.

Tepid tap water will suffice. Occasionally, one finds it necessary to adjust its warmth or coolness for a more effective irrigation, but hot water should *never* be used. A small amount of baking soda or soap will soften very hard water. However, soap solution generally is not necessary, and can be harmful by causing tiny hemorrhages in the bowel.

Catheter Insertion

The catheter should be inserted far enough so that the bowel can retain the inflow of fluid: approximately 4 to 8 inches, or half the length of the catheter. It is inserted with a rotating motion, and it is gradually moved back and forth while the water is flowing. Rarely is it necessary to insert the catheter its full length. It should never be forced, since local swelling or engorgement might be preventing the catheter's entry, and forcing might cause perforation. (In those instances where bowel perforation has occurred, the person had forced the catheter despite difficulty during insertion.)

Occasional difficulty of insertion may be due to the catheter size, or there may be an obstruction due to a hard mass of stool at the colostomy opening. Distension of the bowel or constriction of the stoma are other causes of difficulty.

The catheter sometimes curls back on itself when one tries to insert it. This means that it may be too small, too soft, or too old. Or there may be hyperactivity of the bowel, or it may be due simply to improper insertion technique. When there is difficulty replacing the catheter after initial insertion, one can lubricate it well and then gently move it back and forth a few times, rotating it at the same time. Dilation before catheter insertion may help. To do so, one lubricates and gently inserts a covered finger into the colostomy.

Spillage and Backflow

"Secondary spillage" is caused by inadequate cleansing of the bowel at time of irrigation, or by insertion of the catheter to its full length, causing fluid retention. In either case the bowel will continue to seep throughout the day. Adjustment of the length to which the catheter is inserted and an irrigation until clear should correct spillage.

Backflow may occur during the time the water is flowing in if the catheter has not been inserted far enough, or if the reservoir has been hung too high, causing water to enter only the beginning portion of the bowel. Or there may be excessive flatus in the bowel which prevents inflow. If the bowel will not retain water despite adjustment of the catheter length and the height of the bag, the enema technique can be tried, using a catheter threaded through a baby bottle nipple, half a hand ball, a flange, or one of the commercial devices to prevent backflow during inflow.

Cramps

Several factors may cause painful cramps during the irrigation: failure to expel air from the irrigation tubing before inserting the catheter; hanging the reservoir higher than shoulder height, causing a too-rapid inflow; a catheter which is too large, causing the fluid to flow in too rapidly and under too much pressure; or, water which is too cold, causing overstimulation of the bowel. However, cramps may simply be a signal that the bowel is preparing to empty. If cramps occur, we advise the patient to close off the tubing, sit up straight, and take a few deep breaths. When they disappear, he can release the tubing and continue the irrigation.

Retention

Water is sometimes retained in the bowel after irrigation because the body may be in need of fluid and may absorb it; or there may be a spasm of the bowel which prevents the water from returning; or the catheter may have been inserted to its full length, which would cause the water to be retained temporarily. When the patient is unable to expel the fluid, he can insert a well-lubricated catheter into the stoma and siphon the fluid back. Change of position (raising the arms above the head and twisting one's trunk from side to side) or gentle massage to the abdomen may also initiate a return flow. In instances where a person is very dehydrated, very little water may be returned. In this event, the water will later be eliminated by the urinary system. Another cause of temporary fluid retention may be emotional upset, causing bowel spasm.

Clear Returns

An ineffective irrigation—that is, the return of water without stool—may occur if there has been a movement prior to the irrigation, and the bowel is free of stool. Or, the bowel may be ready to be irrigated less often. Clear returns also occur if the catheter is not inserted far enough, so that water runs in and out simultaneously, or if insufficient water enters the bowel to stimulate evacuation.

In general, freedom from spillage, from odor, and from gas are directly related to the effectiveness of the irrigation.

DIET

A low-residue diet has been described in the literature as being of major significance in colostomy control, but I have found the need for a special diet an individual matter. In the last 250 colostomy patients with whom I have worked, the patient has remained on the low-residue diet for approximately a week and then has resumed his usual regular diet, thus eliminating his being different from the rest of his family. However, he is taught to avoid foods which are known to cause gas or odor, such as onions, peas, beans, cabbage, cauliflower, pork, nuts, and those foods which have never agreed with him. I have also observed that green leafy vegetables (such as spinach), uncooked fruits, and fruit juices may cause diarrhea in many patients, although in many others they do not. And other foods, such as beets, may change the color of the stool. We tell a patient to add new foods in moderation, one at a time. Then he can identify for himself those foods he needs to avoid (those which cause gas, diarrhea, or constipation) and those foods he can tolerate well. If he remembers to eat slowly and chew his food well, with his mouth closed to avoid swallowing air, his dietary restrictions can be largely eliminated. The patient's fear of trying new foods is minimized if he knows how to control the diarrhea, constipation, or gas which may occur. For example, a potential gas-producing food can be tried on the scheduled day of irrigation.

PROBLEMS IN CONTROL

Diarrhea and severe constipation are two of the greatest problems. These can be managed satisfactorily by retraining or reestablishing bowel control through irrigation and diet modification.

Diarrhea

Every patient should be given a prescription for antidiarrheal medication such as kaolin and pectin (Kaopectate) or paregoric when he is discharged from the hospital, so he can stop diarrhea promptly and avoid the anxiety caused by this loss of control. However, such medication should not be taken regularly unless the physician has prescribed it with the intent to help curb a persistent loose stool.

The cause of diarrhea should be determined as soon as possible, because the loose stools will persist, despite temporary measures, until the cause is determined. Most commonly, it is due to eating spicy or irritating foods; taking medication such as some antihypertensives, antibiotics, tranquilizers, or diuretics; drinking large quantities of fluids, especially beer; generalized illness, such as a virus condition; and overexcitement or emotional upset. The colostomate needs to be warned about these causes, especially about the effect of the emotions on bowel function. And when a patient understands that drugs prescribed for unrelated conditions may disturb bowel control, he will understand why he should tell any new physician about the colostomy.

Conversely, one colostomate developed severe diarrhea which later was determined to be caused by his failure to take his prescribed medication for Parkinson's disease.

As a temporary relief for loose stools, the patient can try irrigating the bowel, even though it is not the usual time for irrigation. Generally, the irrigation itself will eliminate the cause. In other instances, the irrigation plus an oral antidiarrheal mixture has been utilized for better control. The very hyperactive bowel may benefit from the use of such prescribed drugs as diphenoxylate (Lomotil).

Constipation

Increasing the fluid intake, adjusting the diet to include bulk, irrigations, and a mild laxative at night (such as prune juice) will control constipation. Medications can cause constipation as well as diarrhea. Narcotics and even aspirin can be constipating to some people. Stool softeners which increase bulk do relieve constipation, but they are generally undesirable for the colostomate because they increase the amount of stool and cause evacuation between irrigations, thus further disrupting control.

When temporary measures for alleviating diarrhea or constipation fail, the physician should be consulted promptly, since the problems may be a clue to impending complications.

Gas and Odor

Most intestinal flatus is due to swallowed air. In addition, certain foods, food combinations, and drinks produce gas. Highly spiced foods, carbonated drinks, and beer are chief offenders. And a too hurried irrigation or constipation may cause gas. Gas can be controlled by eating habits as well as by irrigation. The patient may find he needs to revert to a more frequent irrigation schedule. Or, he may need medication for a hyperactive bowel.

The gas-forming foods are likely to cause odor as well. Most important, a clean bowel will eliminate odor. Commercial products, available from ostomy supply services, are effective for some odor. Derefil, chlorophyll or charcoal tablets, Odo-Way, even aspirin tablets may be used in the bag; aerosols such as Turgesept or Lysol can be sprayed in the room, on a tissue and placed in the bag, or on a dressing covering the stoma (but not on the stoma directly). Other liquid preparations such as Banish or Nil Odor can be used in the bag or on a dressing. Personal cleanliness and the use of clean, odor-free equipment are paramount for control of odor.

PERSONAL ADJUSTMENT

I cannot overemphasize the patient's need to gain *control*, because his personal feelings about himself and his fears of relating to others are due mainly to his helpless feeling of "being dirty" because he cannot predict or control his stools. He loses his self-esteem. He constantly fears a fecal accident. Even when control is established, spillage, gas, and odor remain major concerns.

He may be ashamed, and confine himself to his room. He may avoid contact with family and friends, fearing rejection. He feels humiliated, degraded, unworthy, and unlovable with this physical blemish [2]. This may lead to feelings of self-rejection and despair.

The patient's original attitude toward his colostomy is in part due to the amount of discomfort he had prior to surgery. When the symptoms are few and cause little discomfort, the procedure appears to be out of proportion to the disease. The patient is usually irritable and demanding and complains constantly of many things. But when he has had weeks and months of agonizing pain, or frightening bouts of rectal bleeding or diarrhea, he looks forward to the procedure as a welcome relief, and thus he is able to accept the colostomy as helpful. This patient is usually cooperative, willing, eager to learn self-care, and grateful for his survival.

Staff

After surgery, the patient's attitude toward his colostomy will be greatly influenced by the attitude and the ability of the medical and nursing staff who care for him. If they show they are not only skillful in handling the procedure, but also are interested, sympathetic, and understanding in a consistent caring manner, his burden is lessened and his feelings of helplessness and isolation are dispelled.

In addition, the staff must have a willingness to openly share information about care, drugs, and other treatment if the patient is to have an active part in his recovery. Ironically, successful rehabilitation frequently depends on the very information which was so carefully secreted from patients in the past.

Family

The attitude of the patient's family is very important in shaping his feelings about himself. It may be the patient who is the cause of negative attitudes because he excludes his family from his confidence, creating tensions which increase unless interrupted.

On the other hand, there may be actual rejection on the part of the marital partner and an expression of disgust at the sight of the stoma. Frequently, problems which arise in marital relations are due to lack of understanding or lack of information. The partner may fear injuring the stoma, and therefore will avoid reestablishing a satisfactory relationship, without explanation. But the colostomy may be used by either partner as an excuse for abstinence when there is a desire to avoid marital relations for other reasons. Both partners need to know that sexual relations can be resumed without fear, unless they are otherwise advised by the physician.

Much of this misunderstanding is prevented if the partner is included in the plans for recovery. She or he should learn what the colostomy is, and what limitations if any will ensue. Some one member of the family should be taught the irrigation technique so assistance can be given at home if and when necessary. However, the family should understand the danger of taking over—assisting too much. The family can best assist by showing understanding of the patient's predicament and thoughtful provision of privacy. Unrequired assistance, although accepted, not only may not be appreciated by the patient, but may create bigger problems by placing him in a dependent role, causing self-rejection and despair. The dependency relationship together with the fecal incontinence may change a husband's perception of himself from partner to child.

Colostomy Society

Both the patient's and his family's attitude to his colostomy can be favorably influenced by their referral to the local colostomy society. This gives them an opportunity to meet others who have a colostomy and to get answers to questions and helpful advice. Attending such meetings can affect the nurse's attitude, too. It is here she can learn of the unmet needs of her posthospital patient, and gain insight into approaches she can use in the future.

Family members are encouraged to attend these meetings and to ask questions. Through their increased knowledge and understanding, the colostomate is relieved of the need to explain or to make repeated requests (concerning diet, bathroom, and so forth). Some cities have special group meetings for the women members and for wives of colostomates.

Finally, much of the adjustment will depend on the nature of the family—its strengths and weaknesses, its ability to handle crises, the concern of the members for each other, and their ability to support each other.

Notes on Traveling

Besides the irrigation equipment, the patient will want to take along colostomy coverings, such as large square adhesive patches; a supply of temporary ostomy bags and adherent, such as karaya gum powder, for emergency use; an extra length of tubing, a plastic hook with adhesive backing, or an ample supply of string so the irrigating bag can be adjusted to varying heights; a rubber or plastic sheet for protection at night; and an undershirt to wear in poorly heated bathrooms. The equipment should be placed in a small separate bag so he can carry it with him.

If traveling in another country, he will need to check the water supply: if it is unsafe to drink, it will be unsafe to use for irrigation, and should be boiled. The United States Public Health Service will give necessary information about contamination or safety factors to be aware of in specific locations. The colostomate should be encouraged to continue his established routine, to avoid overexcitement and fatigue, to take a small supply of antidiarrheal preparation as prescribed by his physician for emergency use, to be discreet in food and beverage intake, and—to enjoy himself.

REFERENCES

1   Katona, Elizabeth A. Nurse-initiated and -conducted clinic for colostomy patients, in *Maintaining the Integrity of the Individual: A Nursing Responsibility* (Convention Clinical Sessions, 1964, No. 6). New York, American Nurses' Association, 1964, p. 22.

2   Meyers, Bernard. Some psychological aspects of the colostomy. Paper presented at a meeting of the Colostomy Society of New York, Martinique Hotel, Oct. 4, 1963.

Section D

Amputation Conditions

Amputation involves the loss of a body part. The loss is usually mutilating and frequently disabling. Both of these effects are highly significant in the meaning of amputation to the patient and to those who work with him. Wholeness is given a high value in our culture, and being whole is an important factor in self-esteem. As several of the articles that follow emphasize, self-esteem is a very important factor in the rehabilitation of the amputee.

Amputation frequently deprives the individual of a body part that has served an important role in his body functioning, which, in turn, depends on motor acts based on coordinated contractions of muscle groups. Complex actions are based on sequential steps, each being shaped and influenced by feedback from the previous one. This constant flow of sensory and neurological information provides for in-process correction and adequate coordination. As the sequential steps become mastered and instrumental, they become automatic.

Loss of a body part has effects that are further-reaching and more complex than the immediate mechanical problem. The loss tends to interrupt the feedback-type communication process upon which the total structure depends for coordinated movement. In light of this it appears that rehabilitation of the amputee might be well advised to take a systemlike approach rather than a missing-parts approach. Moreover, the total body functioning, depending as it does on the feedback contribution of all its orchestrated parts, may appear to the observer to be disproportionately affected or disabled by an injury that might otherwise seem of minor importance.

The term "unaffected side" sometimes used by professional persons to refer to the uninjured part is probably an unwarranted oversimplification. The high probability is that amputation results in an affected person, not a person with an affected and an unaffected side. The dependence of the dominant hand on the nondominant hand for feedback as to progress through stabilizing, holding, pushing, and so forth should provide a case in point. Another obvious example is the precision that is programmed into walking. Walking proceeds with the body weight being shifted from one foot to another, and with weight shifted from the heel of one foot to the toe of the same foot and to the heel of the other foot. The body's position in space, the relation of the center of gravity to the ground, the rate of speed, and other facts represent the feedback that provides for the purposeful and coordinated walking we take so much for granted. The loss of the mechanical function or the source of communication feedback necessitates a difficult period of relearning if walking is to be resumed.

Learning is a conscious process. Relearning involves unlearning the former pattern of behavior as it is replaced with the new. The former behavior may have persisted for a lifetime, but it was dependent upon feedback which either does not exist any longer or is distorted. The important fact to remember is that the total person is affected.

In addition to a thorough knowledge of the principles of kinesthesia and their application, the nurse must understand the nature and significance of body image and self-image in rehabilitation. One is not necessarily predictable from a knowledge of the other. Fishman has studied the amputee for many years, and his observations are highly appropriate in providing a basis for the nurse to fill conceptually the gap that exists between amputation and overt behavior. He illustrates that in actuality the paradigm might appear as follows: amputation—perception of amputation—needs—frustration—emotional reaction—defense mechanisms—adjustive behavior—covert and overt behavior.

Recognizing and dealing with the interim conditions is necessary if the nurse is to assist the patient toward rehabilitation. The scheme personalizes each patient's disability and its meaning to him. Loss of an incisor may take the patient through the same sequence of events, although the steps may be shorter, but the loss of function, feedback, and threat to the body image must all be coped with.

The articles by Fishman and Kirkpatrick are particularly effective in throwing into sharp relief one of the key principles in working with the amputee, i.e., the whole person is the true object of the nursing care, not the pathology. Pathology, in a sense, is only as important as the effect it has on the total functioning of the individual, and the proper arrangement of priorities in the nursing care can minimize this effect very considerably.

The relationship established between the nurse and patient at the time of their initial interaction can set the stage for the rehabilitation process. The nurse, if she is sensitive to cues, will be able to build and nurture a relationship based on trust and hope. The nursing care plan will consider realistic long-range goals based on accurate assessment and nursing history, and the plan will carefully articulate and implement these goals through short-term steps. The assessment will include as many of the relevant factors as possible which are important in stump healing, such as personal hygiene, nutritional state, skin condition, activity level, susceptibility to fatigue, and others. It will also include all the factors that might bear a relationship to the patient's motivation. Kirkpatrick is properly concerned with the maintenance of ability as well as the prevention of disability through loss of independence. Her article demonstrates the application of nursing principles in an actual situation, the young amputees from Vietnam fresh from the battlefield. The article emphasizes the importance of careful hygiene to prevent secondary problems. Stump care is practiced from the beginning to prevent swelling and infection and to develop a well-shaped stump to fit a prosthesis.

Every amputee should be treated as if a prosthesis will follow. While Kirkpatrick's patients were young with life ahead, the geriatric patient has the same need for mobilization and balance during his shorter life expectancy. Stump revision to develop a proper shape may never be necessary if good wrapping is initiated. For this reason the section on stump wrapping for compression and shaping is included.

Before physical therapy and the prosthesis become a part of the patient's rehabilitation, every effort must be made to maintain the full range of motion in the joints proximal to the amputated part. Proper exercise and stump hygiene are musts in amputee rehabilitation. One of the simplest and best statements of stump hygiene, including diagrams of bandaging, is provided by Levy and Barnes. Careful attention to the important guidelines they provide will move the rehabilitation process ahead and help prevent secondary problems of a complicating nature.

The cosmetic problems of a metal prosthetic device, as pointed out in the article, may appear to the patient as a hideous collection of bolts and ropes. Each amputation is a personal, and often a family, crisis. Both patient and family need help with procedures, referrals, problems of image, perception of future possibilities, and all the rest of the complicated process of rehabilitation of the amputee. Fortunately, through our modern technology and good nursing procedures, such help is available.

Reading 33

Amputee Needs, Frustrations, and Behavior

Sidney Fishman

Amputations are most frequently viewed in terms of the amount of physical loss involved. The functional consequences of the varying amounts of physical loss related to above-elbow, above-knee, below-elbow, and below-knee amputations are real and measurable, and theoretically it should be possible to make reasonable predictions concerning the amount of function that can be restored on the basis of the extent of physical amputation, the individual's physical condition, and the adequacy of the prosthetic appliance. However, this is not always true.

PERCEPTION OF DISABILITY

In many instances, predictions based upon these physical considerations prove to be quite inaccurate, overshadowed as they are by a psychological factor, namely, the patient's individual perception of his disability. It is this perception, in many instances, that has a greater influence than the physical extent of the disability on the rehabilitation process and its result. Another term for *perception* of the disability is *estimate* of the disability, which consists of the mental picture of the consequences of the disability as it appears to the amputee himself. It may be considered the personal meaning of the loss to the individual and the major influence of the person's self-concept.

It is most unusual to find this perception an accurate one. In most cases, relatively unrealistic and distorted self-perceptions result. This is not a surprising assessment, since the patient does not normally have access to any considerable experience with amputees. He does not know what to expect in living as an amputated person, and, in view of the rather significant trauma associated with his loss, he tends to focus his anxieties on the amputation and to consider the disability a more central factor in his future life than is realistic. In view of these considerations, it is perhaps more correct to say that a person "must learn to live with his perceptions of his disability" rather than "with his disability."

Since the amputee acts in terms of his perceptions, and not necessarily reality, the consequences of a highly distorted estimate of one's disabled condition are reflected in the increased difficulty in accepting the challenges of the rehabilitation process. If these perceptions are not corrected prior to the prescription and fitting of an artificial limb and training in its use, these

Reprinted from *Rehabilitation Literature*, vol. 20, no. 11, pp. 322–328, November 1959.

latter processes are almost impossible to accomplish successfully. When they do proceed, however, they do so only haltingly and with great resistance and difficulty.

It seems therefore that, in the rehabilitation process, we are as much concerned with trying to effect a change in the individual's perceptions as we are in trying to change the realities themselves. If this be the case, the treatment of the amputee assumes two foci: (a) diminution of physical loss by appropriate medical care and introduction of prosthetic devices and training in their use; and (b) revision of unrealistic ideas and attitudes through continuous re-education. Both these approaches are designed to increase the effectiveness of the patient's functional and psychological resources.

AMPUTEE NEEDS*

Having indicated that the problems of being an amputee arise from both physical and psychological considerations, it seems appropriate to identify specifically the areas of human behavior and functioning in which these difficulties manifest themselves.

It is sometimes overlooked and seldom fully appreciated that every human being has a diversity of needs of varying intensity that must be satisfied to maintain his adjustment to the environment. These needs may be considered as being either biogenic or sociogenic in nature. Examples of the first type relate to those evolving from the biology of the organism, such as hunger, sexual desire, avoidance of pain, while examples of the latter relate to those that evolve from our social structure, such as needs for status, achievement, and respect. Although the terms motive, drive, desire, and need have certain technical differences in meaning, for the purposes of this discussion we will overlook these differences and will consider these terms as being synonymous. Because of the intimate and complex overlapping, it becomes fruitless to speak of an amputee's physical and psychological needs separately, since the problems involved tend in most instances to become combinations of both factors in an almost indivisible manner.

The thesis that I should like to propose is that a number of very specific psychological, social, and physiological human needs are thwarted when one becomes physically handicapped as a result of amputation, and, because of the permanency, finality, and irrevocability of the loss, a unique readjustment problem evolves. Only when the limitations imposed by the amputation are realistically accepted and integrated by the individual does the adjustment process proceed. The significance of each one of these frustrated

---

* This paper is primarily concerned with unilateral amputations of noncongenital origin in the adult. The discussions would be applicable to child amputees or to bilateral or other special amputee types only with appropriate modification. Furthermore, we are concerned with the long-range permanent adjustment patterns of the amputee and are viewing him after the period of immediate postoperative shock has passed.

human needs is great and deserves detailed identification. These needs are as follows.

Physical Function

Although the psychological satisfactions concomitant with physical activity have not been clearly detailed or understood, it is clear that there is an inborn drive to use one's physical resources. This is evidenced by the baby's unlearned determination to walk, crawl, and handle things and the child's and adult's natural participation in physical activities. Although we have some difficulty in precisely defining the nature of this drive for physical activity, it is perfectly clear that associated with it are significant psychological satisfactions and that, with amputation, the need for these gratifications associated with physical activity is inhibited.

In addition to the gratifications evolving directly from the use of one's physical faculties (as in walking, dancing, or engaging in sports), there is a host of additional satisfactions that can be achieved only through the use of prehensile or ambulatory function as an intervening step. In this latter instance, the pleasures do not grow out of the physical activity itself but from the results of its application, such as in climbing to the balcony of a theatre, holding a drink, or going to lunch in a desirable but somewhat inaccessible place.

In approaching physical tasks, both for the direct satisfactions involved and for the related pleasures, the alternatives open to the amputee are (a) to avoid performing the task, (b) to compensate for his loss by the greater use of the remaining extremities, (c) to perform the function by utilizing an artificial replacement for the missing member, or (d) a combination of all of these. But no matter which course the amputee chooses, his desire to perform a variety of physical acts without restriction, limitation, or special consideration remains frustrated.

Cosmesis

Visual Considerations The word cosmesis, which Webster's Dictionary defines as pertaining to adornment, beautification, or decoration, is widely used in the field of prosthetic restoration as a synonym for problems associated with one's visual appearance.

It is perfectly clear that when one suffers an amputation, his overt appearance is changed, both in his own eyes and in the eyes of others. It is interesting to note that there is a group of disabilities, similar to amputation, which have this external badge attached to them. All people afflicted with this kind of disability are automatically identified as being different. Of course, the majority of diseases are primarily internal in nature and may be completely secreted unless the individual cares to confide in someone concerning his illness.

These "external" disabilities all tend to set up a single problem related to the fact that we live in a society where great emphasis is placed on the quality, adequacy, and conformity of one's physical appearance. There are all sorts of evidences for this fact; we all tend to groom ourselves according to a pattern—great emphasis is placed on dress and make-up—automobiles and homes are all designed with good looks as a predominant goal.

It is clear that the values associated with appearance are important, and when members of our society do not meet these standards, they are regarded differently. Since the need to have one's appearance congruent with that of the group is a significant one, a problem develops.

It is interesting to point out in this connection that at least one important surgical technic (e.g., cineplasty) for the prosthetic rehabilitation of the upper-extremity amputee has never received acceptance here in the United States. We may attribute this lack of enthusiasm in considerable measure to the cosmetic problems associated with this surgical procedure, since there is little question about its functional adequacy.

Auditory Considerations Although the primary cosmetic problem for the amputee is the adequacy of his visual appearance, there are also frustrations connected with the noise-producing characteristics of the conventional prosthetic device. For lack of a more suitable method of referring to this latter problem, I propose thinking of it as the auditory aspects of the cosmesis problem. Since the prospect of being conspicuous by virtue of some inadequacy in one's make-up is a threatening one, the matter of adapting to a substitute extremity that produces noise becomes an additional cause for concern.

An artificial limb is essentially a simple machine, and, as one considers the matter, most man-made machines have some type of sound associated with them—the artificial limb is no exception. Some amputees will be concerned with noise caused by air escaping around the rim of the socket or in the articulation of the prosthetic knee or ankle. Others are even sensitive to the atypical sound of the prosthetic foot hitting the floor. Upper-extremity amputees may react to the noise associated with the prosthetic elbow locking in position or the terminal device closing on an object. It is important to point out that these noises are on a very low level of intensity and probably go unnoticed by most people with whom the amputee associates. However, a very significant percentage of the amputees are aware of these sounds and because of this awareness tend to believe that other people are conscious of them.

Since cosmetic values, both visual and auditory, are threatened by amputation and attendant prosthetic restoration, the need for minimizing another area of difference resulting from disability is frustrated.

Comfort

Certainly a basic difficulty in adjustment stems from the body's need to be as free from pain and tension and as physically comfortable as possible. It is not ordinarily pointed out, however, that all prostheses are inherently uncomfortable appendages. I should hazard a suggestion that even the most skillfully made prosthesis cannot be considered really comfortable and cannot be taken for granted by the wearer. What we have come to regard as a comfortable prosthesis is simply one that offers a minimum and tolerable degree of discomfort.

Although not widely expressed, the above point of view should not be surprising since, in fitting a prosthetic device for the lower-extremity amputee, tissues and muscles are being used for functions quite different from their normal use, i.e., primarily weight-bearing. Until the tissues become acclimated, desensitized, and/or calloused to these new functions, considerable discomfort, as a result of skin irritations, pressure points, and the like, is the rule. Even after prolonged periods of prosthetic usage, the desensitization is not complete and some discomfort is continuous. Although the problem of weight-bearing does not exist in the case of devices for upper-extremity amputees, the musculature is still used for unusual functions, e.g., humeral flexion or scapula abduction for prehension or elbow flexion, humeral extension and/or abduction for the control of the elbow. For both lower- and upper-extremity amputees, the body tissues are encased in relatively rigid, impermeable materials (wood or plastics) that interfere with normal ventilation of body parts and also cause discomfort due to heat and perspiration.

The ability of the amputee to tolerate the various degrees of discomfort is connected with the wide variation in individual capacities to tolerate pain. It is well known that this ability to tolerate pain and/or discomfort is dependent upon both physical and psychological considerations, although the exact importance of each in the case of an individual patient is ofttimes difficult to ascertain. In any event, the fact that an amputee must continuously tolerate some discomfort and/or pain tends to violate his need for bodily security and absence of tension and thus develops into another problem area for the individual.

Energy Costs

Although research has not yet given us final, reliable data concerning the amount of energy expended in typical tasks by the various types of amputees as compared to normals, preliminary studies tell us that these differences are significant. For example, an above-knee amputee performing a given ambulatory task expends considerably more energy than does his nonhandicapped counterpart.

Since the evidence indicates that the amputee is called upon to expend more effort and energy, he is in the position of having to divert effort that once went to other activities and apply it toward his disability. He is also likely to experience fatigue more rapidly than the nonhandicapped person. Since both phenomena (expenditure of effort and the early experience of fatigue) are alien to the desire of most people, we once again have a significant instance of need frustration.

Another aspect of this problem is concerned with the fact that the operation of prosthetic devices is for the most part *not* automatic. In other words, the amputee needs to pay considerable continuous attention to the activation, control, and use of his prosthesis. This requirement for increased attention may be viewed as making greater demands on the psychological resources of the patient. It serves to divert his attention from other concerns and to focus attention on the problems of prosthetic function. We cannot translate this at the moment into terms of physical energy. However, its role as an additional and consistent drain on the amputee's resources cannot be argued.

Achievement

It may be pointed out that our society has relatively unsympathetic attitudes toward people who fail in the process of performing various activities, whether this be in the realm of school, vocation, sports, or social affairs. Failure in a business or in a spelling bee, an error in a ball game, or failure to get ahead in one's job are all subject to society's criticism.

The use of a prosthetic appliance, however, inevitably implies a reasonable amount of failure as an outgrowth of two facts. Bearing in mind that the prosthesis is a machine: (a) any inadequacy in the design or construction of its parts and/or fitting to the amputee will cause a failure in function; (b) unless the artificial limb is perfectly controlled by the amputee, it again will fail to provide proper function.

In view of these conditions, the amputee, especially the new wearer, must anticipate a reasonable number of instances when he will fail in the simple act of ambulation by falling down or will fail in the simple act of prehension by having something drop from his artificial hand. These failures of essentially elementary human functions are a source of concern and embarrassment for the individual. Even when the individual becomes expert in the use of the artificial appliances, a reasonable possibility of malfunction and failure always exists. Depending upon the individual's need for presenting an appearance of perfection to his peers, this anxiety concerning public failure further tends to inhibit the person's proper use of the appliance.

Economic Security

Any threat to an individual's ability to earn his own way in our competitive society must also be considered as a threat to an important human need. Our understanding of this problem may be aided by referring to the so-called socioeconomic scale, which in a general way categorizes people in terms of the social status accorded them. Generally, an individual's position on the scale is intimately tied in with his occupational pursuits.

Some insight concerning the amputee's economic problem may be gained by referring to this "scale." One notes that the occupations that are highest in status are professional, managerial, and executive in nature, while those that are lowest are termed unskilled labor. It is further to be noted that the duties of the professional and the executive group are primarily dependent upon intellect and personality (ability to think, speak, write, persuade, or make decisions), while those in the unskilled group are primarily dependent on manual resources (carry, pull, push, stack, or load). As a consequence, the potential employability of an amputee depends on the extent to which the individual is involved in intellectual or manual contributions to society.

When people in the former group suffer an amputation, there are perhaps no significant threats based on economic considerations at all. With the exception of the small group in the performing and fine arts, their ability to pursue their occupation is essentially unaffected, as is their position as a wage earner. The only economic problems faced by this group are the medical and prosthetic expenses associated with a chronic illness. On the other hand, those who earn their livelihood primarily by the performance of physical duties involving the use of hands and legs, and who do not have intellectual and personal resources for training in other fields, suffer a very severe economic handicap as a result of amputation.

The empirical fact is that the large majority of unemployed and marginally employable amputees come from this low socioeconomic group. They cannot compete with their full-bodied peers, and unless selective placement is introduced or special arrangements are made on the job, these people remain unemployable. We see then that, for this significant segment of the amputee population, the socially approved need to be economically self-sufficient is frustrated.

Respect and Status

Perhaps the single most important psychological prerequisite for a well-adjusted, productive life is the respect and the status that one earns from his associates and peers. Over and above the physical niceties and amenities of existence, the satisfactions received from the respect and affection of people close to them (friends, family, coworkers) are all-important. With regard to the amputee population, this status is threatened and the possibility of loss of acceptance by one's peers becomes very real. The amputee is not ordinarily obliged to guess how others feel about him. He can (except in the case of the congenital amputee) simply reflect upon what he thought about other handicapped people before he himself was afflicted. These attitudes, which he held toward other disabled people, are now directed toward the self.

It is likely that, early in these reflections, the word cripple comes to the amputee's mind along with its various connotations of inadequacy, charity, shame, punishment, and guilt. Obviously, when an individual views himself or feels that he is being viewed by others in these terms, he considers himself an object for lessened respect and will react to this changed social status accordingly. Since these attitudes are not at all likely to enhance the self-concept, but rather devalue it, the patient may be expected to undertake defenses against these attacks on his integrity.

Social prejudices with regard to the disabled are further reflected in our literature, with such villainous characters as Captain Hook, Captain Ahab, Long John Silver, and others being identified with amputation. These characterizations tend to continue unsatisfactory attitudes toward the handicapped by virtue of their influence on youngsters during their formative years.

It is, of course, true that there are very significant educational programs afoot attempting to change the social attitudes toward the handicapped and teaching that the loss of an extremity does not automatically devalue a person. However, attitudes toward the disabled that have been centuries in the making are not changed by one or two lectures at the outset of a rehabilitation program. For the time being, we must face the reality that significant loss of social status accompanies amputation and that the human need to retain the respect of one's associates is threatened.

The seven above-listed human needs seem to be thwarted when one becomes an amputee and a potential wearer of a prosthesis. The conflicts and frustrations consequent to these considerations cannot be erased. They perhaps can be modified, perhaps can be compromised, but cannot be negated. The problem of rehabilitation of the amputee becomes, therefore, one of assisting the patient to incorporate these limitations into his pattern of life so as to assure minimal interference with the large variety of other functions and activities of living.

It would, of course, in planning a rehabilitation program for amputees be most helpful to determine which of the above seven problem areas are most important. If this decision could be made reliably, emphasis and attention could be paid to the more important aspects of the patient's problem. This is not possible, however, and the difficulty may be attributed to the following. First, with relation to the seven problem areas discussed, a different pattern of significance emerges for each patient, depending upon his personal characteristics and background. Second, prosthetic devices are products that have evolved from a long series of significant compromises in design and, as a result, assist in reducing a number of problems but do not completely resolve any one of them. In the reduction of certain problems (cosmesis, function) new ones are introduced or old ones aggravated (comfort, energy costs).

Wherever one is concerned with human behavior, the often-expressed thought that each patient must be treated in terms of his own system of values remains uppermost in one's thinking. The proper weighing of each of the above seven factors as part of the process of diagnosis and prognosis for each patient is a prerequisite in developing a sound differential management concept.

CONSEQUENCES OF FRUSTRATION

The previous discussions have dealt at some length with the number of significant human needs that cannot be completely gratified as a result of the loss of an extremity. We have suggested that these circumstances tend to frustrate the individual and to generate psychological conflict because of permanently unobtainable goals. Furthermore, it has been pointed out that the extent of conflict is more dependent upon the patient's perception of his disability than its real limitations. Consequently, the more inaccurate the patient's perceptions are, the greater the anticipated psychological distress.

Conflict and frustration are theoretical ideas that have been developed to explain the processes of human adjustment. These constructs are best identified and understood in terms of their causes (which are the unobtainable goals) and their consequences (which are the emotional reactions they induce). As a matter of fact, if no emotion is aroused it may be said that there is no frustration or conflict. Psychologists further tell us that the emotions resulting from conflict and frustration are not of the positive variety (love, affection, joy), but rather of a negative quality (anxiety, fear, jealousy, hate).

In order to re-establish equilibrium within the person, the negative emotions being experienced must be dissipated. This normally is accomplished through the vehicle of some variety of overt or covert behavior. The type of behavior resulting seems to be dependent upon three factors: (a) the way the individual perceives or interprets the situation; (b) the intensity and variety of the emotions experienced; and (c) the individual's adjustive habits and mechanisms. As we have indicated previously, the overt behavior exhibited is dependent to a considerable extent upon how the patient appraises himself and the situation in which he finds himself.

As a result of the frustrations involved, the emotions aroused may be fairly specific ones such as fear, hostility, or shame, or they may be quite unprecise and diffused such as generalized anxiety or tension. Strong negative emotions like anger and fear tend to be expressed rather directly through overt behavior, while less strong and less specific emotions tend to be more easily inhibited. In any event it is not likely that all the amputee's strong tensions will be relieved through the expression of any single type of emotional response.

The ultimate behavior exhibited by the individual is also modified by his previously learned adjustive patterns. As a consequence, he may express his emotions freely, modify or inhibit expression, or utilize substitute reactions—the so-called defense mechanisms, such as compensation, rationalization, projection, and identification.

The manner in which people respond to disaster, the death of a loved one, the destruction of their home, or the illness of a child varies in a myriad of ways. Similarly, the reactions to amputation tend to follow the same variable pattern. In the light of present knowledge, the most that can be said is that the method of adjusting psychologically to an amputation is primarily a function of the preamputation personality and psychosocial background of the person. We therefore see amputees who display behavior typified by depression, resentment, anxiety, defiance, resignation, indifference, perfectionism, impulsivity, dependency, aggression, or withdrawal. As a matter of fact, almost any type of behavioral response can be seen following the expected frequencies of normal, neurotic, and psychotic behavior in the population as a whole.

For the purpose of simplicity, the entire process may be charted as follows:

Amputation/perception of amputation → "Needs" → Frustration → Emotional reaction → Defense mechanisms, Adjustive habits → Covert or overt behavior

[It is interesting to note that only the first and last steps in this process ("amputation" and "overt behavior") are apparent to the unsophisticated observer—yet the interim considerations must be recognized and dealt with if the patient is to be rehabilitated.]

The psychological process described above may well result in a diminution of the amputee's motivation to regain his lost functions and willingness to compromise to unnecessarily limited restorative goals. The consequences of poor motivation are particularly devastating in this instance because the amputee is called upon over and over again to expend greater effort and energy than is normally demanded of a nonhandicapped person for the accomplishment of the task at hand. Also the variety of "secondary gains" that society makes available to certain groups of amputees tends to curtail further the necessary expenditure of effort.

The empirical evidence verifies the theory, in that the single most important problem facing the rehabilitation worker concerns the ways and means of implementing the marginal motivational and rehabilitational patterns of so many patients. Since the rehabilitation process is clearly re-educational in nature (and since it is properly said that no one can teach, only create a situation that is conducive to learning), the question arises as to what type of management procedures will help stimulate the patient's learning during the rehabilitation process.

SUGGESTIONS

Seven important areas of human functioning were described as being frustrated by virtue of amputation, namely: (1) physical function, (2) cosmesis, (3) comfort, (4) energy costs, (5) achievement, (6) economic security, and (7) respect and status. It is clear that in order to assist the amputee these seven reality problems, as modified by the amputee's perception of them, must be dealt with so as to diminish the frustrations and conflicts involved. A number of suggestions for doing this follow.

First, the actual process of physical restoration (providing a prosthesis with training in its use) assists the individual in partially meeting a number of his needs. When the amputee uses a prosthesis, he does not walk as well as a nonhandicapped individual, but his gait pattern more closely approximates that of the normal than it does when crutches are used. The prosthesis does not look exactly like the normal extremity; however, if properly fabricated it can meet the needs for good cosmesis to a great extent. The prosthesis will probably not be completely comfortable but can be designed to fit within the pain tolerance limits of the individual. The advantages obtained by restored function and appearance are most often sufficient to warrant the increased expenditure of energy on the part of the amputee. If he learns to utilize and control his prosthesis, the frequency with which it fails him diminishes. By appropriate rehabilitation counseling and placement procedures, the economic insecurity associated with re-employment can be reduced, and, lastly, one learns to accept himself and thereby the attitudes of others.

Along with these real improvements in the amputee's situation goes the process of correcting and clarifying the patient's perceptions, so that he comes to understand what the goals of the rehabilitation process are, what he may anticipate in the future, and what he must learn to live with.

Therefore, the first rehabilitative step for the amputee may be said to begin with the actual process of prosthetic restoration and the continued verbal explanations thereof to the amputee.

A second significant approach revolves about the ability of the rehabilitation personnel to suggest substitute life goals in the place of those being pursued prior to amputation and around the patient's ability to accept these new goals. For example, if the patient's occupation prior to amputation involves considerable use of the affected extremity, one can achieve significant psychological progress by providing training in another occupation that makes significantly lesser demands on the extremities and yet is equally appealing to the patient. When the substitute goal is offered and accepted, an important factor developing frustration and conflict is thereby eliminated.

Third, a problem frequently exists in preparing the patient to be amenable psychologically to the process of prosthetic restoration and to the acceptance of other rehabilitation goals. In the early postoperative stages an amputee may be viewed as undergoing an emotional reaction not dissimilar to those of people who suffer the bereavement associated with the death of a loved one. In this latter instance, it is well understood that the emotional reactions of the bereaved operate in somewhat of a circuitous fashion that must be interrupted at some point if the individual is to re-enter normal life activities. The individual may not be permitted to "stew in the juice" of his own nonproductive emotions. Following the analogy, the circumstances dictate the involvement of the amputee patient in some purposeful activity, at the earliest psychologically suitable moment, which will tend to divert him from a continuous preoccupation with his loss.

In this connection, the process of prosthetic training fulfills the extremely important function of involving the patient in challenging and important activities, so that the individual's preoccupation with his loss is reduced. In addition to the obvious primary purpose of prosthetic training—that of teaching one to use the prosthesis—the secondary purpose of requiring physical and mental concentration and involvement is significant. It is important to note that ordinarily only the occupational or physical therapist spends sufficient time with the patient to provide a continuous and important supervision and stimulation along these lines.

Fourth, a technic that is sometimes helpful in motivating the amputee patient involves placing him in contact with previously rehabilitated amputees. This is a particularly important procedure to be used with those amputees who find it impossible to relate to or identify with the nonamputated professional worker. In fact, he is unable to receive instruction or reassurance as a result of his attitude that no one who has not lost an extremity can really understand his situation.

In those instances, the use of previously rehabilitated amputees, as persons with whom the new patient may identify and from whom he may learn, cannot be overestimated. A word of caution must be made, however, concerning the qualifications of the amputee to serve as a model. An individual of considerable quality and substantial personal adjustment must be used so that the new amputee does not simply become an outlet for the mentor's problems and anxieties.

Lastly, the continuous expression by rehabilitation personnel of appropriate concern, attention, reassurance, and respect tends to assuage the troublesome emotions being experienced by the patient. Negative destructive emotions simply do not flourish as well in an atmosphere typified by the professional climate described above.

These several suggestions, though by no means exhaustive of what can be done, should tend to reduce the frustration and conflict as well as the strength of negative emotions being experienced by the patient. In turn, the individual's motivation to restore himself as a functioning member of society will tend to increase.

CRITERIA OF SUCCESSFUL REHABILITATION

By what criterion can we gauge the success of the rehabilitation of an amputee? Does the answer lie in the apparent perfect restoration of lost function, or in the ideal cosmetic replacement, or in the most comfortable prosthesis? Partially, success lies in all of these, but it may, in some cases, exist within a minimum of these accomplishments.

We cannot expect the same standards of performance from patients of dissimilar physical and psychological characteristics. We can accomplish only that which the individual's preamputation physical and psychological potentials permit. It is therefore sometimes possible to have a more successful result in the rehabilitation effort with people who use their prostheses less, than with those who use them more.

In view of this fact, success in rehabilitation may be defined in terms of psychological rather than physical criteria. Rehabilitation may be said to be successful when the amputation and its related considerations are no longer the central adjustment problem for the individual. As the ability to use the prosthesis more automatically, or subconsciously, increases; as the client's awareness of being physically limited and different becomes less threatening; and as the amputation becomes a minimal source of interference in his life activities, the elements of successful rehabilitation have been approached.

Reading 34
Battle Casualty: Amputee
Sandra Kirkpatrick

Arriving: battle casualty from Vietnam.

He is a combination of Pseudomonas, rice-paddy mud, and dried blood. His fingernails are black. He is sweating and needs a shave. His hair is long, matted, dirty. His dressings are bulky and nauseatingly foul-smelling. His face and arms are peppered with small shrapnel wounds. He is pale and exhausted after the long flight.

But he manages to look up at you with a faint smile as he says, "Hi, I'm home." He is an amputee.

He has arrived at the U.S. Naval Hospital, Oakland, California, location of the Naval Prosthetic Research Laboratory (NPRL), one of the Navy's two amputee centers, where, before July 1965, the amputee census averaged five to ten patients, usually older men. But with the escalation in Vietnam, our census quickly changed: In the last 24 months we have cared for over 200 amputees, young Marines between 18 and 25 years of age.

On the average, we receive the casualties within three to seven days following injury. Ninety to ninety-five percent of our patients have lost one or both lower limbs by stepping on a land mine or a booby trap. Frequently, the leg had not been totally amputated by the injury itself but impaired circulation, severe nerve damage, or extensive soft-tissue damage had called for immediate amputation on arrival at the field station.

From Vietnam, the men are flown to Clark Air Force Base in the Philippines, where they remain for a day, undergoing debridement and dressing changes under anesthesia. Sixteen to twenty-four hours after leaving Clark they arrive in the United States at Oak Knoll.

At first glimpse, a 40-bed ward of amputees is a depressing sight, and as a young Navy nurse fresh from school, I wondered whether I was capable of caring for an amputee, a battlefield casualty! But before too long I became so involved in the multiphasic amputee program that I had little time for my own thoughts.

Initial evaluation of the amputee usually reveals multiple needs. Rarely is the amputation his only serious problem. Often, continuous intravenous therapy, an indwelling catheter, a temporary colostomy, stump traction, and

---

Reprinted from *The American Journal of Nursing*, vol. 68, no. 5, pp. 998–1005, May 1968. (The photographs and line drawings in the original article have not been reproduced in this book.) This paper reflects the views of the author and not necessarily those of the U.S. Navy.

multiple fractures are present, too. Beginning chronologically with A.M. care, consider what the nursing care of the amputee entails.

PERSONAL CARE

Sergeant Brown was admitted five days after injury with a left below-knee and right above-knee amputation. He was febrile (102°F), had an I.V. running, and a Foley catheter in place. Because of severe soft-tissue damage to his buttocks, he had a temporary colostomy so that the buttock wounds and skin graft could heal without fecal contamination. (Most amputees accept such a colostomy with little difficulty because they know it is temporary, more convenient, and less painful than a bedpan.)

Sergeant Brown, like many critically injured "aerovacs," had required so much medical attention en route that a complete bed bath had been impossible. Before that, he had been in battle: he had not had a hot shower or washed his hair in fresh water in several months. (I have been told that for a long time the only "bath" a fresh pre-op casualty received at the aid station in Da Nang was—if he could tolerate it—a washing down with a hose!)

In view of this, giving a complete and thorough bath is one of our priorities. It often takes several days of gentle scrubbing to get through the layers of grime and dirt. We encourage our patients to do as much of this for themselves as possible, because this is where their independence begins. Unless both his hands are injured and bandaged, the new casualty still can do almost all his own bath. An Ace bandage wrapped over an I.V. needle replaces the arm board, allowing him freer use of his arm.

Sergeant Brown began his morning care by exchanging his colostomy bag. The first day the staff did this for him, explaining the procedure. In two days he was able to care for his own colostomy and bathe himself about the face, neck, chest, arms, and perineum.

Then the nursing staff tackled the job of his back care. For Sergeant Brown, as for many of the amputees, turning from side to side was often difficult and painful. However, with encouragement and help both from the other patients and from the staff, he soon learned to turn in bed with relative ease.

Each of our patients has a bed equipped with a Balkan frame and trapeze bar, which he uses to lift and turn himself while one corpsman supports his stump and a second corpsman gives back care. This includes a thorough washing, followed by a good back rub with alcohol. Because the typical new casualty is febrile, the alcohol serves to cool him as well as to help toughen his skin and prevent breakdown.

Care of the buttocks often involves care of massive open wounds. The combination of continuous purulent drainage and wet Betadine (povidone-iodine) dressings is a constant source of frustration to both the patient and the staff. If the back and buttocks are not kept dry, maceration of healthy skin will occur very quickly. Applying powder to the unbroken skin after the alcohol rub helps keep down some of the moisture.

To minimize the patient's discomfort, his sheets are changed after back care while he is still lying on his side. Use of drawsheets depends on the amount of drainage from the stumps. Frequently, properly placed Chux are used in place of a drawsheet. These must be changed frequently, but the patient stays drier and is more comfortable. Often, too, extra linen means added wrinkles and discomfort, and limits the effectiveness of the alternating-pressure mattress.

When one side of the bed has been made and protected with Chux, the amputee is rolled slowly to his opposite side. When the bed is made and if the patient can tolerate it, he might be left on his side supported with pillows.

Within a day or two, he is ready to be turned onto his abdomen. This proposal is typically countered with groans, but after some positive reinforcement—again, from other patients and staff—the patient gives in, turns onto his abdomen, and promptly falls asleep for one or two hours.

If necessary, a Stryker frame or CircOlectric bed is used to help the bilateral or triple amputee turn successfully.

Completion of the bath is not the end of A.M. care. The patient's fingernails, toenails, hair, and teeth also require attention. Nailbeds often are so dirty that it takes several days of soaking and scrubbing to remove the months' accumulation. And, although a shampoo can be time-consuming and difficult, the smile of comfort afterward makes the effort worthwhile. Shampoos are given at the high, large treatment room sink, where the patient is taken on a stretcher.

P.M. care is similar to A.M. care, but on a somewhat smaller scale. It includes complete back care, oral hygiene, and water for washing the face and hands. Due to drainage and diaphoresis, the linen may need to be changed. If no change is necessary, the sheets are tightened and fresh Chux are placed under the stumps.

Proper nutrition is rarely a problem! The first few days after admission, we have to encourage a high fluid intake because, due to temperature elevation, pain, and repeated surgery, the patient's appetite may be minimal. But within a few days his appetite equals that of any other young adult male. As he improves, Red Cross volunteers often help both his appetite and morale by bringing in special foods.

Initially, constipation can be a problem. Frequently, the casualty has not had a bowel movement since the day he was injured. In addition, he often fears using the bedpan, especially if he has buttock wounds. Often a Dulcolax suppository or a Fleet enema is necessary at first, and, if at all possible, the patient uses a commode. This if often physically more exhausting and painful, but psychologically it is much easier. Further difficulty with elimination is then prevented by giving Colace twice daily and a glass of prune juice every morning.

The Vietnam amputee must undergo multiple surgical procedures, depending on the extent of infection and injury. Almost all his wounds are infected. The organisms found on culture run the gamut, but the majority are Pseudomonas. This is due to the environment at the time of injury, and not to neglect or poor technique on the part of medical personnel.

Our pre-op care is simple. One factor carefully watched is the patient's hematocrit. An amputee usually needs several transfusions to bring his "crit" to at least 35 percent, the required minimum for surgery.

Our psychological preparation would probably evoke cries of protest from nursing instructors everywhere, because very little of the standard sort is necessary. All the amputees have had surgery at least two or three times previously—in Vietnam or prior to arriving at our hospital. In addition, they receive a great deal of encouragement from each other, and their universal concern is "getting that stump closed" and beginning to walk again.

SURGICAL CARE

Debridement with dressing change is done under anesthesia every few days. For some of these patients, only one or two procedures in the operating room are required. For others, especially for the bilateral amputee, it may take six to ten operative procedures to prepare a satisfactory stump.

In the operating room, a fluff dressing of 4 × 8's soaked in Betadine provides coverage over the open end of the stump. Skin traction is accomplished by securely fastening a roll of tubular stockinette to the limb with liquid adhesive and an Ace wrap. Upon return to the ward, traction on the stockinette is maintained by weights and a pulley system. This helps to draw the skin down over the raw surfaces and to prevent contraction of the skin and muscle away from the end of the bone.

Edema and flexion contractures are prevented by placing shock blocks under the foot of the bed rather than by elevating the stump on pillows. The remainder of the postoperative care is the same as that of any other patient who has had major surgery.

Once healthy granulation tissue has replaced all necrotic, infected tissue, the stump is ready for closure. Two methods of stump closure are used. The most desirable closure, suturing two skin flaps over the stump end, requires fewer operations and provides a far stronger surface for weight bearing than the second method of closure, which uses skin grafts. When a patient is to have skin grafts, we scrub and shave the donor site on the morning of surgery, and we also prepare him for the annoying burning sensation at the donor site which follows the grafting. We tell patients this will feel like a severe sunburn, and one young man, awakening from anesthesia, said that next time he wanted to take his suntan lotion.

Because it is hard to find patent veins on a shrapnel victim, the I.V. fluids are usually continued for a bare minimum of 24 hours, so as not to exhaust the supply of patent veins. We also anticipate further use of the I.V., knowing that, if the post-op hematocrit is below 35 percent on the morning after surgery, another transfusion will be given. And, depending on the extent of infection, the I.V. fluids may be used to carry antibiotics as well.

The complications incurred by these amputee casualties are numerous and varied. In the past two years, every service in the hospital has been involved in their treatment. Men involved in land mine explosions often have suffered bilateral perforations of the tympanic membrane. Some have lost an eye. Others have had genito-urinary involvement, including renal failure, or orchiectomy, or ruptured urethra. A few develop septicemia. Many have skin rashes or other dermatologic problems. Most need to see the dentist. Complete care, in other words, is never limited to the orthopedic service.

Of all the complications, there are two we must be alert for constantly. The first is hemorrhage. Most hemorrhages are due to necrosis of minor vessels, and a pressure dressing is sufficient treatment. Application of such a dressing to an amputee's stump is no different than applying one to a severe cut.

Second, and of far greater concern, is pulmonary embolism. In 24 months, three of our amputees died—two from massive pulmonary embolus. Fortunately, in the others, the majority of the emboli were very small and did not totally obstruct a major vessel.

Pulmonary embolism results largely from the extensive damage to the extremity and its vessels at the time of injury. Some of the men were up and about in wheelchairs, while others were still confined to bed when the embolism occurred. There was never one pattern of warning, just a sudden onset of symptoms—marked anxiety and restlessness, diaphoresis, chest pain, dyspnea, tachycardia, and a drop in blood pressure.

Initial nursing care is solely related to the symptoms. The patient is placed in semi-Fowler's position and given oxygen. An accurate record is kept of his vital signs and an I.V. is started. Heparin is given by I.V. drip in a ten-day course of gradually decreasing doses, depending on prothrombin time.

MORALE

Our staff takes great pride in maintaining in the patient a level of morale that astounds both visitors and new ward personnel. However, several very influential circumstances foster and further such morale. The most significant is that the amputee is very, very glad to be alive and back in the U.S.A., away from the war, the death, the filth. Most amputees are relieved to have survived the four obstacles a combat soldier fears most—paralysis, loss of manhood, loss of sight, and loss of life. As documented in a study of World War II amputees, men injured in combat considered themselves lucky to have survived [1].

Second, and equally important, is the group interaction. Forty men on one open ward, mostly Marines, amputees whose injuries occurred in similar ways, form a natural group. Their esprit de corps is difficult to describe—but heartwarming to see. They boost each other's spirits and give encouragement. The new admission is quickly and voluntarily welcomed by one of the older casualties. This is a real help to us, too, because the "older" patient serves as another set of eyes and ears in our observation of the new casualty, and insures that his needs will be communicated to us. Also, seeing others like himself is real, tangible proof for the new amputee that he, too, can expect to function normally once again.

TOWARD INDEPENDENCE

Another essential factor is the program of early ambulation and rehabilitation. As soon as a stump is closed, the amputee is up walking. It is important for the patient to get up and walk about; therefore, fitting him with a temporary prosthesis or skeletal pylon is often a great advantage [2].

Before a nurse can interact usefully with a group of amputees, she must first recognize and deal with her own feelings. It is both traumatic and heartbreaking to see a young man of 19 or 20 missing two legs and an arm. However, tears and sympathy won't cheer him and won't help him walk again [3]. But a smile and some enthusiasm will, and both these attitudes are contagious.

The best psychologic medicine for the amputee is a hopeful yet realistic attitude. Along with this attitude, a firm nurse-patient relationship is necessary so that, along with recognizing that we are there to help him, the patient recognizes our belief that he is required to do his part. Unlike a quadriplegic, who will always be dependent on someone else, the amputee will become independent. No matter how severely injured or how many extremities are involved, there is always something, some one function, he can do for and by himself. The nurse must expect—almost demand—this of her amputee patient if he is to take this first step toward independence.

The ultimate goal of ambulation and independence, particularly for a bilateral amputee, may appear to be far off, very involved, difficult, and therefore futile. But, through the use of a series of short-term goals, we can establish an attitude conducive to adjustment and rehabilitation. Such goals are set up throughout the basic daily routine. For some casualties, completion of their own entire A.M. care, or learning to turn over from back to abdomen without assistance, is a great achievement.

Throughout this period of adjustment, and in order to achieve even these short-term goals, the amputee must learn to handle frustrations, develop patience, and begin to recognize his own limitations. The nurse and her staff sometimes make the amputee wait for a time when he requests something. It sounds harsh and creates grumbles, but a brief reminder that he is not the only patient on the ward is often sufficient. Before too long a demanding introvert becomes cognizant of others and much more patient with both himself and us. (This patience-stretching exercise can be helpful when used judiciously and when the purpose is clearly to teach the permanently handicapped person to put up with frustrations he will have every day of his life. I do not say it is an appropriate maneuver with all acutely ill patients.)

The proper use of narcotics is a prime tool for helping the amputee deal with frustration and pain. On admission, many of our casualties—depending on the extent of injury—receive morphine 15 mg. every three hours. The patient's first goal is to try and wait three and one-half hours, then four, and so on. After 48 to 72 hours the dosage is decreased, until gradually he can take Empirin or Darvon compound instead. Frequently this takes several weeks, because the amputee needs medication for repeated surgical procedures. This is definitely an area requiring careful consideration and sound judgment on the nurse's part. The easy way out would be to administer the narcotic instead of instituting simple nursing measures to increase comfort. Needless to say, the challenge also lies in the nurse's ability to inspire, encourage, and teach.

Along this same line, we learned that we have to consider proper timing in the use of narcotics. For example, our amputees do not receive any narcotic after 6:00 A.M. until their A.M. care is completed, because we found that patients were more alert and were more willing and able to help themselves when they were not under the influence of a recent dose of narcotic. Consequently, holding off on this dose becomes one of the first short-term goals a patient is able to set and achieve for himself. The very realization that he no longer needs the narcotic is a very real affirmation of his returning independence.

One facet of amputee care continually written about is phantom sensation, formerly called phantom pain. Although it has been a problem, it has not been as great as it sometimes appears to an outsider. First, it is one more difficulty the amputee must adjust to. Yes, he does have a sensation that his big toe itches or he has sharp pain at the site of injury. And he can expect to have such sensations for three months, six months, or a year. But the early ambulation and early weight bearing on the stump seem to decrease these sensations [1].

The best proof to me of the value of weight bearing came several weeks ago, while we were working with an amputee who had not been able to go to NPRL. He was having severe phantom sensations which he could cause to disappear by applying pressure to the end of his stump.

We also capitalize on another factor in the environment to help the amputees—their Marine background. Such slogans as, "The Marine Corps builds men," and "Pain builds character," or "Are you a man or a mouse?" when applied with finesse evoke an emotional response reminding the amputee that he is not inferior, not a part of a man, but rather a whole man, a Marine who has done his job! This recall to the military discipline also summons his esprit de corps, and reinforces the extrovertive and independent part of his personality.

Needless to say, we do not always succeed. Those patients with severe and extensive wounds who remain bedfast while their neighbors are up and about in a wheelchair or the amputee who almost reaches his final goal and then suffers a stump breakdown are among those whose former levels of patience and cheerfulness decline rapidly. They become increasingly irritable, frustrated, demanding, and often on the verge of giving up. There seems to be no real answer for this syndrome; but continued encouragement, hopefulness, determination, and diversional activities often play a major role in helping these patients over this hurdle.

PHYSICAL ACTIVITY

Often the psychologic and rehabilitative phases of amputee care are difficult to separate. Programs in both areas are instituted the day the casualty is admitted and never cease until he is discharged. Each reinforces and furthers the other. Getting the amputee into a wheelchair as soon as he is able also increases his independence. Inactivity wastes not only the body but the mind as well. It is appalling to read publications of the last decade in which an amputee was kept in bed two to four weeks until stump closure and healing were complete. He should not be confined to his bed until his stump is healed!

As soon as possible, the amputee gets out of bed, even if it means rolling into a prone position on a stretcher and pushing his stretcher about the ward using two canes. For some patients, it means getting up in a wheelchair. Often the stump has not been closed and skin traction is still necessary. Therefore, special boards with a traction apparatus to keep the stump extended were devised for the wheelchairs. Occasionally, men in CircOlectric beds or Stryker frames were simply moved outside in nice weather—bed, patient, and all.

Many medical people who work with amputees seem to put too much emphasis on the development of contractures, and therefore often advocate keeping the amputee flat in bed rather than sitting in a wheelchair. With continuing effort, however, an amputee can be in a wheelchair almost all day without developing hip flexion contractures. As a part of A.M. care, he should be encouraged to suspend his stump over the edge of the bed and go through full range of joint motion, extension and abduction being particularly stressed. While he is in bed, alignment of the stump to avoid external rotation and abduction is of great importance. Also, the amputee should be encouraged to lie on his abdomen as soon as possible and whenever he can, especially while sleeping. This counterbalances the tendency toward hip flexion contractures.

Very little is impossible for the amputee, and keeping him constructively busy from reveille to taps is a primary principle of our program. Other authorities agree that "activity in any form is the best therapy for the dissolution of anxiety and fear" [4]. For the bed patient, the morning is taken up with A.M. care and various paperwork tasks such as compiling blank charts. In the afternoon, civilian and Red Cross volunteers come to the ward to teach ceramics, leather craft, collage, and painting.

When the amputee is able to tolerate prolonged periods in a wheelchair, he becomes responsible for making his own bed and keeping his own area clean. On a military ward, cleanliness is handled by the patients. Our ward details run the gamut, and include collecting empty soft drink bottles, dusting, folding clean linen, and sweeping the floor. The amputee soon proves to himself and those around him that he is capable of performing productive tasks for others as well as for himself.

The day the stump is closed in surgery is usually a red letter day for the amputee. A specially designed rigid plaster dressing is applied in the operating room and the next morning the patient is taken to the prosthetic research laboratory, where a pylon or aluminum peg leg is applied to this cast. That afternoon he returns, and for the first time walks on both legs. From then on he goes to NPRL twice a day, seven days a week for gait training, prosthetic fitting, physical and occupational therapy.

The rigid plaster dressing serves several functions. It helps to shrink and shape the stump for the prosthesis a great deal faster than an elastic bandage. It accustoms the stump to a constant covering, helps condition it for weight bearing, and provides a suitable surface for attachment of the pylon.

The physical facility at Oak Knoll is extremely conducive to exercise and rehabilitation, for it consists of many one-story buildings spread over several rolling acres, all connected by ramps. The dining hall, physical and occupational therapy, and NPRL are all a good 10- or 15-minute up and downhill trek by wheelchair from the ward. Consequently, by evening our amputee has had a very full day and is physically tired. He has also accomplished things that truly surprise him. There is little time left for worry, introspection, and self-pity. Those who do tend toward this are helped out of it by group influence.

LOOKING AHEAD

What about the future? We rarely see fear, anxiety, or insecurity about the future. This, too, was documented by World War II experience [1].

Today the amputee has not only the financial security of an armed forces pension, but also numerous benefits available through the Veterans Administration and Social Security programs. Representatives of these offices visit the ward and NPRL every week, helping each amputee take advantage of the assistance to which his disability entitles him. Those patients who have not completed high school take special tests and courses and receive their diplomas, while others are aided in selecting and preparing for college.

Transition from a protected environment to the outside world is facilitated by individuals and organizations alike. Fishing and hunting trips, dinners at a large restaurant, an afternoon at a football game, and many other such activities are planned. Thus the amputee can gradually become accustomed to the curious glances and whispered comments of the public before he leaves us.

The nurse who works with amputees will find it an excellent chance to practice her best nursing skills and techniques. Her main tools will be patience, enthusiasm, a creative imagination, and a determination to help her patient attain always just one further goal. And the nurse who works with these men soon finds that, though working with amputees is hard work, it is not depressing. Her long hours and days are abundantly rewarded when an independent man says good-bye—and walks away.

REFERENCES

1 Knocke, F. J., and Knocke, L. S. *Orthopaedic Nursing*. Philadelphia, Pa., F. A. Davis Co., 1951, pp. 84-87.
2 Robert Jones and Agnes Hunt Orthopaedic Hospital, Oswestry, England. *The Oswestry Textbook for Orthopaedic Nurses*, ed. by Robert Roaf and Leonard J. Hodkinson. Philadelphia, Pa., J. B. Lippincott Co., 1964, p. 160.
3 American Medical Association, Council on Physical Therapy. *Handbook on Amputees*. Chicago, Ill., The American Medical Association, 1942, p. 7.
4 Morrissey, Alice B. *Rehabilitation Nursing*. New York, G. P. Putnam's Sons, 1951, pp. 48, 215-217.

Reading 35
Stump Hygiene
S. William Levy
Gilbert H. Barnes

INTRODUCTION

After amputation, the skin of the stump is subject to irritation and often to injury and infection. Care of this skin is therefore a vital part of rehabilitation.

This [article] offers some basic rules to be used in the care of the stump. Although the illustrations show leg amputees, the rules of stump hygiene are also applicable to arm amputees.

In the first section, a daily routine of skin hygiene is shown. Since the socket of the artificial limb may in itself produce a disorder, care of the socket—and of the sock and bandages that come in contact with the skin—is also illustrated.

Some of the common skin disorders of the stump are discussed briefly in the second section.

Correct ways of bandaging the above-knee and below-knee stump are illustrated in the third part of the [article].

An ounce of prevention is worth a pound of cure. If a simple routine of stump care is followed consistently, the amputee can avoid many of the disorders that might force him to stay off his prosthesis. The first and most important rule for the health of the skin of the stump is

Keep the stump clean

A daily routine for keeping the stump clean should become as regular as the habit of brushing one's teeth.

The skin of the stump is confined in a socket all day long. The air does not circulate around it, and the sweat is trapped against the skin. If the stump is not kept clean, its skin may become infected easily and it may develop a bad odor. Small irritations from the rubbing of the socket may become so serious that the artificial limb cannot be worn.

From the Biomechanics Laboratory, University of California, Berkeley and San Francisco, and the Division of Dermatology, University of California School of Medicine, San Francisco. This study was supported by research grant RG-4856, National Institutes of Health, and research grant RD-459 from the Office of Vocational Rehabilitation, Department of Health, Education, and Welfare. The publication of this pamphlet was made possible by the Office of Vocational Rehabilitation. (Illustrated by Thomas B. Harris.)

CLEANSE THE SKIN

HERE IS WHAT SHOULD BE DONE EVERY EVENING TO PROTECT THE HEALTH OF THE STUMP SKIN.

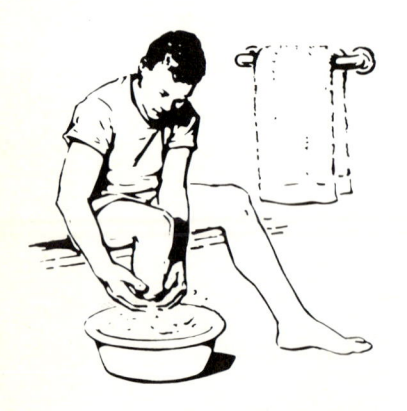

Wet skin thoroughly with warm water.

Add one-half teaspoonful of liquid antiseptic cleanser containing hexachlorophene (pHisoHex and Tod'l are two examples), or else use cake soap such as Gamophen or Dial. All these cleansers can be bought in a drug or grocery store.

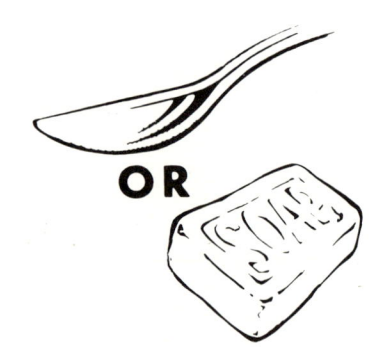

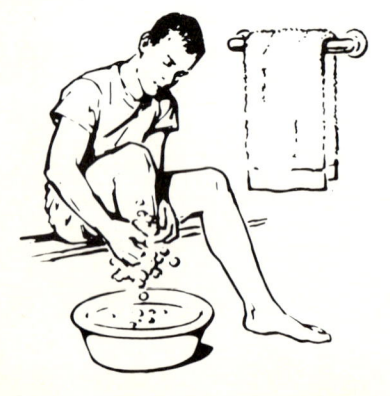

OR

Work up to a foamy lather. Use more water for more suds.

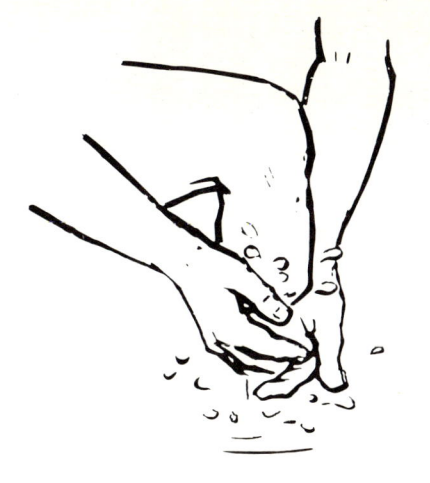

Rinse with clean water.

Dry skin thoroughly. Do not let soap dry on the skin. A soapy film left on the skin may be irritating.

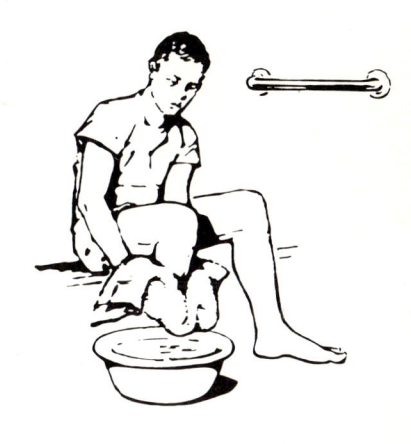

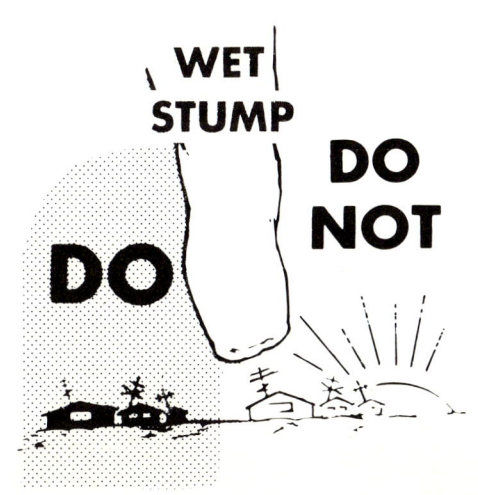

WET STUMP

DO

DO NOT

Usually the stump cleansing should be done at night. The stump should not be washed in the morning unless a stump sock is worn. The damp skin may swell and stick to the prosthesis and may be irritated by rubbing.

...THE SOCKET

THE SOCKET SHOULD BE CLEANSED OFTEN—EVERY DAY IN WARM WEATHER. THE BEST TIME TO CLEANSE THE SOCKET IS AT NIGHT.

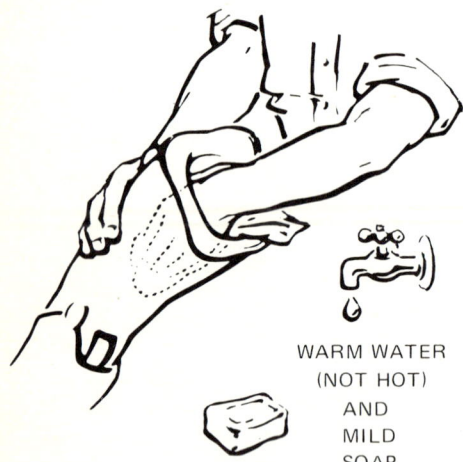

Wash with warm water and mild soap.

WARM WATER
(NOT HOT)
AND
MILD
SOAP

Wipe out with cloth dampened in clean warm water.

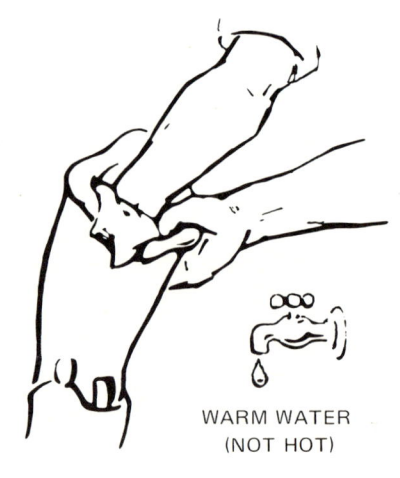

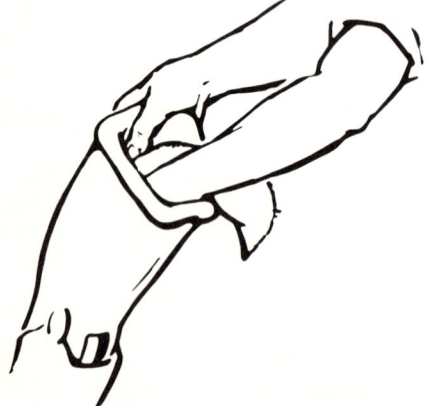

WARM WATER
(NOT HOT)

Dry thoroughly before putting on.

...THE SOCK

THE STUMP SOCK SHOULD BE CHANGED EVERY DAY. IT SHOULD BE WASHED AS SOON AS IT IS TAKEN OFF, BEFORE THE PERSPIRATION DRIES IN IT.

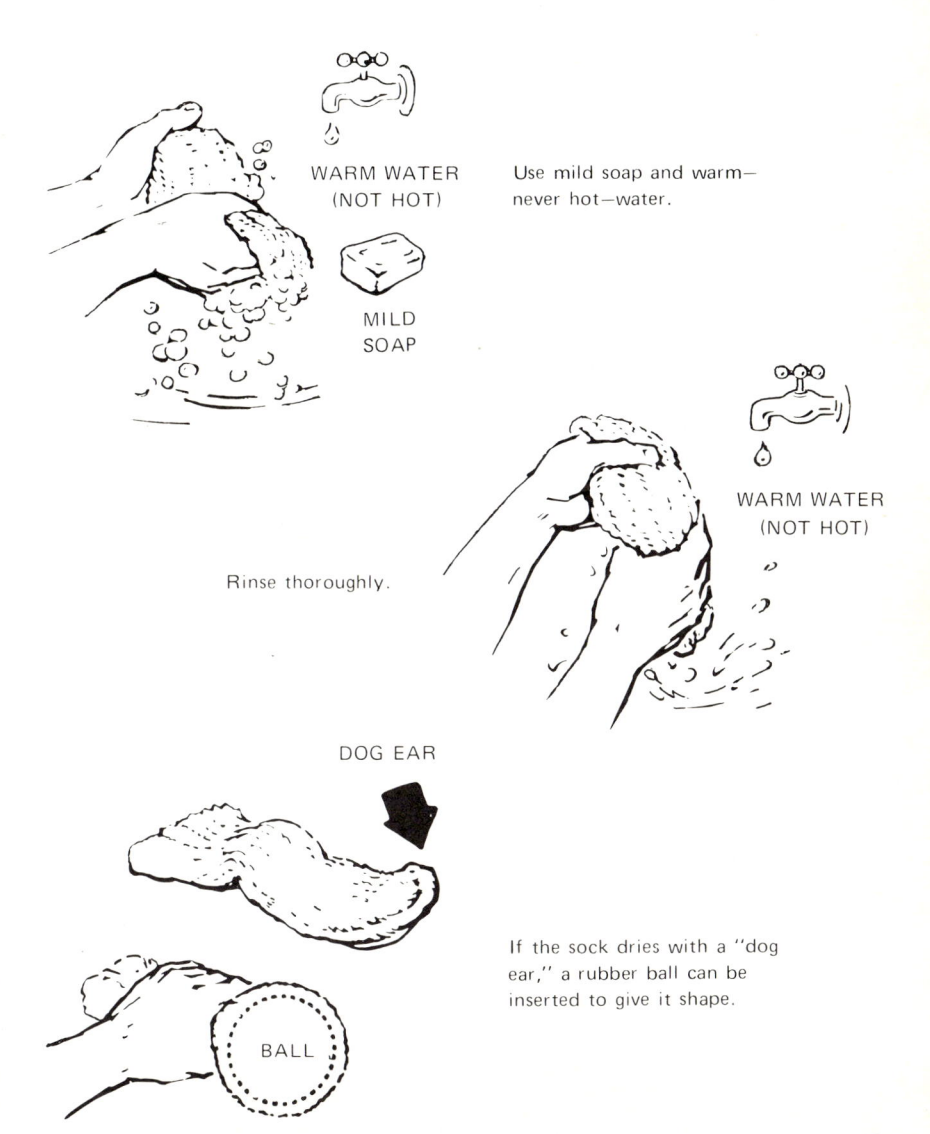

WARM WATER (NOT HOT)

Use mild soap and warm— never hot—water.

MILD SOAP

Rinse thoroughly.

WARM WATER (NOT HOT)

DOG EAR

If the sock dries with a "dog ear," a rubber ball can be inserted to give it shape.

BALL

...THE BANDAGE

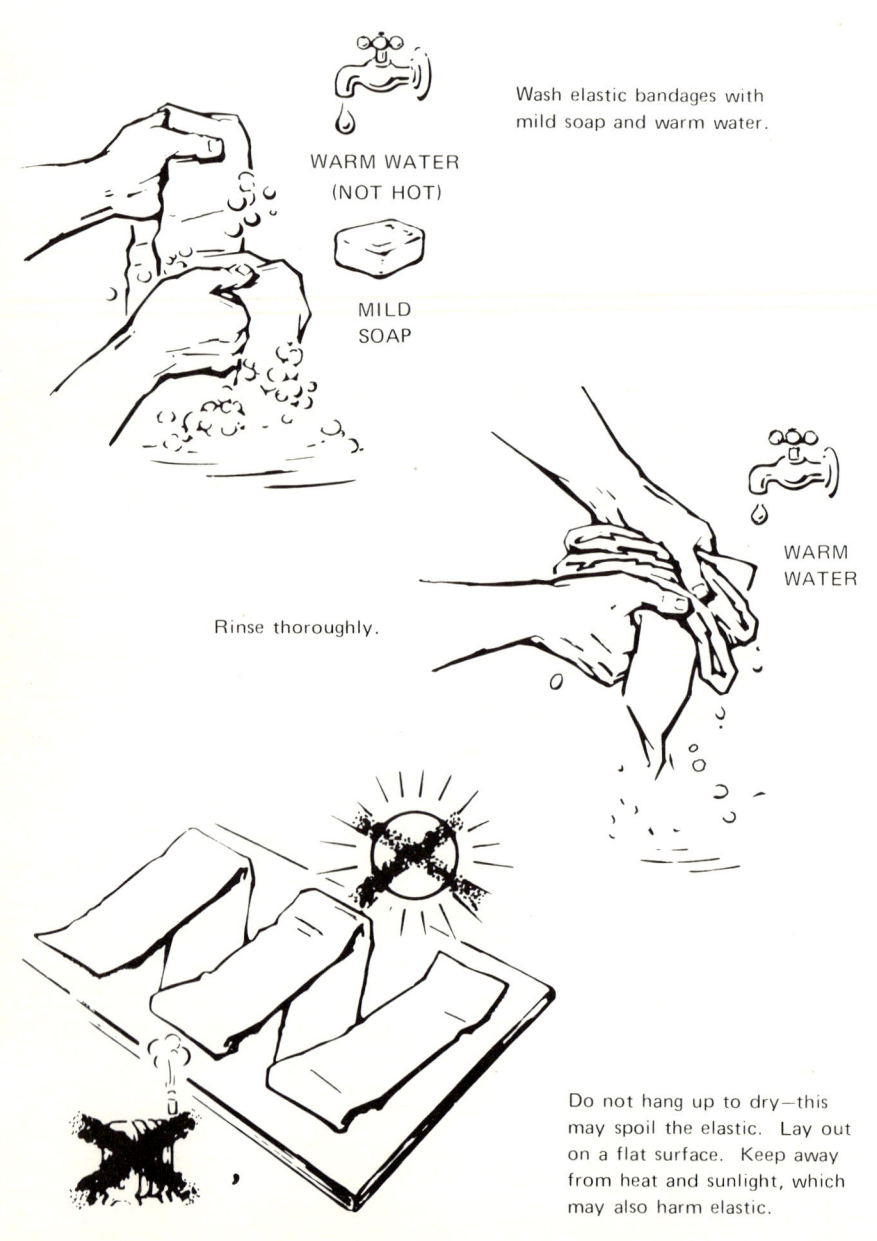

Wash elastic bandages with mild soap and warm water.

WARM WATER (NOT HOT)

MILD SOAP

Rinse thoroughly.

WARM WATER

Do not hang up to dry—this may spoil the elastic. Lay out on a flat surface. Keep away from heat and sunlight, which may also harm elastic.

REMEMBER

MINOR IRRITATIONS, IF NEGLECTED, MAY LEAD TO SERIOUS DIFFICULTY.

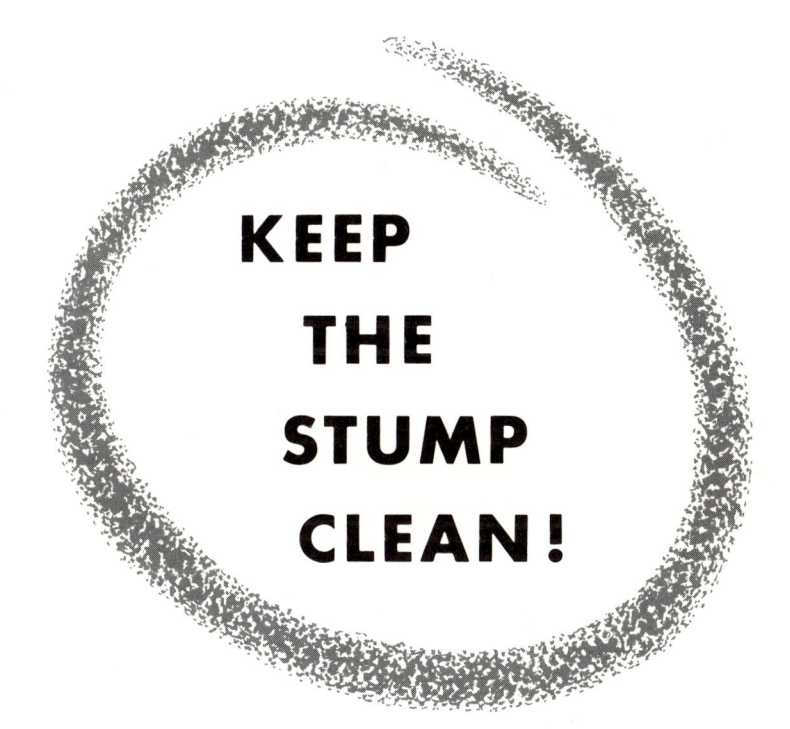

KEEP THE STUMP CLEAN!

SKIN TROUBLES

Here are three general rules if skin disorders develop:

SEE YOUR PHYSICIAN for treatment. A minor disorder may become disabling if incorrect treatment is used.

SEE YOUR PROSTHETIST. Adjusting the prosthesis may do away with the cause of the skin disorder.

NEVER use strong disinfectants, such as iodine, on the skin of the stump.

ABRASIONS.

The skin is sometimes abraded (rubbed raw) by the socket.

- Gently wash skin with liquid or cake cleanser and warm water. Cover with a mild antiseptic, such as bacitracin ointment, and sterile gauze.
- Make sure prosthesis is dry before it is put on.
- If abrasions occur often: SEE YOUR PROSTHETIST.
- If any abrasion shows any sign of infection: SEE YOUR PHYSICIAN.

BLISTERS.

If a blister is small and does not hurt:

- Wash it with antiseptic cleanser and leave it alone. Opening a blister without proper precautions and sterile instruments may cause infection.
- If it is large, painful, and recurs often: SEE YOUR PHYSICIAN

BACTERIAL INFECTIONS

may become serious and should be treated without delay.

HAIR-ROOT INFECTION is a common minor bacterial infection. To treat:

- Clean area daily with liquid antiseptic cleanser.

- Keep dry at other times.

- Allow air to circulate freely over infected area.

BOILS AND ABSCESSES are two more serious types of bacterial infection.

If they occur: SEE YOUR PHYSICIAN.

Until then:

- Rest as much as possible, with prosthesis off and stump raised.

- Apply hot compresses (cloths soaked in hot water) for 30 minutes every 3—4 hours.

FUNGUS INFECTIONS

are usually not serious but may be annoying.

For prevention or treatment:

- Follow rules of stump hygiene.

- Leave area of infection exposed to air as much as possible.

- Keep skin dry.

SWELLING

After amputation, during the healing phase, there is usually some swelling of the stump. This swelling is called edema. Later, a badly fitting prosthesis may cause similar swelling.

What can be done to prevent or treat this edema of the stump?

- The physician and the limb fitter may recommend that outside support should be given to the stump by socks or elastic bandages. (See the next pages.)

- If the prosthesis fits badly, SEE YOUR PROSTHETIST.

- Sit or lie for short periods with stump resting on a pillow. This will improve circulation and decrease the swelling.

- For the below-knee stump, avoid keeping the knee bent for long periods of time.

BANDAGING

To shrink and shape the stump so that the artificial limb can be fitted, elastic compression bandages, such as Ace bandages, are frequently used. Often bandaging must be continued after discharge from the hospital. The physician and the limb fitter should decide whether this should be done and for how long.

Using a well-fitted prosthesis will help prevent swelling. For this reason, the bandaging may be discontinued after the stump is fitted. Again, the decision when to stop bandaging should be left to the physician or limb fitter.

Elastic bandages are also used to treat the temporary edema that is caused, for example, by standing for too long or by gaining too much weight.

The following pages show methods of bandaging both above-knee and below-knee stumps.

HOW TO BANDAGE THE

THE HELP OF A SECOND PERSON IS OFTEN NEEDED IN BANDAGING THE ABOVE-KNEE STUMP. A GOOD METHOD IS SHOWN IN THE FOLLOWING ILLUSTRATIONS. HOWEVER, SOME PERSONS PREFER TO DO THE BANDAGING ALONE, WHILE SEATED.

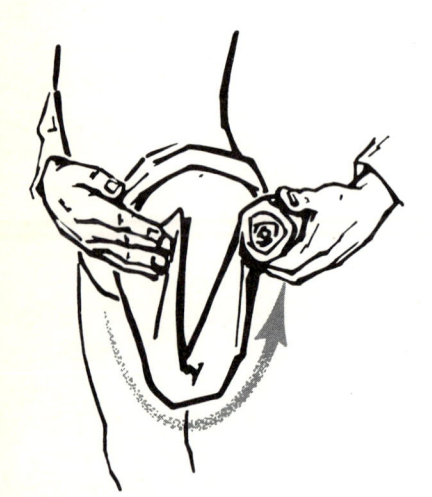

Make two or three turns over end of stump with a woven cotton or elastic bandage 4 or 6 inches wide.

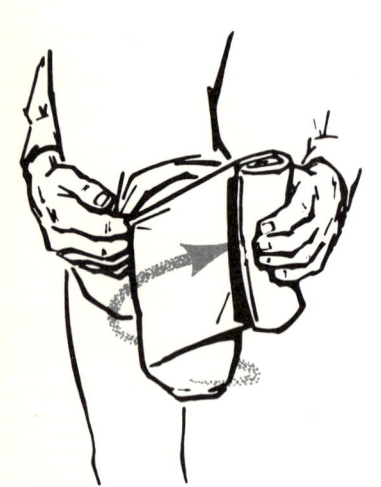

Anchor with one or two loose circular turns.

Wrap with spiral turns upward, making sure that end of stump is wrapped more snugly than the rest.

ABOVE-KNEE STUMP

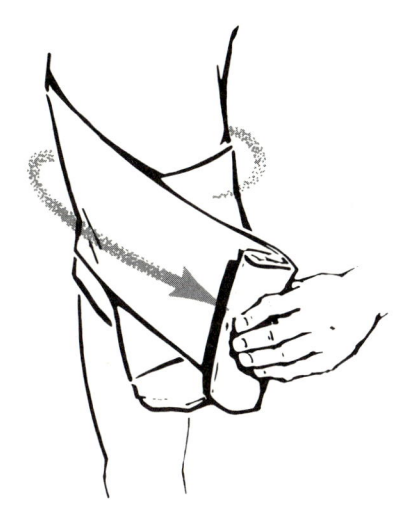

Secure bandage with "figure-of-eight" turns including pelvis and stump. These turns should cross on the outer side of the stump—not in front.

Make at least two turns, and be sure bandage extends full length of stump. Keep stump in relaxed position while bandage is being tightened.

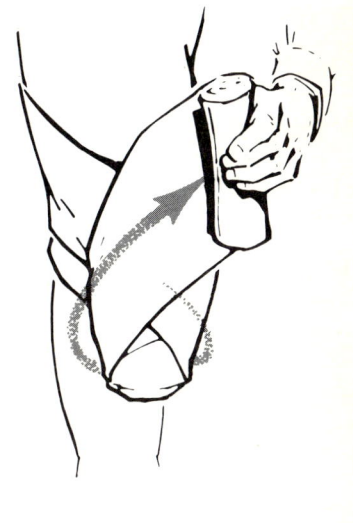

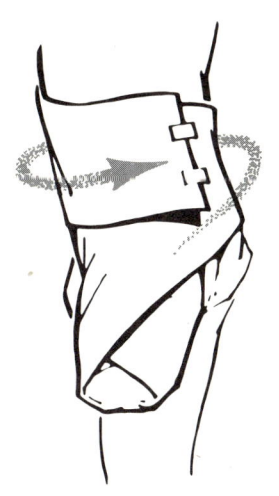

Fasten bandage on side of hip. Bandage should be reapplied if it becomes loose.

HOW TO BANDAGE THE

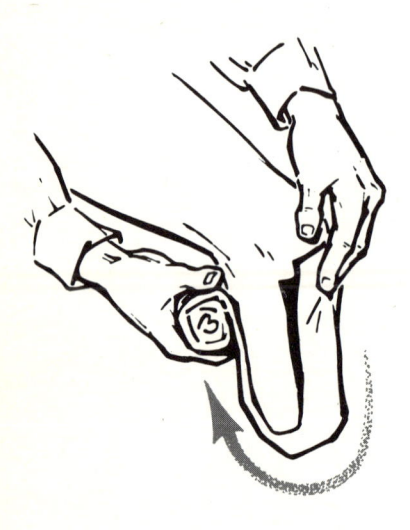

Make one or two turns to cover front, end, and back of stump as shown in illustration. Pull bandage upward so that it presses firmly against end of stump.

Anchor loosely at top with one or two circular turns and continue downward, still loosely, to end of stump.

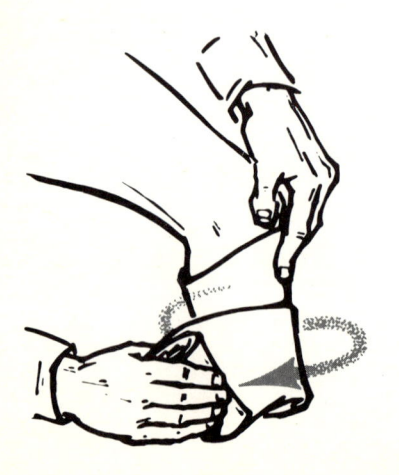

Wrap with spiral turns from end of stump upward. Be sure to make bandage more snug at end of stump than at any point above.

BELOW-KNEE STUMP

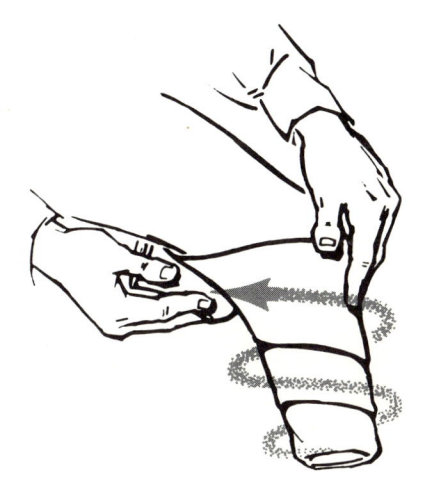

The bandage may be continued above the knee to prevent slipping, but often this is not necessary.

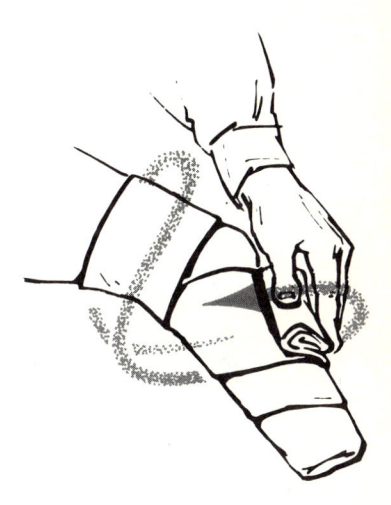

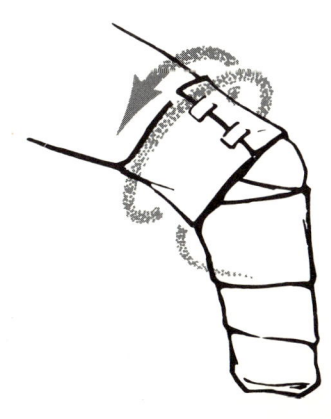

Anchor bandage loosely, making another turn below knee.

Fasten bandage.

Section E

Sight and Hearing Disorders

Man relates to his environment in terms of his ability to perceive it accurately, and much of his life is spent in refining and developing his sensory perception. Consequently, the loss of ability to receive the steady stream of stimuli with which he is bombarded because of a partial or complete sight or hearing problem is a severe handicap. If the loss occurs suddenly, the impact on the person is generally more severe than when it occurs gradually. Gradual decrements can be accompanied by corresponding compensatory adjustment if properly handled. In evaluating needs and planning care, the nurse must be aware of the extent of loss and the time of its acquisition. The deaf person who has never heard and the person who has partial hearing with the use of a device do not have identical problems. This is also true of the blind. A person may be legally blind and still have some ability to see. The extent of the disability has relevance for the patient care personnel in formulating realistic goals.

The loss of sight or hearing seriously impairs the individual's sense of control over his environment. At the same time his sense of dependency is heightened. The person so afflicted may develop a state of depression as he struggles to cope with his loss. The therapeutic task is to enable him to interpret and react to environmental cues through alternate means, and thus to regain a sense of personal adequacy. One of the first steps is to cope with one of life's basic necessities—the establishment of effective communication with others from a somewhat different vantage point. It is with such tasks that the nurse should concern herself at the earliest possible moment after meeting the patient. Basic personal adequacy undoubtedly underlies the learning of higher-order skills and competencies.

Most nurses will not be working with the sensory problems per se but with the person who requires nursing care for some medical or surgical intervention concerning their sensory disadvantage. The patient care personnel's problem is to find ways of communicating with these patients in such a way that their care can be facilitated and they will feel themselves surrounded by an understanding environment. The patient's ability to become actively involved in his own recovery is correspondingly increased. The family members should be valuable resources in interpreting the communication system which has been established and has worked for the patient at home.

It might be very well for the nurse who is teaching the newly blind to try to walk in his shoes for a time. She might, for example, eat her meals with covered eyes in order to learn what eating without visual clues is really like. There is always available to the nurse the experience and accumulated wisdom of many who have gone before. In this sense she does not have to start at the beginning each time; each patient, however, does. They can proceed more quickly and surely with the kind of assistance the rehabilitation nurse can offer.

Blind persons generally elicit great sympathy and consideration from the public. The deaf person's handicap is not so obvious. While his communication problems may be much greater than that of the blind, he is often made to feel inadequate because his problem is not so readily perceived. The nurse who is aware of both types of disability must be sure to use her personal concern to strengthen the patient's independence rather than to increase his dependency.

The article by O'Neill provides valuable suggestions for the person about to confront his first blind patient as well as a check for the more experienced. Much of the specific general information given is about Canada. The nurse functioning in the United States will be interested that, as in Canada, the precise number of blind persons is unknown, but it has been estimated that there are about half a million. The practitioner of nursing in any state may be able to obtain information regarding resources to help the blind from the State Department of Health or from the public rehabilitation agency. Some states have much richer resources than others. The nurse may find it simpler to write to the Vocational Rehabilitation Administration, Department of Health, Education, and Welfare, Washington, D.C., 20201. The American Foundation for the Blind, Inc., 15 West 16th Street, New York, New York, 10011, makes available a *Directory of Agencies for the Blind* which could be useful in locating a needed resource. Patients who are denying their disability may not be ready to make use of resources, but the nurse should be able to provide the necessary information when they are ready to make use of it.

Branson speaks with the authority of personal experience and is extremely practical in suggesting adaptations for the care of the blind. The nurse must not allow her own embarrassment and sense of inadequacy to prevent her from utilizing the resources hidden within the patient to assist with planning realistic care.

Jackson stresses the attitudes of nurses that may be conveyed to the patient through communication. The patient is a total person without vision. The integrity of his personality, his thinking, and his feelings have not been lessened by his handicap; they may have been sharpened. It is imperative that those who would assist the sensory deprived learn to understand their psychological needs.

The person who has been deaf from birth usually does not learn verbal communication but must make use of sign language. His communications are limited to those who know the sign language or are willing to enlist the services of an interpreter. The person who was born deaf or acquired deafness before he learned vocal speech differs from those whose hearing loss developed after vocal language was learned. Many persons, including nurses, find it embarrassing or difficult to raise their voices to the volume required for communication with a deaf person. Others seem to confuse the type of deprivation and tend to shout when communicating with the blind.

Since much of rehabilitation nursing is concerned with prevention, some articles are included which deal with the prevention of hearing loss. In today's noisy world there are few places that afford the quiet and peace of the African jungle, where tribesmen have the most acute hearing known to man. Factory clatter, jet plane noise, traffic, household appliances, and the amplification of rock music bombard the ears continuously with a dangerous level of sound. Sound pollution is under study along with other forms of pollution. Nurses have a place in demanding action to reduce the environmental threats to hearing. Both in her practice and in her life as a citizen the nurse has a responsibility to be aware of the problems of hearing loss as related to environmental pollution. Perhaps the modern hospital is one of the worst offenders. A place that is expected to be restful and therapeutic has become a setting where peaceful rest is impossible. Some hospitals are located on busy thoroughfares with noisy trucks and screeching fire engines and ambulances rushing by. Added to the outside noises is the clatter of clicking heels, clanging carts, and clattering dishes, to say nothing of public call systems and the noisy television sets operated indiscriminately by patients.

A discussion of deafness from the standpoint of employment and training is provided by Vernon. Valuable information concerning educational programs and referral possibilities is included. Silverman defines deafness in a nontechnical, functional way. He discusses diagnostic techniques and the concepts and aids fundamental in the rehabilitation process with this form of sensory loss.

Guberina of Yugoslavia makes a new approach to deafness which promises to change the prospects of those afflicted in a significant way. Certain premises underlie his work—the deaf still have some residual hearing left which can be tapped by finding the person's best level or frequency of sound. His method has the advantage, not presently found in hearing aids, of selectively filtering out frequencies which interfere with hearing. Even the body can receive sound vibrations, and this principle is used in the sound vibrator. Early referral helps in reestablishing the communication possibilities. Acquired deafness is the type which yields successfully to this type of assistance.

Murphy provides a detailed guide for the nurse whose responsibilities include the safeguarding of those who are exposed to dangerous noise levels as a part of their working conditions. She discusses audiometrics, record keeping, referral procedures, and preventive education.

Perhaps because of the horrendous problems related to the education of sensory deprived persons there has been a tendency to develop segregated schools for the education and training of the deaf and the blind. They are often boarding schools which take the child out of his home environment at an early age. The recent emergence of special education programs seems to be a more suitable approach. Sensory deprived individuals must learn to live and compete in a world with normal people. The adjustments after leaving school seem more difficult than they need be in the handicapped child who is educated in a segregated school. It must also be remembered that these young handicapped children will develop into adolescents and then into adults. They have all of the confusions, ambitions, and drives experienced by normal individuals of like age. It is normal for them to have sex interests and a desire to establish a family. In the segregated school they meet and marry persons with handicaps similar to their own. If their sensory loss is genetic, they would have an increased chance of producing sensory deprived offspring through a double genetic deficit. Young handicapped persons and their potential marital partners need a great deal of realistic counseling in order for them to make suitable decisions about both their vocational and their marital choices.

Reading 36

Understanding Your Blind Patient
Paul C. O'Neill

The young blind man paused at the foot of his bed to gather his dressing gown around him. Then he gave a spring lightly upwards and landed full tilt on a dinner tray that had been placed in position while he was out of the room. In a split second, the place was a shambles. White sheets turned red with tomato soup while mashed potatoes embedded themselves in the blankets. Dishes flew. The startled patient jumped off the bed, stepped on a chunk of ground steak and slithered across the floor.

Such accidents do not happen often, but almost every time a blind person goes to hospital, some similar experience adds difficulties to his convalescence. It even slows down the get-well process. Half-open doors strike him as he walks across the room. He gets annoyed when he falls over clean-up gear left in the corridors. The unexplained equipment in his room worries him. Perhaps the most retarding factor of the whole procedure is the endless time with nothing to do and few people to talk to.

The tragedy is greater because none of it needs to happen. With a little common sense on the part of the nurses, a blind person's hospitalization can be a pleasant experience that he will want to remember. The secret of the whole thing depends on the nurse. She should take a positive instead of a negative approach.

A good beginning is a thorough understanding of blindness. It is more confusing than it looks. Blindness does not always mean total loss of sight. In fact, more than half the blind people of Canada can see a little. Some can distinguish only the difference between light and darkness. If you close your own eyes, put your fingers over them, and turn towards the window, you will get a good impression of light perception vision. Others see in a mist as if a thick, white curtain were always in front of their eyes. Still others have peripheral sight, seeing the world around the edges of a great dark mass in the centre of their eyes. They never see the whole shape of anything, but only the top and bottom or the ends. Another group have pinhole sight, with everything blocked off but a tiny speck of light. In the low vision levels, the different ways people see are almost as varied as the people.

I know one man who can read a theatre sign from across the road, yet will stumble over a garbage can on the sidewalk at his feet. The confusion clears up when you examine the definition of blindness. In Canada, a person

Reprinted from *The Canadian Nurse*, vol. 61, no. 9, pp. 728-730, September 1965.

is legally blind if the visual acuity in both eyes with proper refractive lenses is 20/200 or less with Snellen Chart or equivalent, or if the greatest diameter of the field of vision in both eyes is less than twenty degrees. If you can read no more than the letter "E" on the Snellen Chart, you are a blind person.

When you discover your patient is blind, begin the positive approach by finding out whether he is totally blind or whether he sees a little. Once you know this, you need only observe the common courtesies to ensure a pleasant, successful relationship with him. When you first meet, take his hand or touch his arm. This physical contact gives the person some sense of your personality and suggests your interest in him. Speak directly to the blind person, but do not shout. He is not deaf. It is not enough to nod or shake your head. Give it words, give it expression. He cannot see your smile, but he can hear it in your voice. Keep your conversation natural, without consciously avoiding the word "blind" or changing "see" to "hear." When addressing a blind person, speak his name, otherwise he has no way of knowing that you are talking to him. When you leave him, tell him you are going. It is most disconcerting to suddenly find yourself talking to thin air.

Naturalness, real kindness and an inherent human respect will result in the most successful relationship. This will avoid an overdose of assistance that makes a handicap more noticeable and damages the value of your contact.

Tell him where his glass of water is and locate the position of the bell button on the bed. Keep his personal things, such as cigarettes and ash tray, easily accessible—a blind person enjoys a smoke as much as the sighted. His shaving kit is an important item. Once the male patient is well enough, he can shave himself. There is no need for anxiety because he cannot see. If you move his gear, make a sound so that he will know what you are doing. In this way you will prevent annoyance when he does not find his belongings in the old place.

Meal time can be a real problem for blind persons. Even those with a little sight have trouble cutting meat, and those with misty vision cannot recognize the vegetables on the plate. Not long ago a blind man spent 10 days in hospital. Just 24 years old, he had lost two fingers on his right hand. He had suffered a hearing loss and was totally blind. He did not complain, but one afternoon as a visitor was leaving, the nurse's aide brought in his tray. She placed it on a side table, threw a helpless look at the patient, and went out without saying a word. If the visitor had not been there, the blind man would not have known his dinner had arrived. The meal consisted of soup, roast beef (uncut), and a preserved pear (again, uncut).

Now let us restage this scene, assuming the nurse's aide knew what to do. She enters with the tray. "Hello sir," she says clearly, "I'm bringing your dinner. It's soup and roast beef with a nice half pear for dessert." She places the tray on the table as the young man prepares to eat. "You can drink the soup right out of the cup," she suggests, "and I'll be glad to cut your meat. If you like, I will cut the pear too."

Eating is frequently a problem, but this kind of help removes the worry. When vegetables are on the plate, simply think of the meal in terms of a clock. Blind people are taught this arrangement as a part of their rehabilitation program. You simply say, "Potatoes are at twelve, peas at nine and meat from two to five."

When the blind patient reaches the point where he can get out of bed and walk around a little, he should receive some orientation training. This is not difficult and shouldn't take more than 10 minutes, but it will save hours of anxiety and extra time for the nursing staff. Explain where his bed is—the second from the door—and show him where the bathroom is. If there are other doors in the room, tell him where they are and try to keep them completely open or completely closed. A blind person will not hurt himself on a closed door. Take him out in the corridor and explain what is going on in the immediate vicinity. Show where the telephone is and, once he has the idea, let him make his way to it alone. If there is a stairway nearby, explain where it is. Once the blind person knows its location, he will avoid it without difficulty.

Sometimes hospital personnel will insist that a blind person use a wheel chair, simply because he is blind. This only annoys him and accentuates his handicap. If he is well enough, let him walk. He does not need a wheel chair unless he is seriously ill. Do not push a blind person into a seat. Place his hand on the chair and he will be able to seat himself. It is simply a question of knowing where the chair is.

When guiding a blind patient around the hospital, always offer your arm. With his hand lightly on your arm, he feels the movement of your body and because you will be slightly ahead of him he will have a feeling of confidence with each step. To be propelled from behind can be most awkward and unnerving.

Another area where the blind patient needs help is in the passing of time. A sighted man will watch television, read the paper, or talk to the other patients. A blind person, even those who see to some extent, cannot read, does not notice the other patients, and cannot watch television. You can help him without adding greatly to the burden of your own daily duties. Introduce him to the other patients in his room. This will break the ice and make conversation easy for the whole group. Instead of television, offer him a radio. Find out if he reads Braille or would prefer to listen to "talking books" from the Canadian National Institute for the Blind. These books are recorded editions of printed books read by professional people. Prepared for a special tape play-back machine, the talking book brings the printed page to the blind listener in all parts of Canada.

Every day, more than two tons of Braille and recorded books are mailed across Canada from the CNIB library, Toronto. Covering every subject from the Bible to Perry Mason, the library caters to all readers. A children's library serves blind boys and girls. Your patient will be sure to find a book from this selection that will interest him. Your own hospital social service staff can help here with a call to the CNIB.

When it is time for medication, do not spring it on your patient without advising him. If you are about to give him a needle, tell him. Remember, he will not see you approach, and you can avoid a sudden shock by telling him what is going to happen. If you are giving him a pill, or medicine, warn him in advance and explain the purpose of the medicine. If he asks questions, answer them. Some blind people like to know as much as possible about what is happening to them.

When you discharge your patient, make sure he knows the doctor's instructions about medication. Do not be satisfied by merely asking him if he knows. Go over the instructions with him. In this way there can be no slip-up through lack of reading written instructions. If he obtains his medicine from the hospital pharmacy, see that someone goes with him to pick up his package. If there is need for a prosthesis, it is advisable to provide it while he is still at the hospital.

Visiting nurses who call on the blind patient at home can do a special service by observing housekeeping procedures. If the person is living alone, there may be assistance which CNIB would be glad to provide. Sometimes a CNIB volunteer can make a world of difference. She reads letters, sews on buttons, and serves as the blind person's contact with the community. She helps with shopping by escorting a blind woman to the shopping centre. She drives people to the doctor or dentist. She serves as a guide in a year-round recreation program for the blind. In short, the volunteer service brings the blind person who lives alone out of the confines of his own four walls into a world of activity and companionship.

The public health nurse should contact the nearest office of the CNIB, particularly if she is in a rural area. By discussing her blind patient with the CNIB field secretary, she will be able to set in motion a constructive program.

In large communities, blind persons are earners. Through the employment service of the CNIB, they are placed in industry and commerce, the professions, CNIB canteens, and executive posts with the CNIB. For the elderly, CNIB's sheltered shops provide part-time employment in light assembly work to supplement government allowance. This year, 90 blind Canadians are attending university in preparation for a professional career. Others are housewives and mothers fulfilling the regular role of a woman in a modern household. Nurses who handle prenatal and well-baby clinics can expect to find blind mothers among their clients. Here, the secret of service is a thorough explanation of each point and a demonstration, where necessary, to convey to the blind mother those ideas which usually come through seeing.

Encourage the patient to be as independent as he ought, but be ready to supply a pair of seeing eyes when vision is essential. Too often pity takes over. Sympathy is good, but understanding and the right kind of assistance will have your patient on his feet again in record time. You solve the problem when you concentrate more on the person and less on the handicap.

Perhaps the whole approach can be reduced to a single thought—put the accent on *ability,* not disability, and the blind will thank you.

Reading 37
Caring for the Blind Patient
Helen K. Branson

The relationship which the newly blinded person has with nursing personnel can be the beginning of acceptance and adjustment, or bitterness and self-pity. This is particularly true of the largest group of visually handicapped persons—those over 60.

Perhaps it would be helpful at the outset to define "blind." Most states accept the federal statute definition as acuity of 20/200 and below, thus not necessarily totally blind. In this paper when the word "blind" is used, it means vision so seriously impaired that the person lacks sight perception in mobility. The words visually handicapped, visually disabled, or visually limited mean much the same.

The adjustment to a serious visual handicap, particularly that of total blindness, is a series of traumatic processes. Few individuals who lose their sight after 20 achieve adequate emotional adjustment or physical compensation. Most make a compromise of some kind, both with themselves and with the circumstances which force limitations on them.

When I was younger and adjusting to visual limitations myself, I had the feeling that my compromise must be very small; and further, that it must not be readily apparent to my friends or, especially, my fellow workers.

Possibly that attitude accounts, at least in part, for my having been able to continue, to some extent, in professional activity. But now, after many associations with other visually handicapped persons, I do not encourage this approach.

Reprinted from *The American Journal of Nursing,* vol. 63, no. 10, pp. 98-100, October 1963.

First of all, continual pretense leads to never being accepted as I really am. People have been known to view me with suspicion and think that I can see more than my medical records indicate. Or they may surround me with uncertain restrictions which I must continually violate, either by subterfuge or by outright deceit.

The nurse dealing with a person who has suddenly or even gradually been forced into blindness must consider such emotional reactions. Especially if the prognosis for residual vision is uncertain, there will be alternating depression and attempts at compensation, some of them faulty.

As an emotional and physical tool, compensation can be valuable, provided it is not carried too far. If in the beginning I had been encouraged to move toward the restrictions that might come to me, rather than away from them, the dynamics of rehabilitation might have been much less traumatic. But because neither my family nor I could entertain the idea that my visual problems would be permanent, I kept living in the expectation that improvement would come. I feel now that, while hope should never be destroyed, it should be realistically tempered. I have heard nurses make such remarks as, "Well, you never know what will be discovered in the future, but as things stand now, why don't you try walking around the room?"

Cruel? No, not in the end. For if better vision comes, the patient will quickly discard his compensatory methods. If his situation stays the same or grows worse, he has taken the first steps toward becoming independent.

The nurse is in a good position to sow the seeds of motivation. For instance, to me the most difficult and embarrassing aspect of visual limitation is table manners. Elderly people, whose motivation is not great, often prefer to be fed, and many nurses would rather feed a blind patient than accord him a "sloppy" independence. For some very ill, elderly patients, this may be justified. But if a person is going to live with visual limitations for more than a few months, he should be encouraged to maintain as much independence as possible.

At first he will need help. When he is given his tray, the nurse can indicate which is salt and which is pepper, but she would do well not to use the shakers for him. She might tell him what is on the menu and place his plate so that his meat is in an accustomed position. She might see that his glass is not filled too full with milk, or that his tea is poured. If he is in the room with others, she can cut his meat—taking care to be unobtrusive about it. If he indicates he prefers to cut his own, so much the better. The first few times he eats without being able to see, she might stay long enough to see that he gets started, chatting about something pleasant. Then she might drop in once or twice during the meal just to see how he is managing. Her acceptance of the situation, her faith in his ability, her willingness to modify a situation to his limitations will give him the courage to try other things.

The pleasant chat while he gets started helps with the task at hand; it also has a further-reaching purpose. As the nurse tells him about the weather, describes some funny incident, relates some experience of inspiration or beauty, he can begin to enjoy the world through the experiences of others—a valuable asset which he now must develop to a high degree.

"Seeing through one's ears" is a compensation which has many valuable assets but which the elderly blind frequently fail to develop. The nurse can help with this, too. For instance, I was once night nurse for a blind patient in her late sixties who had undergone surgery. Hemorrhage made the outcome almost certainly total blindness. Even before her bandages were removed, we made a game of identifying people's footsteps. I shall never forget her profound satisfaction when she told me that she could recognize the hospital administrator—a nun—by the sound of a crucifix swinging against her habit as she walked.

Actually, the great curse of blindness is not the blindness itself, hampering as it is at times. The enforced idleness and social isolation it can entail are the two forces that cause the most emotional disintegration. Only the most aggressive among the blind can compromise with these two factors. And they do not come about because of a lack of good will or public sympathy. It is just that, among professional and lay people alike, this good will is not always—or even usually—channeled by an acceptance of the limitation for what it is.

Blindness is regarded as one of the catastrophic disabilities, synonymous with helplessness. Often relatives are less able to accept the visual limitations of the blind person than he is himself. They do not want him to learn to walk with a cane for fear he will "get ideas" about going around the block or downtown. They find it difficult to refrain from helping him with his clothes, rather than merely drawing an error to his attention and letting him remedy it himself. They may avoid the use of the word "blind," instilling in him their own shame and insecurity. Well-intentioned but emotionally confused, they impose on the blind person the role of complete disability.

The nurse is frequently the only one, aside from the doctor, who can overcome this misconception and create in the patient, by degrees, a self-confidence that will make it possible for him to surmount the hurdles which others will unwittingly put in his way. And it is she, along with the doctor, who can help relatives, by both example and precept, to understand that the blind person must be allowed to orient himself, be encouraged to venture and develop new interests, and be accorded as many opportunities to make decisions and choices as possible.

Even so small a thing as ordering a meal at a restaurant may illustrate the point. Waitresses often say to someone accompanying me at lunch, "Does she want sugar in her coffee?"

I always feel like shouting "hurrah" to the companion who says, unobtrusively, "Ask her." This may seem a little blunt or tactless, but it does vest the individual with his own rights as a person—and thus begins his rehabilitation.

Further than this, it helps destroy the misconceptions about blindness. This destruction can come about only when the sightless themselves, and those who speak for them, are able and willing to demonstrate proper attitudes.

Essential to independence is getting about by oneself. The elderly often seem unwilling or unable to accumulate that cluster of perceptive sensitivities referred to as "facial perception." We do not really know whether facial perception is strictly hearing, or a combination of tactile and auditory reactions, but most blind children and many blind adults make use of this echo interpretive factor which allows them to recognize such solid obstacles as high fences and walls. However, cane travel should be learned by every person whose vision is defective enough to interfere with his moving about safely. Even if the individual is elderly, so long as he is well-oriented mentally, he should be taught the use of a cane. Some feel that there is stigma to this, and I once shared this feeling. But I have learned that it is unfair to myself and to motorists who have no way of knowing whether a person has seriously impaired vision.

Training for cane travel can begin in the hospital during the first orientation after surgery. It is, however, usually only the exceptional person who can develop skill enough to travel safely in unfamiliar surroundings without at least one month of orientation in a specialized setting such as a training center or school. It takes time to learn to use hearing and cane travel to the fullest, but the nurse plays an important role when she accepts and encourages the use of a white cane.

Guide dogs serve a valuable purpose to many of the younger blind. Even some older persons can use a dog safely. But many blind people are neither temperamentally nor otherwise adapted to the use of dogs. Furthermore, the person who relies on a dog may be limited in place and type of work. The nurse might encourage her patient to investigate the possibility of a guide dog, but she should help him look on this as only one of many possible solutions. Once a person has gained the confidence of cane travel, he will find that training with a dog is easier. And when his dog is ill, or when he must wait to train with another after the death of a dog, he still has a means of independent movement.

Talking books (recordings of fiction and nonfiction) can be used by every well-oriented blind person, old or young. Many who are neither motivated nor capable of learning Braille can benefit from these records. Using earphones, the "reader" can use them even in a rest home or hospital, and they help him avoid the long, dreary hours that make the newly blinded tend toward depression. The nurse can put the individual and his family in touch with the local distributors of the players, lent without charge by the U.S. Library of Congress to eligible, reliable persons. If no information is available locally, it can be secured by writing to the Library of Congress, which will refer one to the closest local facility.

Finally, the way to guide a blind person might well be taught to all student nurses. There is nothing more devaluating or awkward than being "pushed" about by someone. The blind person can follow best when his hand rests on the arm of the individual who is leading him. This puts him just slightly behind his guide, whose body movements tell him direction and changes of surface. A pause before steps, curbs, or other step-downs is usually all that is necessary. If a ramp slopes up, however, a word might be helpful. And, when the blind person is just learning to sense body movements in his guides, exaggerated pauses before changes in the walking surface are very helpful.

It is only good manners to inform a visually handicapped person by a word of greeting that you are entering the room. He may or may not be able to recognize your voice. If there is any doubt, the name of the person entering should be spoken. I have frequently been at meetings and other places where people whose voices I would have recognized did not speak. I feel sure they meant no offense, but it is this sort of thing that creates the feeling of isolation and discourages blind people from developing friendly attitudes. It is also a pleasant bit of consideration to inform a blind person when someone is leaving. This kind of thing helps overcome the feeling, which the newly blind in particular are likely to have, that unseen people are observing them, invading their privacy.

All these things can help overcome the stereotype, as well as help the patient to realize that he is still a person, capable of independent thought and action.

Reading 38
The Needs of the Visually Handicapped
George D. Jackson

"Please stay in your room so you won't get hurt." This firm, though well-intentioned, order was given me by a nurse at the nurses' station where I had gone to ask directions to the smoking lounge. Her judgment was the outcome of a conference that my inquiring presence had precipitated among the nurses who were at the nurses' station.

I did not expect the nurses to know that I had already obtained a fair impression of the layout of the floor (a technique often used by blind people

Reprinted from *Nursing Outlook*, vol. 13, no. 9, pp. 34–37, September 1965.

to increase their mobility in new surroundings). I did, however, expect that the nursing staff of a reputedly good metropolitan hospital would offer to get assistance for me as they did for a friend of mine in another hospital. Upon his admission the nurse advised him to feel free to ask for any help he needed. She told him that in time other patients would be available to help him to the smoking room and other places. Another nurse offered to telephone the Red Cross for Braille literature to help him pass the time. Hospital staffs are very busy and the above considerations may be impossible in many settings. However, understaffing and overwork cannot explain the following examples of treatment accorded blind persons whom I have known.

A blind friend and his wife were standing at the bedside of their hospitalized child when a nurse on seeing them offered to get a chair—for the father, not the mother! A blind mathematician, in the process of being admitted to the hospital, was asked by the nurse who had taken his history if he could undress himself—this after she had been told that he was a mathematician and the father of two children, whose care he shared with their mother. A blind musician was never consulted directly about his physiological needs; rather, the other patients in his room were asked, "Does he need a bedpan?"; "Does he need a urinal?"; "Does he need fresh water?"

The way in which the nursing staff related to me as a blind patient and the collective experiences of associates lead me to suspect that there is a significant number of nurses who have not learned how to deal with blind patients.

As a scientist I am keenly aware of the dangers inherent in making generalizations from a small number of experiences. The discussion which follows is not intended as a scientific report. I am not an authority on blindness and I do not purport to speak for all blind people. I hope, however, that my experiences, observations, and impressions will encourage the kind of learning that leads to greater understanding and more positive attitudes.

Some readers may find it incredible that nurses could be guilty of some of the practices cited above. It is not shocking to me, for I have found very little correlation between education and positive attitudes toward the visually disabled. Many of my colleagues become anxious when dealing with blind persons—socially and professionally. Recently, a psychiatrist and I conducted a joint interview with a patient. The psychiatrist was so traumatized by my blindness that he could not concentrate on our patient. Finally, the patient asked the psychiatrist, "Gee, doctor, haven't you ever seen a blind person before?"

How does it happen that educated persons, such as nurses, fall so short when relating to blind persons? A profound answer to this question would be unmanageable within the confines of a single article. However, a discussion of relationship of attitudes of nurses and those held by the public and derivation of public attitudes may be helpful.

GENERAL ATTITUDES

On the whole the attitudes and conduct of nurses and other professionally trained persons toward the visually disabled do not differ significantly from those of the general population.

The incident of offering a chair to the blind father instead of his wife has its parallel in the frequency with which blind men are offered seats on transportation facilities. Although the gentlemanly act of offering a woman a seat has become practically outmoded, we still find women offering seats to blind men. Blind men with dates are embarrassed when waiters ask their sighted companions, "What does he want?"

Within the past ten years I have noticed an increasing number of people who know how to assist blind persons in crossing streets and in getting on or off public transportation. Many social agencies have helped to educate the public on the proper way to relate to blind persons. However, there are psychological variables and historical factors which will not be dissipated by mere dissemination of public information.

Many agencies which seek to foster the well-being of the visually disabled and which, by and large, have done an excellent job, nonetheless contribute to the public's confusion and to the aura about blindness through their public education and public relations techniques. Their use of such terms as "seeing eye," "lighthouse," and "second sight" tends to perpetuate the traditional image of the blind. On the one hand, these agencies seek to promote the notion that the blind are equal. On the other, their workers stand in public places shaking containers to attract handouts from the public for the support of projects designed to assist the blind.

Last year at the New York World's Fair a group of blind persons were placed in a cage in the "Better Life Building" to demonstrate their proficiency in handling industrial equipment. How much better it would have been to have employed blind persons in various capacities throughout the Fair so that the public could have seen them as average people making a living.

FRAME OF REFERENCE

The number of blind persons in our society is quite small and is declining steadily. This reduces the probability of experiences that sighted persons can have with the visually disabled. When people are confronted with persons possessing characteristics unfamiliar to them, they are usually compelled to rely upon their own subjective frame of reference as a basis for intuitively executing the relationship.

The life experiences and education which contribute to the images that sighted persons have of blind persons are many and varied. Many people have or have had elderly blind relatives who lost their sight in the aging process. When meeting a younger blind person, they sometimes, although usually unconsciously, generalize from their experiences with the older person to the younger one.

Literature, folklore, and superstition also play a role in attitudes toward the blind. Few systematic studies in this area have been conducted, but I think one can speculate that the written word and hearsay continue to wield a profound influence on the general population's attitudes toward blindness.

In the literature, blindness is invariably associated with above-average talent, as in the case of Homer, or with villainous or mysterious qualities, like those of Pugh in *Treasure Island.* The degree of deprivation which the concept of blindness connotes is reflected in its use in the literature as punishment—Oedipus, in Greek mythology, and *Sophocles' Oedipus Rex.*

The Bible states in verses one to three, ninth chapter, Book of St. John:

> And as Jesus passed by, he saw a man which was blind from his birth.
> And his disciples asked him, saying, Master, who did sin, this man, or his parents, that he was born blind?
> Jesus answered, Neither hath this man sinned, nor his parents; but that the works of God should be made manifest in him.

I am neither finding fault with the theological or religious connotations of the Bible, nor is it my intention to offend anyone's religious sensibilities. From a psychological point of view, however, I contend that many people reading this passage derive the notion that blindness can be some sort of a blessing in disguise. The fact of the matter is that blindness is *not* a blessing; it is a disability. To be sure, it is a disability to which one can make a wholesome adjustment. But the blind person can make a superior adjustment to it only if he recognizes it as a liability, not a blessing.

Not to be overlooked is the use which various authors have made of blindness in constructing fables and analogies. The fable of the five blind men and the elephant and H. G. Wells's *Country of the Blind* are examples in point. To be sure literature of this type can effectively communicate positive thoughts to its readers, but simultaneously, and on another level, it exploits and fosters the aura which has come to surround blind persons. In short, our literature has contributed to the image in the minds of people that blind persons, be they bright, stupid, industrious, or beggars, are some sort of "freaks" and never simply average persons.

I have decided that there must be more blind people in the country than Census Bureau records show. Almost every person I've met has told me about a blind friend, a blind relative, a relative who has a blind friend, or a relative who has a friend who knows a blind person. In all instances, these blind persons, although practically nonentities, were "marvelous," "ingenious," "incredible," and "fabulous."

Using "blind" as an adjective to modify "rage" or "stupidity" results in expressions which are pictorial and which, while not offensive to the blind person, help promulgate improper attitudes toward the blind, especially among persons whose contact with the sightless is infrequent.

In short, there is a tremendous discrepancy between the image which blindness connotes and the way blind people usually are. When a person's frame of reference or image is not congruent with the real situation, temporary anxiety is generated. The person whose expectancies are not realized will use the defensive posture which has become characteristic of his personality. The blind person may perceive this defensiveness and will handle it in terms of his own degree of social adjustment. If he perceives hostility or threat, he may react in a manner which will intensify the discomfort of the sighted person.

VISION IN COMMUNICATIONS

As a blind psychologist, I am keenly aware of the tremendous role that vision plays in human communications, particularly in situations in which dialogue is intimate or emotionally charged, both parties anticipating and relying on feedback from the expressions they see in the other's eyes.

Once I was in a science class with nine other blind students. The teacher suddenly stopped and, without warning, said, "You know it's awfully hard and frustrating teaching you fellows. I can't see what you are thinking and I can't tell whether you know what I'm saying. You always have the right answers to my questions, yet when I look at you, I don't know if you are asleep or awake." This, of course, is an extreme example, but I think it points up the anxiety which can be aroused when persons are not able to communicate in the customary manner. This may explain to some extent why many people, in addressing questions to a blind person, direct them to his companion. Sighted people can overcome any anxiety they may have in their relationships with the visually handicapped if they use a little empathy, and a little flexibility.

FEELINGS OF INADEQUACY

To persons beset with strong feelings of inadequacy, there is nothing so disarming as the specter of seeing an apparently disabled person functioning on an average or above average level. Although some of them are sincere in extolling the virtues of their blind acquaintances, they unconsciously seek to place them in an inferior position, thereby protecting their own status. I once had occasion to train a woman counselor in group therapy techniques. She frequently told me and other persons how wonderful she thought it was that I was able to be a psychologist despite my blindness. One day I showed her a picture of my 9-year-old daughter. She remarked, "Gee, I bet she's the apple of your eye—if you had an eye."

Still other persons with feelings of inadequacy react with hostility toward a blind person. It is my impression that many employers and personnel directors who resist hiring blind persons are motivated not so much by wish to protect the company as they are by the need to protect their own damaged egos. To such persons, statistical evidence, such as the fact that the number of gainfully employed blind persons has increased significantly in the last 20 years, and other arguments are not sufficient to dissuade them from refusing to hire the blind.

FEAR OF THE UNKNOWN

It is extremely difficult, probably nearly impossible, for a person with sight to comprehend sightlessness. Psychoanalytic literature holds that something unknown can assume as much negative valence as a known threat or feared object. While this analytic principle may or may not be valid for all situations, it seems to me that many people adorn the unknown quality "blindness" with all manner of fears, superstitions, and social stereotypes. They believe that the blind person can see more things than they can; that because he is extrasensitive, he can read their minds and ferret out their guilt.

I have seen this happen in my own psychotherapeutic work. I once had a patient who was terrified of me because he thought that I knew what he was going to say even before he said it. I was, in his mind, extrasensitive. Blindness, as such, neither brings with it special powers of concentration or special talents, nor, from a scientific point of view, does it lower the threshold of other sense modalities. Successful blind persons do organize their activities so as to minimize their handicap. They are forced to use other modalities to compensate for their deficiency. Some blind persons concentrate a good deal of effort on specializing in a given area so as to compete successfully with sighted persons. But there is nothing mysterious or supernatural about these processes.

IMPLICATIONS FOR NURSING

I have endeavored to point up some of the reasons why nurses do not relate in a wholesome manner to their blind patients. In saying that the attitudes of nurses are not unlike those held by other professionals and the public at large, I tried to temper my criticism of nurses. Yet, I would hope that in their education they would be taught how to relate more effectively to patients who are blind. To help nursing students understand the visually disabled better, instructors might contact state agencies for the blind to arrange field trips to schools, camps, and places of employment. If nursing students could see blind children swimming, playing baseball, and wrestling, it would do much toward giving them a positive image of the blind. These agencies provide speakers competent to answer questions.

Films, literature, and bibliographies are available from various voluntary and official agencies. In short, what I am suggesting is that contact and experience with the visually handicapped should be part of nursing education.

Blind persons are by no means homogeneous in terms of their personality characteristics or their adjustment to blindness. Blind people differ in their degree of mobility, independence, and values. It therefore becomes difficult to make any hard and fast generalizations as to how one should relate to a blind person. Despite the heterogeneity, there are some commonalities.

The blind person, it should be assumed, knows his limitations and capacities better than the nurse. The nurse should, when in doubt, consult the blind patient or ask him in a dignified manner if he needs a service she has in mind. Generally speaking, blind persons will want to do everything which is feasible for them. Sometimes if the nurse renders assistance, she may facilitate the patient's execution of an act. This is often desirable, but she should help him directly without being clumsy and without getting in his way. The nurse should address the blind person himself. If she doesn't know his name and wonders if he will be aware that she is addressing him, a slight touch on the arm while asking the question will do the job.

Blind persons, like all other people, are entitled to dignity and respect. Thus blind patients should not be subjected to nursing practices which undermine their dignity.

A nurse who is sensitive, able to empathize, and capable of using common sense will not be greatly troubled when dealing with a blind patient. If she has learned how to recognize and cope with feelings and reactions, if she has learned to be aware of her own positive and negative interpersonal attitudes, she will be able to intuitively relate to the blind patient in a wholesome way.

SIX COMMANDMENTS FOR THE SIGHTED[1]

1 Do not think that blind people are abnormal because they cannot see. Their every interest in life is similar to yours. Blindness is a disability but does not necessarily mean lack of ability.

2 There is nothing "wonderful" about a blind person lighting his own cigarette, cigar, or pipe, dialing the telephone, counting out change, or consulting his watch.

---

[1] Adapted from *Our Ten Commandments for the Sighted,* Associated Blind, New York.

In dialing the phone various methods are used by blind people. The most popular one is committing to memory the three letters corresponding to each hole on the dial.

Counting out change is easy since coins are distinguished by size, thickness and edge. For example, the penny is larger than the dime, which is thinner and has a milled edge. The nickel is larger and thicker than the penny—it is smaller than the quarter, which has a milled edge. The half dollar is the largest and heaviest of the coins, with the exception of the silver dollar. . . .

3   Do not hesitate to use the word "blind" in the presence of a blind person. It is not necessary to substitute the words "sightless," "unseeing," "unsighted" or other euphemisms. It is also unnecessary to avoid using the word "see." The well-adjusted blind person accepts the reality of his handicap and does not object to the use of the words "blind" and "see."

4   Do not hesitate to offer help to a blind person who is walking in your direction. Although he can arrive at his destination by himself, your assistance is always appreciated as it minimizes the extra time and nervous tension involved when traveling alone.

5   Once you have started to help a blind person to cross the street, never leave him until he is safely on the opposite sidewalk. Never say "You're all right now" when you have just reached the middle of the crossing and leave him stranded while you make a dash for your bus. . . .

6   When assisting a blind person to cross the street, helping him onto a vehicle, or to mount stairs, do not push, carry, or drag him. Merely let him take your arm when crossing, or place his hand on the door handle or rail, as the case may be. When escorting a blind person to a seat, put his hand on the arm or back of the chair, or, when this is not possible, walk with him up to the seat which he naturally will be facing.

Reading 39

Available Training Opportunities for Deaf People
McCay Vernon

Rehabilitation counselors and other specialists are often at a loss as to what to do for deaf clients. What training programs are there to meet the unique needs of these clients? In what types of employment have deaf people succeeded in the past?

Reprinted from *Hearing and Speech News,* vol. 38, no. 1, January–February 1970. This investigation was supported, in part, by a research and demonstration grant (RD-2-2407-S) from the Rehabilitation Services Administration of the United States Department of Health, Education, and Welfare, Washington, D.C. Sections of this article were drawn from a paper entitled "Vocational Guidance for the Deaf" (Williams, B., and Vernon, M.). This paper will appear as a chapter in the upcoming edition of *Hearing and Deafness* (Davis, H., and Silverman, S. R., Holt, Rinehart, and Winston, New York).

The Rehabilitation Services Administration has cooperated with state divisions of vocational rehabilitation to develop a number of programs. Ironically, despite the demonstrated need for these programs, many counselors are unaware of them. Thus, deaf clients in need of training may not get it.

This [article] describes available programs and gives basic orientation to problems of deafness and present and future employment trends. It is written for general counselors, speech and hearing specialists, and other professionals who work with deaf people. It should aid in delivering effective services and in alleviating the present under-training and the resultant under-employment found among deaf people [1].

EMPLOYMENT TRENDS

What happens to deaf people in the world of work? They have approximately the same range of vocational and professional employment hearing persons do. There are deaf scientists, teachers, accountants, Ph.D.'s, and entrepreneurs—just as there are deaf welfare recipients, ditch diggers, and peddlers.

While the range of employment for deaf people is as wide as for hearing people, there is a centering of from 60 to 85% of employed deaf persons in unskilled or semi-skilled work. This is two to three times the percentage for the total hearing population. Stated differently, five-sixths of deaf adults are manual laborers of varying skills, as contrasted to one-half of the hearing population [2]. Conversely, 17% of the deaf population are employed in white-collar jobs, including professional, technical, managerial, clerical, and sales positions, as compared to 46.8% of the general United States population [3-7].

Among the employed deaf there is a strong relationship between educational attainment and both income and level of work. However, the percentage of deaf students able to attain college entrance is only about one-tenth the percentage of those with normal hearing who are admitted to college [8]. This figure may decline with decrease in post-lingual deafness and increase in multiple handicaps in deaf youth [9-10].

Deaf employees are stable in job tenure, and employers report satisfactory work records [4,5,11-13]. Despite this exemplary work history, it is not uncommon to find employment practices that discriminate against deaf applicants [6,14].

The American Federationist, official publication of the AFL-CIO, points out that automation is eliminating many of the unskilled, semi-skilled, and manual jobs in which the overwhelming majority of the deaf have worked in past years [15]. Jobs in technical areas, service industries, professions, and management are expanding, and this is where the deaf are currently least well represented and presumably least well prepared by aptitude and by training [16].

Frequently these facts about the vocational adjustment of deaf adults are unknown to professionals who counsel deaf youths and to the families of these youths. Without this basic information, appropriate educational and vocational planning and counseling are impossible.

A note of caution comes from John Sessions, an AFL-CIO labor authority. He states that if present trends are not reversed, within ten years unemployment among deaf people will approximate 70% and most of the remaining 30% will be dead-ended in unskilled menial jobs [17]. To avoid this, careful steps must be taken by counselors, by parents, and by deaf youths early in education planning.

LANGUAGE SKILLS

Most young people who are deaf were born with hearing loss or acquired it early in life, before they were old enough to have learned to talk and use language [18]. Under these circumstances, normal speech cannot be developed. Sometimes intelligible speech can be acquired, but in many cases the prelingually deafened are not able to talk in a way that is understandable to parents, rehabilitation counselors, or potential employers. Many of the best lipreaders understand only 25% of what is said. Most deaf youths grasp about 5%. Problems in mastering vocabulary and syntax compound the overall difficulty.

Because of the problems deaf persons have with speech, lipreading, and writing, many find they achieve greatest communication skill in the language of signs and finger spelling. Often deaf persons who lack any appreciable ability in oral or written communication can express and receive complex ideas in the language of signs.

In years past, most deaf youths attended residential schools—at least during their high-school-age years. Consequently, those who could not communicate orally were able to communicate manually. This is no longer true.

Today many deaf young people attend day classes with hearing students. This works out fairly well for a few. They develop partially intelligible speech, can read and write, and are able to use lipreading for limited communication purposes. However, a large proportion of these youths do not learn to speak intelligibly. They cannot lipread and write enough to convey more than rudimentary daily needs, and they have not learned to speechread.

UNPREPARED YOUTH

Vocational counselors see more and more of these cases, especially in larger cities. Counselors and parents react with righteous indignation, but metropolitan school systems have done little to improve this deplorable situation. Deaf youths are often turned out of school at age 16 to 18 with no adequate means of communication, despite 10 to 12 years of "schooling."

It is necessary with these persons to start almost from scratch. They need intensive instruction in the language of signs before vocational counseling and planning are possible. As it takes a year or more of close exposure to manual communication, these youths represent an unfortunate, frustrating group. Rainer et al. discussed the seriousness of this problem in New York [13]. I see many such clients from Chicago and neighboring suburbs.

To maximize the future of a deaf youth in the world of work, it is important that counselors, the deaf youth, and his parents have full communication—which usually means skill in finger spelling and sign language. When the counselor lacks this skill, an interpreter should be used unless communication by other methods is fully satisfactory.

The Rehabilitation Services Administration and state divisions of vocational rehabilitation recognize the problems faced by deaf people in today's highly technical, rapidly changing, and tremendously demanding world of work. Programs at state and national levels attempt to meet these needs. Several colleges provide for deaf students specialized services needed to maximize their chances for academic success. There are also junior colleges, vocational technical schools, and various special educational facilities which make special efforts to meet the needs of deaf youth.

PROGRAMS AVAILABLE

Gallaudet College—For many years higher education for a deaf person meant attendance at Gallaudet, the world's only liberal arts college for the deaf. This accredited college has served deaf youth for more than one hundred years, offering majors in fields such as chemistry, mathematics, education, biology, literature, and psychology. Admission is based on academic entrance examinations administered throughout the United States and in Canada and other countries. In recognition of the tremendous educational lag which often accompanies deafness, Gallaudet has a Preparatory Department where students of college potential who are not academically ready for college work are given a year of intensive advanced academic courses.

Any educational guidance for deaf youth of college potential should include strong evaluation of the possibility of attending Gallaudet. Unfortunately, many deaf young people who do not attend residential schools or large day programs are never told of Gallaudet. For information write: Registrar, Gallaudet College, 7th & Florida Ave., N.E., Washington, D.C., 20002.

National Technical Institute for the Deaf—The limitations of a liberal arts curriculum and its inappropriateness for many deaf college students led to the recent establishment of the National Technical Institute for the Deaf. The first deaf students entered in 1968. Deaf students may earn baccalaureate degrees in many technical fields, e.g., engineering, graphic arts, and commercial photography. Some courses are taken with other deaf students, but much of the program involves classes with hearing students. Extensive tutorial and adjunctive educational assistance is provided to aid the deaf student in overcoming problems of deafness. For information write: Registrar, NTID, Rochester Institute of Technology, Rochester, N.Y., 14608.

San Fernando Valley State College—A grant has been received from the California Department of Rehabilitation, with supporting funds from the Rehabilitation Services Administration, to add special services for the deaf to the four-year undergraduate program. The funds will be used for remodeling, equipment, interpreters, and additional staff. For information write: Department of Special Education and Rehabilitation, San Fernando Valley State College, Northridge, Calif., 91324.

Other Colleges—Some deaf students attend colleges where there are no special programs for them. Education under these circumstances is an especially demanding process, not only academically but socially and psychologically. The price paid in stress and in missing out on aspects of social and intellectual interaction makes attending regular college a dubious procedure for deaf students. Generally, deaf students who succeed in graduating from regular colleges are exceptionally bright and aggressive—and have good command of language. Often they also have understandable speech and family members who offer intensive support and help as note-takers, interpreters, or tutors.

Junior Colleges—Delgado Junior College in New Orleans is a new institution designed to take deaf students with a fifth-grade achievement level or higher and provide them with either a vocational-technical education, an academic program covering the first two years of college, or combination of these. Students live off campus, but excellent tutorial and supplementary education services are provided. For information write: Registrar, Delgado Junior College, New Orleans, La., 70119.

St. Paul Technical Vocational Institute has launched an outstanding post-secondary vocational technical school program. Like the program at Delgado, the St. Paul T.V.I. aims at vocational, technical, and academic education for deaf people. For information contact: St. Paul Technical Vocational Institute, St. Paul, Minn., 55104.

Community College of Denver—The program for the deaf is under the Division of Business and Management Occupations. There is a full-time professional teacher of the deaf and a part-time tutor-interpreter. Most students are working for a general clerical certificate. They attend classes with hearing students when possible. Included in classes offered are such courses as introduction to business, business machines, typing, keypunch, business math, office practices, and clerical recordkeeping. Students who wish to take classes outside the program or in other areas are encouraged to do so. In addition there are several adult deaf education classes, in cooperation with the Colorado Hearing and Speech Center, which the students have the option of taking for credit.

Regional junior colleges with services for the deaf are now being established in Seattle, Wash., and Pittsburgh, Pa., and possibly in other areas. They will take deaf students for vocational-technical or academic study and will provide supportive specialized educational services. For residents of California, the Riverside City College has such a program.

Many of the junior college programs are new. For information it is best to write to: Chief, Communication Disorders Branch, Division of Disability Services, Rehabilitation Services Administration, Dept. of Health, Education, and Welfare, Washington, D.C., 20201.

Graduate Schools—There has been a recent growth of opportunities for graduate work. San Fernando Valley, Gallaudet, and the University of Arizona are forerunners and have graduated a number of deaf students at the master's or doctoral level. New York University and the University of Pittsburgh are following this pattern. For information write: Chairman, Dept. of Special Education & Rehabilitation, San Fernando Valley State College, Northridge, Calif., 91324; Chairman, Rehabilitation Center, Univ. of Arizona, Tucson, Ariz., 85721; Director, Program in Deafness & Communication Disorders, Dept. of Education Psychology, New York Univ., Rm. 51, 80 Washington Square East, New York, N.Y., 10003; Director, Program in Deafness, Dept. of Special Education & Rehabilitation, Univ. of Pittsburgh, Pa. 15213; and the Gallaudet College Registrar (address given earlier).

Hot Springs, Arkansas, Rehabilitation Center—This institution offers intensive vocational training and evaluation for deaf persons 16 years of age and older. Over 30 vocational skill training courses are taught in 20 vocational areas. Special emphasis is given to needs of multiple handicapped deaf students and those who may have had difficulty in school or job settings in the past. Among courses taught are television repair, watchmaking, laundry work, secretarial skills, body and fender repair, drafting, and custodial skills.

This center is residential and accepts hearing students as well as those who are deaf. Counseling on work habits and practical aspects of daily living is emphasized in addition to the vocational and academic coursework for which strong supportive services are available. Recreational activity is encouraged, and rehabilitative medical services are available. Students usually stay six to eighteen months. For information write: Director, Program for the Deaf, Hot Springs Rehabilitation Center, Hot Springs, Ark., 71901.

Michigan State Technical Institute & Rehabilitation Center—This residential vocational-technical school is of high standards and offers preparation in many trades and technologies, including machine skills, tile-setting, drafting, design, and office machine repair. It is limited primarily to Michigan residents but has taken out-of-state students. For information write: Director of Services for the Deaf, State Technical Institute & Rehabilitation Center, Plainwell, Mich., 49080.

Northern Illinois University Rehabilitation Program—This program helps deaf persons from 16 to 24 years of age bridge the gap between the end of school and a realistic vocational objective. Offerings include job training, vocational exploration, diagnostic services, business courses, and basic reading, writing, and mathematics. Students must have Performance IQ of 80 and a third-grade or better academic achievement level—some exceptions are made in regard to achievement. The students live in college dormitories and are given guidance in activities of daily living and work.

There are two basic programs. One runs for nine months, during which students get a half-day of academic remedial work and a half-day of work experience on a job. Practical courses include check-writing, work habits, sex education, manual and oral communication, insurance, etc. The other program runs during the summer and involves diagnostic testing, communication skills, academics, recreation, counseling, reading, and writing. For information write: Director of Program for the Deaf, Speech & Hearing Center, Northern Illinois University, DeKalb, Ill., 60115.

Jewish Vocational Service (Chicago)—Vocational evaluation, counseling, workshop training, and placement are provided for deaf persons in Illinois. Diagnostic and counseling services can serve a wide range of deaf youth and adults. Workshop programs are primarily for those who have difficulty finding and keeping work and/or have psychological or other problems in addition to deafness. Clients must make their own living arrangements in Chicago. For information write: Director, Program for the Deaf, Jewish Vocational Services, One South Franklin, Chicago, Ill., 60606.

Jewish Employment & Vocational Service (St. Louis)—Similar to the Chicago service, this program consists primarily of workshop training, diagnostics, counseling, placement, and some on-the-job training. There are no official living accommodations, but special arrangements are made with local boarding houses. Many clients have limited educational achievement, sporadic work histories, and other problems. For information write: Director of Services for the Deaf, Jewish Employment & Vocational Service, 8200 Exchange Way, St. Louis, Mo., 64144.

In addition to the major centers described, there are smaller facilities offering varying degrees and types of services. Almost every year new programs develop. Information on changes and recent developments is available from the Rehabilitative Services Administration (address above). Apart from specialized services for deaf persons, existing general vocational-technical schools and colleges are often used with supportive services for deaf students provided through state divisions of vocational rehabilitation.

REFERENCES

1. Williams, B. R.: *Rehabilitation of the deaf* (Workshop for Baptists on Deafness and Rehabilitation). Vocational Rehabilitation Administration, Department of Health, Education, and Welfare, Washington, D.C., 1965.
2. Babbidge, H. D.: *Education of the Deaf: A Report to the Secretary of Health, Education, and Welfare by His Advisory Committee on the Education of the Deaf.* U.S. Department of Health, Education, and Welfare, Washington, D.C., 1964.
3. Crammatte, A. B.: The adult deaf in professions. *Amer. Ann. Deaf,* **107**:474-478, 1962.
4. Lunde, A. S., and Bigman, S. G.: *Occupational Conditions among the Deaf.* Gallaudet Press, Washington, D.C., 1959.
5. Rosenstein, J., and Lerhman, A.: *Vocational Status and Adjustment of Deaf Women.* Lexington School for the Deaf, New York, 1963.
6. Vernon, M.: What is the future for the deaf in the world of work? *Silent Worker,* 1962, pp. 7-12.
7. Vernon, M., and Fischler, T. G.: Vocational needs in educational programs for deaf youth. *Amer. Ann. Deaf,* **111**:444-451, 1966.
8. Schein, J. D., and Bushnag, S.: Higher education for the deaf in the United States—A retrospective investigation. *Amer. Ann. Deaf,* **107**:416-420, 1962.
9. Vernon, M.: The brain-injured (neurologically impaired) child: A discussion of the significance of the problem, its symptoms, and causes in deaf children. *Amer. Ann. Deaf,* **106**:239-250, 1961.
10. Vernon, M.: Multiply handicapped deaf children: The causes, manifestations, and significances of the problem. *E.E.N.T. Digest,* **31**:40-58, 1969.
11. Boatner, E. B., Stuckless, E. R., and Moores, D. F.: *Occupational Status of the Young Adult Deaf of New England and Demand for a Regional Technical-Vocational Training Center.* American School for the Deaf, West Hartford, Conn., 1964.
12. Furfey, P. H., and Horte, T. J.: *Interaction of Deaf and Hearing in Frederick County, Maryland.* Catholic University, Washington, D.C., 1964.
13. Rainer, J. D., Altshuler, K. Z., Kallman, F. J., and Demings, W. E. (eds): *Family and Mental Health Problems in a Deaf Population.* New York State Psychiatric Institute, New York, 1963.
14. Craig, W. N., and Silver, N. H.: Examination of selected employment problems of the deaf. *Amer. Ann. Deaf,* **111**:544-549, 1966.
15. Tally, N. L., and Vernon, M.: The impact of automation on the worker. *Amer. Federalist,* **72**:20-23, 1965.
16. Lowell, F. L.: *Higher education for the deaf* (Cutter, D., ed.) (Workshop for Baptists on Deafness and Rehabilitation). Vocational Rehabilitation Administration, Department of Health, Education, and Welfare, Washington, D.C., 1965, pp. 28-36.
17. Sessions, J. A.: *Automation and the deaf.* A paper presented to the Leadership Training Program in Deafness, San Fernando Valley State College, June 3, 1966.
18. Vernon, M.: Current etiological factors in deafness. *Amer. Ann. Deaf,* **113**:106-113, 1968.

Reading 40
Rehabilitation for Irreversible Deafness
S. Richard Silverman

In the past three decades, many factors, not wholly unrelated, have stimulated interest in education and rehabilitation of persons with impaired hearing. They include development of refined electroacoustic instruments, particularly audiometers, to measure hearing loss; improvement of hearing aids; evolution of surgery for otosclerosis and of reconstructive surgical procedures for the middle ear [1]; development of promising investigative techniques in psychoacoustics, auditory biophysics, physiology, and microanatomy [2-5]; recognition of the problem of noise-induced hearing loss in industry and the armed forces [6]; awareness of hazards to hearing such as heredity, unfavorable prenatal conditions, or perinatal stress or injury; and a growing public appreciation of the rehabilitative needs and the economic and social potential of handicapped persons.

Forward-looking management of persons with impaired hearing requires (1) dissemination of information about hearing impairment and acoustic hygiene, (2) early identification through a "high-risk register," through screening programs in clinics for babies and in schools, and through audiologic examinations prior to employment, (3) complete diagnoses, (4) appropriate medical and surgical treatment, (5) thorough assessment of hearing after completion of all indicated medical and surgical procedures, with particular attention to educational and rehabilitative needs, and (6) appropriate measures such as hearing aids, lip reading, speech correction and conservation, special education, vocational planning, and psychological guidance [7].

WHAT IS DEAFNESS?

This simple statement of the important facets of the management of deafness should not cause us to underestimate its complexity, particularly when normal hearing is medically or surgically unattainable. We realize this when we ask the question, "What really is deafness?" Is it a number on a decibel scale that describes the severity of hearing impairment? Is it a disease like mumps or measles or meningitis? Is it an ankylosed stapes? Is it a piece of tissue in the auditory system that would be judged to be abnormal if viewed under a microscope? Is it an affliction to be conquered by the ingenious

Reprinted from *The Journal of the American Medical Association*, vol. 196, pp. 843–846, June 6, 1966. Copyright 1966, American Medical Association.

scientist? Is it the burden of a child whose parent hopes persistently and fervently that the scientist will be successful, and soon? Is it a special mode of communication? Is it something that is encountered occasionally in the man or woman whose fingers fly and whose utterances are arrhythmic and strident? Is it a cause to which diligent, skillful, and patient teachers have committed themselves for generations? Is it the agony of isolation from a piece of the real world? Is it the joy of accomplishment that mocks the handicap? Is it the bright mind and the potentially capable hands for which the economy has no use because they are uncultivated? Is it a crystallization of attitudes of a distinctive group whose deafness modes of communication and other associated attributes, such as previous education, that they have in common cause them to band together to achieve social and economic self-realization? Of course, it is all of these and more, depending on who asks the question and why.

In seeking the answer to the question, each one of us has his own motives, his own purposes, and his own responsibilities. The public official is concerned with the magnitude and severity of the problem, ways of organizing to solve it, legislative needs, and costs; the physician and the investigator study causes and pathology of deafness, its "psychology," and its management; the educator considers the physical plant, personnel requirements, and methods of instruction and communication; the rehabilitator is sensitive to training and job opportunities; and the deaf person himself and those close to him seek the opportunity for him to be all he can and wants to be [8]. As in the legend of the five blind men, it is difficult to perceive and comprehend the whole elephant. Time does not permit the grand synthesis here. The focus of this presentation is on the management of irreversible deafness.

THE AUDIOGRAM

The audiogram is the most commonly accepted measure of hearing loss. It indicates loss of sensitivity of the ear in decibels for the six frequencies (sometimes seven) from 125 to 8,000 cycles per second. For the purpose of this discussion it is sufficient to express the overall hearing loss as the average of the losses at 500, 1,000 and 2,000 cps, as these are frequencies most important for hearing speech.

Knowledge of losses at other frequencies aids in diagnosis, but this is not pertinent to this paper. Of course, patterns of audiometric losses may vary even in the frequencies of 500 to 2,000 cps and influence the types of communicative difficulties encountered by the listener. For example, persons who have better sensitivity at 500 than at 2,000 cps may hear but not understand and may ask the talker to speak clearer. The reverse situation may cause the listener to ask the talker to speak louder. In the former instance the primary difficulty is with discrimination, while in the latter it is sensitivity.

Despite the possible variations, the outline in Table 1 is useful in understanding the relation of the amount of hearing loss to communicative efficiency. In general, the critical points are a loss of 30 db, where communicative difficulty begins, and perhaps a little more than 60 db, where the visual system supplemented by hearing is likely to be the primary channel of communication. Persons in groups 1, 2, and 3 in Table 1 would be termed hard of hearing, and all in group 5 would be considered deaf. Group 4 represents a transitional stage and is likely to contain both hard-of-hearing and deaf persons.

Critical, of course, in rehabilitation is time of onset. An important point in life in regard to time of onset of hearing loss is roughly from 3 to 5 years of age. A child born with a hearing loss of more than 60 or 70 db or a child in whom such a loss occurs before the age of 3 to 5 years is not likely to develop the expressive and receptive skills of communication a hearing child does. It will be difficult for him to initiate language through speech, nor will he understand the speech of others unless he receives special education. Early identification and immediate institution of educational measures improve the prognosis.

If hearing loss occurs after early childhood, the teacher or therapist must determine the individual requirements according to the amount of residual hearing and memory the person has retained for language and speech.

Table 1 Relation of Amount of Hearing Loss to Communicative Efficiency*

Group	Amount of hearing loss	Effect
1	Less than 30 db	May have difficulty hearing faint or distant speech. Is likely to "get along" in school and at work requiring listening.
2	30 to 45 db	Understands conversational speech at 3 to 5 ft. without too much difficulty. May have difficulty if talker's voice is faint or if face is not visible.
3	45 to 60 db	Conversational speech must be loud to be understood. Considerable difficulty in group and classroom discussion and perhaps in telephone conversation.
4	60 to 80 db	May hear voice about a foot away. May identify environmental noises and may distinguish vowels, but consonants are difficult to perceive.
5	More than 80 db	May hear only loud sounds.

* Adapted from Silverman [9].

REHABILITATION AND EDUCATION

The most helpful and generally acceptable measures for hard-of-hearing persons are hearing aids, including auditory training; instruction in lip reading; speech conversation and correction; and educational, vocational, and psychological guidance.

Hearing Aids

This term refers to the modern electronic hearing aid rather than mechanical or obsolete electric types. Essentially a hearing aid is a miniature telephone. It consists of a microphone, an amplifier, batteries (most hearing aids now have one battery), and a receiver. The voice of the talker impinges on the microphone and is converted to electric energy supplied by the battery. The amplifier delivers a stronger current to the receiver, which converts it back to sound. Advances in telephony and radio have influenced the design of hearing aids.

What factors influence the performance of a hearing aid? First, it should have sufficient gain, i.e., ability to increase the intensity of sound to overcome the loss of sensitivity. Generally, the gain should be at least 30 db, and in some cases it should be 60 db. Second, it should have an adequate frequency range. Our main interest in helping persons who are hard of hearing is to improve their communication by speech, and we are not concerned with the more difficult problem of providing the listener with symphonic music. The frequencies from 200 to 4,000 cps contain all the necessary speech energy, whereas music contains energy from 20 to 15,000 cps. A hearing aid need only reproduce sounds in the frequency band from 200 to 4,000 cps, except for certain special cases. Noises that contain energy in lower or higher frequencies then do not distract the listener. A third and important factor is the maximal acoustic intensity the hearing aid will generate. Studies made to determine the maximal intensity of sounds we are able to hear without discomfort and pain have shown that for most persons a sensation of pain may occur at sound intensities of 130 db and greater. A hearing aid should limit the sound intensity it will produce.

Hearing aids have had a phenomenal acceptance in the past decade, probably largely because of the advent of the transistor, a substitute for the larger vacuum tube. It has been possible to reduce the size and weight of hearing aids without affecting electroacoustic performance seriously. The transistor also has eliminated one of the batteries. Emphasis on cosmetic features has stimulated the development of hearing aids built into the temples of spectacle frames. However, acoustic feedback or "squeal" resulting from placement of the microphone close to the receiver may limit the value of such instruments for persons with severe hearing impairment. This type of hearing aid introduces the possibility of providing true binaural hearing, i.e., one complete instrument for each ear. Investigations are under way to determine the conditions under which amplified binaural hearing is advantageous.

All too frequently the promotional literature on hearing aids emphasizes the concealment of hearing loss. From the standpoint of rehabilitation, this may be one of the major abuses in the field of hearing impairment. A cardinal principle of good mental health is recognition of reality and adjustment to it. It is a disservice to handicapped persons to encourage them to evade reality. Some dealers are to be commended for emphasizing that the wearing of a hearing aid is a demonstration of courtesy, since it spares the wearer's associates and family from having to shout or repeat.

Lip Reading

Lip reading, sometimes called speech reading because it involves observing more than the lips, is the process through which a person understands speech by carefully watching the speaker. For hard-of-hearing persons it is an essential supporting skill. The eye and the ear together apparently are better than either one alone, and for this reason there has been emphasis in recent years on associating lip reading instruction with hearing and with auditory training.

Speech Correction and Conservation

The major speech problem with hard-of-hearing persons is correction and conservation of speech. They do not hear speech and speech patterns clearly and therefore have a poor model for imitation. Furthermore, defective hearing prevents adequate monitoring of articulation and phonation.

Educational, Vocational, and Psychological Guidance

We need to know the interests, aspirations, aptitudes, abilities, and limitations of the individual. To provide guidance for hard-of-hearing children and adults, one should be aware of the possibilities of education and rehabilitation to reduce the limiting effects of the hearing handicap.

Educational guidance for hard-of-hearing children should recognize the particular needs listed in Table 2. With proper recognition of the difficulties and with appropriate auxiliary aid, children whose hearing impairment is from less than a 30-db loss to a 60-db loss (groups 1, 2, and 3 in Table 2) and some in group 4 may be placed in a special class for the hard of hearing within a public school system or in a regular classroom. Where the child is

Table 2 Educational Needs of Children with Impaired Hearing*

Group	Amount of hearing loss	Educational needs
1	Less than 30 db	Lip reading and favorable seating.
2	30 to 45 db loss	Lip reading, hearing aid (if suitable) and auditory training, speech correction and conservation, and favorable seating.
3	45 to 60 db loss	Lip reading, hearing aid and auditory training, special language work, and favorable seating.
4	60 to 80 db loss	Probably special educational procedures for deaf children with special emphasis on speech, auditory training, and language, with the possibility that the child may enter regular classes.
5	More than 80 db loss	Special class or school for the deaf. Some of these children eventually enter regular high schools.

* Adapted from Silverman [9, p. 326].

placed depends on the amount and time of identification of his hearing loss and the availability of special help. The latter includes special classes, itinerant teachers, and speech and hearing clinics in a university or hospital or provided by a society for the hard of hearing.

There is no agreement as to the existence of a set personality structure for hard-of-hearing children, but in general, as already stated, they need to be made aware of their handicaps, and as Ramdell [10] suggested, "The most successful adjustment is the one that overrides and submerges the handicap in normal activities centering outside one's self."

DEAF CHILDREN AND ADULTS

Deaf Children

When we consider deaf children, we must realize special techniques are necessary to build the skills of communication. The essential and primary channel for receiving the acoustic symbols we call speech is either absent or severely restricted. All the skills of communication that depend on learning over this channel are adversely affected. From infancy to early school age, the chief mode of communication for the normal hearing child is auditory. The child hears and learns to talk from what he hears. Furthermore, he not only learns how to communicate; he also learns what to communicate.

For a child who does not have daily experience of listening to language, its acquisition is indeed difficult, if not impossible for some, even with instruction. The teacher is confronted with the task of communicating language to a child in the absence of the sensory system considered to be essential for its acquisition.

The educator, therefore, must seek ways to manipulate information so that it can be transmitted over whatever sensory system or combination of systems is indicated: vision, touch, residual hearing. At the same time, we are concerned about the content of what we communicate—language and subject matter, as it is influenced by the demands of society and the child himself.

Vocational and Psychological Guidance for Deaf Adults

A deaf adult may differ from his deaf acquaintance as much as or less than he does from his hearing friends. It would be desirable if those who counsel deaf persons who cannot speak or read lips were familiar with the manual alphabet and the language of signs. Studies are under way to explore the occupational activities and the problems of psychological adjustment of deaf adults. In general, society now understands that deaf persons not only can be educated but also can, with proper guidance and opportunity, become economically and socially productive. Their accomplishments in industry, the arts, certain professions, and in community activities attest to this.

I cannot improve on a previous contribution as an appropriate conclusion to this discussion.

> Although man has traveled a long tortuous road from the pre-Christian era in evolving an enlightened understanding of the social problems of deafness, a large portion of society still looks upon the deaf and hard of hearing as queer, dependent, and, sometimes, ridiculous. We are all familiar with the cheap humor of which they are often the target. Since their handicap is not as visible as that of the blind and the crippled, the deaf often find themselves in embarrassing and humiliating situations because others do not understand their special problems.
>
> The answer of the deaf to such misunderstanding is to continue their social and economic achievements as self-respecting and productive individuals. Our social action for the deaf, therefore, should not aim for special privileges for them, but should constantly strive to provide opportunity without discrimination for the deaf to help themselves.
>
> The achievements of the deaf in the United States since the founding of the first school for the deaf in Hartford in 1817 have been good, but the record can be improved. This is the conjoint task of the teacher, the parent, the scientist, the physician, and of course, the deaf person himself.

REFERENCES

1. Schuknecht, H. F. "Otosclerosis," in Schuknecht, F. H. (ed.), *Henry Ford Hospital International Symposium,* Nov. 12, 1960, Boston: Little, Brown & Co., 1962.
2. Hirsh, I. J. Hearing, *Ann. Rev. Psychol.,* **6**:95-188, 1955.

3 Wever, E. G., and Lawrence, M. *Physiological Acoustics,* Princeton, N.J.: Princeton University Press, 1954.
4 Davis, H. Biophysics and Physiology of the Inner Ear, *Physiol. Rev.,* **37**:1-49, 1957.
5 Galambos, R. Some Recent Experiments on the Neurophysiology of Hearing, *Trans. Amer. Otol. Soc.,* **54**:133-139, 1956.
6 Glorig, A. Guide for Conservation of Hearing in Noise, *Trans. Amer. Acad. Ophthal. Otolaryng.,* suppl. revised 1964.
7 Hardy, W. G. *Children with Impaired Hearing,* publication 326, Children's Bureau, Government Printing Office, 1952.
8 Silverman, S. R. "What Is Deafness," in *Proc. of a National Workshop on Improved Opportunities for the Deaf, The University of Tennessee, Knoxville, Oct. 18-22, 1964.* Vocational Rehabilitation Administration, Department of Health, Education and Welfare, 1964, pp. 52-53.
9 Silverman, S. R. The Hearing Handicapped: Their Education and Rehabilitation, *Postgrad Med.,* **23**:321-330, March 1958.
10 Ramsdell, D. A. "The Psychology of the Hard-of-Hearing and the Deafened Adult," in David, H., and Silverman, S. R. (eds.), *Hearing and Deafness,* rev. ed, New York: Holt, Rinehart & Winston, Inc., 1960, pp. 459-473.

Reading 41

Deaf Patients Learn to Listen on a New Wave Length

An entirely new approach to the re-education of the deaf, known as the verbo-tonal method, has been developed in Yugoslavia by Prof. Petar Guberina, director of the Phonetics Institute of the University of Zagreb. The technique is applicable to deafness from various causes.

Deafness, whatever its etiology, is seldom complete, says Dr. Guberina. He believes that there always remain one or more audible frequencies along which sound reaches the brain's hearing centers. In essence, his technique is to find each patient's best frequency and then to filter speech through a device that takes out all the other frequencies. The Yugoslav researcher has found that filtered words with some component frequencies strained out are easier for the deaf person to understand than a full range of sound at high volume.

The increase of sound volume is frequently useless and may even inter-

Reprinted from *Journal of Rehabilitation,* vol. 31, no. 6, pp. 20-21, November-December 1965.

fere with the understanding of speech, Dr. Guberina says. Just as turning up the volume on a radio makes the static even more bothersome, so a hearing aid may increase the volume of interference, drowning out significant frequencies and decreasing intelligibility.

A linguist as well as a phonetician, Dr. Guberina was teaching at the University of Zagreb when he became interested in intonation and rhythm as factors in the understanding of languages. He enlisted the aid of electronics engineers to develop the first audiometer to filter the frequencies used in spoken words. With this instrument, they are able to study the perception, not of pure frequencies, but of those in actual speech.

The patient is told to listen to a series of taped words filtered through different frequency bands and to identify words that he understands. The tester checks off the words that are understood and notes the frequency through which they have been filtered and the minimal intensity required for intelligibility. By the end of a 40-minute test, the patient's optimal verbotonal field of understanding is identified.

PERSONAL UNITS EFFECTIVE

In order to test conversational intelligibility along selected frequency ranges, Dr. Guberina and his engineers developed another apparatus, SUVAG (System of University Verbo-Tonal Audition, Guberina), that can be adjusted to each patient's range of understanding. For instance, it can eliminate all frequencies above 8,000 cycles per second, or all frequencies below 500 cycles per second.

After testing numbers of deaf persons, Dr. Guberina found that their understanding improved if the voice reaching them was filtered to include only their optimal frequency range. "Then we started to make hearing aids that were miniaturized SUVAGs, each adapted to a particular patient. We discovered that deaf or partly deaf persons, after working for a while with their personal filters, learned to select their optimal frequencies from unfiltered speech. Some eventually became able to understand speech without any hearing aid at all."

This learning is most effective in a person with acquired deafness, the phonetician says. Earlier in life, such a person has been conditioned to hear the full range of speech frequencies. When his hearing deteriorates, there is no longer a correspondence between this conditioning and the altered stimulus he receives. Re-education must re-establish a link between the new stimulus and the old conditioning.

At best, results become apparent after three or four one-hour sessions, although 20 to 40 sessions are needed for optimal results. The improvement persists, says Dr. Guberina, because "the normal brain has adapted itself to the abnormal ear."

Even if the ear is completely useless, many patients can learn to perceive sound vibrations through their bodies, Dr. Guberina says. "This is different from bone conduction, which is only another pathway to the auditory receptor. Verbo-tonal research has shown that the body as a whole is involved in sound perception. This body perception seems to be especially well developed in patients who have severe defects of the inner ear."

The body is known to vibrate at low frequencies, around 7 to 12 cycles per second, and different parts of the body vibrate at different frequencies. SUVAG is so designed that it can attenuate speech frequencies down to a few cycles per second, within the range of body vibrations.

"Each person has a preferential area for perceiving vibrations most clearly—the chest, the hand, sometimes the fingertips," says Dr. Guberina. "A person with normal hearing can also understand speech reaching him through a vibrator held in his hand. It is a strange experience to understand words that do not reach you through the ear.

"The surprise of a totally deaf person first exposed to the voice-vibrator is even more striking. Children, especially, often have awed or delighted expressions on their faces when words they still do not understand reach them for the first time."

Reading 42

A Guide for Nurses in a Hearing Conservation Program

Anne J. Murphy

In many plants, employees in certain areas are exposed to noise of harmful intensity. Continuous exposure to noise of 90 decibels (db) or above in any octave bands between 600 and 2400 cycles per second (cps) may produce irreversible hearing loss. The greatest loss occurs during the first few years of exposure. It is the joint responsibility of management and labor to protect employees from this hazard.

A program to control exposure to hazardous noise should be allied with

Reprinted from *American Association of Industrial Nurses Journal*, pp. 21–25, October 1963.

the company's safety program and the preventive medicine program. It should provide for:

1 Identification of work areas where noise is a hazard.
2 Elimination of noise at its source, whenever possible.
3 Prevention of hearing loss among employees through:
   a Providing for the detection of hearing loss before it becomes disabling.
   b Seeing to it that employees who work in areas where noise is of potentially harmful intensity utilize protective devices.

The third portion of this program, which relates to work with individual employees, is largely the responsibility of the industrial health unit, where one is available. Where plant medical facilities are not available, an appropriate local service should be established.

Much of the success of a hearing conservation program depends upon the competence and enthusiasm of the nurse in carrying out her responsibilities under the supervision of the plant physician or the consulting otologist. These responsibilities may include:

1 Making audiometric measurements.
2 Maintaining the records of audiometric findings.
3 Referring employees who have abnormal measurements to a physician.
4 Participating in the education of personnel about the need for ear protection.
5 Instructing employees in the use and care of protective devices.

AUDIOMETRIC MEASUREMENTS

Schedules for Testing

Preplacement audiometric measurements should be taken on all new employees and on those being transferred to new work areas. Such measurements establish a base line and serve as a protection to both employer and employee. Approximately 25 per cent of all new employees have some degree of hearing loss at the time of employment. The causes are varied and numerous; noise is one cause. New employees with hearing impairment who are to be employed in noisy areas should be referred to the plant physician and should have their hearing rechecked after 30 days and after 60 days.

Periodic audiometric measurements should be taken on all employees exposed to noise levels of 90 db or above in any octave band between 600 and 2400 cps. The interval between examinations is governed by the length of daily exposure, as follows:

> For 5-8 hours of steady exposure, recheck every 12 months; if the noise is of extreme intensity, every 6 months. For 4 hours or less of steady exposure, recheck every 18 to 24 months. For anyone showing distinct loss, regardless of exposure, every 24 months.

The subject should be free of acute respiratory infection and should have been away from a noisy environment for at least 16 hours.

Personnel

Audiometric tests should be made by a nurse or a technician who has been properly trained and certified by a qualified person or center of learning.

Environment

In audiometry rooms, noise should not exceed the allowable noise levels suggested by the American Standard Association. The allowable background noise levels are:

   300 to 600   cycles—40 db
   600 to 1200 cycles—40 db
   1200 to 2400 cycles—48 db
   2400 to 4800 cycles—57 db
   4800 to 9600 cycles—67 db

If there is doubt about the existing levels, noise levels should be determined by surveys in the area.

Equipment

Consists of a pure-tone audiometer with frequencies at 500, 1000, 2000, 3000, 4000, 6000, and 8000 cycles, as recommended by the American Academy of Ophthalmology and Otolaryngology.

An audiometer is a precision instrument which produces tones by means of a complicated electric network. It must be handled with care. It should be accurately calibrated, in good working order, and checked daily on someone with known hearing acuity—that is, someone who has a number of recent measurements recorded, usually another nurse. It should be calibrated only when it is known to be out of calibration, not routinely every two years. A daily record of calibration should be kept. Care should be taken not to drop the earphones, since this may alter the accuracy of the calibration. The headbands should have sufficient tension to hold the earphones snugly over the ears.

Procedure

Measurements should be taken of the thresholds at frequencies of 500, 1000, 2000, 3000, 4000, and 6000, according to the following procedure:

1. Turn the power switch to "on" at least 5 minutes before starting the examination.
2. Explain the procedure to the subject in a pleasant, positive manner, and demonstrate sounds on the audiometer. Answer questions. Be clear, concise, complete. For example: "The object of this hearing measurement is to determine how weak a tone you can hear at certain pitches. Each ear will be tested separately. When you hear the tone, regardless of how weak it sounds to you, please raise your finger as soon as you hear it, hold your finger up until it stops, then put it down. (If an electric device is used, instruct the subject to push the button rather than raise his finger.) To eliminate visual distractions, close your eyes while listening. Listen for the sounds in your right ear first."
3. Place the subject so that:
    a. He cannot observe the audiometer panel or your hands.
    b. You may observe his facial expression.
    c. The cord is not rubbing against clothing, thus making background noise.
4. Check all panel controls. Set the frequency selector at 1000 cps and the attenuator at 10 db. The interrupter switch is in "off-on" position; the tone is produced only when the interrupter switch is pressed down.
5. Place the earphones over the subject's ears so that they fit snugly and are properly aligned. Be sure that the earphones are on the correct ear and adjusted comfortably. Remove the subject's glasses and any jewelry worn on ears, and pull the hair well back.
6. Take the measurement on the right ear first, except when it is known to have greater hearing loss than the left ear.
7. When giving the test tone to a new subject, avoid making it too loud; this may produce temporary auditory fatigue.
8. With the frequency dial set at 1000 cps, start the first tone at an intensity of 20 db above the estimated threshold; then reduce the sound intensity progressively, avoiding a rhythmic pattern of signals.
    a. Avoid making a clicking noise with the interrupter switch. Interrupt the tone for each change. Do not make changes in the db or frequency dials with the tone "on."
    b. The 1000 frequency is presented at 20 db for a second or two.
    c. The subject responds.
    d. Reduce in steps of 10 decibels and again present the tone in the same manner.

- **e** If the subject responds at 0 db, reduce to −5 or −10 db.
- **f** If he definitely hears one of these weak tones for three responses, this is threshold at 1000 cps.
- **g** If he cannot hear at −5 db, recheck at 0 db. (Taking too long to determine whether the threshold is −5 or −10 db is unjustifiable because, in calculating loss, the minus numbers are not considered.)
- **h** If he responds properly, then record 0 as the threshold. If he does not respond at 20 db, increase the intensity to 40 db. If he responds, then presume that the threshold lies between 40 and 20 db.
- **i** Present the next tone at 30 db and proceed as above, reducing the sound intensity progressively until the threshold is determined. Allow sufficient time for the subject to respond to every stimulus presented; usually a second or two suffices.
- **j** When the threshold for the 1000 frequency has been determined, and recorded for the right ear, move the frequency selector to 2000. Repeat the procedure for frequencies of 2000, 3000, 4000, and 6000. When threshold for the 6000 frequency has been determined, return to the 1000 frequency and recheck. Record both the first and the second responses; then turn to the 500 frequency and determine the threshold. After this is done, say "Now listen for the sounds in your left ear."
- **k** Starting at the 500 frequency, determine the threshold for each frequency—500, 1000, 2000, 3000, 4000, and 6000. The last decibel to which the subject responds with three "yeses" is considered his threshold.
- **l** If a threshold cannot be determined in the usual manner because of tinnitus (ringing in the ears), try several short interrupted bursts of tone two or three times instead of the single tone usually presented.

9. Compare the findings with those of previous tests. To avoid being influenced by previous records, it is best not to review them until you have finished the present measurement.

   Anyone showing a marked change in measurement since his last audiogram should be given a repeat audiogram on a different day, under similar conditions. A good practice is to recheck the threshold for those frequencies where the loss is greater than 20 db. If the repeat audiogram agrees within a plus or minus 5 at four frequencies, the two tests are consistent, and referral to the plant physician or to another designated physician is in order.

10. Interpret the audiogram findings to the subject. Explain that the 500, 1000, and 2000 cps are the speech range of frequencies and that any loss of 15 db or less is considered within normal range. If the subject has a loss of significance, explain that this could be for many reasons—heredity, infections, injury, age, and so on—that further evaluation by a physician is needed, and that the plant physician or other designated physician will discuss this finding with him.

To a great extent the acceptance of the hearing conservation program will depend upon the skill of the examiner in her explanation of the audiogram to the subject. She should be positive in her approach, willing, and competent to answer questions intelligently and allay misconceptions which may exist.

Records

Audiogram record forms should be completed by the nurse or technician; date and signature should be included. The audiogram may be an important medico-legal record at some future date, and comments about anything pertinent or unusual may be vital. Trauma, such as may result from a direct blow to the auditory region, or certain drugs, such as Neomycin, are among the many causes of hearing loss. If the subject has had previous exposure to noise, his previous work history is extremely important.

The history and the threshold number at each frequency should be carefully recorded in ink, and all other pertinent information should be *without erasures.* If an error in recording has been made, the incorrect number should be crossed out with a single line and the correct number placed near the canceled number.

REFERRALS

The nurse or technician who takes the audiogram should refer to the plant or other designated physician for further evaluation any employee:

    1 Showing, in his first measurement, an *average* loss, in either ear, of 15 db or more at 500, 1000, and 2000 cps.
    2 Showing any unusual irregularity, particularly an abrupt loss beginning at 2000 cps.
    3 Showing a shift of 15 db or more at the 3000–4000 cps level.
    4 Showing a loss in excess of 35 db at any two frequencies beyond 2000 cps since his last audiogram.
    5 Making responses that are so varied that an accurate threshold is not obtainable. This may indicate a functional hearing loss, an organic condition, or malingering.
    6 Showing widely fluctuating threshold levels, with hearing loss in the low frequencies. The ears should be checked for cerumen or another pathological condition.
    7 Complaining of an abnormal increase in loudness, out of proportion to the actual increase in intensity (recruitment). This may be indicative of labyrinthitis (Meniere's disease).

EMPLOYEE EDUCATION

Since the elimination of noise at its source involves a number of considerations, it is often necessary to protect employees who are exposed to excessive noise by fitting them with ear defenders, either plugs or muffs or both, until noise elimination can be achieved.

Individual ear protection may not be readily accepted for many reasons. Some of them are:

1 Ear plugs may be uncomfortable, especially when first worn.
2 Since noise does not hurt, an employee may become accustomed to it.
3 Hearing loss is gradual and may therefore not be noticed until it is severe and permanent.
4 Employees may consider the fitting and cleaning of ear plugs a nuisance.
5 Employees may feel that ear plugs will interfere with their work performance.
6 Previous warning never to put any foreign object into the ear may cause fear of injury.

Education is essential for a successful program. Knowledge helps to win acceptance. Repeated explanations by the nurse of the "why" of the program are essential.

The following are among the methods she may use to gain acceptance for ear plugs:

Meeting with company supervision in which she explains the problem, shows different types of plugs, and answers questions.

Soliciting the cooperation of selected members of the safety committee and getting them to wear ear protection for one month, then report back to safety committee. One sold person sells others.

Encouraging members of management and medical personnel to wear ear plugs when they go into noisy areas. (Carry an extra set and have an employee wear them while conversing with you.)

Demonstrating with the audiometer at 3000 frequency that properly fitted ear plugs reduce noise from 20 to 35 db.

Publishing, in the company magazine or newsletter, a letter to employees that explains the reasons for wearing ear protectors.

Using posters, brochures, films, and notices on bulletin boards.

Visiting those departments where the noise is in excess of 90 db in any octave bands between 600 and 2400 cps and counseling with the employees of these departments at every opportunity.

Demonstrating to employees the degree of protection by having them suddenly remove the ear plugs in a noisy area.

Using each visit by an employee to the medical department as an opportunity to discuss the ear protection program; to give the employee straight facts on noise, audio measurements, and ear protection devices; and to shape proper attitudes, clear up misunderstandings, and combat prejudices.

Explaining the hazards of excessive noise to new employees and fitting them with ear plugs at the time of the preplacement audiogram.

THE EAR PROTECTORS

The following are some suggestions to the nurse who fits ear plugs:

1 Provide a choice of types and a range of sizes. The size is critically important, as ear canals are different, even in a person's two ears. The elongated type will not fit in some ear canals, while shorter types may fit comfortably.

2 Carefully fit the plugs. Self-fitting should be discouraged. It is a good rule to overfit slightly.

3 To insert the plug properly, grasp the upper portion of the ear and draw it upward and backward. This procedure tends to straighten the canal. When the ear is released, the angulation of the canal will hold the protector firmly in the ear. The plug will tend to remain in place when an attempt is made to withdraw it.

4 The individual's voice should sound amplified to him when he has a properly fitted plug.

5 If the employee feels that he will have difficulty in becoming accustomed to the plug, suggest that he try the following schedule:

   1st day—30 minutes in A.M., 30 minutes in P.M.
   2nd day—1 hour in A.M., 30 minutes in P.M.
   3rd day—2 hours in A.M., 1 hour in P.M.
   4th day—all A.M., 2 hours in P.M.
   5th day—all A.M., 3 hours in P.M.
   6th day and thereafter—all day

Invite him to return in one week to report whether the device is satisfactory. If it is not, try other available kinds.

SEVEN POINTS ABOUT EAR PLUGS

Plugs should be pliable and fit tightly.
Ear protection must be fitted by trained personnel.
Plugs work loose and must be reseated.
Plugs do not cause infection.
Plugs must be kept clean.
Ear protectors make it easier to understand speech and warning signals in noisy situations.
The only ear protector is one that is worn.

DEFINITIONS

Audiogram A written record of an individual's threshold of hearing at certain specified frequencies.

Cycle Cycles per second—the number of sound waves set up by any vibrating body. They travel through the air at approximately 1,120 feet per second. They are much the same as water waves produced by dropping a stone in a pond.

Decibel The unit for measuring the loudness of a sound. A level of 0 decibels represents, roughly, the average weakest sound that can be heard by a person of good hearing.

Frequency The number of vibrations in cycles per second; pitch; the highness or lowness of a sound. Middle C on the piano is approximately 250 cycles per second. The top note on the piano keyboard is 4,000 cycles per second.

Threshold The average weakest tone which the subject's ear can detect in a given frequency.

Section F

Pain

Pain in one form or another and in some degree is one of the universal experiences of mankind. The complex nature of pain requires a multidimensional orientation to the subject. While everyone "knows" what it is, pain nevertheless has been difficult to define, and attempts to do so go back many years. Aristotle considered pain as an emotion which was the opposite of pleasure. Livingston has characterized some of the conceptual problems attending attempts to provide a satisfactory definition of pain.[1]

> One reason pain is so difficult to define is that it has so many aspects. The interpretation varies with the point of view of the investigator or the sufferer. To the sociologist pain and the threat of pain are powerful instruments of social learning and social preservation. To the biologist, pain is a sensory signal which warns the individual when a harmful stimulus threatens injury. To a man with an incurable cancer, pain is a destructive force which does not stop after the warning has been given. To the psychologist pain is a sensation like sight or

[1] Livingston, W. K., "What Is Pain?" *Scientific American Reader,* New York: Simon and Schuster, 1953.

hearing, but he tends to ignore its conscious, perceptual aspects, because consciousness has, as yet, no physiological equivalent; one might say that he is studying the pain signal. To the physiologist, on the other hand, the important thing about pain is the brain's translation of the signal into sensory experience. He finds pain, like all perceptions, to be subjective, individual, and modified by degree or attention, emotional states, and the conditioning influence of past experience.

The patient who requires rehabilitation nursing will frequently also be a patient who experiences pain in relation to his disability. The pain may be a physiological manifestation of tissue injury or it may be a symptom of an inability to cope with stresses that disability causes. In rehabilitation nursing, the nurse must make judgments which have a clinical import for the future. Such judgments go beyond the commonplace "PRN" order which the physician has left. McCaffery and Moss suggest two prior steps, i.e., ascertaining the nature of the complaint and utilizing nursing intervention, and only then giving medication if it seems indicated.

The nursing intervention described by McCaffery and Moss is based upon the programmed instruction for pain which was printed in the *American Journal of Nursing* (May and July 1966). The substitution of nursing care for the use of analgesics when possible helps prevent the patient from becoming dependent upon chemical relief. Its principal value, however, is in helping the patient to understand himself and his pain.

In order to implement successfully some of the indicated procedures (rotating a painful joint, for example), it is essential that the patient's trust be gained. The exercise may keep function intact, but it may cause the patient considerable distress. Rehabilitation may not take place unless the patient makes the decision that the pain he bears is worth the promise of the effort. Effective communication may be more important than the hypodermic syringe and the pill to assist the patient to tolerate the discomfort which accompanies the stress of indicated effort.

In spite of the universality of pain, the reactions to pain on the part of individuals can be noticeably different one from the other. Some of the reaction or response differences are thought to stem from genotypic determinants. Others are believed to have been learned as a result of intervening variables of a sociocultural nature. Christopherson discusses the bases for differential response to pain. His discussion helps sharpen perception by introducing comparative data for contrast. The importance of the nurse gaining as complete an understanding as possible of the cultural base of pain response is clearly brought out.

The section is concluded with a discussion by Melzak of one of the oldest and most persistent problems facing both patient and therapist in the area of pain, that of phantom pain. Melzak suggests some alternate and *productive* ways to approach the problem.

Reading 43
Nursing Intervention for Bodily Pain
Margo McCaffery
Fay Moss

Patients, as well as nurses, ask themselves what they can do about pain. But what a patient is capable of doing is greatly influenced by many factors in his past experience, as well as, to a certain extent, by what the nurse chooses to do. We know it is no longer sufficient for us simply to give an analgesic; we are responsible for many other types of intervention.

Our personal clinical experience (M. McC.) has led us to believe that the nurse's pain-relieving activities tend to fall into nine somewhat overlapping categories: administering pharmacologic agents, administering placebos, altering the pain stimulus or source, assisting the patient to utilize physical activity, providing distraction, suggesting psychotherapy, discussing pain with the patient, remaining with the patient, and providing touch. We shall discuss only these last three activities here, with mention of the overlapping areas.

The nurse who plans to use one of these activities to intervene between the patient and his pain may consider that his pain experience has three parts: the anticipation of pain, the experience of pain, and the period immediately following pain. In this discussion we are not separating the anticipation and experience phases, because the three nursing activities we shall discuss are adaptable to either phase.

DISCUSSING PAIN WITH THE PATIENT

A discussion about pain may be carried out in several different ways and may achieve various related purposes. These purposes are: to obtain the patient's trust and to convey concern, to mobilize the patient's adaptive mechanisms, to enforce and stabilize his adaptive mechanisms, and to change his attitude toward pain-related stimuli.

Perhaps first the nurse should strive to obtain trust and convey concern. Many studies of the placebo phenomenon suggest that the type of

Reprinted from *The American Journal of Nursing*, vol. 67, no. 6, pp. 1224–1227, June 1967. The authors are elaborating on three of the six nursing interventions mentioned in the *Journal's* two programmed instruction units on pain (May and July 1966): decreasing pain perception, modifying pain interpretation, and decreasing pain reactions. They would like to stress to the reader that the activities suggested here are merely hypotheses from their observations of successful types of intervention, and that both the activities and their stated purposes require further investigation and are subject to revision in the light of ongoing and future research.

communication as well as the subsequent method of alleviating or preventing pain are probably significantly affected by the patient's perception of the nurse's intentions, trustworthiness, and expertness [1]. If the patient's perceptions are positive, he tends to evaluate what is done as favorable and to accept what is said.

One method of communication which helps to obtain trust and convey concern is to maintain the essence of a "one-person situation" [2]. As originally conceived, the one-person situation involved a lack of communication between the experiencer of pain (the patient) and another person (the observer, or nurse in this case). When the experiencer does not communicate his pain, there is no observer except himself, and, therefore, there is no question of validation of his pain. If he does communicate, he risks disagreement between himself and the nurse about whether the pain is real or even exists at all. We are in no way advising the nurse to prevent nurse-patient communication, but rather to communicate in a manner that promotes the patient's goal in the one-person situation. If the patient senses that the nurse does not believe in the existence or severity of his pain, he will obviously have difficulty trusting her or believing her concern.

Mrs. K. illustrates the different results obtained by using the one-person and two-person approaches. Mrs. K. was alternately watching television and talking on the phone when she reported to the nurse that she was having abdominal pain. This nurse replied with a two-person approach by saying, "It couldn't be too bad. You seem to be enjoying yourself." The patient said no more, but continued her activities and then reported her pain to a second nurse. This nurse asked Mrs. K. to describe the pain. This one-person approach, which did not question or disagree with the patient, resulted in several minutes of informative conversation which enabled the nurse to relieve Mrs. K.'s pain by repositioning.

Discussing pain with the patient also helps him mobilize his adaptive mechanisms—those behaviors which assist him in handling pain with minimum physical and mental discomfort. This purpose may be accomplished during pain, but it is preferable that it be achieved prior to pain [3]. Sometimes the patient is not aware that a painful situation is imminent, and therefore he is unable to prepare himself to mobilize his defenses. Under these circumstances the patient needs to be informed of what will occur. Initially this information tells him what he may expect to happen. It includes not only what he may feel, but also when, who will do it, why, how long it will last, and what equipment will be involved. For children (and, in some situations, for adults) this information is best imparted by letting them handle the equipment.

The nurse will need to be as honest as possible about what pain the patient will feel. Otherwise it will be difficult for him to mobilize appropriate adaptive mechanisms. Just to mention that pain will or may be felt is often not enough. The patient may choose to ignore or deny this, or the word "pain" may convey to him a greater or lesser meaning than was intended. The word need not be avoided, but other descriptive words may be more useful, such as sting, prick, or pressure. It may be helpful for the patient to know what the specific pain stimulus or source will be. For example, when seven-year-old Timmy was asked by the nurse to go with her to the treatment room to see the doctor, he began to cry, saying, "What's he going to do? I don't want him to hurt me." Timmy stopped crying when he was told the doctor would prick his finger, a procedure familiar to Timmy.

Sometimes the decision is made not to forewarn the patient of pain, or the warning is given immediately preceding the pain or during the pain. This kind of professional judgment, or decision, is worthy of thorough consideration. The reasons most often given for making this judgment are related to believing that the patient will only become upset and worry about it. This does not seem to be adequate reasoning, since worry is a necessary part of mobilizing defenses [4]. However, if the nurse ascertains, after careful investigation, that the patient is incapable of constructively mobilizing his defenses, then perhaps he should not be forewarned of pain.

Janis suggests that forewarning the patient about intrusive procedures gives him time to visualize a horrible ordeal and to develop vivid fantasies. Therefore, the best time for giving an explanation to reduce the patient's fear might be at the time such a procedure is performed [4]. Janis's suggestion seemed to apply to Mr. J., who was having numerous intrusive diagnostic procedures. It was observed that forewarning him resulted in such symptoms of anxiety as dyspnea, vomiting, and random movements. When the decision was made not to forewarn him, these symptoms were eliminated, and he underwent the procedures with less apparent anxiety.

The length of time the patient needs to mobilize adaptive mechanisms is subject to great variation and is difficult to assess. He should have enough time to ask questions and to think about the expected experience; yet the longer he anticipates a stressful situation, the higher his anxiety may become. Therefore, the period of anticipation of pain should extend only until the patient has reached a comfortable and constructive way of handling the situation [5].

A further purpose of discussing pain with the patient is to enforce and stabilize his adaptive mechanisms. This, too, can be accomplished both before and during pain, but the changing characteristics of the pain make it an ongoing process. Unfortunately, very little is known about the specific adaptive mechanisms patients may utilize, nor have these mechanisms been categorized.

One specific way to elicit the patient's adaptive mechanisms is to ask him how he has handled or reacted to pain in the past. These mechanisms are dependent on many aspects of the patient's past experiences and are influenced by the particular pain situation—the same patient may use different mechanisms for different types of pain. For pain of severe intensity accompanied by high anxiety, the patient may prefer to control his behavior by lying quietly and perhaps by having an "expert" nurse present. Another patient may be more comfortable if he expresses his feelings by crying out and flailing about or by controlling his external environment through ordering others around. For prolonged pain of low to moderate intensity, the patient may utilize distraction in the form of games, visiting, or television.

Some of the possible adaptive mechanisms just described may be difficult, initially, for certain nurses to tolerate and work with. Of course some adaptive patterns, which tend toward denial and self-destruction, are not worthy of enforcing and stabilizing if the patient can be assisted to develop more constructive behavior. However, it is well to remember that an individual establishes his adaptive mechanisms within the limitations of his culture and personal experiences. Such behavior is not easily changed, and an attempt at change may be very disruptive to him. Whether or not the behavior needs to be altered is probably best judged on the basis of the degree of the patient's anxiety, denial, or self-destruction, not on the basis of the nurse's personal cultural expectations.

A fourth purpose of discussing pain with the patient may be to change his attitude toward pain-related stimuli, thereby achieving pain alleviation through altered pain perception [6]. It has been shown that a person's attitude toward a particular stimulus may be changed if he is allowed to participate actively in discussing and making decisions about his response toward that stimulus [7]. Therefore, we suggest that a patient's attitude toward pain-related stimuli may be changed if he is allowed to participate in a discussion of his pain and to make decisions about what action he will take in relation to the stimuli. This discussion will overlap the first purpose, that of obtaining his trust and conveying concern, because the nurse who intends to help the patient change his attitude must be perceived as trustworthy, as being capable of helping, and as intending to help him [7,8].

Initial study in this area indicates that the nurse can effect a change in the patient's attitude toward pain-related stimuli. In this discussion, the nurse guides the patient in describing and explaining various aspects of his pain, such as the nature, location, intensity, and duration of the pain. She may ask the patient what nursing measures he feels would alleviate the pain, and she may suggest measures which she believes will help. She then allows the patient to make the decision about which of these measures he will employ to alleviate his pain. When this type of nurse-patient interaction occurs, the result very often is pain alleviation without the use of medication [9].

REMAINING WITH THE PATIENT

Naturally, the nurse must be with the patient if she is to perform any of the activities mentioned. However, when she is not saying or doing anything, but is simply standing by quietly, her presence may serve some important purposes.

One purpose is to prevent or reduce social isolation. The presence of the nurse allows the patient to initiate interaction if he wishes. Even if he chooses to remain quiet, the nurse's presence may lessen his feeling that others do not care.

But, for one reason or another, many persons seem too often left alone to experience and handle pain without assistance from anyone else. The nurse probably tends to avoid patients who are experiencing pain for many of the same reasons that she avoids the dying patient [10]. Long-lasting, intense pain which does not readily respond to measures intended to alleviate it may cause her to feel helpless and guilty. In addition to her self-blame, the patient, especially if he is a child, may blame her for the pain. At other times the nurse may be afraid she will inflict more pain. Or, as mentioned before, the patient's pain reaction may be difficult for the nurse to accept.

There are, of course, situations in which the presence of the nurse may be quite undesirable to the patient. For example, a male patient who is undergoing an embarrassing procedure or a patient who momentarily loses control of his behavior may prefer to have as few witnesses as possible.

Remaining with the patient is in itself an appropriate response to his anxiety. The desire to be with another person appears to increase as anxiety increases [11]. Just being with the patient may imply that someone else shares his experience and is available to help him, thus assisting him to control his anxiety. The presence of the nurse may be especially important during the latter stages of pain anticipation, since anxiety seems to increase as the time approaches to engage in a stressful activity.

PROVIDING TOUCH

Touch can probably convey as wide a variety of meanings as verbal communication. Some kinds of touch may be helpful to the person experiencing pain.

Touch may be used for the purpose of communicating to the patient that dependency is allowed during stressful periods, such as during intense pain or high anticipatory anxiety. The nurse, of course, must be discriminating about how and when she uses touch. Patients who are striving to maintain their independence may reject touch because it involves a certain degree of dependence [12]. However, under suddenly stressful situations, these same patients may reach out for the nurse's hand. A firm touch seems effective at such times. When a patient is experiencing less acute anxiety, a tender, stroking touch may be helpful.

Touch may also be used for the purpose of controlling anxiety through relaxation. A well-timed back rub may do much to relax the patient's tense muscles and to curb his mounting anxiety. There appears to be a relationship between increased relaxation and decreased pain, and preliminary studies show that a back rub during pain often reduces signs of tension [13-15].

Perhaps touch could be used for the purpose of giving the patient a pleasurable orientation to his body. Pain tends to draw attention to itself, causing increased preoccupation with the body [16]. Touch can be a localized, pleasant sensation providing the opposite of the unpleasant sensation of pain. For example, a patient experiencing generalized discomfort associated with a high fever may again view his body as a source of pleasure when the nurse's cool hand lightly strokes his forehead.

THE AFTERMATH

The period immediately following the painful experience seems to be a neglected area of nursing intervention. While many of the already mentioned nursing activities and purposes pertain at this time, the most important is that of talking with the patient to achieve two major purposes. First of all, he needs to realize that all or part of the course of his pain has been partially or completely altered. Some situations make it difficult for the patient to obtain this information for himself, particularly if a procedure has been done out of his range of vision. Unless the patient knows he need not anticipate or experience any more pain, his level of anxiety may be sustained or increased, or he may misinterpret other stimuli as painful.

Second, the patient needs to assimilate his painful experience. His comprehension of the situation may affect his future reactions to pain. Intellectual and emotional incorporation of the painful period may be facilitated by reenacting the event. With an adult, verbal discussion, including what actually happened, what he felt physically, and what his emotional feelings were, may be sufficient. For a young child, assimilation may be best accomplished through playacting with the equipment and the people involved.

In summary, it seems that in many instances how well the patient is able to handle his pain is dependent on what his nurse does. It appears that when the nurse is confronted with a patient who anticipates or feels pain, there are several activities she can perform, which, when varied appropriately, assist him in coping with his immediate experience, and may influence his future pain experiences as well.

REFERENCES

1. Liberman, Robert. An analysis of the placebo phenomenon. *J. Chronic Dis.,* **15**:761-783, August 1962.
2. Szasz, T. S. Language and pain. In *American Handbook of Psychiatry,* ed. by Silvano Arieti. New York, Basic Books, 1959, vol. 1, pp. 982-999.
3. Smith, Margo M. Nursing knowledge and activity in relation to the period of anticipation of pain in the adult. In Solving "Difficult" Problems in Nursing

Care, *ANA Convention Clinical Papers, No. 20,* New York, American Nurses' Association, 1962, pp. 25-34.
4   Janis, I. L. *Psychological Stress.* New York, John Wiley & Sons, 1958, pp. 374-394.
5   Aasterud, Margaret. Explanation to the patient. In *Social Interaction and Patient Care,* ed. by J. K. Skipper and R. C. Leonard, Philadelphia, Pa., J. B. Lippincott Co., 1965, pp. 82-87.
6   Allport, F. H. *Theories of Perception and the Concept of Structure.* New York, John Wiley & Sons, 1955, pp. 215, 412.
7   Sherif, Muzafer, and Sherif, Carolyn W. *Outline of Social Psychology,* rev. ed. New York, Harper and Row, 1956.
8   Hovland, C. I., and Weiss, W. The influence of source credibility in communication effectiveness. *Public Opin. Quart.,* **15**:633-650, 1951.
9   Moss, Fay T., and Meyer, Burton. Effects of nursing interaction upon pain relief in patients. *Nurs. Res.,* **15**:303-306, Fall 1966.
10 Menzies, Isabel E. P. A case-study in the functioning of social systems as a defense against anxiety. *Hum. Relations,* **13**(2):95-121, 1960.
11 Schachter, Stanley. *Psychology of Affiliation.* Stanford, Calif., Stanford University Press, 1959, pp. 12-19.
12 Fenichel, Otto. *Psychoanalytic Theory of Neurosis.* New York, W. W. Norton and Co., 1945, pp. 65, 159.
13 Wenger, M. A., and others. *Physiological Psychology.* New York, Holt, Rinehart and Winston, 1956, p. 103.
14 Bunten, Judith. *Effect of Touch on Patients in Pain.* Los Angeles, Calif., University of California, School of Nursing, 1966. (Unpublished undergraduate paper for honors seminar.)
15 Hellwig, Karen. *The Use of Supportive Touch with Patients in Pain.* Los Angeles, Calif., University of California, School of Nursing, 1966. (Unpublished undergraduate paper for honors seminar.)
16 Pain, Part 1. *Basic concepts and assessment* (programmed instruction supplement). *Amer. J. Nurs.,* **66**:1085-1108, May 1966.

Reading 44
Sociocultural Correlates of Pain Response
V. A. Christopherson

Pain is a highly subjective sensation which cannot be seen, felt, or denied by any other than the one who reports it. We all know what it is, for it is a near-universal experience, and it is almost always a nuisance to everyone con-

The investigation upon which this discussion was based was supported in part by a research grant, No. 1390, from the Vocational Rehabilitation Administration, Department of Health, Education and Welfare, Washington, D.C., and in part by the Agricultural Experiment Station, the University of Arizona, Tucson, Arizona.

cerned. On the other hand, pain is probably as vital to the health and welfare of an individual as his daily bread. Some pain warns of disease and injury; however, other pain is apparently useless and pernicious—that which accompanies trigeminal neuralgia, for example. Inasmuch as pain is so frequently instrumental in patient behavior and so often a point of contact between the nurse and patient, all effort made to comprehend pain and its implications should be time profitably spent.

Pain is a difficult and elusive concept when it comes to definition, and attempts to evolve standard and adequate concepts go back many years. The word "pain" is derived from the Latin "poena" which means punishment. Aristotle considered pain an emotion which was the opposite of pleasure. More recent definitions are grounded more soundly in science, perhaps, but it would be difficult to improve much on the Aristotelian concept.

Pain response is a secondary or derivative phenomenon as opposed to the primary sensation of pain per se. The response, however, may be more significant than the sensation, for it colors and affects the way the sufferer relates to his world. When different individuals suffer the apparent same degree and kind of tissue damage or noxious stimuli, the most casual observation reveals differences in response. The question has been raised as to what it is to which the individuals are responding. Does a certain amount of tissue damage "feel" different to different individuals, or do individuals respond differently to the same feeling?

LEARNING FACTORS IN PAIN RESPONSE

Without consideration of physiological determinants of differential pain response, there is ample grist for the mill with regard to determinants of a learning type. Learning approaches to pain response and pain management might succeed not only in providing a basis for greater insight into patient behavior, but the learning approach might provide the nurse with tools which have a more permanent impact than any analgesic. At the present time, however, learned responses to pain sensation represent an area somewhat less well developed than such areas of pain study as physiology of pain, classification of pain, and relief of pain.

That cultural patterning can affect and possibly reverse what is considered common and appropriate pain response is indicated by the widely read anthropological novel by Ruesch entitled *Top of the World*. The culture of the Polar Eskimo described in this book encourages laughter as the most acceptable response to pain.

Keel [3] cites the French surgeon René Leriche's observations of Russian Cossacks in World War I. The surgeon, by invitation of some Russian officers, dislocated the joints of the hands and feet of Cossack soldiers without an anesthetic and without complaint from the men.

Pain is undoubtedly influenced by a number of variables in addition to tissue damage. E. G. Poser [5] suggests ethnic origin as one of the possible sources of response variation. Mark Zborowski's study [9] is perhaps the best known and most frequently cited study relating sociocultural background to pain response. He compared pain responses of Jewish, Italian, Irish, and Old American groups. The last of these consisted of individuals who were predominantly of Anglo-Saxon stock and who had lived in the United States a number of generations. Other studies of sociocultural variables were carried out by Sternbach and Tursky [8], Sherman and Robillard [7], and Lambert, Libman, and Poser [4]. In each case it appeared that the ways in which people responded to pain had been influenced by their backgrounds and previous experience—in effect, pain response is a learned response.

SITUATIONAL DETERMINANTS

In some situations response to tissue damage (and presumably pain) seems to transcend national and subcultural patterns in favor of cogent situational determinants. Beecher's well-known studies [1,2] of seriously wounded soldiers in a combat zone hospital vis-à-vis male civilians who had undergone major surgery revealed sharp differences in response to comparable tissue damage. Beecher attributed the difference in response to the significance of the wound to the men in question. The soldier perceived his wound as a blessing. It enabled him to escape the battlefield and leave with honor. It was his ticket out. The civilian, on the other hand, perceived his "wound" as a calamity. It was painful and disabling. Only one-fifth of the postoperative patients refused medication for the relief of pain, whereas two-thirds of the wounded soldiers refused medication.

Another example, well known to nurses, of the influence of context or situational determinants was the common observation during World War II concerning the bravery of soldiers suffering from severe wounds. In contrast, they were observed to respond emotionally to the point sometimes of tears over the unwelcome prospect of daily antibiotic injections.

It is all well and good to learn about the Polar Eskimos or the soldiers of World War II, but once the concept or principle has been established, it is important to make application in one's own area of operation. Consequently the author undertook a study comparing pain response of the three dominant ethnic groups in Southern Arizona, i.e., Mexican-Americans, Anglo-Saxons, and Papago Indians.

ETHNIC COMPARISONS

There were a number of very significant differences in pain response found on the part of all three groups when considered in relation to one another.

The nurse who works with Mexican-American patients could scarcely afford to ignore or remain ignorant of the pain orientation of this subculture. Pain, for example, may have a meaning to the person involved which has little or no bearing on the medical or prognostic implications from the Anglo-Saxon point of view. Even among the dominant culture groups it may be that much of the reported pain is not as important as the patient thinks it is; it may, however, be a good deal more important than the nurse or physician thinks it is.

An excellent reference to help the nurse appreciate and understand the significance of the differences between the Anglo-Saxon and Mexican-American pain cultures would be *Cultural Differences and Medical Care* by Lyle Saunders, 1954. A few points made by Saunders that provide an excellent backdrop for our findings in differential pain response are the following recurring behavioral responses on the part of the Spanish-speaking patients.[1]

1   Delay in seeking medical aid
2   Failure to keep appointments
3   Ignoring dietary recommendations, particularly those applying to the feeding of infants
4   Failure to follow instructions
5   Resistance to suggestions for hospitalization
6   Resistance to sanitarium treatment for TB
7   Leaving institutions against medical advice
8   Failure to obtain prenatal care
9   Resistance to surgery
10   Failure of communication in history taking

Underlying these problems are a number of areas in which the perceptions and points of view developed by "Spanish-speaking" and "Anglo" cultural bases may be in sharp opposition. Illustrative of these areas are the following contrasts in cultural perspective.

1   *Anglo:* Disease and (pain)[2] result from known, predictable, and (frequently) controllable causes. *Spanish-speaking:* Disease and (pain) are manifestations of the will of God, of fate, of the actions of enemies, of punishment for moral deviations, or of the whimsicalities of chance. There is not much that one could or should do to avoid or prevent these things.

---

[1] These two series of points were made by Mr. Saunders in a conference address made at the University of Arizona in 1961. See Report of Southwestern Conference of Cultural Influences on Health Services and Home Economics Programs, School of Nursing and School of Home Economics, in cooperation with the Arizona State Department of Health, Arizona Dietetic Association, and State Department of Vocational Education, 1961, pp. 70-72.

[2] Saunders used death in his example.

SOCIOCULTURAL CORRELATES OF PAIN RESPONSE

2 *Anglo:* A person may be ill regardless of how he feels. *Spanish-speaking:* Illness is a matter of subjective feeling. A person is not ill if he feels well.

3 *Anglo:* The presence of disease requires surrendering the patient to professional healers who, for his own good, may require that he be separated from his family during the treatment process. *Spanish-speaking:* The presence of disease requires that the family surround the patient even more closely than usual and that the role of the healer, if one is consulted, be subordinated to that of the family group.

4 *Anglo:* One should be alert to future possibilities of present conditions and take steps to avoid undesirable consequences. *Spanish-speaking:* The future is nebulous and distant; one will do well to cope with problems of the present.

5 *Anglo:* Contagion can be transmitted by anyone. *Spanish-speaking:* One cannot inadvertently harm someone he loves.

The characterizations are but a small portion indeed of the considerable amount of available information to assist the nurse in successful interaction with Spanish-speaking Americans. Inasmuch as the Papago Indians are much less acculturated with respect to the dominant Anglo-Saxon society than are the Mexican-Americans, their pain response might be expected to vary more considerably from the Anglo-Saxon norms. The investigation proved this to be the case.

The several Papago Indian reservations are very near Tucson and together occupy an area of almost three million acres. In spite of their geographical proximity to major population centers, the Papagos' concepts of health, disease, and significance of pain are far removed from the norms of middle-class America. An inquiry into the pain responses of the Papago is a venture into another world. The Papago world is served by principles of causality that are not only completely foreign and naive from the Anglo-Saxon viewpoint, but they are determinative of a great many phenomena of ceremonial and everyday life that come into conflict with the educational objectives and health goals established by the dominant culture.

Dreaming of a certain animal, crossing its track, or showing some form of disrespect can bring about a disease and/or painful condition. In the event the Papago suffering a painful condition is unable to obtain relief from a fetish with magical curative properties, help from a shaman or medicine man may be sought. When the Papago feels himself to be "out of harmony" with the established order of things, he expects to be sick or have some misfortune befall him. Much of the medicine man's success is due to his bringing the person back into harmonious relation with his environment. As such the shaman's medicine is highly charged with a practical psychology.

From the Anglo-Saxon point of view, the Papago's response to pain is stoical indeed. Keeping in mind, however, that an individual's behavior is a product of his assumptions, attitudes, and knowledge, the inference that a Papago responds better or less well to pain than the Anglo-Saxon is an oversimplification. The contributory factor is that the Papago simply does not know about and consequently does not consider available alternatives to pain. The examples of pain response we discussed with the physician and nurses at the Papago Indian Hospital, Sells, Arizona, led one of the nurses to comment, "We have learned from experience that when a Papago complains of pain or requests medication, such requests should receive prompt attention, for he is usually in serious trouble."

A LEARNING MODEL FOR PAIN MANAGEMENT

The relief of pain is one of the most cherished of all blessings born of modern medical technology, and it is now an important and rapidly growing edge in pain research. One of the recent developments to come out of one of the most progressive research centers for pain in the country, the Pain Clinic of the University of Washington Medical College, Seattle, Washington, is a learning-type model in pain management. The underlying assumption in this approach is that if pain response is to some extent at least learned behavior, it follows that the individual can also learn to respond in certain predetermined ways to pain as a result of a training or learning process. Application of the learning approach yields a set of strategies and premises different from those derived from the medical model.

The learning approach to pain management is utilized principally in the case of chronic pain, and it consists essentially of an application of the operant conditioning technique, i.e., desirable behavior is rewarded immediately by reinforcement, and undesirable behavior, on the other hand, is followed by undesirable consequences.

Medication for pain under usual conditions is given following the patient's request or expression of discomfort. The first step in the operant procedure, following the orientation of patient and family, is to shift medical prescriptions from a pain schedule to a time schedule. This results in medication being administered according to time intervals rather than according to the patient's requests or complaints. Next the analgesic components of the prescriptions are put in a masking substance which permits variation in dosage without the patient's knowledge. Finally, the time interval is extended until the amount of medication received is minimal or inconsequential.

Apparently this method, although somewhat oversimplified in this description, when applied consistently and knowledgeably by the entire therapeutic team and followed by appropriate continuation in the patient's normal or home environment, has produced very promising results. Further details and/or reprints of articles dealing with the learning-type model in chronic pain management can be obtained by directing inquiries to the Pain Clinic, University of Washington, Seattle.

In addition to the cultural determinants of pain response there are the idiosyncratic factors which influence each individual within a general cultural or learning situation. Much of the idiosyncratic response to pain appears to hinge upon the individual's self-concept—how he sees himself. An orthopedic surgeon recently related to the author many examples of the remarkably short recovery periods of university athletes to major and painful surgery resulting from athletic injuries. He said, referring to the athletes, "The image they have of themselves simply does not include or permit physical disability or incapacity. They are usually up making passes at the nurses when most people would still be stretched out flat feeling sorry for themselves."

Understanding the role that learning and cultural influences have with regard to how the individual responds to pain, and then applying some of the learning techniques now being utilized in elementary psychology classes, should help maximize the effectiveness of all attempts to deal with what is perhaps the most distressing and universal symptom of mankind, pain.

REFERENCES

1 Beecher, H. K., "Pain in Men Wounded in Battle." *Annals of Surgery,* **123**:95-105, January 1946.
2 Beecher, H. K., "Relationship of Significance of Wound to the Pain Experience." *Journal of the American Medical Association,* **161**:1609-1613, August 25, 1956.
3 Keele, K. D., "Pain: Past and Present." *Yale Review,* **49**:43-50, September 1959.
4 Lambert, W. E., Libman, E., and Poser, E. G., "The Effect of Increased Salience of a Membership Group on Pain Tolerance." *Journal of Personality,* **28**:350-357, September 1960.
5 Poser, E. G., "Some Psycho-Social Determinants of Pain Tolerance." Paper read at the XVI International Congress of Psychology, Washington, D.C., 1963.
6 Saunders, Lyle, *Cultural Differences and Medical Care.* New York: Russell Sage Foundation, 1954.
7 Sherman, E. C. and Robillard, E., "Sensitivity to Pain in the Aged." *Canadian Medical Association Journal,* **83**:944-947, October 29, 1960.
8 Sternbach, Richard A., and Tursky, B., "Ethnic Differences among Housewives in Psychophysical and Skin Potential Responses to Electric Shock." *Psychophysiology,* **1**:241-246, 1965.
9 Zborowski, Mark, "Cultural Components in Response to Pain." *The Journal of Social Issues,* **8**:16-30, 1952.

Reading 45
Phantom Limbs
Ronald Melzack

In 1956 I was privileged to attend the late Dr. W. K. Livingston's pain clinic at the University of Oregon Medical School. Among the patients was a Mrs. H., a remarkable woman of about 70. Because of persistent circulation problems and, finally, gangrene, she had just undergone amputation of both legs above the knees.

After the amputations, Mrs. H. could still "feel" the missing portions of her legs. At unpredictable intervals she suffered excruciating pain in both phantom limbs—intense pain that made her scream out in helpless agony.

Despite her suffering, Mrs. H. tried to maintain a happy home for her devoted husband, continued many of her household activities, and occasionally painted pictures to amuse herself. The pain persisted.

In 1958 I suggested to Mrs. H. that she try painting with a long brush strapped to one of her stumps. She soon showed remarkable talent and dexterity. Gradually her pain decreased to tolerable levels—perhaps because painting distracted her, but more likely because her use of the stump muscles evoked increased levels of sensory input.

In the majority of cases, an amputee reports feeling a phantom limb almost immediately after surgery. He describes the limb as having a definite shape. It moves through space the way a normal limb would when he walks, sits, or stretches out in bed. At first the phantom limb feels perfectly normal in size and shape—so much so that the amputee may reach out for objects with a phantom hand, or try to get out of bed by stepping onto the floor with a phantom leg. Amputees also report that they can clench missing fists and even try to scratch missing fingers that itch.

As time passes, however, the limb begins to change shape. The leg or arm becomes shorter, and may even fade away altogether, so that the phantom foot or hand seems to be hanging in midair. Sometimes the limb slowly telescopes into the stump until only a hand or foot remains at the stump. Over the years the phantom may become less distinct and disappear. If the patient wears an artificial limb, however, the phantom usually remains vivid and may correlate perfectly with the movement and shape of the artificial limb.

An amputee generally reports a tingling sensation in the phantom limb, but many also report other sensations, such as pins-and-needles (which we

Reprinted from *Psychology Today*, vol. 4, no. 5, pp. 63–68, October 1970. Copyright © Communications/Research/Machines, Inc.

all feel when we block a limb's circulation), warmth or coldness, heaviness, and many kinds of pain.

About 30 per cent of amputees report pain in phantom limbs. Fortunately the pain usually tends to decrease and eventually to disappear. In about 5 to 10 per cent of the amputees, however, the pain is severe, and may even become worse over the years. While the pain usually starts just after the surgery, sometimes it does not appear until weeks, months, or years have passed.

The pain may be occasional or continuous, but it is felt in definite parts of the phantom limb. A common complaint, for example, is that the phantom hand is clenched, fingers bent over the thumb and nails digging into the palm of the hand, so that the whole hand is tired and painful. Sometimes the pain is described as shooting, burning, or crushing.

Phantom-limb pain is more likely to develop in a patient who had pain in the limb before it was amputated. Even minor pains associated with a limb may continue. Thus, a patient who suffered from a bunion on the day that he lost his leg in an accident reported that he could still feel the bunion on the side of his phantom foot.

The study of phantom-limb pain can teach us much about pain in general, and it forces us to take a second look at many accepted theories of pain. For example, phantom-limb pain continues for more than a year after onset in about 70 per cent of patients. It endures long after the injured tissues have healed, even when the stump itself is perfectly formed and not painful or sensitive.

Sometimes *trigger zones* develop—spots that, when touched, produce intense pains in the phantom limb. Trigger zones may appear in the stump, but they may also develop at distant areas, such as the head or the opposite healthy limb. Sometimes a pain in another part of the body, such as the heart, may evoke intense pain in a phantom limb, even one that in 25 years or more had never produced pain.

Once phantom-limb pain is under way, almost any kind of stimulus will make it worse. Even gentle brushing of sensitive areas can evoke severe, prolonged pain. Paradoxically, increased sensory input may sometimes bring relief. Salt solution ejected into the tissue around an amputee's spine produces a sharp, localized pain that radiates into the phantom limb. It lasts only about 10 minutes, yet it may produce dramatic relief for hours, weeks, sometimes indefinitely.

On the other hand, *decreasing* the sensory input is a more reliable method of relief. Local anesthetic in the stump tissues or nerves may stop the pain for days, weeks, sometimes permanently. Anesthesia can also change the pain without reducing it: one subject who had painful phantom toes said he could barely feel his toes after an injection of anesthetic into the tissues near the spine. But now he had pain in his phantom heel, a pain that persisted for more than two months.

Traditional theories of pain cannot easily explain phantom-limb pain. For example, many theorists say that pain is merely the result of stimulation of pain receptors in the skin—but they have a hard time finding pain receptors in a foot that isn't there.

These theorists may then look at the severed ends of the nerves at the stump and claim that big-toe pain is the result of stimulating the end of the pain nerve that *would* be coming from the big toe if the leg were intact. They may point out that pressure on tender neuromas, the abnormal neuron growths in damaged nerves at the stump, can evoke severe, prolonged pain. But how can this theory explain a trigger point that develops on the other leg? And phantom-limb pain can occur spontaneously, or it can be triggered by vibration or by light touch, which are too weak to stimulate pain receptors.

Besides, the peripheral nerves can be cut completely—without stopping the pain. Even when the dorsal roots are severed in a rhizotomy, which cuts off the only sensory-input path into the spinal cord, the pain may persist. One recent neurosurgical text describes the case of Henry B., who suffered agonizing, stabbing pains in the phantom fingers that protruded from his upper-arm stump. Physicians cut the dorsal roots that carried all sensory information from his chest to his brain. After the surgery he could feel nothing from his shoulders to his navel, but the pain persisted in his phantom fingers, sharp as ever.

We can therefore rule out irritation at the stump as a major cause of pain. Mild irritation certainly can contribute to the pain—anesthetizing the area can sometimes bring dramatic relief—but it is not the whole story.

Since cutting sensory nerves often does not work, some theorists attempt to salvage the specific-receptor theory with another hypothesis. It is assumed that pain fibers travel through the sympathetic ganglia—part of the autonomic nervous system that controls such body functions as blood flow and digestion. Part of the reason for this belief is that the stump shows abnormal sympathetic signs, such as excessive sweating. It is also known that some autonomic functions such as urination or orgasm can induce phantom-limb pain. Sympathectomy, cutting the sympathetic ganglia, should relieve the pain.

Sympathectomy does relieve some kinds of pain, but, unfortunately, not phantom-limb pain: fewer than 10 per cent of cases report complete pain relief one to four years after surgery. In the few successful cases it probably works by cutting down the total amount of activity entering the spinal cord. Sensory nerves from the stomach, blood vessels, and other deep tissues converge into some of the spinal-cord cells that receive inputs from the skin.

Together these impulses produce the nerve-impulse patterns that eventually lead to the sensation of pain. Cutting the sympathetic ganglia cuts down on the total amount of activity in these spinal cells, and would therefore reduce the pain.

Surgeons have tried almost every conceivable operation to relieve phantom-limb pain. Results have been discouraging. As Sydney Sunderland wrote: "Operations have been performed for pain at nearly every possible site in the pathway from the peripheral receptors to the sensory cortex, and at every level the story is the same—some encouraging results, but a disheartening tendency for the pain to recur."

Some dismiss the whole dilemma by proposing that phantom-limb pain is psychological. The pain, they say, is simply a manifestation of pathological personal need. In support of this view, they note that pain is often triggered by emotional disturbance, and is sometimes diminished by psychotherapy, hypnosis, or simple distraction. Patients suffering from phantom-limb pain are often anxious and have worrisome social adjustments. Indeed, the intense, unrelenting pain may itself produce marked withdrawal, paranoia, and other personality changes.

It is clear that all phantom-limb pain cannot be ascribed to psychological factors. Anesthetics injected into the wrong nerve will not relieve the pain, but, injected in the right nerve in the same patient, they may have dramatic effect. Moreover, reliable studies have shown that patients with phantom-limb pain do not have greater incidence of neurosis than amputees who do not have pain. Emotional problems undoubtedly contribute to the pain, but they are not the major cause.

If the pain is not strictly psychological, and if we cannot assume that there are specialized nerve fibers that carry pain to the brain, then other theories of pain must be considered. One of these other approaches is the pattern theory of pain, which assumes that it is the pattern and frequency of nerve impulses, carried by nonspecialized fibers, that the brain interprets as pain.

W. K. Livingston proposed that there might be self-sustaining *reverberatory circuits* in the spinal cord—closed loops of nerve fibers in which one fiber stimulates another, which in turn stimulates others that eventually restimulate the first, and so on. These reverberatory circuits would send volleys of nerve impulses up the spinal cord, and the brain would interpret them as pain.

Such circuits might be started by the initial injury to the limb, or even by the amputation itself. After that, even minor irritations of the skin or nerves would feed into the circuits to keep them abnormally disturbed over a period of years. Impulses that would ordinarily be interpreted as touch may then stimulate the neuron pools to send more impulses to the brain, resulting in still more pain, pain that will persist even after the touch stimulus is gone.

Once the abnormal spinal-cord activity has become self-sustaining, removal of the source of stimulation may not stop it. Since the source of the persistent pain is in the spinal cord itself, this would explain why traditional surgery—neurectomy, rhizotomy, sympathectomy—may have little effect.

If Livingston is correct, it would appear that in order to cure phantom-limb pain, we would have to cut fibers in the spinal cord itself, somewhere between the reverberatory circuit and the brain.

These pathways *have* been cut by optimistic surgeons, at nearly every level from the spinal cord to the thalamus, sometimes on both sides and at successively higher levels—yet pain often returns. Indeed, new pains may arise to make the patient even more miserable than before.

Working with several colleagues—Kenneth Casey, Bernardo Dubrovsky, and Karl Konrad—I have made some discoveries with cats that suggest a new approach to the problem. Gentle rubbing of the skin of a normal cat for 10 or 15 seconds produces short-lasting changes in the electrical activity of the sensory system in the brain. In anesthetized cats, the same brief stimulation may produce changes in the brain that last 10, 15, even 30 minutes.

Apparently there is a natural inhibiting influence that normally shuts off the brain activity as soon as a stimulus is removed. Moderate anesthesia removes this inhibiting force so that a stimulus that usually has only momentary effects may produce persistent activity. The mechanism for this long-lasting activity might be a group of nerve fibers similar to Livingston's proposed reverberatory circuits. In fact, Sir John Eccles and other physiologists have found evidence for a simple two-neuron closed loop that can produce sustained rhythmic activity for prolonged stretches of time.

These observations allow us to propose a model to explain at least some of the phenomena of phantom-limb pain. Nerves from a limb contain fibers that activate pools of neurons in the spinal cord. Some of these fibers are relatively large and conduct impulses quickly; other fibers are small and conduct impulses more slowly. We know that after a limb is amputated, about half of the cut nerve fibers still in the stump die. The rest regenerate and grow into the stump tissues. These fibers are usually small and slow-conducting.

Thus, stimulation of the stump tends to produce synchronous volleys in the small fibers, rather than the complex, dispersed patterns seen in a normal nerve that contains the full range of fiber sizes.

The sensory neurons in the spinal cord project upward to the thalamus and cortex of the brain, of course, but they also send impulses to the reticular formation in the brainstem. On receiving these impulses, the reticular formation acts primarily to inhibit nerve transmission in the spinal cord, the thalamus, and the cortex—at all the levels of the sensory system.

Since the inhibitory influence of the reticular formation is partly maintained by sensory inputs from the skin, any decrease in the number of sensory fibers from an area would mean that there would be less inhibition at all levels of the sensory pathway from the spinal cord to the brain. Consequently, inputs from the skin or deeper tissues would tend to produce sustained, uninhibited activity in neuron pools in the spinal cord, thalamus, and cortex.

Even if this activity stopped spontaneously, the volleys of impulses from the remaining small fibers at the stump would again reactivate it. These neuron pools have widespread connections, and it would be only a matter of time before the sustained, rhythmic activity would spread to adjacent areas of the nervous system. The pain-signaling pathways in the spinal cord could be cut, but activity patterns in the thalamus and cortex would continue: the pain would persist. Indeed, some cells in the thalamus and cortex have very large sensory fields, sometimes half or more of the body surface, so that stimuli from distant skin areas could cause sustained activity at these levels. This could explain how trigger zones can develop far from the stump.

This model is, of course, highly speculative. However, it can explain many facts of phantom-limb pain. For example, an anesthetic injection of several hours' duration would block all sensory input from an area; it would stop the sustained activity and would bring relief from pain. The relief would sometimes outlast the anesthesia, because as the anesthesia wears off a certain amount of time would be required before the sustained activity could spread to a sufficiently large number of neurons within the pool. Moreover, while the patient is relieved of pain he would be able to use the stump. This would produce patterned, temporally dispersed activity that would be out of phase with the rhythmically firing neuron pools and would disrupt their activity. Massive, continuous inputs, such as those produced by salt-solution injection, could bring relief by interrupting the rhythmic activity and also by raising the level of inhibition. In contrast, cutting a sensory pathway in the spinal cord would decrease the inhibition still further and would tend to enhance rather than decrease the pain.

The model also proposes new approaches to the relief of phantom-limb pain. It suggests a search for drugs that enhance the inhibiting influences of the reticular formation. It also proposes that sensory inputs of moderate or high intensities, applied to widespread areas of the body, should increase inhibitory levels and decrease pain. Because the reticular formation is also influenced from above, by activity in the cortex, it also suggests that manipulation of psychological attitudes toward pain may have powerful effect.

Part Four

Rehabilitation Nursing Care in Life-threatening Conditions

Section A

Cardiovascular Disorders

No one can have heart disease in the United States today and not be aware of its implications. Volunteer agencies like the Heart Association offer continuous information, and the federal government is sponsoring programs to reduce the mortality rate. Still, heart disease remains the number one killer, and more people die from heart disease than from all other causes.

Since the concept of heart disease is so inextricably associated with disability and death, the heart disease consciousness is a morbid one. Although there are many instances of people living satisfactorily with their impaired hearts, even Presidents of the country, the association of death and disability has made the connotation a fearful one. Each must start anew with his own situation and his attitudes and knowledge. It is necessary to begin with the gaps in the patient's knowledge, the meanings of heart disease to him, experience with his family and friends, and finally with the feelings he has. Perhaps one of the most important guides of the planning for the care of the patient with heart disease is the fact that each attack is personal and solitary. No one learns from the experience of others but only from his own experience, and he may need assistance with the interpretation of this matter.

The invention of electronic devices to monitor the patient allows care to be divided into two types: the mechanistic, in which the patient becomes a series of observations confirmed by electronic and chemical scans, or the humanistic, in which the devices are used as an adjunct to the personal care which can be given since the highly reliable monitoring system allows close supervision of the patient. In the first, the nurse is a colleague of the machine; in the second, the machine is used as a servant of the nurse, who is concerned with monitoring the whole patient, his feelings, and his fears, as well as the conduction systems, pressures, and chemistry of the body. The mechanistic approach denies the patient as an individual except as he registers on the indices used. The second approach requires awareness that the patient as a person may be affected by the very treatment and diagnostic devices. The resultant threat may serve as the trigger for "cardiac cripple" symptoms.

Kos, in her article on "Rehabilitation of the Patient with Myocardial Infarction," is aware of the threat which exists. She has developed a tool for "decompressing" the patient from his experience with the life-saving equipment and testing which treatment involves. The fact that the experience may be as threatening as the disease is not understood or often considered by the health professional to whom it is the commonplace and everyday experience. Only through consideration of the fact that heart disease is a solitary and personal experience can the role of the patient with heart disease be understood. The index described by Kos offers such a tool for assisting the health professional.

The nurse who cares for the patient with myocardial infarction is faced with assisting the patient prepare for his home care. He is frequently given the ambiguous and quick response that he will have to "take it easy" for a while. How easy and for how long is not explicit in the statement, and frequently the understanding is confused. The index devised by Kos starts with a good teaching principle—start where the patient is and determine his readiness to learn and his understanding. While this is being done, the nurse has the opportunity to help the patient link together the elements of knowledge which he has, but which he may not have developed into a framework for relationships as a whole. Determining where the patient wants to go defines the realism of his present knowledge and the strength of motivation. Finally the index suggests that the patient develop his own plan of progress, but with assistance where he has gaps in his knowledge or is unrealistic in his expectations of himself.

The article by Trigiano expresses a plea for allowing more activity for the cardiac patient on the basis of good clinical judgment. It has implications for the development of a body image consistent with the care being given. It is easy for the nurse caring for the amputee to understand the change in body image which occurs with physical mutilation. She may forget that the patient with heart disease has an altered view of himself as a functioning individual also. This may or may not be consistent with reality. Continuity of the familiar helps to develop a congruent picture of the present and the future when one is incapacitated by heart disease.

Trigiano has given definite principles based on the presently accepted knowledge about rehabilitation of the cardiac patient. The fact is that healing in the myocardium (or any condition which changes the finely tuned equilibrium of the compensated heart), proceeding at a relatively slow rate, must be considered in any resumption of activity. He also stresses the necessity for clinical judgment to precede any planned program. The nurse can relate the activities in the program for graded exercise to the activities for daily living. For the patient in the hospital, time tends to pass slowly. Diversional activities are advised. They should be part of the nurse's plan for care; however, there are a number of other factors which should be taken into consideration and which the nurse must call to the attention of the physician.

One of the most important of these factors is the meaning of the person's illness to him in relation to his image of himself as a functioning person. The submission by an adult to another person for the very intimate tasks of personal care is frequently emotionally traumatizing in itself. Trigiano says that emotional stresses may be more important than the physical ones. The first learned tasks of personal care are the ones which are delegated to another with reluctance. Proper toilet habits, achieved early in development, form one of the crucial points. Trigiano refers to the earlier study by Benton, Brown, and Rusk showing that the bedpan involved more expenditure of energy than the use of the commode for a bowel movement. How much of this is physical energy and how much is related to emotional distress is not stated, and perhaps cannot be measured. Feeding oneself is another task learned early in childhood. This is a task that is probably never accomplished satisfactorily by another person. The frustration in submitting to being fed is energy-consuming. The childlike relationship of dependency for feeding destroys the adult's image of himself as a well and functioning person. It is likely to produce an incongruent picture, as he may be assured that he is progressing satisfactorily, yet he is not allowed to do this task which was learned at some long-forgotten period.

Most future actions are rehearsed. Planning takes place on the basis of these rehearsals, and such planning is realistic only as the rehearsals are based on actual fact. The patient with heart disease goes through all the grief processes as he goes from one stage to another in developing a way of coping with his heart disease. He will be depressed and look to others to give him the signals which relieve that depression. He will deny the illness, and there are many ways of doing this. However, the patient will eventually develop his coping mechanisms. The crippled leg and the crippled heart have much in common.

An article on rehabilitation of the patient with a pacemaker is included. As the population of the aged increases, so too will the use of pacemakers to help the heart perfuse the brain and vital organs for living. The change in ability to live a normal existence is so marked that their use will increase. Few nurses outside cardiac units will become acquainted with the nursing care during the immediate period following implantation. But nurses in every field except maternal and child health nursing will be concerned with the care of the patient with a pacemaker who is hospitalized for the numerous illnesses and disabilities which occur with aging. The nurse should have at hand a reliable source of information concerning the functions of the different pacemakers. One type of pacemaker is set to deliver impulses at a set rate. The one which is being used increasingly delivers impulses when the patient's own heartbeat is not forthcoming. There is a difference in rhythm between the two. The nurse must also be conscious of the change in rate which occurs when batteries are losing their period of usefulness or the electrode tip in the heart is corroded. If the patient is committed to her care, such knowledge will be expected of her. Since pacemakers are being improved, changes are occurring. Inservice programs and her professional journals and books will help the nurse update her knowledge. Kos and Culbert discuss one of the most important aspects of all concerning pacemakers: that of adequate patient instruction.

Reading 46

The Nurse's Role in Rehabilitation of the Myocardial Infarction Patient

Barbara A. Kos

Perhaps no other illness, with the exception of cancer, has the multiple causation implications or the emotional impact of the illness broadly referred to as heart disease, including the continuum of atherosclerosis through massive myocardial infarction. Its increasing rate of occurrence with the advance in civilization, and despite modern technologic and scientific advances, is a frightening reality. Prevention is the hope for the future; today we are involved with the vast numbers of those afflicted in an attempt to cure, rehabilitate, and restore to optimal function.

The focus of this article is the long-range care and rehabilitation of the myocardial infarction patient. The United States Conference on CardioVascular Disease defines rehabilitation as "the return of a person disabled by accident or disease to his greatest physical, mental, emotional, social, vocational and economic usefulness, and if employable, an opportunity for gainful employment." White states that "primary among the needs of a person with a cardiac disability is doing something constructive and purposeful. We live in a society which emphasizes man's constructive and creative role" [15]. If we do not provide for this rehabilitation in medicine, we leave the patient little more than an empty shell. He feels frustrated, anxious, and rejected, all of which does more damage to his heart than proper, purposeful activity.

THEORIES OF CAUSATION OF HEART DISEASE

Most of the various theories as to the etiology of heart disease have been well publicized and are familiar to us. Among the many societal factors that have been correlated with coronary artery disease are stress, an overabundant diet and obesity, smoking, and decreased physical activity. The American diet, often rich in cholesterol and beta-lipoproteins, is frequently implicated in the pathophysiologic process. Russek describes the high-fat diet in conjunction with stress as "the lethal combination" [2].

A look at the hereditary aspects of coronary artery disease reveals many interesting theories. Gertler has discovered an inverse relationship between height and incidence of coronary artery disease. He has also determined that the occurrence of heart disease in both mother and father greatly increases the possibility of incidence in the offspring [7].

Reprinted from *Nursing Clinics of North America*, vol. 4, no. 4, pp. 593–603, December 1969.

The hormonal influence has long been recognized through the higher incidence of heart disease in men in their thirties and forties, and a lower incidence in women of the same ages, but with a sharp increase in women after the menopause.

A LOOK AT THE PATIENT WITH CORONARY HEART DISEASE

Personality type is a highly controversial factor in the incidence of coronary artery disease. A cause and effect association has not definitely been shown. Whether or not genetic and environmental determinants that influence personality and behavior also predispose the heart and vascular system to faulty performance has yet to be determined. Whatever the relationship may be, there seems to be a bond of similarity in the personalities of those afflicted.

Dunbar found that the cardiac patient is a compulsive, striving, self-disciplined, hard-working type. He feels that these patients have had childhood problems of identification with authority and have a present inability to face their sense of insecurity and weakness, despite even considerable accomplishment [5]. Kemple describes the patient as aggressive and self-driven [5]. Russek and Zohman report, in a study of 100 patients under 40 with similar personalities, that the emotional stress of their occupations is far more significant than a positive heredity, a high-fat diet, obesity, tobacco, or lack of exercise [5].

In his review of the previous findings, Fisher hypothesizes that if the cardiovascular stress response (increased blood pressure, increased peripheral resistance, increased blood viscosity, clotting time, and cholesterol level) is sustained for a period of time, it will influence the onset or course of coronary artery disease [5]. To support this hypothesis, Fisher has found that patients very frequently report a history of a gradually increasing stress situation before the occurrence of a myocardial infarction.

In an attempt to clearly identify the personality type, and to recognize patterns early enough for possible preventive intervention, Friedman and Rosenman developed the following "stress-coronary profile" [6].

                                                                Yes   No

I have an intense, sustained drive to get ahead.
I'm anxious to reach my goals, but am uncertain what they are.
I feel a need to compete and win.
I have a strong desire for recognition.
I am always involved in too many things at once.
I'm always clock-racing—on edge about meeting deadlines.
I have a drive to speed things up—get them done faster.
I'm extraordinarily alert, mentally and physically.

Researchers have found a strong position correlation between persons scoring a high number of yes responses on this profile and incidence of coronary heart disease [3].

MAKING THE REHABILITATION PROGRAM EFFECTIVE

Despite the beginning shift of emphasis in medicine over the last several years from the cure to the person being cured, most patients with heart disease today still report that they are sent home after hospitalization with the meaningless advice to "take it easy." It is apparent in talking to recuperating patients that they want and need to know more definitely the activity prescribed.

White has outlined the following program of rehabilitation based upon Osler's 19th-century concept of medical treatment—"Learn not only what kind of sickness this man has, but what kind of man has this sickness" [16].

1   Evaluate the patient's medical, psychological, social, and vocational status.
2   Individualize management, including diet, drugs, physical activity, emotional stress, and environmental stress.
3   Discuss with the patient the nature of his disease, the treatment and prognosis, as well as the assessment of his capacities, and how he can best arrange his life to fit his needs.
4   Make every effort to eliminate fear of heart disease.
5   Encourage him to live the best life possible within the limits (if any) imposed by disease [15].

Some hospitals have cardiac evaluation units where tolerance and ability are measured physiologically. Heart rate, respiratory rate, oxygen consumption, blood pressure, ballistocardiography are all employed in determining the functional capacity of the patient. In addition to this, the physician must estimate the amount of physical and emotional stress produced by the patient's work, the climate and temperature, the effort involved in traveling to and from work. It is interesting to note that the majority of jobs in the United States today require an energy expenditure of only 3 to 4 times the basal metabolic rate. This is especially encouraging to cardiac patients, as this expenditure is equivalent only to climbing a 9-inch step 20 times a minute for 10 minutes [18].

Energy costs, however, are only one indication of whether the patient can do the job. More important is an assessment of his temperament, emotional make-up, reactions, skill, experience, and his *attitude toward returning to work*. This attitude can be measured by the degree to which he attempts to pursue his former job or look for others, and is the prime factor in his rehabilitation to work [19].

White urges those involved in the care of cardiac patients to realize that, to most, work is extremely important. They are highly charged, and "action absorbs this anxiety" [20]. Idleness breeds unhappiness and is actually bad for the health. It is a rare patient who is fit for nothing. Even when there is cause for doubt, the physician and evaluation team should lean in favor of work!

Meanwhile, the patient is hopefully being taught the principles of prevention by the health team. As is the case in many areas of medicine, the question of a regime to be suggested is open to some controversy.

It is agreed by many authorities that to lower the dietary intake of fat from 45 per cent to 30 per cent is advisable [11]. Others suggest limiting saturated fats to minimal levels, while increasing amounts of unsaturated fats, in order to reduce cholesterol levels. But a recent seven-year study by a committee of the British Medical Research Council indicates that diet-watching after a myocardial infarction is like shutting the barn door after the horse is gone. American cardiologists commenting on the study indicated that it is still advisable to cut down on fats. They emphasized, however, that it is far more important to adopt and adhere to a low-cholesterol diet all through life, as autopsies have shown that the atherosclerotic process often begins shortly after birth [4].

All medical authorities agree on a program of weight control, especially when a patient exhibits hypertensive tendencies or increased cholesterol or uric acid levels. Rusk urges that optimal weights be individually determined, taking into account body types [11].

The best insurance offered to date against recurring myocardial infarction, for many patients, is a systematic program of specified exercise. Exercise results in an increase in the number of collateral vessels to the heart, dissolution of thrombi, increased serum plasmin levels, and a decreased incidence of atherosclerotic changes [12]. Evidence is available to show that "patients who participate in an exercise program can be trained to do more work with fewer heart beats, lower heart rate and blood pressure, and greater stroke volume. Further, even during sleep, fewer heart beats are required" [9]. These cardiovascular changes, it is hypothesized, are the result of decreased serum triglyceride levels, increased permeability of the skeletal muscle membranes for glucose, and an alteration of the catecholamine stores and availability, affecting adrenergic receptor sites in the brain, and consequently the patient's mood [9].

Each individual exercise program is determined by an evaluation of the structure and function of the coronary arterial circulation. In the beginning, exercises are mild and of short duration, and are gradually increased, with tolerance. Along with the program itself, time must be spent on motivation [9]. Robert Frost has said, "The world is full of willing people; a few who are willing to work and many who are willing to let them." This applies so well to the attitudes of people toward becoming more physically active.

Results of cardiac rehabilitation programs are very striking. In one study, 70 to 75 per cent of all cardiac patients returned to their former employment within three to six months. Of these cardiac patients who returned to their jobs, 54 per cent had unblemished attendance records for one year or longer. The overall absenteeism rate was one-fourth that of regular workers. Among other patients classified as severe cardiacs, 30 per cent were able to hold a regular job and 70 per cent returned to limited work [13].

A REHABILITATION INDEX FOR NURSING ASSESSMENT

Throughout a period of research into literature related to coronary heart disease, myocardial infarction, rehabilitation, nursing care, adjustment to illness, and the various coping mechanisms involved, the role of the nurse in the long-term care of, and planning with, the cardiac patient loomed larger and larger. This role was confirmed in clinical experience. Theory continues to be abysmally separated from practice, and the patient suffers from the gap. The question of paramount importance seemed to be: What can the nurse do, *practically*, to gain a clearer understanding of the individual patient, including his family, environment, work and health concerns, what his plans are, how he will carry out the plans, and how she can help him along the way? This question nurtured the development of a tool for patient appraisal—a rehabilitation index from which the nurse can take her cues for problem solving and teaching. At the same time, use of the index allows the patient to formulate, express, and hear his feelings toward his health problem, and his plans for the future.

The rehabilitation index is a data-gathering and classifying tool, serving the same purpose as a nursing history form in a specific instance. It provides a springboard for inferences and hypothesis formulation, and for nursing diagnosis and intervention. The questions asked incorporate many of the most recent research findings and are geared toward obtaining the most meaningful and complete picture of the patient possible. Many areas, however, are not amenable to immediate evaluation and must, of necessity, be left in the prediction phase.

REHABILITATION INDEX OF THE MYOCARDIAL INFARCTION PATIENT

A Determining where the patient is:
1 How do you picture what has happened to your heart?
2 What are the factors in your life which you feel may have contributed to your problem? (Diet, smoking, worry, weight, overexertion, underactivity?)
3 When you overdo, do you have any warnings?

      4 Do you know what causes them?
      5 Do you take medication for these symptoms?
      6 Do you know what causes relief with the medication?
      7 Are there any other measures that relieve them?
      8 What has your doctor discussed with you about activity and exercise when you return home?
      9 What are the meals and snacks you normally eat and enjoy?
     10 What are the types of worry or aggravation that bother you?
     11 What are your immediate concerns?
     12 What type of personality do you feel you have?

B Determining where the patient wants to go:
      1 What has your doctor told you about your future?
      2 How do *you* see your illness?
      3 What is your plan for gradually increasing activity and exercise?
      4 What do you feel would be desirable changes in your diet?
      5 How do you feel about returning to work?
      6 How do you usually release pent-up energy? (Physical activity?)

C How the patient will get there [8]:
      1 What are your plans for the future? Do they go along with your doctor's suggestions?
      2 Are there any changes you can make in your work pattern to make it easier or more efficient?
      3 What is your plan for strengthening your heart?

Beland has said that cooperative patient and family motivation, as well as the program outlined by the rehabilitation team, is needed for successful rehabilitation. The plan will not succeed until the patient, family, and team are all working toward the same goal—at the same time [1]. The patient appraisal form provides an opportunity to look at the patient from all angles and to determine any obstacles to realization. It allows opportunity for the patient to verbalize current needs as well, which must be met if he is to progress to the level of rehabilitation.

Before demonstrating the use of the index in two clinical instances, it is important to explain that the patients who shared in this experience were beyond the critical post-myocardial infarction period. They had progressed from the coronary care unit and intermediate care unit to the unique facilities at Loeb Center for Nursing and Rehabilitation, Montefiore Hospital and Medical Center. They were all semi-ambulatory and looked forward to discharge within a two-week period.

In the interim between infarction and their Loeb experience, each patient had begun the process of adaptation to illness and acceptance of what his illness meant to him. The variety of physiologic coping mechanisms including anginal pain, fatigue, syncope, dyspnea, vertigo, and diaphoresis had largely given way to the more insidious psychologic coping mechanisms of anxiety, regression, anger, apprehension, frustration, egocentricity, dependency, hypochondriasis, and some degree of denial [10]. It was determined that these patients were at a point in their adaptation to illness where they were able to begin to work through these coping mechanisms and see their health problems in perspective. This decision was made on the basis of the arrest of the pathogenic process of myocardial destruction, continuing progress in recuperation, and ability to think in terms of the future [10].

ASSESSMENT AND INTERVENTION WITH TWO PATIENTS

Mr. A.

Mr. A., a 55-year-old route deliveryman for a pharmaceutical firm in New York City, was stricken with a myocardial infarction while on the job. He realized that the severe chest pain was unlike any symptom he had ever experienced. "Heart attack" occurred to him for a fleeting moment, but he reacted almost immediately with disbelief and denial. Nausea, vomiting, diaphoresis, and weakness followed shortly after the onset of pain. Each of these physiologic coping mechanisms was the result of the crisis of coronary inability to satisfy the heart's demands for oxygen, followed by rapid myocardial tissue destruction and the release of monoamine oxidase, stimulating pain receptors. This parasympathetic reaction to pain and resulting reflex vasoconstriction is a fairly common pattern, and, in combination with decreased cardiac output, often produces some degree of shock.

Mr. A.'s knowledge of the pathophysiology of his cardiovascular system was partial and somewhat confused. He had a vague notion that there was a lack of blood to his heart, but stated that the blood was seeking a new course. He felt that his medication was somehow creating new channels to his heart. Mr. A.'s knowledge of contributing factors to his illness was equally sketchy. He was aware of the dietary, weight, and smoking components of heart disease, and vigorously assured me that he had given up smoking. He did not relate underactivity or psychologic stress to his illness.

Mr. A. listed his worries and aggravations, which centered mostly around his work situation—schedules, irritating and difficult customers, and a demanding boss. As he put it, "They never leave me alone—just none of them. If it's not the boss bossing, it's the drug store on the other side of town wondering where I am." He readily identified his own driving, perfectionistic personality and a tendency to contain his frustrations and aggressions.

From all of the data that Mr. A. so willingly shared with me, I inferred that knowledge of his illness and contributing factors was inadequate. From this followed the hypothesis that for him to move toward a positive goal, he would need a better understanding of the disease process. He did seem to know himself well—his evaluation of his reactions, attitudes, and personality make-up was supported in later discussions.

Nursing intervention included careful explanation, in a very basic way, of what Mr. A. would need to know in order to move forward. He expressed an interest in reading further, and readily accepted my suggestion to read Townley's *Heart Disease and Common Sense,* which he later described as an "excellent experience."

Mr. A. gave many clues to the fact that his primary concern was whether or not he would be successful in returning to work. He employed psychologic coping mechanisms of apprehension, self-doubt, and anxiety, and previously, on the occasion of two proposed discharge dates, had reverted to physiologic coping, with anginal pain. In addition, Mr. A. called in a staff nurse to watch a television program in which the nurse succeeded in helping the patient to talk about and find a solution to his "returning to work dilemma." He suggested that "real nurses learn to do that for patients," and followed this by wondering aloud about the cause of his pains. "If they keep up, I'll never be able to get back to work," he mused.

After reading this account in the nurses' notes, and summarizing information obtained during our discussion, I could infer that Mr. A. was afraid to return to work. From his self-description, I could also infer that he valued work very highly. The two are seemingly incompatible. Several hypotheses were derived from these data. First, in light of Mr. A.'s personality type, if he were unable to return to work, the inactivity would actually cause additional heart damage. Also, if Mr. A. could devise a plan to return to work, gradually increasing to his full load over a period of time, it would serve to decrease his anxiety about work and prevent a repeated episode of anginal pain, delaying discharge. (He had originally seen as impossible hiring anyone to help with the driving and lifting, because of union regulations.) Finally, if Mr. A. could direct his energy toward successful rehabilitation, with his new knowledge and persevering, goal-directed behavior, he would succeed.

Mr. A. was encouraged to try to devise a plan for easing back into work. A chat with his boss about the newly learned relationship between pressure and demands and repeated illness resulted in a more relaxed schedule and more efficient ordering system. Help with lifting and driving for the first six to eight weeks by a relative or friend was suggested, thereby getting around union hiring regulations. During my next visit, Mr. A. introduced me to a retired friend with whom he was making plans for assistance for the first two difficult months.

To summarize, Mr. A.'s diagnosed nursing needs for knowledge, support, reassurance, and guidance in job difficulties were met by appropriate nursing intervention, determined through use of the nursing process. As had been predicted, Mr. A. was discharged without incident.

Mr. B.

Despite the variability of the behavioral response in individuals, I found a remarkable similarity in the personality patterns and physiologic and psychologic coping mechanisms of several cardiac patients. This similarity can be demonstrated by a look at Mr. B.'s clinical history. Mr. B. is a 56-year-old salesman with mild anginal attacks occurring over the past two years, and culminating in a myocardial infarction. He, too, had some vague conception of the pathophysiologic process and contributing factors, adding "fast living," which he described as "too much drinking and running around."

Over the past few months, Mr. B.'s body was responding to increasing myocardial ischemia, with anginal pain on slight exertion. He began to observe this coping mechanism occurring with emotional states and overindulgence in food. He felt exactly the same work pressures as Mr. A. had, and responded in much the same manner. In addition, Mr. B. has a wife who upsets him with her emotional outbursts, and who is extremely dependent upon *her* family, apparently threatening his masculine strivings. As he says: "Whenever my wife has a problem with anyone, even our son, she heads straight for her mother's. What does she think I'm there for? But that's the way she's always been."

Finances are a serious problem. The only income during Mr. B.'s illness and hospitalization was compensation of 60 dollars weekly. Mrs. B. had begun to complain to her husband about finances, which only weakened his already poor self-concept.

Mr. B. wanted to return to work, despite some doubt of his ability, in order to reach his goal of retirement in four years, at 300 dollars a month. His attitude toward work, too, typified adherence to the Protestant ethic of hard work, conscientiousness, and self-discipline. He expressed a desire to "do anything" to improve his health situation, but hadn't the slightest idea of how to proceed. Finally, Mr. B. confessed not having verbalized any of these concerns to the staff because he felt they were his problems.

The following hypotheses were formed from these inferences, obtained from the rehabilitation index:

The services of the social worker are essential in assisting the patient with his financial problems.

A conference between the social worker, the doctor, and Mr. B.'s wife will help her to understand the patient's problems, and help her to adjust to his illness.

If the staff encourages Mr. B. to verbalize his concerns, his anxiety will be reduced, and he will receive help in problem solving.

With knowledge of the principles of rehabilitation, Mr. B. will readily participate and be able to return to work, in at least a partial capacity.

The nursing diagnosis, then, was the patient's need for financial assistance, understanding from his wife, opportunity to verbalize, and knowledge of a rehabilitation program.

In carrying out the derived nursing intervention, I spoke to the physician and the senior and staff nurses, alerting them to Mr. B.'s needs. The senior nurse arranged for social work consultation which resulted in temporarily increased weekly payments through a related social organization. Mr. B.'s wife met with both the physician and social worker to discuss her husband's problems, particularly those involving threats to his masculinity. The staff nurse spent increasing amounts of time with him, allowing him to talk about whatever his present concerns were. And finally, after a discussion with the doctor, I worked with Mr. B. in a teaching program, including pathophysiology of coronary heart disease, and principles and methods of rehabilitation.

Mr. B. was discharged with a realistically optimistic outlook and a plan for the future. Although neither his nor Mr. A.'s progress since discharge has been evaluated, it is with some certainty that I can predict that both men are adjusting to their lives, after experiencing myocardial infarctions, with a better understanding, direction, and a degree of satisfaction.

REFERENCES

1. Beland, Irene L.: *Clinical Nursing: Pathophysiological and Psychosocial Approaches.* New York, The Macmillan Co., 1945, p. 1246.
2. Blumenfeld, Arthur: *Heart Attack: Are You a Candidate?* New York, Paul Ericksson, Inc., 1964, p. 58.
3. Ibid., pp. 56-57.
4. Brody, Jane E.: When it's too late to diet. *New York Times,* Nov. 13, 1968, p. E9.
5. Fisher, S. H.: Psychological factors and heart disease. *Circulation,* **27**:113-117, January 1963.
6. Friedman, Meyer, and Rosenman, R. H.: Association of specific overt behavior pattern with blood and cardiovascular findings. *J.A.M.A.,* **169**:1286, Mar. 21, 1959.
7. Gertler, M. M., et al.: The candidate for coronary heart disease. *J.A.M.A.,* **170**:149-152, May 9, 1959.
8. Hall, Lydia, and Alfano, Genrose: Myocardial infarction—Incapacitation or rehabilitation? *Am. J. Nursing,* **64**:C20-25, November 1964.
9. Hellerstein, H. K.: *Exercise Therapy in Coronary Disease.* Conference on Coronary Heart Disease: Preventive and Therapeutic Aspects. New York Heart Association, 1968, p. 1045.
10. Lederer, Henry: *How the Sick View Their World.* In Jaco, E. G. (ed.): Patients, Physicians and Illness. Glencoe, Ill., Free Press, 1958, pp. 247-256.
11. Rusk, H. A.: *Rehabilitation Medicine,* 2d ed. St. Louis, C. V. Mosby Co., 1964.
12. Ibid., p. 578.
13. Ibid., p. 590.
14. Townley, Rex: *Heart Disease and Common Sense.* Sydney, Angus and Robertson, 1966.

15 White, P. D.: *Rehabilitation of the Cardiovascular Patient.* New York, McGraw-Hill Book Co., 1958, p. 21.
16 Ibid., p. 116.
17 Ibid., p. 115.
18 Ibid., p. 118.
19 Ibid., p. 123
20 Ibid., p. 125.

Reading 47
Move That Cardiac Early
L. L. Trigiano

Cardiac disease, whether it be the result of mechanical defects, metabolic disturbances, or extracardiac maladies (such as increased peripheral arterial pressure), tends to decrease heart efficiency and function. The manifestations of this decrease in function are either the acute myocardial infarction or cardiac failure. With newer methods of diagnosis and therapy (thiazides, etc.), failure does not present the problem of treatment that it once did. On the other hand, coronary infarction still remains a pressing problem.

Since 85 percent of patients with acute myocardial infarction survive the first three weeks [1], it is apparent that active programs are needed for their rehabilitation and return to work. The same is true of many cases of cardiac failure.

The normal heart in healthy, young males has been estimated to be able to increase its output to about nine times its basal level [2]. The capacity of the heart to do work above basal conditions is referred to as cardiac reserve. This cardiac reserve can be decreased by normal activities or by disease states.

In the normal individual at high levels of energy expenditure, the heart muscle placed under stress experiences fatigue. With fatigue, cardiac reserve diminishes. With rest, however, the myocardium recovers as does any other muscle. Once the myocardium has recovered, the cardiac reserve is restored.

In disease, the cardiac reserve may be so decreased that even with minimal activity the capacity and demand may be so close that decompensation can occur easily. A diseased heart may be able to meet the demands placed upon it by ordinary activities but will decompensate under stress. This may be either physical or emotional. In addition to the physical problems of heart disease, patients experience extreme anxiety. This alone can

Reprinted from *Pennsylvania Medicine*, pp. 52–55, January 1969.

cause increased adrenal stimulation which, in turn, will speed up ventricular contraction, decrease diastolic filling of the heart, and demand more energy output of an already-taxed heart. This patient with disease then requires more actual work by the heart than the disease-free individual. Increases of respiratory rate and blood pressure, frequently seen in disease states, again may need more cardiac work. The rehabilitation of the heart patient then becomes a program dedicated to sparing of cardiac reserve.

If preventive techniques fail, acute episodes transpire. Although management of the acutely ill cardiac patient lies within the province of the internist or cardiologist, the rehabilitation specialist may be of service during the periods of early care, convalescence, and eventual return to employment.

The treatment of the acute coronary by armchair methods was described in 1952 by Levine and Lown [3]. The basis for this treatment has sound physiological principles. Postural attitudes have a definite effect on heart output. Studies have demonstrated that a patient in a sitting position has a cardiac output of only 85 percent of that when lying supine. This difference of only 15 percent or so decrease in effort imposed upon the heart is highly significant considering the probable decrease in cardiac reserve and other influencing factors of disease [4].

Positions other than supine also influence cardiac output. Dangling on the side of the bed with feet supported requires 95 percent of the supine cardiac output. A semi-reclining position in bed with knees flexed and back flexed to 45 degrees increases cardiac output to 110 percent of supine. It, therefore, becomes obvious that it is necessary to take full advantage of a dependent posture in order to decrease cardiac output. Full protective efforts of posture are best in the sitting position with the legs dependent. This allows pooling of blood in the lower extremities, thus reducing cardiac output.

Chairs with a head and arm rests are recommended. Some authors [5] are advocating electric chairs with fingertip toggle switches so that patients may change positions with ease. They can be placed in a chair early in their rehabilitation program. Good clinical judgment is needed to determine when a patient may get out of bed; however, it is felt that if he is medically stable (blood pressure, respirations, EKG, absence of angina and arrhythmias), he is ready to begin chair-bed activities. One should take into consideration the fact that stress of both physical and emotional origin must be kept at a minimum for the first three critical weeks following an acute coronary attack. Patients with decompensation should increase their activities according to their clinical progress.

When convalescence begins (as determined by the clinician in charge), so should mobilization. The armchair-bed method of treatment is strongly advocated. Getting a patient from the bed to a chair can present problems.

Patients lifted from a bed to a chair expend more energy than if a semi-help transfer technique is used. Attendants, nurses, or physical therapists can help a patient learn to sit in bed and transfer to the chair with little effort to the patient.

Once the patient is sitting on the side of the bed and the bed is at chair height, it is a simple matter to assist him by allowing him to pivot on one leg into the bedside chair. The same technique is used to transfer to the bedside commode. With use of the bedside commode, less energy is expended by this transfer procedure than having the patient use the bedpan. Using the bedpan expends up to 50 percent more energy than using a bedside commode [6]. Once the patient has started treatment in the chair and is using the bedside commode, activities are started. Activity is started as chair activity. Chairs are equipped with cutout tables in order to carry out hand tasks.

Light activities which increase cardiac work 0.5 to 1.5 times that of basal requirements, even though carried out for long periods of time, are not strenuous enough to decrease cardiac reserve. Moderate activity that increases basal cardiac work 1.5 to 3.0 times can decrease cardiac reserve if carried out for long periods of time (hours). Heavy activities that increase heart work three to five times the basal requirements cause considerable reduction of the cardiac reserve in an hour or less. Extensive heavy activity that increases heart work five to ten times the basal will reduce cardiac reserve significantly in a matter of minutes [4,7]. Thus, it becomes obvious that a program of graded activities should be instituted, upgrading the activity as convalescence progresses.

Several methods of grading activities have been described using calories utilized per minute for a given task, increase in cardiac output over basal requirements, or increase of metabolism over basal. Oxygen uptake/min. is determined by spirometric methods. Most studies use the factor of 200 cc./min. O_2 uptake as equaling 1 Cal/min. Basal metabolic rates in males and females range between 0.9 and 1.3 Cal/min. The literature is quite prolific in describing tasks of self-care, exercise, locomotion, recreation, and the demands of various occupations expressed in calories used per minute of each activity [8,9]. This method of expression of physical activity is chosen here for the grading of tasks.

With the help of the occupational and physical therapist, a program of "training" can begin. Care is taken to start each activity for only short periods of time at first (two to five minutes) and then increase the time as endurance is acquired. Chair patients are started on activities that utilize 1.5 to 2.0 Cal/min. Psychologically, diversional activities certainly allay many fears and anxieties that could be detrimental to cardiac function. When a heart patient is doing something, he is able to realize progress and thus alleviate undue tensions.

Eating, sitting, light hand activities, such as leather lacing and tooling, writing and reading are some activities that fall into this category. Although some self-care activities are below the 2.0 Cal/min. level, many are considerably above. Showering, for instance, requires 4.6 Cal/min., dressing and undressing 2.3 to 2.5 Cal/min. Thus, several self-care activities require more energy than many types of occupations (Table 1).

Table 1 Energy Output of Some Given Tasks and Self-care Activities

Up to 2.0 Cal/min.			
1. Sleep	0.8 to 1.2	7. Leather tooling, lacing	1.4
2. Rest, supine	1.0	8. Link belts	1.4
3. Eating	1.4	9. Writing letters	1.8
4. Conversation	1.4	10. Sewing, machine (pedal)	1.8
5. Hand sewing	1.4	11. Typing, 30-40 wpm	1.8
6. Knitting	1.5		

Up to 3.0 Cal/min.			
1. Dressing & undressing	2.3	11. Abdominal exercise	3.0
2. Washing hands, face, brushing hair	2.5	12. Sitting painting	2.0
		13. Playing cards	2.2
3. Washing & shaving	2.6	14. Car driving	2.8
4. Washing & dressing	2.6	15. Canoeing, 2.5 mph	3.0
5. Peeling potatoes	2.9	16. Ceramics	2.6
6. Brushing shoes	2.2	17. Tailoring	2.2
7. Polishing furniture	2.4	18. Photography	2.6
8. Washing clothes	3.0	19. Sawing, power	2.6
9. Wheelchair, 1.2 mph	2.4	20. Sanding, power	2.2
10. Bending at waist sideways, 13/min.	2.2		

Up to 4.5 Cal/min.			
1. Bedside commode	3.6	8. Hanging wash	4.5
2. Showering	4.2	9. Walking, 2.5 mph	3.6
3. Kneading dough	3.3	10. Cycling	4.5
4. Scrubbing floor	3.6	11. Playing with children	3.5
5. Making beds	3.9	12. Volleyball	3.5
6. Ironing	4.2	13. Bowling	4.4
7. Wringing by hand	4.4		

Over 4.5 Cal/min.			
1. Ambulation, braces & crutches	8.0	4. Sexual intercourse	6.0 plus*
2. Walking downstairs	5.2	5. Masters 2-step test	5
3. Walking, 3.75 mph	5.6		

* Estimated.

Above activities are affected by training and pace of work. Emotional stimuli represent the greatest possibility of error.

The rapidity of upgrading of activities is, of course, influenced by the severity of the patient's particular heart problem. Ultimately, activities requiring 4 to 5 Cal/min. should be attained before the patient leaves the hospital. This may include ambulation, which requires 3 to 6 Cal/min. or more, depending upon variables of speed of walking and types of walking surfaces.

The timing of the increase in activities is a clinical decision. Gordon, in 1963 [10], showed that convalescent cardiac patients could be taken to their capacity for work by observing clinical signs such as dyspnea, fatigue, palpitations, angina and pulse rate. A tachycardia of twenty beats above resting or sustained high rate after two minutes required stopping or slowing of activities. Patients in this series were able to do most graded activities during their convalescent hospital stay without distress at between 2 to 3 Cal/min. Some patients were able to tolerate activities requiring up to 4 to 5 Cal/min. for short periods of time without symptoms. Most coronary infarctions have a critical period from onset to fourteen days. Here, activities would be kept at a minimum (less than 2.0 Cal/min.). From the fourteenth to the twentieth day, an increase in activities is started (2 to 4 Cal/min.). After the first three weeks following an acute coronary infarction, ambulation, including going down stairs, is started (5.2 Cal/min.). During the weeks of convalescence at home, activities are held at the 4 to 5 Cal/min. level. Patients with cardiac failure will vary in these programs according to their response to treatment.

During any treatment program, activities, calories expended per minute by the body, or the known metabolic increases for certain tasks, of course, do not preclude good clinical judgment. The physician must be aware of the previously mentioned parameters; however, he must remember such things as the need for rest, allaying of anxieties and emotional fears, posture, oxygen consumption as related to digestion, and oxygen consumption related to the part of the body doing work.

It is interesting to note that most occupations in American industry, with the exception of heavy work such as foundry workers, longshoremen, heavy laborers, farmers, etc. require a caloric output of about 4.0 Cal/min. or less (Table 2). Certainly one would not send cardiac patients back to the heavier occupations; however, most cardiac patients who are able to do activities requiring 3.5 to 4.0 Cal/min. output without distress or symptoms are able to return to most jobs.

Employment of the cardiac patient is not as easy as the previous statement may lead one to believe. Stress periods in performance of occupational tasks affect cardiac status and energy expenditure. The physical stresses, such as sudden, short periods of pushing, pulling, lifting, and dragging, and emotional stresses may influence the return to a former job. These physical stresses may be more easily controlled than the emotional problems that

Table 2 Occupation-Energy Output Examples, Cal/min.

1	Clerical work		6	Pick, shovel, & wheelbarrow	
	a. Typing, 40 wpm, mechanical typewriter	1.5		a. Shovel—8 kg. load less than 1 M lift, 12 throws/min.	7.5
	b. Miscellaneous office work: standing	1.8		8 kg. load from 1 to 2 M lift, 12 throws/min.	9.5
	sitting	1.6		b. Shoveling, 16 lb.	8.5
2	Light bench work			c. Wheelbarrow, 115 lb., 2.5 mph	5.0
	a. Watch repair	1.6		d. Hewing with pick	7.0
	b. Light assembly line	1.8	7	Building	
	c. Armature winding	2.2		a. Light work laying brick	3.4
	d. Radio assembly	2.7		b. Making wall—bricks & mortar	4.0
3	Shoe repair			c. Plastering	4.1
	a. Polishing shoes	1.8		d. Mixing cement	4.7
	b. Fixing soles	2.4		e. Sawing hardwood	7.5
	c. Shoe manufacturing	3.0		f. Planing hardwood	9.1
4	Tailoring			g. Heavy hammering	6.3–9.8
	a. Hand sewing	1.9–2.0	8	Miscellaneous	
	b. Cutting	2.4–2.7		a. Tractor	4.2
	c. Pressing	3.5–4.3		b. Plowing	5.9
	d. Ironing	4.2		c. Mowing by hand	7.3
5	Postman—climbing stairs			d. Felling tree	8.0
	a. Load—11 kg.	9.8		e. Tending furnace	10–11.0
	b. Load—16 kg.	9.8–13.8		f. Ascending—carrying 22 lb. 54 ft./min.	16.2

arise in everyday work. The emotional tensions seem to be more important than the sudden bursts of physical activity in determining what kind of work the heart patient can do. Emotional tensions on or off the job plus the "cardiac anxieties" are far the most variable factors in determining success of returning to work. The type of work to which the patient returns is a critical decision based on a thorough knowledge of each specific job. For instance, a recovered coronary patient may be able physically to climb a roof. If another coronary attack were to strike while he is on the roof, he may be able to survive the coronary but not survive a twenty- to thirty-foot fall. A crane operator would be a poor risk to return to his former occupation following a coronary infarction. A second coronary occurring during operation of the crane could jeopardize many lives of men below on the ground. Decisions to return to work depend upon not only the safety of the patient himself but what hazards he may present to his fellow workers. The return to work then requires a more practical clinical decision rather than a purely scientific approach.

It has been shown by Karpovich et al. [11] that soldiers with cardiac disease (rheumatic fever) were able to return to full duty when placed on graded exercise programs. Hellerstein and Goldston [12] also showed that 76 percent of cardiac patients were able to return to their same vocation following recovery. This program suggests that patients treated in this more aggressive way would be able to return to society as productive citizens much sooner and more comfortably than if this program were ignored.

SUMMARY

1 Cardiac disease can manifest itself as coronary infarction or cardiac failure.
2 Early armchair-bed method of treatment is advocated.
3 Upgrading of physical activities is started early based on caloric output for given tasks.
4 Upgrading of activities is carried on thru the home convalescent period.
5 Over 75 percent of cardiac patients can return to their former employment.
6 Both physical and emotional stresses determine ability of patient to return to work and remain on the job.
7 Emotional tensions and cardiac anxieties are by far the most variable factors in determining success of returning to work.
8 Return to work requires a practical clinical decision by the physician based upon knowledge of the specific job details.

REFERENCES

1 Wright, I. S.: The pathogenesis and treatment of thrombosis. *Circulation,* **5**:161–188, 1952.
2 Asmussen, E., and Nielson, M.: Cardiac output during muscular work and its regulation. *Physiol. Rev.,* **35**:778–800, 1955.
3 Levine, S. A., and Lown, B.: "Armchair" treatment of acute coronary thrombosis. *J.A.M.A.,* **148**:1365–1369, 1952.
4 Kottke, F. J., Kubicek, W. G., Danz, J. N., and Olson, M. E.: Studies of cardiac output during the early phase of rehabilitation. *Postgrad. Med.,* **23**:533–544, 1958.
5 Lewis, L.: Convalescence: A positive approach. *J. Rehabilitation,* **32**:35–38, 1966.
6 Benton, J. G., Brown H., and Rusk, H. A.: Energy expended by patients on the bedpan and bedside commode. *J.A.M.A.,* **144**:1443–1447, 1950.
7 Kottke, F. J.: Prescription of physical activity during acute stage of cardiac disability. *Arch. Phys. Med.,* **48**:126–132, 1967.

8   Passmore, R., and During, J. V. G. A.: Human energy expenditure. *Physiol. Rev.,* **35**:801-835, 1955.
9   Gordon, E. E.: Energy expenditure in health and disease. *Arch. Intern. Med.,* **101**:702, 1958.
10 Gordon, E. E., and Anderson, Mary: Work prescription for cardiacs in the convalescent stage. *J.A.M.A.,* **183**:2:137-139, 1963.
11 Karpovich, P. V., Starr, M. P., Kimbro, R. W., Stroll, C. G., and Weiss, R. A.: Physical reconditioning after rheumatic fever. *J.A.M.A.,* **130**:1198, 1946.
12 Hellerstein, H. K., and Goldston, E.: Rehabilitation of patients with heart disease. *Postgrad. Med.,* **15**:265-278, 1954.

Reading 48
Teaching Patients about Pacemakers
Barbara Kos
and
Pamela Culbert

"Is there anyone here who can tell me about my pacemaker?"

This seems such a simple question to many of us who work almost routinely with modern scientific devices like the pacemaker. Yet it too often goes unanswered. The time spent in thoughtful explanation can, and often does, make the difference between merely life-saving medical intervention and a reorientation to "living." As Rusk puts it, ". . . responsibility does not end when acute illness is ended. . . ." [1]. This is especially true when the patient's understanding, motivation, and participation are vitally involved in determining whether he returns to a full, active life or dies meaninglessly.

It was this question and others like it that prompted us to assess the learning needs of patients with newly implanted cardiac pacemakers, determine appropriate nursing intervention derived from a review of current medical literature, apply this information, and evaluate the results in terms of the patients' abilities to resume safe, independent, satisfying lives.

Several recent nursing articles have covered, quite thoroughly, the indications for pacemaker implantation, types of pacemakers available, the surgical procedure itself, and the immediate postoperative care [2,3,4]. But little information in the way of health teaching or long-term rehabilitative care is available for the nurse, and literature for the patient is even more conspicuously absent.

Reprinted from *The American Journal of Nursing,* vol. 71, no. 3, pp. 523-527, March 1971.

Our review of medical literature revealed that the elderly are most often afflicted by atherosclerotic changes which affect the heart and blood vessels. These changes result from years of lipid buildup in the form of narrowed, fibrosed vessels and plaque formation. The resulting decreased circulation produces anoxia and infarction of parts of the myocardium which heal by replacement with fibrous tissue [5]. This granulation tissue cannot assume the conductive function of healthy myocardium and, thereby, causes a disturbance in the normal rhythmicity of the heart. This disturbance manifests itself in varying degrees of heart block. When second-degree block approaches complete atrialventricular dissociation, the life-sustaining pacemaker is most frequently used to counteract this change in conduction.

It is the sudden, dreaded Adams-Stokes attacks characterized by inadequate cerebral blood flow and syncope which must be avoided. These attacks occur when impulses from the atria to the ventricles are blocked. The ventricles then fail to contract from 4 to 10 seconds before a slower idioventricular focus assumes the pacemaking role [6]. Episodic fibrillation or standstill and bradycardia with resultant inadequate tissue perfusion are indeed indications for surgical intervention [7]. The cardiac pacemaker with its ventricular electrodes supplies the much-needed assurance of regular cardiac rhythmicity.

How, then, can the nurse help to insure that patients whose lives have been saved, lengthened, or improved by pacemaker implantation are able to use their new-found "gift" optimally?

An assessment of each person's previous knowledge about his cardiac problem, the pacemaker itself, and his plan, or lack of one, for when he returned home provided the take-off point for teaching.

As far as possible, factual material was presented, and the patients were able to make their own connections between this material and their particular situation. Allowing this sort of flexibility in applying the knowledge to themselves and in joint goal-setting seemed to evoke enthusiastic responses in the learners, which was noted in a text by Klausmeier and Goddwin [8]. Learning was also facilitated by simplicity in the presentation, frequent repetition of important points, a slow pace, and encouragement of active learner participation. Many times, questions which were asked were so pertinent that we included them in subsequent teaching.

Perhaps the most important learning aid was the booklet which we prepared as part of this instructional program and which could be used for future reference. This booklet was written at a fourth- or fifth-grade reading level, a level determined to be an optimal one for reaching the greatest number of people in a study done by Mohammed [9]. Large print and generous spacing accommodated diminishing vision. Sentence structure was simple and concise. Important information was emphasized by diagrams, pictures, and repetition [10]. Although this booklet was primitive by most standards, its appeal was far-reaching. It has now been improved and expanded by the American Heart Association and will shortly be ready for general distribution to "pacemaker patients."

Our study included 26 patients, both male and female, over 65 years of age. We felt that specific learning needs would be met best by maintaining a homogeneous group. These patients spoke, understood, and read English at the fourth- and fifth-grade level and had adequate visual and auditory acuity. All patients had been hospitalized in one of three selected community hospitals of approximately 300 beds for permanent pacemaker implantation to correct heart block. Consent to participate in the study was obtained both from the patients and from the cooperating thoracic surgeons and internists caring for them.

Our purpose was to determine whether there would be a difference in knowledge related to pacemaker therapy and application of that knowledge to daily living between a group of patients who had participated in our teaching program and a similar group of patients who had not participated.

We had previously defined six areas of content—simple cardiac physiology and pathology, pacemaker functioning, pulse taking, medication taking, dietary requirements, and activities and restrictions. Accordingly, learning objectives were geared toward demonstration of basic understanding in each area and of ability in actual pulse taking along with recognition of significance of the rate and appropriate action based upon it.

In order to determine whether or not such a teaching program would, in fact, make any difference in the lives of these patients, we assigned them alternately to either the teaching or nonteaching group. All patients in both groups were given a 25-question true-false pretest to determine levels of knowledge. Because it was not always possible to know about impending surgery before the fact, we pretested patients on their third or fourth postoperative day. At this time, heart action was reasonably stable and general physiologic and psychologic equilibrium was returning.

Following the pretest, the patients in the teaching group participated individually in the learning program. The program was divided into two sessions and took place in the patients' hospital rooms. Families could be present during these sessions if they wished. The nursing staff members involved were asked to continue caring for these patients as they had previously cared for similar patients to avoid introducing additional variables.

The basic content of the program was constant for each patient in the teaching group. At this time, patients in the nonteaching group were uninvolved. An ongoing record was kept of unusual concerns, questions, and desirable new areas which were then added to the teaching content.

In teaching, we described the heart as a pump which delivers oxygen and nutrition to all parts of the body. We said that there are electrical impulses which cause and control ventricular contraction. We confined pathophysiology to saying that there are "changes in the heart cells which disturb the regular electrical waves. These cause uneven or slow heartbeat and pulse" [11]. In all instances, the patients were able to comprehend this description and began to make associations between this theory, their problem, and the pacemakers' action.

We found that the use of an actual pacemaker model provided a valuable adjunct to teaching. The patients were able to handle it and, because it was encased in clear plastic, examine the working parts, which they found both a satisfying and exciting experience in all instances. By directly visualizing the batteries and components, the patients were able to understand the concept that the batteries could "wear out like any electrical appliance" and the need for replacement.

At the time of our teaching, the estimated life for most pacemakers was 24 months. Recent experimental advances in pacemaker design, however, promise longer, if not indefinite, operating time in the near future. Power, according to an article in *The New York Times*, might possibly be supplied by components of body fluid [12].

From the discussion of heart and pacemaker action, we went on to discuss ways of determining when replacement of the batteries might be necessary. Now that the patients understood the relationship between heart rate and pulse rate, we could teach them how to take their pulses daily—one way to detect pacemaker failure.

Teaching patients how to take their pulses was done in three discrete steps: locating the pulse, recognizing its rhythmicity, and counting it for a full minute. They were also taught the range of rates normal for them, the meaning of these rates, and what action should be taken when this range showed a significant deviation. It was important that the patients understood that a drop in rate with either a fixed-rate or a demand pacemaker warns of impending failure [13]. Sometimes, an increase in heart rate, too, is indicative of failure, but this increase must be distinguished from a rise in rate during increased activity, which is possible with demand pacemakers [14].

We encountered four patients who were unable to assume responsibility for taking their own pulses. In each case, a reliable family member took on this aspect of care.

Instruction about medications and dietary concerns is not unlike what is taught cardiac patients in general. The underlying pathology of pacemaker patients has not been corrected by the pacemaker, although cardiac action has been improved. Therefore, digitalis and diuretics are commonly prescribed to improve heart action and decrease the work load [15]. We stressed why it was important to maintain this medical regimen. The dietary discussion included information on a well-balanced intake of all vital nutrients with concentration on food high in potassium to compensate for this loss through diuretic action.

Activities and restrictions seemed to generate the most interest and the greatest number of questions. We told patients that, in general, household appliances could be used quite safely. According to some of the literature, there is some reason for caution in the use of an electric razor. Shaving with a safety razor was encouraged whenever possible.

Related precautions stressed avoiding contact with high-frequency signals, electrocautery and ungrounded power tools, and large electrical devices [16]. Most physicians warned against leaning over a running car, boat, or lawnmower engine.

On the other hand, each patient was encouraged, with approval of his physician, to participate moderately in activities which were not terribly strenuous. Walking in gradually increasing amounts was recommended. Each patient was taught that he could evaluate his own tolerance for activity by using common sense and remaining free from symptoms which would indicate overindulgence or impending pacemaker failure. He learned that these symptoms included any of the following: chest pain, dizziness, shortness of breath, or excessive fatigue [17]. Frequent rest periods throughout the day were encouraged.

In addition to this list of reportable symptoms, patients were urged to report prolonged hiccoughs to their physicians. Although it rarely occurs, the catheter tip can perforate the heart and extend to the diaphragm, resulting in spasmodic contraction [18]. Patients were also encouraged to report swelling or drainage from the incision.

Patients were assured that bathing and showering were safe activities because the electrical system was completely enclosed. In most instances, patients resumed driving with their physicians' permission and were free to participate in air travel.

Sexual activity was a concern of many. Several held on to the notion that pacemaker implantation would cure long-standing impotence, while others were more realistically concerned with a cessation of heart action during sexual relations. Interestingly, most of the patients, including the males, asked us questions about sexual activity and hesitated in questioning their physicians. Here again, there were no hard and fast rules and no medical precedents to fall back upon. Moderation and tolerance were the guides.

Approximately two weeks after being discharged from the hospital, all of the patients in both groups were visited and retested with a true-false test. At the same time, we used a questionnaire to determine how well the knowledge was being applied in their daily living. Answers were verified by talking to the patients' families and by contacting their physicians.

Briefly, the statistics used to analyze data obtained from the teaching group of patients strongly indicated that they knew considerably more about pacemaker functioning and related self-care four weeks after the completion of teaching than before. The score reflecting this difference was less than .005, far less than the present level of .05, indicating little probability that this difference in test scores was due to chance. The tests given at the same intervals to the nonteaching group indicated that this group had approximately the same amount of knowledge one month after discharge as they had at the first meeting.

Post-test scores of both groups indicated a high positive correlation between knowledge and application of knowledge in the teaching group and only a moderate correlation with the nonteaching group. It seems fair to say that teaching did make a difference in the lives of these patients. As soon as all the data were collected, the patients in the control group were given the opportunity to participate in the teaching program as well.

Perhaps more important than the statistical significance was the exciting and rewarding personal experience which we encountered. It was fascinating to observe patients' interest and motivation in learning about the pacemaker and its effect on their individual lives. Ausubel has stated that motivation can be derived from anticipation of future satisfaction [19]. This was evident, in most instances, in the careful way in which they studied the teaching booklet, their questions, and the requests for us to visit friends or acquaintances of the study groups who also had pacemakers. Their motivation was also evident in the carefully kept logs of daily activities and in articles which they clipped from newspapers and magazines. It was evident also in the interest shown by family members who requested to be present during the teaching sessions and in the thoughtful and pertinent questions they asked. Finally, it was evident in the way in which these patients made the small modifications in their daily activities necessary to insure safe living.

Some of the more human touches were revealed in their questions, such as one 80-year-old gentleman who wondered if his rate of sexual activity might be vastly improved by the pacemaker. Another of approximately the same age wondered if he could resume his 10-hour work day at the women's dress shop which he owned. Several of the women, aged 70 and older, were concerned about the appearance of the pacemaker "bulge" in the upper chest area and then came up with their own solutions on how to disguise it. One woman suggested using a folded gauze pad under bra and slip straps to relieve pressure on the pacemaker site.

The most interesting report came from an elderly man living with his son's family. "They had it all wrong," he told us. "They told me I shouldn't do anything—just take it easy. I had to teach them all about the pacemaker and now they make sure I get my exercise."

Our greatest concern in teaching had been for the safety of the patients in preventing recurrent heartblock or in reducing the chance of ventricular tachycardia or fibrillation. Beregovich and Fenig emphasize that the incidence of complicating features is indeed high and that strict follow-up observation and readily available corrective facilities are essential [20].

Each of the complications which we encountered was well documented in all the pacemaker literature. The incidence of wound infection and drainage prompted us to include information about this in the teaching booklet as one of the things to report to the physician. On one of our home visits to a patient in the control group, we found that he had a rapid pulse rate. His physician was notified. We learned that a visiting nurse had seen this patient the previous week, but she said she knew little about pacemakers. A decision was then made to develop a hospital-based teaching program on pacemakers and nursing care for all public health nurses in the area.

As a result of our study, requests for booklets, information, and assistance in the teaching of other nurses have been quite overwhelming. Some of the physicians involved have been instrumental in planning the establishment of pacemaker clinics at local hospitals to provide out-patient care for these patients. Again, this was, in part, an outcome of the demonstrated need and results of teaching. Finally, continuity in teaching new patients with pacemakers has been assumed by clinical nurse specialists at two of the hospitals.

This study, in summary, has shown that there is need for nurses' involvement in newer technical advances in medical therapy and practical application of this information. There is room for both collaboration with the physician and for creativity in translating research into nursing practice. With such a life-sustaining advance as the pacemaker, the involvement becomes an obligation.

REFERENCES

1. Rusk, Howard. *Rehabilitation Medicine,* 2d ed. St. Louis, C. V. Mosby Co., 1964, p. 20.
2. Hunn, Virginia Kliner. Cardiac pacemakers. *Amer. J. Nurs.,* **69**:749-754, April 1969.
3. Jenkins, Adeline C. Patients with pacers. *Nurs. Clin. N. Amer.,* **4**:605-614, December 1969.
4. Moore, Sister Mary C. Nursing care of a patient with an implanted artificial pacemaker. *Cardiovas. Nurs.,* **2**:19-22, Winter 1966.

5. U.S. Public Health Service. *Working with Older People: A Guide to Practice.* vol. 1: Practitioner and the Elderly (Publication No. 1459). Washington, D.C., U.S., Government Printing Office, 1964, p. 16.
6. Guyton, Arthur. *Textbook of Medical Physiology,* 3d ed. Philadelphia, W. B. Saunders Co., 1966, pp. 170-232.
7. Furman, Seymour. Fundamentals of cardiac pacing. *Amer. Heart J.,* **73**:261-281, February 1967.
8. Klausmeier, H. J., and Goddwin, William. *Learning and Human Abilities.* New York, Harper and Row, Publishers, 1961, p. 65.
9. Mohammed, Mary F. B. Patients' understanding of written health information. *Nurs. Res.,* **13**:100-108, Spring 1964.
10. Allport, G. W. Teaching-learning situation. *Public Health Rep.,* **68**:876, September 1953.
11. Kos, Barbara, and Culbert, Pamela. *Teaching Geriatric Patients with Implanted Cardiac Pacemakers.* Adelphi University, 1969 (unpublished master's thesis).
12. Schmeck, H. M. Using the body to run pacemaker. *New York Sunday Times,* May 17, 1970.
13. Taber, R. E., and Webb, D. F. Lessons from 118 pacemaker implantations. *J.A.M.A.,* **194**:1133-1134, Dec. 6, 1965.
14. Ibid.
15. Thind, G. S. Ventricular arrhythmias in a patient with artificial pacemaker. *Amer. J. Cardiol.,* **20**:730-734, November 1967.
16. Germain, Carol H., and Hanley, Sister Maureen P. Metronome for a music teacher. *Amer. J. Nurs.,* **68**:502, March 1968.
17. Sowton, Edgar. Cardiac pacemakers and pacing. *Mod. Conc. Cardiovasc. Dis.,* **36**:31-36, June 1967.
18. Ibid.
19. Ausubel, D. P. *Psychology of Meaningful Verbal Learning.* New York, Gruen and Stratton, 1963, p. 225.
20. Beregovich, Jonas, and Fenig, Sidney. Complications with permanent transvenous pacemakers. *New York J. Med.,* **70**:766, Mar. 15, 1970.

Section B

Pulmonary Disorders

At one time a reasonable goal for patients with severe and chronic respiratory problems might have been that of maintaining the status quo. The all-consuming task of breathing from minute to minute was the primary concern, and the hope of significantly improving the level of respiratory status was seldom considered as feasible. There is now hope for the latter.

Regardless of the severity of the symptoms, there may remain some health which can be mobilized to improve one's clinical status. The principles are relatively simple, but the facts show that the process is a very complex and complicated one. Adequate gas exchange takes place across a membrane, and the greater the area of membrane the more adequate the ventilation. The problem for the patient with respiratory disease is to free a larger area of membrane. This means removal of secretions which interfere with access to membrane, and exchange of trapped air for a fresh air supply.

First, both the nurse and the patient must be convinced that the effort of trying will be rewarding. Unless the nurse is thoroughly committed to the idea that the effort to be made by the patient will achieve a better health status, the patient may have lost one of the most cogent incentives toward trying. In many instances, a totally new breathing pattern must be learned. The old is not readily changed for the new. The patient must be oriented or conditioned to think of each action in light of its utility. That utility, of course, will be measured in terms of his own values, and long-range goals for increased respiratory efficiency may not seem to be feasible. The nurse also must be convinced of the value of long-range measures, since her enthusiasm will be an important part of the change in the patient's behavior.

The idea that rehabilitation starts with prevention is no longer held in question. The nurse as a citizen will concern herself with all the problems of environmental pollution, especially those forms of smoke and dust which lead to emphysema and pneumoconiosis. Chronic bronchitis should not be allowed to progress to the problem of chronic obstructive lung disease. Perhaps the best method of teaching is by example; the example of the nurse should point to positive health.

There are a few procedures which the nurse can use to remove secretions from the patient with chronic obstructive lung disease, but at times a surgical intervention is necessary. Bronchial and pulmonary toilet are the patient's own responsibility and he must be involved if they are to be successful. Coughing, postural drainage, and retraining for breathing can be taught; however, they necessitate some assistance from another person in the beginning. However, the individual can be motivated to assume an active role. In addition to the patient's own faith in the procedures, there must be faith in the competence of the physician, the nurse, and other therapists who work with him. Only then can he relax and allow the minute-by-minute problem of obtaining oxygen to be amenable to retraining.

The person who is struggling for air does not easily relinquish the system which is working for him even though inadequately. While retraining, it may be expected that moments of panic over obtaining air will upset the entire program as the patient returns to the behavior which sustains his life, however inefficiently. One patient said, "I know what to do when I have trouble breathing, but when I am having trouble, I forget that I know what to do."

The newly learned behavior must become as habitual as the former behavior before it is part of the patient's repertoire. The nurse who can gently help a patient remember, during his first moments of panic, increases the likelihood that learning will occur. As the patient is rewarded with success in controlling his breathing problems, he will learn to control his reactions and he will panic less often. Decreasing the intervals of excitement reduces the need for air. When a panic situation is perceived by the patient as life-threatening, he may not be certain of its consequences except that lack of air for a few minutes is fatal. This fear leads to overreaction to obstruction of his airway. The nurse, though aware of the panic of the patient, can help most with her own calm and deliberative action. Life is threatened, but perhaps not to the extent that the patient believes, and his total reaction increases the threat.

This kind of nurse-patient cooperative relationship must be predicated on a feasible and factual basis. The nurse as a teacher contributes to the growth processes of the individual and helps him strengthen his own resources. The nurse must be well grounded in the theories behind each concept and procedure, and she must be able to adapt techniques to the unique situation which each patient with a respiratory problem brings to her care. She defines the areas of health remaining in the individual and works to sustain and maintain those areas which will be used to work with the problems of disability.

Coulter discusses the implications and necessity of achieving optimal physical condition under the limitations imposed by chronic respiratory situations. Suggestions as to how to proceed are presented, and the nurse's role in helping the patient progress is characterized. She calls the reader's attention to a successful experimental program in physical conditioning at the University of Colorado Medical Center. The reference is provided for the complete account.

Hoffman describes retraining for the patient who has problems with respiration. Much of the article is devoted to procedures which nurses have practiced for many years. Hoffman retells the procedure in a new and fresh manner which invites the nurse to test her practice against that which is described. Perhaps no one factor is as important as that of motivation. The world which is centered on taking the next breath and avoiding dyspnea, must be enlarged to include other people and other sites. Inactivity not only leads to boredom, but causes deterioration of the patient's physical status. Medical management is usually centered on relief of symptoms, but a new way of living can also frequently result in their amelioration. Such a new way of living cannot be prescribed and followed—it must be taught to a patient who will have to be convinced that treatment is sound.

The final article in the section deals with the rehabilitation of patients with chronic obstructive lung disease (COLD). Kinney provides an informative case history and brings the reader into the decisions and procedures that were made and utilized in dealing with a severe respiratory problem. Kinney goes on to describe in detail and in a general way the problems involved in the COLD condition and also the procedures to be employed toward the amelioration of the symptoms. COLD emerges as a pathological condition having serious repercussions for the patient and presenting the patient care team with challenging opportunities.

Reading 49
Physical and Muscular Reconditioning
Pearl Parvin Coulter

A general physical reconditioning program is fundamental to rehabilitation in emphysema and chronic bronchitis, since these patients tend to become more and more sedentary as their illness progresses. They will tend to sit at home doing nothing, and eventually their muscles will become wasted and flabby. A graded exercise program is therefore necessary.

Studies made at the University of Colorado Medical Center and elsewhere have shown that after proper physical reconditioning, patients can exercise and walk further with a slower pulse rate, a slower respiratory rate, and a need for less oxygen than before physical reconditioning. Many even gained weight during the program.

After patients have learned the new breathing technique they can learn to walk and exercise using the same controlled breathing pattern. They should walk at a slow pace, in a relaxed fashion, to the limits of their tolerance. Mild or moderate shortness of breath which may occur is not harmful and does not mean the lungs are being damaged. Once the patient knows and accepts this fact, he can pursue his regimen of physical reconditioning without apprehension or fear.

In this reconditioning program the patient should be encouraged to walk more often and greater distances on a planned schedule. This can be done by setting goals with him in the room, the house, the yard, and finally outside the confines of his home. He should be encouraged to go to the same place each time and then a little bit beyond. These exercises can be repeated with more and more frequency as the reconditioning program advances.

When the patient has become familiar with this pattern of exercise, more advanced ones can be started. After he has walked a block, a stair step should be included in the regimen, and more difficult physical barriers of a like nature should be attempted. In this way, by advancing in slow stages, the patient can easily overcome many physical problems connected with the disease and go on to a normal active life within the limitations the disease actually exerts on his body, rather than with the limitations psychologically imposed.

These exercises have been extremely beneficial even with very ill patients. Seldom were actual physical limits reached beyond which the patient could not go.

OXYGEN USE IN PHYSICAL AND MUSCULAR RECONDITIONING

Seriously ill patients may experience shortness of breath even while sitting in a chair. They may need oxygen to relieve breathlessness caused by a sedentary existence and to provide oxygen which is needed more during exercise than at rest. These patients can begin their physical reconditioning by walking around the room with the oxygen supplied from the conventional metal cylinder and increase their exercise in this manner. Portable oxygen equipment is now available which provides the patient with a unit that he can carry away from home. These portable units are extremely good in providing oxygen during the exercise program and help the patient attain more exercise than would be possible if he were confined to supply from a fixed unit.

The major gain reported by patients participating in this rehabilitation program is marked relief of symptoms and the ability to function at a higher activity level. This occurs in spite of the fact that marked improvement in lung function does not occur. As a matter of fact patients were selected in this study on the basis of severe irreversible emphysema and chronic bronchitis. Despite their pathology, most patients are at least temporarily benefitted and are able to perform necessary and pleasurable tasks in comfort.

Breathing retraining, reconditioning exercises, and bronchial hygiene are extremely important in the rehabilitation of the emphysema and chronic bronchitis patient. It is, in many cases, the nurse's task to see to it that all three are carried out as effectively as possible so that these patients can return to the normal world. The ability of the nurse (1) to instill within the patient the awareness of how important all these factors are and (2) to help patients learn to help themselves cannot be stressed too strongly. Some pulmonary diseases which were formerly considered "irreversible" can be reversed effectively with the application of techniques and programs that have developed out of research and study such as that conducted by the University of Colorado Medical Center.[1]

The Director of the Respiratory Unit, Dr. Petty, emphasizes both mental and physical aspects of the care of patients with chronic bronchitis and emphysema. An increasing number of persons suffer from these disorders, and the results of air pollution now constitute one of the most serious threats to the nation's health.

Briefly described, the bronchial hygiene program consists of the following treatment sequence:

---

[1] "Rehabilitation of Emphysema and Chronic Bronchitis Patients," *Bedside Nurse,* March-April 1969, pp. 23-27. Portions are quoted by permission.

Inhalation of bronchial dilators
Inhalation of moisture
Expulsive coughing

When the airway is severely obstructed, an IPPB (intermittent positive-pressure breathing) device is used. A simple, inexpensive one was developed and evaluated as a part of the study. It has made possible individual equipment for use of patients in hospital or home. After the medical plan has been established, the nurse plays a major role in assisting the patient with his self-help regimen, which he performs with increasing independence and confidence in the hospital and continues at home under the guidance of the public health nurse.

Medical management is usually centered on relief of symptoms, but a new way of living may have to be found if the symptoms are to be kept under control. This new life-style is not followed in response to a prescription—it must be taught to the patient in such a way that he will become actively involved in his own restoration. "After patients have learned the new breathing technique, they should learn to walk and exercise using the same controlled breathing pattern. They should walk at a slow pace, in a relaxed fashion, to the limits of their tolerance. It should be noted that mild or moderate shortness of breath which may occur is not harmful and does not mean the lungs are being damaged. Once the patient knows and accepts this fact, he can pursue his regimen of physical reconditioning without apprehension or fear."

"These exercises have been extremely beneficial even with very ill patients. Seldom are actual physical limits reached beyond which the patient could not go."

Even patients who required supplemental oxygen were encouraged to exercise. Portable equipment was made available which could be carried on walks. It seems likely that the presence of the oxygen equipment may have helped the patient psychologically. If he knows it is available he tends not to use it, but when separated from it his anxiety level becomes so high that a need for oxygen is created.

The Colorado study was described as "a total care program." It can be regarded as a model for the nurse who is (1) well versed in the physiological mechanism of breathing, (2) understanding enough to help patients gain insight into these basic principles and their application to individual pathology, and (3) sufficiently able to help patients manipulate their environment sufficiently to protect themselves from such air pollutants as dust and smoke; she can anticipate a gratifying degree of success with its use, but she must realize that a model, even a very good one, is not necessarily the final answer. Appropriate modifications will have to be penciled into every nursing care plan to make it functional for the individual concerned.

Industrialization with accompanying urban living as well as personal habits and life-styles have contributed to a degree of atmospheric pollution that is hazardous to human life and is responsible for an increasing number of persons with varying levels of respiratory obstruction. The ultimate solution to the widespread environmental problem must gain momentum through official action by national, state, and local governments. In the meantime the patients whose symptoms are the result of environmental hazards must have immediate and often intensive help. There is a great deal already known which patient care personnel can translate into care for individual patients. They include treatment modalities and changes in life-style for the patient which may include the elimination of pollutants in their own immediate environment.

Reading 50

Rehabilitation of Chronic Obstructive Lung Diseases
Frances P. Hoffman

PREVALENCE

Chronic obstructive lung diseases have existed with man for many years. Statistics for these afflictions have increased alarmingly in the past 10 years. The Vital Statistics Division of the U.S. Public Health Service in 1965 indicated a 110 percent increase in the number of cases of lung disease diagnosed in a three-year period from 1961 to 1964.[1]

Cases of emphysema are increasing at a much faster rate than those of all other respiratory diseases. Emphysema now leads the list for respiratory diseases and is second only to atherosclerosis as a disabler. The U.S. Social Security Administration[2] reported nearly 15,000 emphysemic persons under 65 years of age on disability compensation in 1963. Deaths from emphysema increased from 6,707 in 1958 to 15,120 in 1963. This is an increase of 125

[1] As reported in the November 19, 1965, issue of *Medical World News*, in a news story titled "Emphysema Incidence Paces Other Respiratory Diseases" (**6**:4:40).

[2] National Tuberculosis Association. Report of the Task Force on Chronic Bronchitis and Emphysema, sponsored by the Chronic Respiratory Diseases Control Program, National Center for Chronic Disease Control, Bureau of Disease Presentation and Environmental Control, U.S. Public Health Service, and the National Tuberculosis Association, Princeton, N.J., October 16 to October 20, 1966. *Bul. Natl. Tuberculosis Assn.*, May, 1967. **53**:5:2–23.

Reprinted by permission from *Rehabilitation Literature*, vol. 29, no. 2, pp. 34–39, February 1968.

percent and passes the 90 percent increase of deaths due to chronic bronchitis and the 5 percent increase due to asthma for the same year's report.[3]

Mary E. Switzer, Administrator of the U.S. Social and Rehabilitation Services, stated, "In 1960 alone, 12,374 workers were found with this disease who were awarded social security disability benefits."[4] One out of every 14 workers eligible for social security disability benefits is emphysemic.

DEFINITION OF TERMS

The terms used to describe all of the pulmonary obstructive diseases or chronic obstructive lung diseases vary considerably in the United States and abroad.

The literature in the United States does appear to be heading toward some uniformity of recognition. The general terms obstructive lung diseases and chronic airway obstruction seem to be the preferred headings.[5]

The term obstructive pulmonary emphysema is generally used to describe a nonreversible progressive condition in which there is obstruction of airflow on expiration due to the destructive changes in the alveolar walls. This tissue destruction, leaving holes or windows in the lungs, results in shortness of breath, respiratory insufficiency, a loss of lung compliance, and oxygen-carbon dioxide chaos. Emphysema can be considered the end of obstructive pulmonary disease when the tissue of the lung begins to deteriorate.

The term chronic bronchitis is generally used to describe the presence of a sticky mucous condition, a chronic cough, a narrowing of the airways, some loss of ciliary action, and some mucous plugging of the alveoli. There is ventilatory insufficiency, but unless there is destruction of tissue, chronic bronchitis can be considered reversible.

The term asthma is generally used to describe a reversible condition of paroxysmal obstruction of the smaller bronchi. The terms bronchial asthma and chronic bronchitis seem to remain interchangeable. There is very little differentiation in the literature, and it becomes very difficult to make clear-cut definitions. Further research may serve to clarify these terms.

The term wheeze is used to describe a sound recognizable in airway obstruction. Although it is evidence of obstruction, it is not a diagnostic symptom by itself. Where a wheeze is heard, it is obvious that the obstruction is allowing the passage of some air. In the low lung areas in emphysema there is no wheeze, no sound at all, and no airflow.

[3] Ibid.
[4] New York University Medical Center, Institute of Physical Medicine and Rehabilitation. *The Application of Physical Medicine and Rehabilitation to Emphysema Patients*, by Albert Haas and Aleksander Luczak. New York: The Institute, 1963 (*Rehab. Monographs*, no. 22).
[5] U.S. Public Health Service, Division of Chronic Diseases. *Management of Chronic Obstructive Lung Diseases: Conclusions of the Eighth Aspen Emphysema Conference*, Aspen, Colo., June 10-13, 1965. Washington, D.C.: Government Printing Office, 1966 (Public Health Service Publication No. 1457, May 1966).

Dyspnea, a symptom of respiratory insufficiency, is a sensation experienced by the patient, a subjective symptom. Described by the words of the patient, "I cannot breathe," "I cannot catch my breath," dyspnea is best understood by the physician, nurse, and therapist by carefully watching the face, neck, and chest of the patient.

A fibrocystic lung is secondary to pancreatic disease. Alterations in the tracheobronchial secretions bring cystic fibrosis into this family of obstructive lung diseases. A very viscid, tenacious secretion occurs. Recurrent pulmonary infection, mucosal and submucosal edema, and bronchial spasms are the general symptoms. Fibrosis of the lungs produces a loss of alveolar tissue similar to emphysema.

REHABILITATION

It is the responsibility of the doctors, nurses, and physical therapists to assist in improving the physical condition of all patients with chronic airway obstruction.

It is possible with retraining in breathing and muscular reconditioning to relieve some of the patient's physical distress. The patient can be assisted to become more socially acceptable and to remain in the labor force for a longer period of time. He can be taught to protect himself from environmental conditions and to exercise regularly; he must learn to follow a daily procedure to slow up the physical changes that are taking place and that will eventually incapacitate him. By encouraging the patient to increase his muscular abilities and to retrain his breathing pattern, not only can his physical distress be relieved but also the apathy and hopelessness so frequently seen among patients with chronic airway obstruction will be reduced.

The tracheobronchial tree consists of the trachea and the bifurcating tubes of various sizes. The bronchi are lined with a very fine membrane covered with cilia. This lining under normal conditions remains moist. The amount of moisture increases whenever any source of irritation enters the airways. Irritations can be caused by fine dust breathed in or from smoke inhaled. The lining reacts by producing moisture in an attempt to flood out the irritant, very much like the eye does when grit is blown into it.

Increased bronchial secretions in patients with pulmonary problems must be controlled. Allowed to accumulate, these secretions obstruct the airways and interfere with air exchange and at the same time expose the bronchi to infection. If the mucus can be kept loose, the normal clearing mechanisms can expel it. When mucus becomes thick and tenacious, it is increasingly difficult to move it along for expulsion. Intake of fluids is very important, and the patient should be told to drink sufficient amounts of liquids other than coffee and tea. Coffee and tea are both diuretics and will deplete the fluid content of the body.

Because of indoor heating in winter months, humidifiers should be used to prevent the drying out of tissues during sleep. Secretions tend to accumulate during the night and there will be a period of coughing and dyspnea on awakening.

The goblet or mucous cells in the lungs secrete mucus continually, which is brushed upward by the cilia, to be ejected by the bronchi and swallowed or expelled. This action permits air to pass into the alveoli without taking any of the secretion into the lungs. Ciliated, mucus-coated epithelial cells line the respiratory tract. The cilia beat with an upward motion and are in constant motion, pushing particles along toward the pharynx. This action is similar to the lashing action of a whip. The cilia bend, recover, bend again, like a field of wheat with a light breeze blowing across the area. The whole ciliated surface is not in action at one time, but the movement is wavelike, undulating. This continuous upward sweep, moving secretions from the smaller bronchi to the larger tubes until the particles reach the trachea, is exceedingly important in keeping the airways clear, enabling air to pass freely into the alveoli, where gas exchange must take place.

The changes in the compliance of the lung produce many difficulties because of the interference in the expiration phase. Dyspnea, or shortness of breath, plus an inadequate distribution of inspired air occur. Respiratory insufficiency can result also from a narrowing of the bronchioles due to structural changes. Changes in the structure of the alveoli will result in retained or trapped air because of the loss of recoil of the tiny air sacs. The trapped air causes a buildup of pressure in the alveoli, producing a collapse of the bronchial tubes and making it impossible to release the air. Forced expiration under these conditions will produce only a greater collapse within the bronchial tree. The abnormally high pressures occurring in the overdistended alveoli can of themselves produce a compression of the bronchioles.

Mucosal edema or obstruction of the airways due to tenacious secretion also may interfere with alveolar ventilation.

Since airflow is now definitely obstructed, this leaves the lungs overinflated and expanded. A continuation of this condition frequently leads to a continually expanded chest wall or "barrel chest," so common with emphysemic and asthmatic patients.

PULMONARY HYPERTENSION

With the inefficient air exchange, impaired diffusion results. The capillaries may become thickened and distorted, further compounding the problem of gas exchange. With this disturbance in gas exchange, less oxygen reaches the blood and the tissues. Inevitably there is a retention of carbon dioxide in the blood, with a resultant confusion to the central nervous system. The heart begins an increased drive to relieve this dilemma and to assist with the ventilation. The result is pulmonary hypertension and failure of the right ventricle. Because of the cyanotic aspect of this condition, persons having it are often called blue bloaters. For those who simply huff and puff, do not hyperventilate, do not have a heart reaction, and retain their skin color, the term pink puffers is frequently used.

DRAINAGE

A patient can position himself so that the secretions are aided by gravity in movement toward the trachea; this artificial assistance is called postural drainage. The terms bronchial drainage and pulmonary drainage are also frequently used to describe this assistance in getting the material out of the bronchial tree.

Postural drainage is the oldest of the terms and is most generally used. It simply means placing the patient in various positions to expedite the drainage of all segments of the lungs.

Before drainage is begun, tight clothing must be removed. The patient must be unencumbered, particularly around the thorax and the abdomen. Ambulatory patients should do some light exercise prior to drainage since this frequently loosens the secretions and facilitates expectoration. The drainage routines should last for at least 15 minutes. Percussion, or cupping, on the area being drained is helpful. The therapist can instruct someone in the home in this procedure. All drainage routines must be done prior to meals, since draining initiates the gag reflex and a meal would be lost.

The "tipping" position provides an angle that is very productive for drainage. Tipping from the bed to the floor is not easy, and for the elderly it is muscularly impossible unless they are assisted throughout. For most patients it is a worrisome position to be in and sets up tension and anxiety. Since the patient must be relaxed and at ease for good drainage results, substitute tipping positions should be used.

A low bathtub can be made use of with excellent results. Telephone books or a hard roll of newspapers inside a blanket can be kneeled on to get the hips up, the feet remain on the floor, and the arms and forehead are on the floor. When finished, the patient can push back onto his heels and stand up easily. There is no danger of falling or losing one's balance.

Drainage positions for all areas of the lungs should be carried out daily on an inclined bed. A neighborhood lumber yard will make a pair of 15-inch-high wooden blocks with saucered tops for the feet of the bed to be set in to prevent slipping.

In all of the drainage positions, it is important that gravity be used to help in removing the secretions. If the tissues are very dry and if expectoration is difficult, inhaling steam for about 40 minutes can be very helpful.

COUGHING

Coughing is an essential part of the postural drainage procedure. Therefore, before the positions for drainage are taught, it is important that the cough be practiced until it becomes a productive skill.

A cough is a reflex to clear the bronchial tree, similar to the blinking of the eye to protect against the invasion of particles. It is essential to life, since it is the only way to clear the passageways of all foreign materials. When pollutants, smoke, or other irritating substances enter the trachea, the nerve endings in the epithelial lining of the tract become irritated and a cough is produced.

Since not all people can cough effectively, some must be taught. The sound of a cough very often indicates how good or productive it is. If it is muffled, the mouth is being kept closed. If the sound is high-pitched, the mouth is closing at the end of the cough and the patient is straining. The cough should have a soft, hollow sound for best results.

At the start of the cough, a deep breath should be taken. The glottis and the vocal cords close down tight over the trachea, trapping the air. At the same time the abdominal muscles should contract firmly, pushing against the diaphragm and building up pressure in the thorax. The tongue, pressed against the lower teeth, allows the soft palate to move downward, thereby increasing the pressure. The mouth should be open.

When the glottis and the vocal cords open, the cough will explode the air from the mouth, carrying the materials with it. The mouth must be open to allow for the explosion and the expulsion; if the mouth is allowed to close, real distress will result. The force of the exploding air can deposit droplets halfway across a room. For this reason, tissue should be held in front of the mouth during the procedure.

If the patient is seated, holding the thighs together will help in the process. In this way the pelvis is held tight, and the viscera are kept from moving downward on the explosion phase. Leaning forward while sitting and holding a pillow tightly against the abdominal wall will also assist in the contraction of the abdominal muscles, forcing the viscera upward against the diaphragm and increasing the force of the cough.

Regardless of where the patient is, in bed, sitting, or standing, the head must be forward so that the material to be expectorated can slide out. Keeping the head up or holding it backward simply allows the material to slide backward into the pharynx.

The action of the diaphragm is effective in coughing. On inspiration the diaphragm must contract and descend to allow for the inrush of air. Then it must relax and ascend swiftly to increase the pressure behind the air to be expelled. The abdominal muscles contract strongly. The narrowing of the bronchi, along with this swift relaxation of the diaphragm, which is pushed upward when the abdominal muscles contract, also increases the pressure behind the air to be exploded out. When the diaphragm is paralyzed, atelectasis, a collapse of the lung or portions of it, often occurs.

Frequently not enough time is allowed between the inspiration and the cough, and the patient becomes breathless, red in the face, and exhausted. There may also be some mechanical failure in getting the mucus out of the bronchi. Variations for expulsion should be tried. One successful method is to lean forward, head low, over the basin, breathe in, cough, and then hold the breath momentarily to keep the trachea open and allow gravity to assist in sliding the material out. This same procedure can be followed in the tipping position over the bathtub or on the tipping board. Patients frequently are taught to perform two coughs in rapid succession. It is not uncommon for the second inspiration to pull the mucus backward into the pharynx, making it impossible to expel the plug and clear the tree.

Newly formed mucus tends to remain moist and loose. If infection is present, the mucus becomes thick and the cough may not be effective enough to move the plug upward and explode it out. The bronchioles will block and, if the condition is allowed to continue, the cilia cease to function, the walls of the bronchioles become soft, and the bronchi dilate instead of constrict during the cough, and there will be no pressure behind the air to be exploded. The mucus that fills the tubes becomes stagnant and a very disagreeable odor results. This condition can be reversed with immediate medical treatment.

Failure of the cough may be due to insufficient muscular force. (This is an additional reason for reconditioning.) Atelectasis may exist. Also the ciliary action may be interfered with, as occurs in those who smoke.

RETRAINING IN BREATHING

Man normally breathes at a very regular, easy rate. The rate changes as he changes his activities. Under stress of competitive athletics, it can become very fast and the person can be said to be laboring for breath. The consumption of oxygen then becomes so great that the competitor piles up a tremendous oxygen debt that he must repay. When the activity ends, the competitor must continue his fast breathing for a short time until the entire oxygen debt is paid off.

A person with badly impaired breathing can be compared to this competitor who has been straining to win a race. He is breathing hard and fast and his heart is beating very fast, but, unlike the competitor who is able to repay his oxygen debt in a few minutes, the impaired breather is piling up carbon dioxide.

The primary muscles for breathing are the diaphragm, the abdominals, and the intercostals. Most people tend to use just the intercostals for ordinary breathing. Only under stress and for forced inhalation and exhalation will the abdominals be brought into action. It is imperative that someone with impaired respiration learn to use his abdominal muscles and diaphragm at all times. Instead of resorting to the accessory muscles and panicking when dyspnea occurs, he should be prepared to drive hard, with several piston-type contractions of the abdominal muscles forcing the diaphragm into faster action until the dyspnea dissipates itself and a regular breathing rate is established. Since this person has serious difficulties in the expiration phase, it is of utmost importance that the abdominals be kept working. It is these muscles, along with the intercostals, that will enable him to expel the air.

Most people have to be taught to use the abdominal muscles. To handle heavier work loads, all must strengthen the abdominals so that the muscles can respond adequately. Weights can be used for this particular reconditioning. Sandbags of different weights, from one pound to 15 pounds, can be made from canvas or heavy mattress ticking. The filling should be a sandy-type soil that is dry, or sand if it is available. A small type of bean can also be used. Bags should not be overfilled because they tend to roll instead of sitting flat.

The person using the sandbags should lie supine on the floor or the bed. Place the sandbag directly over the navel and practice lifting the bag up with the action of the abdominal muscles. The rise and fall of the sandbag should be easy and regular with a count of one for the lift and a count of one, two for the fall, with the sandbag settling gently. As this exercise becomes familiar and easy, the sandbag used should be heavier and the exercise should be done on an inclined bed.

Before exercises for retraining breathing are practiced, it is best for the patient to go through the positions for bronchial drainage, so that excess secretions, which accumulate constantly, are removed from the bronchial tree.

PURSED LIPS

In airway obstruction, the air in the alveoli is trapped by edema, secretions, or inflammation and cannot move out through the bronchioles. Hence the sensation of not being able to breathe out. In patients with asthma or very early emphysema, there will be a wheeze on expiration as the air flows around the obstruction on its way out through the bronchial tree.

If force is used at this time to expel the trapped air, the bronchioles collapse due to the uneven pressures, for the pressure in the inflated alveoli has been steadily increasing. When the air is expelled, some pressure from without must be created to equalize the pressure in the air sacs and to slow up the exiting airflow by offering some resistance. If the lips are "pursed," the airflow outward can be controlled to a slow stream. This establishes resistance and will prevent the collapse of the bronchioles. The lips should be pursed into the position of "prisms." This position allows for a steady controlled "streaming" of the expired air.

The length of time for the expelling of the air can be extended to a count of two or three, whichever is most comfortable for the patient. In any case the air is eased out comfortably by steady pressure of the abdominal muscles and the ascending intercostal muscles (the interosseous portions of the internal intercostals), which will maintain the spacing between the ribs until all of the air is expelled.

The purpose behind the altered breathing pattern is to improve the mixing of air in the lungs and to aerate the blood more efficiently, to use the rib cage and diaphragm more effectively, to give the patient a tool by which he can conserve his energy, to reduce the amount of dyspnea he experiences, and to ease the tension and apprehension his condition produces. To this end, as many exercises as possible should be taught the patient to assist him in using and strengthening the abdominals and the diaphragm. He should be constantly reminded to purse his lips during exercise to control the outflow of air, to prevent the collapse of the bronchial tree, and to bring into constant and strong use the abdominals and the diaphragm. The breathing rhythm should always be longer on expiration than on inspiration. The exercises are not an end in themselves; that they have purpose should be understood by the patient.

RECONDITIONING

All patients, regardless of age, who can physically get out of bed should be encouraged to walk. The length of the walks should be increased regularly, and eventually the patient should attempt the stairs unless there is cardiac involvement. The patient who is at home should be cautioned against sitting or lying about. Such inactivity simply leads to more obstructive problems as well as physical problems. With children, there will be a loss in body growth, and with the middle-aged, loss of muscular strength and range of motion in joints.

For those who are not physically incapacitated, a program of daily reconditioning exercises should be followed. The exercise program, of necessity, must be individual and should be worked out by the therapist for each patient. The type of exercise program will depend upon the age, the physical ability, the extent of pulmonary obstruction, cardiac involvement, and the previous physical experiences of the patient. Whatever the program, the difficulty of the exercises should be increased at regular intervals to insure a strengthening of musculature. The principle of overload must not be overlooked.

The purpose of reconditioning is to strengthen all of the musculature and return the person to working status if attainable as soon as possible.

TREATMENT

The treatment for the patient with a chronic obstructive airway condition is always directed toward the reversible problems first. Where conditions are not reversible, prevention of further complications is of utmost importance.

For persons with early emphysema, asthma, and uncomplicated chronic bronchitis, a nebulizer of some sort is indispensable. There are pocket-sized nebulizers and atomizers of several kinds. Regardless of type, they do bring instant and gratifying relief.

With advanced and complicated problems, which in most cases are accompanied by irreversible conditions, there are bound to be oxygen-carbon dioxide disturbances and perhaps some cardiac complications. Careful use of bronchodilators, antibiotics, and assistive respiratory apparatus such as intermittent positive-pressure breathing devices[6] gives excellent results.

Regular use in the home of the intermittent positive-aerosol machine will increase ventilation, assist in making the cough more productive, and relieve dyspnea. With medication in the inhalant, the bronchial tree will be dilated and secretions will be made more moist.

Antibiotics and steroids, formerly used with some regularity, are now used only for emergencies. There are a number of combination tablets containing sympathomimetic amines, expectorants, antihistamines, and buffers that work well in acute management. An increasing number of therapeutic regimes use epinephrine parenterally, aminophylline intravenously, isoproterenol sublingually, and sympathomimetic amines in aerosol form.

Regardless of severity, complications, reversible or nonreversible conditions, all persons with any degree of chronic airway obstruction should give up smoking and protect themselves from unnecessary exposure to smoke, such as being in a room or a car with persons who are smoking heavily. Avoidance of environmental pollutants should be considered in re-employment. Whatever means can be used to keep household dust and pollutants at a minimum should be employed, particularly for the sleeping area.

---

[6] Motley, Hurley L. Mechanical Aids in Respiration. *J. Kentucky Med. Assn.*, vol. 64, pp. 757-769, September 1966.

Reading 51

Rehabilitation of Patients with COLD
Marjorie Kinney

Mr. J., 69 years old, was admitted to the hospital for the tenth time this year. For the past eight years he has had chronic obstructive emphysema and chronic bronchitis. He now has some degree of congestive heart failure and a superimposed respiratory infection, which further aggravates his chronic shortness of breath. Mr. J.'s first symptom of chronic obstructive lung disease (COLD) was exertional dyspnea, which has so progressed that he now is occasionally dyspneic even at rest, and he complains of constant fatigue. Cough has never been an outstanding symptom except during an acute respiratory infection. However, he does retain mucus which he does not cough up.

Mr. J. has smoked 20 to 30 cigarettes daily for the last 30 years, although lately—on his physician's recommendation—he has tried to smoke less. He breathes mostly through his mouth and purses his lips as he breathes out.

Pulmonary function tests show increased residual air volume and decreased expiratory reserve volume. Arterial blood studies demonstrate decreased oxygen pressure and oxygen saturation; arterial carbon dioxide pressure is increased. Mr. J.'s symptoms are representative of a mild hypoxemia with some hypercapnia. A bronchogram shows more involvement in the lower lobe of the right lung than elsewhere. Chest X-rays show the diaphragm to be somewhat flat and depressed on the right side.

In all the years he has been under medical care he has had no rehabilitative measures. Treatment for the most part has been directed toward short-term relief of symptoms.

The current plan of therapy is designed to increase ventilation in order to decrease pulmonary CO_2 and to increase pulmonary O_2. Drugs, postural drainage, and intermittent positive-pressure breathing (IPPB) were ordered to clear trachea, bronchi, and bronchioles. Bronchodilator drugs, administered by various methods, were ordered: isoproternerol hydrochloride (Isuprel) with equal parts of saline to be used in the hand nebulizer as well as in the IPPB nebulizer; theophylline ethylenedramine (Aminophyline) suppositories to be used p.r.n. after an initial intravenous infusion of the same drug; actylcysteine (Mucomyst), a detergent-like drug, to be administered in the

---

Reprinted from *The American Journal of Nursing*, vol. 67, no. 12, pp. 2528-2535, December 1967. The original article contains seven diagrams illustrating beneficial exercises and procedures for the alleviation of respiratory congestion.

IPPB nebulizer along with Isuprel four times a day. An expectorant, saturated solution of potassium iodide, was prescribed to assist in thinning secretions, or lowering the viscosity of mucus. Amesec, an oral combination of aminophyllin, ephedrine, and amytal in one tablet was to be taken twice a day. Tetracycline was ordered to act against the organisms causing the upper respiratory infection.

For his congestive heart failure he was put on a maintenance dosage of digitoxin, hydrochlorothiazide (HydroDiuril), and potassium chloride, as well as a sodium-restricted diet.

Postural drainage, directed toward the right lower lung segments, is being done daily to assist in clearing his airway. Humidification by an ultrasonic nebulizer and an increase of oral fluids has helped to liquefy the mucus. Intermittent positive-pressure breathing is being used to increase alveolar ventilation.

The social worker also saw this patient. She learned that eight years ago, because of illness, Mr. J. was forced to abandon his work as a painter just as he was anticipating the enjoyment of retirement. Previously, he had enjoyed outdoor activities and especially liked walking, an exercise he can no longer tolerate. His daughter, who is married, lives several hundred miles from his home. He would like to be able to see her and his grandchildren, but cannot travel. His wife has been forced to return to work in order to assist with some of the hospital bills, especially drugs, which average about $30 a month. In spite of his obvious disability, Mr. J. is striving to maintain his independence. Although he appears anxious about his breathlessness, his behavior is focused positively and he is actively engaged in doing as much as he is able.

The nurse, assessing Mr. J.'s need for assistance in activities of daily living, found him highly motivated to help himself. He is able to perform grooming, hygiene, feeding, and elimination activities with little assistance. Both he and Mrs. J. were interested in learning how to help conserve his energy. We found that his pulse and respiratory rates did not increase significantly if activities were done slowly and at the proper arm level. However, he could walk only about 40 feet before dyspnea increased.

The physical therapist found that Mr. J. has considerable muscle weakness, but no limitation of joint motion or contractures even though he has spent much of his time just sitting in a chair at home. It is obvious that he uses his upper chest muscles in breathing, and his whole thorax appears somewhat rigid. Rehabilitation goals, planned with Mr. and Mrs. J., are based on evaluations of the various health personnel, and are limited to two closely related goals.

First, increasing his exercise tolerance is a primary goal in view of his motivation and need for independence in activities of daily living. The physical therapist and the nurses worked together with him toward this achievement. Following improvement of the acute infection and heart failure, his daily activities were gradually increased. Instruction in abdominal diaphragmatic breathing exercises was initiated so that breathing could become more efficient through strengthening the muscles of respiration. Mr. J. learned to slow his breathing during increased activities and developed confidence from the relief this gave him.

Walking and other mild exercises were also increased after he had learned breathing control in an upright position. Small amounts of oxygen were given during these exercises to prevent oxygen desaturation.

Over a period of four weeks, the distance Mr. J. was able to walk without increased dyspnea quadrupled. Fluoroscopy of the diaphragm following breathing exercise training showed improvement in the elevation of the right diaphragm upon exhalation.

The second goal for Mr. J. was to help him and his wife acquire more understanding about his illness and the therapeutic measures to be followed at home. First they were given a booklet, written in simple language, which explained pulmonary emphysema and chronic bronchitis. They then joined another patient with COLD for group discussion about the illness. Mr. J. also was taught how to use his hand nebulizer to the best advantage: inhalation during compression of the hand bulb, and the need to pause after inhalation to permit the nebulized particles to be deposited on the mucous membranes.

The social worker was able to secure an IPPB respirator for home use. Mr. J. and his wife were taught how to set up the apparatus, add the medications which were to be nebulized, and observe the color and quantity of coughed-up mucus as one indication of an acute respiratory infection.

The general purpose of drugs prescribed for home use was reviewed with the patient. He had difficulty understanding why several bronchodilating drugs were given in different forms. When we explained the various forms of absorption, he understood.

While Mr. J. was doing his postural drainage, the nurse tested his ability to remember and follow through with this procedure. Since his right lower lobe was involved, we emphasized his need to remain on his left side in various positions in order to drain the bronchial segments. During the period of drainage, Mr. J. was encouraged to practice appropriate breathing and coughing. Vibration and chest clapping were not necessary for Mr. J. as for some patients who have more adherent drainage.

Mr. and Mrs. J. were given a written schedule for the time and sequence of his various treatments. Mr. J. understood the reason for taking the bronchodilating and mucolytic drugs (per hand nebulizer and IPPB) before postural drainage. He also understood that he would derive more benefit from the breathing exercises if these were done after the airways were dilated and drained. The physician reviewed the reasons why he should reduce his smoking.

We also discussed practical measures to avoid infection:

1 Avoid exposure to drafts, sudden changes in temperature, excessively dry air, and excessive wetting of the body.
2 Avoid bronchial irritants.
3 Avoid exposure to groups during epidemics and known infections.
4 Keep up general resistance through a well-balanced diet.

Mr. J. was able to return home feeling more comfortable. He was able to increase his tolerance in activities of daily living; he was able to walk farther and travel to his daughter's home; he has been able to avoid repeated infections and, therefore, has avoided further lung damage.

As was the case with Mr. J., exertional dyspnea is usually the first and most pronounced symptom of COLD, especially if the patient has pulmonary emphysema. Dyspnea usually comes on slowly; the patient complains of increasing shortness of breath upon exertion. It may be present for years before it interferes with ordinary activity, but as it progresses, the patient is unable to carry out ordinary physical activities, or even walk, without increasing dyspnea. In advanced disease, the slightest movement is exhausting and the patient is dyspneic even at complete rest. Dyspnea and fatigue increase as the absorption of oxygen decreases. Airway obstruction, unequal distribution of oxygen in the lungs, and lessened diffusion of oxygen into the pulmonary capillaries may all contribute to diminished arterial oxygen. Eventually, the patient is unable to meet even minimum metabolic needs, and he suffers from chronic arterial hypoxia. Cyanosis may or may not be present.

A history of repetitive bronchial or pneumonic infection is common in patients such as Mr. J. and is considered a causative as well as a complicating factor. Infection produces cough, wheezing, and an aggravation of the shortness of breath. Chronic inflammation of the lungs, if uncontrolled, gradually results in a narrowing and irreversible destruction of bronchioles, pulmonary blood vessels, and alveoli and in a loss of lung elasticity.

Loss of lung elasticity and the downward displacement of the flattened diaphragm interfere with the mechanics of breathing. These two factors, combined with the collapsed, narrowed, and damaged airways, make expiration most difficult. Because of distended lungs, the rib cage becomes fixed as in inspiration. Residual air which becomes trapped in the lungs increases the patient's difficulty in getting fresh air into his lungs. The resulting ventilatory deficiency decreases oxygen saturation and increases carbon dioxide content in the blood. At this stage, the patient uses his shoulder, neck, and upper chest muscles in breathing.

Cough may be a common and persistent sign as the bronchial tubes are ineffectively emptied of secretions. Cough may be absent or inconspicuous as with Mr. J.; cough may also precede or follow the onset of dyspnea.

Other signs and symptoms which add to a patient's disability include loss of appetite and such related signs as increasing weight loss and pallor.

Although direct damage in COLD is to the lungs, there are other effects on the individual's activities as the disease progresses. Not only are there physiologic and physical effects, but complex and interrelated psychosocial and economic consequences occur. The cyclic results of these are summarized by Miller [1]:

> Pulmonary ventilatory or circulatory insufficiency may be responsible for exertional dyspnea which, in turn, causes fear and inactivity. Fear, itself, tends to promote further inactivity. Inactivity promotes diminished muscle tone, decreased muscle efficiency, easy fatigability and progressive physical debility. All of these in turn lead to more inactivity and exertional dyspnea. Eventually, more serious problems of sustained bed rest occur, such as venostasis, phlebothrombosis, pulmonary embolization, and increased bone resorption which may result in fractures.

Many different types of information are needed before a program of therapy and rehabilitation can be planned with the patient and medical, psychosocial, functional, and nursing goals can be defined.

MEDICAL EVALUATION

Appraisal of the type and severity of the pulmonary impairment, including its reversible and irreversible components as well as any complications, is a first step in the determination of rehabilitation goals. The type of disease causing airway obstruction will determine the treatment selected. Mitchell and others, in a study of pulmonary emphysema and chronic bronchitis, found it possible to differentiate clinically between these two diseases. Although they may exist alone or may coexist, discrimination between the two is important in determining therapy [2]. Moreover, differentiating the pathologic lesions in emphysema—whether diffuse or regional—is important even though difficult. For example, regional distribution of emphysema indicates that there are areas of the lungs which are not involved and are still functional.

Assessment of the severity of airway obstruction, the degree of respiratory insufficiency, and the likelihood of progression, or stabilization of the condition, is important in estimating the success of a rehabilitation program. Success is dependent upon arresting or stabilizing the disease process as early as possible before extreme disability and such complications as cor pulmonale, respiratory acidosis, and extreme hypoxia occur. In other words, the reversible components of COLD need to be recognized, assessed, and controlled.

PSYCHOSOCIAL EVALUATION

The psychologic, sociologic, and vocational aspects of the patient's life must also be taken into account. The home environment, the patient's role in the family, supporting as well as disturbing interpersonal relationships within the family, and the patient's reaction to illness all will affect therapy and recovery.

The basic personality of the patient, his reaction to illness, as well as any neurotic aspects of his personality, need to be known if he is to be helped. Hospital personnel often speak of the "typical emphysema patient" as one who is uncooperative, depressed, irritable, anxious, and dependent. These behaviors may well be a result of fear. Such patients, therefore, need thoughtful, understanding care.

As the disease progresses and the patient is unable to perform his usual physical activities, his work habits become irregular. Early retirement, or a new occupation, less strenuous and free from bronchial irritants, may be indicated. Vocational evaluation determines the need for retraining, possible job opportunities, and referral for financial assistance.

Costs of hospitalization, medications, oxygen, and breathing apparatus may reach a considerable amount during a year, causing financial strain on families such as the J.'s.

FUNCTIONAL EVALUATIONS

The relatively inactive patient who sits in a chair or the severely disabled patient who remains in bed will have loss of muscle strength and diminished joint motion through lack of use. Evaluation of a patient's muscle power and range of joint motion will serve as an index of his capacity for physical activity and his need for retraining.

The specific muscles used by the patient in breathing must be evaluated: respiratory muscles used in inspiration as well as the accessory muscles used in voluntary and forced breathing. Abdominal muscles in these patients also need to be strengthened and retrained to assist in expiration.

Exercise tolerance may be measured by such standard forms as walking on a treadmill, climbing stairs, or the step-up test. Exercise is carried out to the point of dyspnea and the following observed: exercise tolerance; respiratory and pulse rates and electrocardiogram at rest, during exercise, and during recovery; and the duration of subjective post-exercise dyspnea.

Energy cost studies may also be done as a basis for determining oxygen consumption needed to perform selected activities on a job or in the home. The length of time required to recover from incurred oxygen debt following various activities is then recorded.

Studies of ventilatory function are needed: forced vital capacity, the rate of expiratory air flow, and the maximum voluntary ventilation. Determining the ratio of residual air to total lung volume is also helpful. These tests may be done before and after the administration of bronchodilator drugs.

NURSING EVALUATIONS

The nurse is usually responsible for assessing a patient's ability to perform such activities of daily living as hygiene, grooming, dressing, elimination, and ambulation. His requirements for assistance with his normal physical needs and daily tasks are noted. The nurse's initial evaluation may be based on information recorded in the functional evaluation as well as on direct observation of the patient in the performance of each activity, or some one part of an activity. Recorded on a special form, this nursing history serves as a basis for planning immediate nursing care as well as for the establishment of rehabilitation goals.

REHABILITATION APPROACH

The patient and family should participate with the staff in determining both short- and long-range goals of care. These goals will, of course, need to be modified periodically in relation to the patient's progress. The broad rehabilitation aim of the patient with COLD is maximum cardio-respiratory function with minimal risk so that he may perform his life role as effectively and efficiently as possible. All patients cannot achieve complete rehabilitation. The attainment of comfort with less effort may be the best some patients can hope for. Other patients will be able to increase their exercise tolerance and participate in more activities at home, thus being spared great dependency. A few may even be able to return to work and achieve considerable independence.

Recognition and assessment of the following six factors facilitate the rehabilitation process; overlooked they negate it.

Extent of Lung Damage and Reversibility of Lung Pathology

The amount of physical activity a patient with COLD can be retrained to do is related to the extent of his remaining normal and reversible lung tissue.

Treatment is directed toward reversible components of the patient's disease in order to restore ventilation of the normal remaining lung and to protect it from further damage.

Motivation of Patient and Family

In a chronic progressive disease such as COLD, which is usually accompanied by fear and depression, the patient's psyche suffers from the constancy and frustration of his illness. He is continually threatened by feelings of uncertainty and helplessness. Success in rehabilitation, therefore, depends to a great extent on the patient's strong motivation to want to do his part in getting better. Encouragement and understanding from a family member is most important. Support from nursing and other health personnel also is needed.

Maintenance of Adequate Physiologic Treatment

Most specialists agree that implementation of a complete physiologic treatment program is the chief prerequisite to a physical rehabilitation program in patients with COLD.

The following program may be considered exemplary of maintenance treatment measures for uncomplicated COLD [3,4,5]:

1. Elimination or reduction of smoking and other bronchial irritants.
2. Prevention and prompt treatment of any bronchial and/or pulmonary infections with appropriate antibiotics.
3. Relief of bronchial edema and bronchospasm with bronchodilator drugs, administered through various routes, including nebulization.
4. Control of bronchial secretions through adequate administration of fluids, expectorants, detergents, deep breathing, and rotary postural drainage, with clapping and vibration.
5. Relief of mental depression through the judicious use of tranquilizers as long as they do not add to the problem of hypoventilation.

Special forms of therapy such as intermittent positive-pressure breathing and oxygen therapy may be included at different times.

IPPB may be ordered for the patient who can no longer breathe deeply and use a hand nebulizer, or when there is persistent retention of carbon dioxide in the alveoli and blood. It is not currently considered useful in the rehabilitation of all patients.

Oxygen therapy is used with caution to avoid further depression of ventilation. It may be used in patients with repeated episodes of right heart failure, such as Mr. J. had, and in patients with secondary polycythemia.

Breathing Exercise Training

Training in breathing is basic since the mechanical difficulty of breathing is responsible for respiratory distress which, in turn, puts limits on physical exercise.

The purpose of breathing training is to increase efficiency in breathing mechanics in order to overcome airway obstruction and assist in efficiently emptying the lungs of trapped air. The patient is taught a new pattern of breathing to substitute for the overuse of his upper chest, shoulder, and neck muscles. Emphasis is placed on complete, but not forceful, emptying of the lungs.

The patient learns to strengthen his abdominal muscles which, in turn, assist the weakened and flat diaphragm to elevate during expiration so that more air can be moved out. First, he exercises in supine, sitting, and walking positions and, eventually, while he is doing various activities of daily living. He also is taught to prolong the expiratory phase of breathing after a short inspiratory phase. This is believed to counteract the over-breathing-in which occurs during dyspnea and helps to rid the lungs of excess air. Learning to breathe through the nose and then to exhale slowly through pursed lips while contracting the abdominal muscles is advocated by some as beneficial in preventing the collapse of diseased small airways during expiration. Others believe this type of breathing is harmful because it further increases resistance to expiratory airflow.

Teaching and supervising breathing exercises are usually the responsibility of the physical therapist, with the nurse reinforcing that instruction. But regardless of who instructs the patient, it is important that other health personnel observe, report, and evaluate the extent to which the patient is successful in controlling his breathing. The patient requires much support and encouragement while he is learning to breathe in a new manner. It is not easy to change a breathing pattern, especially when one has difficulty in breathing. Breathing control should be practiced during breathlessness, moderately strenuous exercise, such as walking up a slope, up stairs, or in walking increased distances, and following the administration of bronchodilator drugs and postural drainage [6,7,8].

Patient and Family Education

Experience has shown that an interested family, oriented to the needs, abilities, and disabilities of the patient, usually shortens the period of disability. Often, it is helpful, and even necessary, for a member of the family to learn to assist with the patient's physical care and treatments.

Since the patient needs to learn how to live with his condition, he and his family must understand the mechanical nature of his breathing difficulties, the extent or limit of breathing function, purposes of the various laboratory tests, general principles and methods of administration of the prescribed therapy, including bronchial hygiene, and prevention of further lung injury. Simple drawings, diagrams, and other visual aids related to the normal mechanics of breathing may be used to explain the disease process and his therapy.

Demonstration of prescribed treatments which are to be continued at home should be initiated early in the teaching program. The patient and a member of his family should administer treatments under a nurse's supervision until they have learned to the extent of their capacities. This approach enables them to ask realistic questions about treatments and care. It also secures their cooperation when they go home.

Especially important is practice in the use of the hand bulb, or mechanical pump nebulization of bronchodilator drugs; in doing rotary postural drainage and chest vibration, directed toward the specific lobes to be drained; and in coughing. For best results, these treatments should be done in the sequence listed. Since bronchial secretions tend to settle and accumulate during sleep, the patient usually is more dyspneic when he awakens and also starts coughing. Nebulization with a bronchodilator immediately upon arising will apply the drug directly to the bronchial tissue, relax the musculature, and relieve the symptoms.

Patients require considerable assistance in the technique of using the nebulizer. Whether the nebulizer is a hand model or has a mechanical pump, the patient should place the nozzle well back into his mouth and, with his mouth open, exhale fully and then pump the nebulizer vigorously, all the while breathing the medication in deeply through his mouth. He should then pause, or hold his breath, to allow the medication to be deposited on the bronchial mucosa and produce its effect. This procedure—full exhalation, deep inhalation of drug, and then a pause—should be repeated until all of the prescribed drug is used. The nebulizer produces greater benefits if it is used at the prescribed time (usually four times daily) rather than when brief "whiffs" are taken frequently.

The IPPB device is sometimes used to administer bronchodilator drugs to a patient, such as Mr. J., who cannot coordinate the nebulizer or cannot inhale deeply. The IPPB respirator, with a special nebulizer attached, supplies controlled pressure which inflates the lung during inspiration. This machine can be set to cycle at a respiratory rate initiated by the patient, or it can be set to cycle automatically at a predetermined rate. It acts by forcing compressed air or oxygen (optional) along with the bronchodilator drug into the bronchial tubes at a pressure greater than bronchial air resistance. It is believed to promote a more uniform distribution of aerosols.

Considerable instruction and guidance is needed when a patient first uses the machine. He is instructed to keep his lips shut tightly over the mouthpiece and to avoid having air escape through his nose. As with the hand nebulizer, he should exhale fully before attaching the machine and then inspire gently to switch the respirator on. From this point on, he should be encouraged to relax, since the respirator will fill his lungs without his assistance. This method thus provides some degree of rest in labored breathing. The patient should be encouraged to remove the mouthpiece whenever he feels an urge to cough and he should be encouraged to cough up secretions as much as possible without straining. For best results, continued supervision by a nurse or inhalation therapist is needed when an IPPB respirator is used.

Rotary postural drainage and chest vibration should follow the administration of bronchodilator and detergent drugs in order to promote drainage from the lungs. By periodically positioning the patient's body on a bed (or tiltboard) in a succession of positions according to the distribution of bronchopulmonary segments, the flow of secretions in the bronchial tubes is promoted through gravity. The patient is positioned in upright, horizontal, and head-down positions in a sequence starting with the uppermost and proceeding to the lowest bronchial tubes.

If secretions are thick or are adherent to the mucosal walls, the chest wall is manually vibrated during expiration or percussed with "cupped" hands over areas to be drained—an additional aid in loosening secretions. (Because this procedure and postural drainage will not be tolerated by the severely disabled dyspneic patient, they will require modification.) In order to elevate the foot of the bed for the head-down position in the home, a straight chair or stool, blocks, or other hard material can be placed under the foot of the bed to raise the bed approximately 14 inches from the floor. Deep abdominal breathing during postural drainage procedures will also help loosen secretions. The frequency and duration of postural drainage depends on the patient's individual need and tolerance [9,10].

There is little agreement in the literature about the amount of coughing which should be done or even how it should be done. Coughing up secretions during postural drainage is necessary to clear the airways of loosened secretions. But coughing at this time should be voluntary and gentle, never strained or forced. Brown and Watts recommend that coughing be preceded by several slow, deep, abdominal inspirations, well controlled and localized, to direct air gently into that portion of the lung from which secretions are to be expelled. The cough on expiration should then be short and double [11]. Color and amount of sputum coughed up each day should be reported to the doctor.

Excessive and ineffective coughing should be voluntarily suppressed since it subjects the lungs to additional trauma and causes collapse of the airways. The presence of bronchial secretions, however, often induces severe coughing. Severe coughing produces bronchospasm which, in turn, decreases the elimination of secretions, thus causing more irritation to the bronchial tubes with resulting spasm and cough. Coughing also is exhausting since it requires muscular energy.

Rehabilitation for COLD patients is not an unrealistic goal, but it does require the combined efforts of the patient, family, physician, nurse, social worker, psychologist, and physical and inhalation therapists.

Success is dependent upon the motivation of the patient and his family, adequate medical management, the extent of lung damage and reversibility of lung pathology, breathing control, patient and family education, and physical reconditioning.

The total rehabilitation goals may not be achieved by the patient; achievement of any part should be considered worthwhile. Most patients feel more comfortable and their symptoms are relieved with rehabilitation efforts. Some learn to conserve their energy and to control breathlessness. Many are able to return home and care for themselves. A few are restored to a more productive home or work life.

To date, the prevention and cure of this serious disease are not yet seen as realistically achievable. But the prevention of disability and maintenance of optimal health should have high priority in the care of patients with COLD.

REFERENCES

1. Miller, W. F., and others. Rehabilitation of the disabled patient with chronic bronchitis and pulmonary emphysema. *American Journal of Public Health,* 53(no. 3 Suppl.):18-23, March 1963, p. 18.
2. Mitchell, R. S., and others. Chronic obstructive broncho-pulmonary disease, IV. Clinical and physiological differentiation of chronic bronchitis and emphysema. *American Journal of Medical Science.*
3. Barach, A. L., and others. Emphysemas, diagnosis and treatment, in *Dyspnea: Diagnosis and Treatment,* ed. by Andrew L. Banyai and Edwin R. Levine. Philadelphia, Pa., F. A. Davis Co., 1963, pp. 95-98.
4. Boren, H. G. Pulmonary Emphysema: Clinical and Physiologic Aspects, in *Textbook of Pulmonary Diseases,* ed. by Gerald L. Baum. Boston, Mass., Little, Brown and Co., 1965, p. 421.
5. Miller, W. F. Treatment of chronic pulmonary emphysema. *Postgraduate Med.,* 39:230-239, March 1966.
6. Livingstone, J. L., and Reed, Jocelyn M. W. *Exercises for asthma and "emphysema."* London, Asthma Research Council, 1962, pp. 4-28.

7 Haas, Albert. *Essentials of Living with Pulmonary Emphysema: A Guide for Patients and Their Families* (Patient Publication No. 4). New York, Institute of Physical Medicine and Rehabilitation, New York University Medical Center, 1963, pp. 27-39.
8 Gaskell, D. V., in *Physical Therapy for Medical and Surgical Thoracic Conditions,* 2d rev. ed. by Jocelyn M. W. Reed. London, Physiotherapy Department, Brompton Hospital, 1964, pp. 26-27.
9 Haas, op. cit. pp. 15-23.
10 Gaskell, op. cit. pp. 7-10.
11 Brown, Gillian, and Watts, Nancy. *Outline of Physical Therapy Programs for Medical and Surgical Chest Conditions.* Based on the original work by E. Thacker, Harefield Hospital, England. Reprinted by the Physical Therapy Department, Institute of Rehabilitation Medicine, New York, 1964 (mimeographed).

Section C

Malignancy Conditions

The patient with cancer poses at least three problems to the nurse whose nursing care includes the goal of assisting the patient to reach his highest potential. First is the problem of rehabilitation of the patient with cancer. The person and his family are faced with fighting a battle against a disease which still has a high ratio of failures in treatment, and when it is treated, there is a long waiting period to determine whether the treatment has in fact been successful in eradication. The physical fact is accompanied by emotional distress for which support is needed to maintain self-esteem and hope. The second problem is that of the treatment itself, which may require mutilation of the body with resulting disability both from loss of one's image of his intact body and from actual functional loss, as in colostomy or laryngectomy. The nurse is most familiar with her role in helping the patient function in a new way, and this problem is the one on which most nursing care plans focus. The third problem is helping the patient face his death.

In rehabilitation nursing the assumption is made that until the moment of death, each person is entitled to as full a life as possible. So long as life is responsive the nurse helps the patient to maximize its meaningfulness, and where the attritional process results in death, she has the responsibility to help the patient and his family face it with a minimum of distress.

For the nursing skills to be effective, it is necessary that the nurse adopt a constructive philosophy regarding the kind of long-term illness which results in death rather than in recovery. She should regard death as the end of a sequence of events and not a result of failure. She tolerates body mutilation in the service of eradicating disease. In order to arrive at a philosophy that will allow her to care for patients comfortably, the nurse will need the opportunity to share her feelings with her colleagues. She needs support in expressing her own discomforts, anxieties, and fears. Discussions will allow her to take a look at her feelings and admit them to herself. Recognition of her limitations gives a starting point for growth. The nurse who feels a sense of frustration and failure in the care of the cancer patient probably will not make long-range goals for her patient, thereby denying him the basis for rehabilitation.

In the care of a patient with cancer, nursing has a unique role in rehabilitation. The patient with a colostomy or ileostomy requires a team of practitioners—the physician, the patient, the family, and the nurse. From the moment the patient presents himself for medical care, the office nurse can be helpful in preparing the way for eventual rehabilitation; she can pave the way for hospitalization by referral to the staff nurse who will care for the patient. The patient's selective hearing may require repetition of instructions. Initial shock may necessitate supportive interaction as the patient gropes with the idea of cancer, which in our culture is still almost synonymous with death.

If surgery or diagnostic tests have confirmed the presence of cancer, the patient is not ready for teaching until he has worked through denial of the illness, anxiety, regression, and depression.

The first article deals with general patient reactions to the diagnosis of cancer and the approaches the nurse can take to enable the patient to negotiate the accompanying shock. Francis discusses the common emotional stages experienced by persons who have cancer. She believes that deliberately keeping the patient unaware of his condition is to participate in one of the "very disrespectful games played in hospitals." She suggests helpful courses of action for the nurse and discusses a number of broad principles that apply to all cancer patients.

Before the nurse can offer any substantial support to the cancer patient, she must learn to be sure of her own feelings. Barckley offers some rare insight into an honest approach to this problem. There are no pat answers, according to Barckley, and the acceptance of this fact allows the nurse to be truly creative in her approach to each patient. There are no punches pulled, but a jolt now and then in the anticipatory period of training may help prevent the overt show of revulsion on the part of the nurse so devastating to the patient.

It is important for the nurse to appreciate in full the crisis nature of cancer diagnoses and treatment. Patient reaction, if not detected and dealt with, can take the form of prolonged depression and possibly even suicide.

In a second article, Barckley discusses the crises in cancer and how to deal with them. The way the nurse helps the patient meet the crisis of diagnosis and treatment—especially in the postsurgery or postradiation period, with the knowledge that metastasis may have closed the door to recovery—can be the beginning of rehabilitative nursing for the patient. She emphasizes the creative aspects of nursing in her statement, "The nurse helps during this difficult period by doing all the ordinary tasks of nursing in an extraordinary way, by adding her own special, personal quality of caring."

The human being prizes his ability to control. The primary control is over the functions of his own body. The person who must surrender one of the earliest-learned control functions—that of elimination—faces a devastating loss of self-esteem as he sees himself as different from other people. Social participation diminishes as control over one's feces and urine diminish. The nurse assists the patient by maintaining a noncritical attitude, and by accepting the patient's grief and depression over his loss of sphincter control. She helps him by establishing a relationship through which he can receive teaching when he is ready.

Dyk and Sutherland studied twenty-nine men and twenty-eight women patients who had undergone colostomy. They had survived for five years after surgery and were free of recurrent disease (cancer). Questions centered on preoperative adjustment in areas of sex, work, and social life, and on postoperative adaptations in similar areas, in addition to information on the stress of the preoperative period, surgery, and its aftermath. Significant relationships were found between the quality of husband-wife relationships prior to the operation and the degree of acceptance of the colostomy.

Frenay has written of the holistic and dynamic approach to the person for whom the experience of an ileal conduit is necessary. The portion of the article concerned with preoperative care indicates the delicate processes in which the nurse must participate with the patient and his family. The postoperative care in particular demands that the holistic approach be completely individualized to help the patient face the reality of his altered body. Rehabilitation follows surgery and must be kept in the forefront of the nursing care plan. Teaching will be required for the care of the ileal conduit, which will necessitate frequent attention. In addition to the skill required in maintaining elimination through this means will be the skill needed to adjust to a social world again without fear or shame. "To foster an optimistic attitude does not minimize the patient's problems or deny their existence." This is a task for continuous nursing care—in the office, the hospital, and the home.

The patient with cancer of the breast usually goes to the physician for confirmation of suspicious symptoms. She faces a possibility before she has allowed anyone else to share her suspicions with her; this possibility is that of cancer and with it, the loss of an important source of feminine identification, or loss of life itself, or both. Treatment involves grave physical problems which require skilled nursing care. Gribbons and Aliapoulios have discussed this area of nursing care in detail as well as referral to the community agencies which can help the patient at the time of discharge from the hospital.

Bard and Sutherland have offered many insights into another area; i.e., the psychological problems of the mastectomy patient. Twenty white women, ages 28 to 58, who had had radical mastectomies were seen during their preoperative and postoperative period. The nurse who cares for the patient during the postsurgery period must listen with the third ear and be very sensitive to nonverbal communication in order to answer the questions the patient must have answered if she is to leave the hospital and assume her usual role in the family and community. While it is true that the patient may need little by way of physical care, she has a real need for an understanding person who can continue to help her when she is in her own home. The nurse who visits in the home can help in the adjustments which will take place at this point. The mastectomy becomes a part of a larger context which is the adaptation of the patient following a crisis—or in facing death.

Two articles on laryngectomy have been included, giving respectively the standpoint of a nurse and of a speech therapist. Pitorak, the nurse, offers an excellent discussion of the postoperative care of the patient with a laryngectomy. It is during this time that the patient sees himself mirrored in the face of his nurse and family as they adjust to his silence. Every nursing event is a teaching process during which a new way of breathing and communicating must be learned. Inherent in every nursing event is the process of rehabilitation—or the converse, which is the nursing-care plan that does not include all the physical and emotional problems with which the nurse must concern herself.

Adler writes from the viewpoint of the speech therapist. His concern is also the patient's foremost concern—communication. Preoperative preparation is the first step. There may be no speech therapist in the team at this particular time, but this lack must not deprive the patient of the necessary information and support which is needed. The family must be prepared for the event and assisted in their adjustment to new ways of communication which will enhance the patient's self-esteem. The section on tracheostomy hygiene—both mental and physical—with the new handicap is especially well written for nurses. As in all the mutilating procedures, it is necessary to remember that few patients are ready to assume full responsibility for their care when they are physically ready to leave the hospital. Continuity of care in the home helps to ensure that rehabilitation will take place.

The care of the adolescent with leukemia offers a challenge to nurses, since frequently they have only recently passed that particular period in their own lives. The prospect of death as the final outcome is ever present, and each exacerbation leads to increased anxiety on the part of the staff. The patient is usually fully aware of the consequences, but youth is youth and each one clings to the fine thread of life, savoring each moment. It is rare that any one institution will have a ward for teenagers such as the one described in Vernick and Lunceford's article. However, the underlying assumption prompting the kinds of care which made life meaningful for the leukemia patient should lead to general principles which underlie the care of any patient with cancer. A normal existence is maintained as far as possible with fun and responsibilities. The patient is encouraged to talk, and his physician is frank in the answering of questions. Most important, the staff is encouraged to discuss their feelings. Death of teenage friends is presented as a problem, and two solutions are offered. While the adolescent is the focus of the article, any nurse caring for a patient will find implications to assist in her own nursing-care plan. The principles of openness and maintaining a normal existence in the face of threat are implicit throughout the article and should be implicit in the nursing-care plan.

In those cases where a patient must have a new outlet constructed to replace the urinary bladder, the nurse's constant presence preoperatively may help to establish a relationship in which the patient can have hope in the complete alteration in a body function. After breathing, elimination is probably the physiological function of which he is most aware. Under cortical control from infancy, this function has social and cultural implications which separate it from the more generally socially accepted processes. Its anatomical proximity with the organs of reproduction acquires for it a perceptual ambiguity which in our culture is often characterized by social taboos.

Reading 52
Cancer: The Emotional Component
Gloria M. Francis

How do people with cancer think and feel? The deceptively simple answer is, it depends. It depends on the answers to a number of questions. Does the individual know he has cancer? If he knows, how long has he known? Has the cancer metastasized? Has there been radical surgery? What characterizes his basic personality? And, what are the attitudes of the attending staff? There are other factors, to be sure, but the point is that the emotional component in persons with cancer is relative.

Although this thesis is widely accepted, there are those who speak of the "cancer personality" and view the emotional component as less relative and more absolute.

The concept of a cancer personality presupposes that persons with certain personalities have a predisposition for cancer. Le Shan, for example, writes that the patient who has cancer has always been concerned with the "establishment of control over things," and is one-sided, rigid, orderly, and relatively inflexible [1]. Disease strikes him when some particular object, over which he has had control, seems to have been irretrievably lost. Those who subscribe to the psychoanalytic school of thought would term this an anal personality. In this basic personality type some characteristics of the first three years of life persist to adulthood in various disguised and sublimated forms. These disguised characteristics are usually observed in the adult as excessive orderliness, frugality and tightness with money, stubbornness, and persistence. One can understand how such a person needs to exercise control over things. He likes to have things his way.

Another idea about cancer and personality is expressed by Dunbar, who says that in cancer "the wrong kind of cells run wild in the body. The patient has lost the ability to have his mind maintain control of his body. . . ." [2]. This may seem far out to some, but there is accumulating evidence that, indeed, the body is the servant of the mind. We humans apparently have an unbelievable and vastly underdeveloped mind potential. This thought, along with the powerful autonomic nervous system that literally connects mind and body, precludes the possibility of taking any mind-body concept too lightly.

Practicing nurses, however, need to be more pragmatic, and in planning care they need to gather facts, analyze and interpret them, and then decide what their action will be. It is best to put aside the cancer personality idea

Reprinted from *The American Journal of Nursing*, vol. 69, no. 8, pp. 1677–1681, August 1969.

and examine the emotional component from a more practical frame of reference—how people with cancer think and feel.

One can never go wrong in applying what one knows to be common psychological reactions to physical illness [3]. Most persons faced with illness, or its imminent prospect, pass through a predictable sequence of behavior.

First there is, almost always, denial of the illness, or at least of its seriousness. This might only be a passing moment, as when an otherwise healthy person coming down with a cold says, "Oh, it's nothing."

When acceptance of the illness does come and one realizes he is sick, denial gives way to overt anxiety. Anxiety is energy and it must go somewhere. Anxiety aroused by physical illness is usually handled by its being channeled into more infantile behavior. One hears, "He's such a baby when he's sick."

The third stage is regression, characterized by clinging and dependence on family, physician, nurse, or all three. Lay persons might describe this regression as "having slipped backwards" or "having given up."

Depression is the fourth stage in the natural sequence. It is seen as lowered self-esteem, insomnia, anorexia, a general loss of interest in family, friends, and the things that usually catch one's interest. Following these natural stages the emotionally healthy person begins to achieve realistic adaptation to the illness and to any limitations imposed by it.

These phenomena occur in all illnesses to a lesser or greater degree. In this respect persons with cancer are not different, emotionally, from other patients. Why do some patients, including many cancer patients, continue to deny their illness, sometimes right up until they die? Why do some remain in an anxious state? Why do some remain regressed, helpless psychological invalids? And why do some become depressed and even attempt suicide? The answers depend in part upon the variables mentioned earlier and will help to explain why some patients remain more or less in one of the four natural stages of physical illness, and others do not.

Of course, the one broad answer is that emotionally healthy persons, even those with cancer, will not remain in one stage but will progress to a realistic adaptation to illness. Man possesses an innate force which moves him toward growth and health. This force is inherent, but can be impeded by an individual's emotional set. As the perceived severity of illness increases, the changes of emotional turmoil increase. Most people view a diagnosis of cancer as one of great severity.

DOES HE KNOW?

In trying to determine the patient's view of his illness, the first key question then is, is he aware of his diagnosis? The answer can be one key to the emotional component in persons with cancer. I believe that, in general, the patient should know he has cancer. The human organism has built-in mechanisms to deal with painful reality; the gaps left by an absence of facts will be put into some kind of believable framework by the patient. Man is a rational being. By nature he tries to make sense out of his environment. Keep the facts from him and he is likely to fill in the empty spaces with something conjured up from his imagination. It is often more frightening than the truth.

"But," asks someone, "isn't it sometimes more kind not to tell patients?" Those "sometimes" are rare. When the rationale is examined closely, it frequently contains a defense for the health worker who must do the telling. The question then follows, "more kind for whom?"

Patients who are kept unaware of their diagnoses are only unaware as far as we know. "Who is the best at pretending," is one of the very disrespectful games played in hospitals [4]. The staff think they are sparing the patient untold misery by pretending, while the patient thinks he is sparing the staff endless discomfort by playing along. And so it goes for weeks and months. Each party carries the same burden when it could be shared, and thereby be reduced for both parties.

Now assume the patient has been given appropriate facts and is aware of his diagnosis. He might cry, become hysterical, angry, depressed, withdrawn. On the other hand, he might call upon his resources and experience a very meaningful personality reintegration at a higher level of emotional functioning than ever before. Most persons are reasonably emotionally healthy individuals. They want to know. They need to know. They have things to do, plans to make, and unfinished business to attend to.

Back to those persons who have less than healthy reactions to an awareness of the diagnosis of cancer. They run the gamut from hysteria to withdrawal; some even commit suicide. Such persons are usually manifesting unresolved conflicts and fears that have been underground all along. The words, "You have a malignant tumor of the stomach," become the precipitating event that triggers a reaction that very possibly had its roots in childhood. It is not too unsound to say that years of bottled-up feelings might welcome an event which will permit its legitimate expression. Such dynamic forces usually operate outside the patient's awareness.

HOW LONG HAS HE KNOWN?

The second of our key questions is concerned with the length of time the patient has been aware of his diagnosis. If he has just learned of it, he may show many of the reactions described above. If he has been aware of his cancer for months, even years, the reasonably emotionally healthy person will have made a realistic adaptation. He will feel good about himself and other people, particularly his family and the attending staff, and he will do whatever everyday tasks of living he is physically able to do. It is likely that such a person views his cancer as a chronic disease, not a death warrant, which is a realistic way to view many malignant tumors today.

What about the emotional component in the less than healthy person who is aware he has cancer? The knowledge that he has cancer will precipitate great anxiety, and he will handle it the way he usually handles anxiety. Depending upon his basic personality he will probably remain in one of the four natural stages of illness.

Denial

If the patient becomes stuck in the otherwise normal period of denial, he will not usually express it verbally since denial operates unconsciously. He will unwittingly act it out. He might refuse surgery, chemotherapy, or radiation. Why should he go through extra stress? There is nothing wrong with him, he thinks. So he could be a general nuisance in the hospital by not accepting his role of patient. How can he be a patient when he thinks there is nothing wrong with him?

What does one do? Generally speaking, accept him. Because denial is an unconscious mechanism, appealing to his conscious mind is useless. If he chooses to exercise his privilege of refusing medical and nursing care, one can only perform what palliative measures are acceptable to him. Denial, like all other mental mechanisms, defends the conscious self; take this defense away and vulnerability to more pathological expression results. Care, therefore, would be based on an analysis of the particular behavior. If unmet needs can be identified, meeting them will diminish the patient's anxiety and his need to deny will begin to dissipate.

Anxiety

The person who becomes stuck in the second psychological stage of physical illness—overt anxiety—may show much motor restlessness and vague apprehension. Free-floating anxiety is not expressed in disguised forms. It remains pure. There might be pacing, continual movement in bed, wringing of the hands, urinary frequency, inability to concentrate, and, often, quite a bit of talking, usually in the form of questions. The feeling of apprehension is also expressed directly. Patients often say, "I'm so nervous. I wish I could relax. I can't stay still."

It is not too common to find patients remaining in this stage for as long as they sometimes remain in any of the other three stages. So-called pure, or free-floating, anxiety is painfully hard to bear, and one's natural defenses against anxiety quickly go to work and channel it into hidden forms.

Regression

A common means of handling the anxiety aroused by physical illness is regression. It is a partial and symbolic return to more infantile patterns of reacting and can probably be remembered from personal illness. One becomes more baby-like, more dependent on others; whether bed rest is indicated or not, one often retreats to bed. It is easy to see the tremendous natural benefit to the reestablishment of physical health in this phase. The individual thinks, "O.K., so I'm sick. I'm going to bed and someone can wait on me. I'll take an extra blanket, two aspirins, hot tea, and it would be nice if you'd sit in here and read so I don't have to be alone." The body is at rest, however, which is the best state for it during illness.

Depression

A feeling of dejection and sadness of a pathologic degree is termed depression. Depression that is not so deep and is not pathologic is grief. Both are reactions to a loss or a threatened loss. The mechanism which channels anxiety into depression is usually thought of as introjection, whereby the meaning a person or thing has to an individual is taken into the self and becomes part of the person. Thus, if the diagnosis of cancer or its treatment means suffering, disfigurement, pain, long hospitalization, separation from loved ones, or death, even though these things have not yet occurred, that meaning becomes part of the individual. Because of the nature of such thoughts now turned inward, the person becomes depressed. Patients pass through this normal illness stage of depression at varying speeds. A common expression from emotionally healthy persons in this stage is, "I'm sick and tired of being sick and tired." One can hear the dejection; but the fact that it is being expressed, along with the subtle wish for better things, is an indication that the person is not going to get stuck in this stage.

The person with cancer is no different from the person with any other physical illness; the difference will be in his perception of his illness. Cancer is viewed by many as a death warrant and herein lies the difference. The person who receives a diagnosis of diabetes mellitus will pass through the same stages of illness, but because diabetes is not viewed as terminal, this person is much less likely to remain in one of the four stages. The other factor, of course, is the emotional health of the person who has the physical illness. The less healthy he is emotionally, the more likely he is to remain in one of the stages.

Like the individual stuck in the period of denial, those who remain in the stages of regression or depression also need to be accepted as they are. This a hackneyed term, but it implies that the patients are not acting like babies or sitting around moping in order to irritate the staff. The behavior is unconsciously motivated and must be accepted. The next step is also the same as with the person who is denying his illness. Observe the behavior, collect data, and search for the cause.

One apparently unmet need of the regressed individual is the need to be dependent. So wait on him and meet some of his dependency needs, thereby helping him toward greater independence. The same applies to the depressed patient. An additional guideline for this stage is that the nurse needs to be decisive, assertive, and matter-of-fact. Depressed persons have little energy. They cannot make decisions and they do not care enough to make them. Do for them whatever they will not or cannot do for themselves. Make decisions for them without asking "what," "how," or "when." Decide what is best and do it.

HAS IT SPREAD?

The third question relevant to how persons with cancer think and feel focuses on whether or not there is metastasis. Assuming that the tumor is inoperable and the patient is aware of it, the question then becomes: what is the meaning of death to this person? Some, consumed by fear of death, disintegrate emotionally; others retain their emotional integrity and face death with equanimity. When I look for a reason for the difference I turn to the concept of the psychoanalyst Erik Erikson. He postulated the well-known "Eight Ages of Man," the eighth being maturity [5].

The mature individual will feel complete, whole, and satisfied; he will have successfully achieved the tasks of the other seven ages. Erikson calls this achievement *ego integrity*. Basic psychologic needs will have been met sufficiently all along the way. As an infant he will have learned to trust; as a toddler he will have experienced autonomy; as a preschooler he will have been freed to experience initiative; and so on through the ages. Having had reasonably healthy emotional development, he will reach adulthood feeling good about himself and will be able to look back on his life and think, "It has been good." The thought of death does not carry a sting for such persons.

Those who are terribly afraid of death, however, look back and realize that they are not ready. Instead of having achieved integrity, they may experience disgust and despair. They may feel they produced little good or happiness in the lives they have touched. They may not have trusted—the very first developmental task of life—and a life without trust is empty. How would they have really loved another person? They feel there is unfinished business in their lives and are simply not ready to die; yet, death is near. When they are threatened they may become hysterical, angry, or depressed or may lash out, depending on their pattern.

One can be sure that the person who does not feel complete and is facing death will also feel indescribably frightened, lonely, and abandoned. For such a person, to have another just spend time with him is probably the most helpful and comforting experience. Abandonment is a particular fear of many persons with terminal illness. However, as he gets to know and depend on visits from another, he will talk about himself. The nurse, when she is that other, can, by listening intently, discern the little things that can be done for him. It might just be helping him to write to a brother whom he has not spoken to for years.

HAS HE HAD RADICAL SURGERY?

The fourth question about how a person with cancer thinks and feels has to do with radical surgery. Somehow radical surgery, such as hemipelvectomy or radical head and neck surgery, does not usually have its impact until after the fact. The depressive reactions that occur frequently as a result of body disfigurement represent a mourning for the lost parts. The reaction is also related to the expectation of rejection and fear of separation from loved ones. Following a loss of anything one naturally feels depressed. Losing a leg, a breast, or half a face is no different, dynamically, from losing a child through death. A loss is a loss. Again, if the person is reasonably emotionally healthy, he will experience transient feelings of depression as part of the normal grieving process. No one should try to talk him out of it or cheer him up.

WHAT IS HIS BASIC PERSONALITY?

The fifth key question is concerned with the patient's basic personality. How a person perceives a stimulus, in this case the diagnosis of cancer, is determined by his or her past experience. An emotionally healthy young man might be thankful that he has had at least one year of married life with the girl he loved all through high school, and may well be able to make a realistic adaptation. He might feel sad, yet thankful. Life, though limited, is still life. A selfish, immature, middle-aged woman might feel this is just one more blow that God has dealt her. She might feel angry. She might punish others, including staff, because she has to be the one.

HOW DOES STAFF ACT?

The last of our key questions is involved with the attitudes of staff toward the patient. Regardless of the emotional health of the patient, the staff can affect him for better or for worse. If the attitude is one of secrecy, the patient has to expend energy in coping with the unknown. The patient should know where he stands, what alternatives he has, and what is coming next. The nurse needs to be careful when she blames secrecy on the physician. More often than not she is in the secret with him. If a nurse has a hunch the patient needs or wants to know more, she should talk with the physician about it. She can offer to help with the difficult task of talking with the patient, as many physicians are no more comfortable at dealing directly with the truth than are many nurses.

Another attitude that is helpful to the patient takes into consideration his desire for a realistic approach from staff. False assurance is one of the most disrespectful attitudes a professional person can have and will hinder the patient in learning to cope with reality. The young girl who is no longer pretty following head and neck surgery will not believe anyone who tells her falsely that she is. It can be indicated to her, however, that reconstructive surgery offers great results, and she can be helped to focus on her remaining assets. If chemotherapy is temporarily halting tumor growth, no one should talk of a cure, but rather, that cell growth has been slowed or stopped as of now. When the truth has been distorted, it is more often to meet the needs of staff than of patients.

A hopeful but realistic attitude will result in the most useful psychological environment for the patient.

Patients also need to feel good about themselves and they need to be as busy as their condition permits. When one is productive, an hour slips by rapidly, but when one has nothing in his mind but thoughts of his own unfortunate state of affairs, an hour is an eternity. Generally, the more real work and the less entertainment for distraction provided, the better the patient will feel about himself. Coming up with the useful job is left to nursing creativity. Are there new charts to be put together? Could he "special" sicker patients? Could he do anything in the utility room? Could the bed patient make favors for the children's trays?

Helping patients to feel better about themselves can also be accomplished through direct work on the patient's appearance. No man should be allowed to go without shaving daily. If he is too depressed to bother, it should be done for him. Nor should a woman go without combing her hair and putting on makeup. As soon as patients can stay up, for instance after surgery, shoes and street clothes can be worn—nothing says sick, weak, and dependent like hospital gowns and paper slippers.

These three approaches—being honest, realistic, and creative in helping patients feel better about themselves—are some of the more useful attitudes of staff caring for patients with cancer. They alone might bring out the best, might accentuate the person's emotional strengths.

The nurse has almost complete control over some emotional components that are manifested by patients who have cancer. Others can be altered through knowledgeable nurse action. Obviously, though one can apply broad concepts, care must be highly individualized.

REFERENCES

1. Le Shan, L. Psychological states as factors in the development of malignant disease. *J. Nat. Cancer Inst.,* **22**:1-18, January 1959.
2. Dunbar, Flanders. *Mind and Body.* rev. ed. New York, Random House, 1955, p. 239.
3. Holland, Bernard C., and Ward, R. S. Homeostasis and psychosomatic medicine, in *American Handbook of Psychiatry,* ed. by Silvano Arieti. New York, Basic Books, 1966, vol. 3, p. 359.
4. Glaser, B. G., and Strauss, A. L. *Awareness of Dying.* Chicago, Ill., Aldine Publishing Co., 1955, p. 64.
5. Erikson, E. H. *Childhood and Society.* New York, W. W. Norton and Co., 1963, p. 247.

Reading 53

What Can I Say to the Cancer Patient?

Virginia Barckley

Mahatma Gandhi once made a speech in the British Parliament after which he was congratulated—with reservations—by Churchill. "Why don't you lighten your talk a little?" he said. "It was so somber." Mahatma Gandhi replied, "Sir, I am the protagonist of people who have nothing to laugh about." The nursing of cancer patients is a somber topic, too, but it has a wealth of interest for us.

How does the patient with cancer feel? What are his worries, his fears, his hopes? First, he is in a dramatic situation. His life is threatened, and often he has surgery of a profound type which, happily, he knows little about. We realize that human beings are capable of tremendous heroism, when confronted by emergencies; to be brave, to be noble in a situation that is not prolonged is within our capacities. To be courageous over a period of years is different, more difficult. Most patients with cancer need to be heroes every day. Small wonder that many of them fail.

Reprinted from *Nursing Outlook* vol. 6, no. 6, pp. 316-318, June 1958.

Often this failure takes the form of regression. Nurses sometimes are baffled by the inappropriate behavior of men or women in their sixties. "They act like children!" they say, and this is true. These patients find the present too hard to bear and so they revert to childishness as a refuge. They turn their backs on today and seek the yesterday when the world was a pleasanter, easier place to live in. If their worlds have become fearful, what are the things that made them so?

Patients fear the loss of money a long illness brings, the loss of their jobs. "Will they want me back at the office with a colostomy?" they ask themselves. They fear the loss of friends, of loved ones. Women may think that after a mastectomy their husbands will no longer admire them, and those with laryngectomies may wonder when they will again participate in a social evening with their old companions. All patients fear disfigurement, for this is a threat to the body image they hold of themselves and it is closely bound up with their feelings of self-respect. Most of us long ago decided to make the best of our far from beautiful faces, but to have onlookers shudder because of extensive head and neck surgery is an experience we would dread.

UNDERSTANDING—THE DIFFICULT ART

How genuine are these fears? Many of them stem from what we call reality situations. It is a bleak fact that many cancer patients will have to endure great physical anguish; it is a fact that often great expense is involved; it is a fact that long periods of not working are especially hard for those with ambition or a profound sense of family responsibility. It may also be true that friends will grow impatient or indifferent, that husbands or wives will find other interests. How, then, can we help our patients?

Not, certainly, by the false cheery assurances that many of us are wont to employ from kind but mistaken motives. "You haven't a thing to worry about—you look just fine!" deceives only ourselves. "Why, you are just a gold brick—you'll be up in no time!" is not what the patient needs either. Although we must not weep with our patients, we should let them know that we realize they are in a hard situation and that we feel for them.

When we respond to patients in any other way we are, in effect, saying their worries are trifling, that we, in similar circumstances would not be affected by them. Belittling any human being never pays off. Even if the fears expressed seem groundless to us, or neurotic in origin as sometimes they are, we must remember that that fear is just as sound and logical to the person experiencing it as any one derived from actuality. The important thing to understand is that it *is* real to the patient.

To nurses, this knowledge has special meaning which may be applied to pain, too. If I have an infected tooth, and you have an ache for which no organic cause can be found, then you are suffering too. This is the difference: my distress can be alleviated in one minute by extraction or drainage, but yours will not yield so readily. If the cause is emotional, relief may be a long process.

We alienate our patients by diverting their attention with a bright quip or a funny story when they are deeply troubled. We make them feel alone in their suffering, that they are surrounded by people who simply don't care about them or try to understand them. This drives them deeper within themselves. Are we, then, to be gloomy? Or worse, are we to be amateur psychiatrists? Neither one. Our role, as the professional person closest to the patient most of the time, is to be kind in a thoughtful way. Sometimes a simple remark, "It *must* be hard," or "I can see that this isn't easy for you" is sufficient, for this in no way robs the patient of his dignity—we are telling him he isn't a complainer, he isn't a bore, he is just a person in trouble.

Refusing to listen to a patient describe his feelings by rushing away, interrupting, kidding, or diverting him may be done from good motives, but it isn't effective. Everyone needs an audience. To listen attentively may sound like elementary advice, but when we let our patients relieve themselves through talking we help them more than we know. Through sharing, we dilute our misery. Is there any one of us who hasn't experienced this in some way? If someone has hurt or ridiculed you, doesn't it ease the pangs to tell your best friend about it? Conversely, let us all try to remember one time in our lives of deepest trouble. Would it have helped then to have had someone tell you a joke? I think you know the answer.

NO PAT ANSWERS, NO PRESCRIPTIONS

If patients have problems, their families cannot escape involvement. To know that a greatly loved relative is doomed to great pain, and eventually to death, is a special dilemma for which there are no prescriptions. Another kind of distress arises from the absence of what families think they should feel at such a time. All people are not equally lovable; some parents do no more for children than to produce them, yet many times the guilt these children feel at not honoring their parents is all-consuming. The solicitude of some families, the complete lack of it in others, are both normal reactions. We can help the families in both groups by accepting their feelings.

Many times doctors and nurses complain that relatives are "always in the way," "forever fussing," or "too demanding." Are they just where they should be—close to a loved person who is suffering? Are their requests exactly what ours would be were the roles changed? Are their "demands" simply clutching at any straw to alleviate an unhappy situation? We lose our irritation when we know why people do what they do. If we see what it is that lies behind the forbidding facade, it no longer stings or goads us so much that we cannot move ahead.

Finally, the nurse who cares for a cancer patient has many problems; the answers are in no book. Most of us respond to the appeal of obstetrics, of sick children, and the intense drama of surgery. We are sustained by a sense of accomplishment in our difficult role when a patient's life is in jeopardy following operation. We know that our prompt reporting, our keen discernment, our accuracy can contribute to the salvaging of a life. In caring for a cancer patient, as with other chronically ill patients, this excitement, this immediate reward is missing. Instead, there is hard work, often with little hope for the patient's recovery.

This can be, however, the most challenging of all nursing. For example, many patients who die at home are cared for by the public health nurse who sees them suffer interminably, go by inches. She must make them comfortable with little help, few appliances, and often a dearth of necessities. What does she do when a man's hand and arm weigh almost as much as his wasted body? She puts his arm on a pillow, but soon he is tired of this. She then places it in a sling, but this, too, is quickly intolerable. Next she devises an overbed table to rest it on—but then what?

Superlative skill is required; the knowledge, experience, and imagination of one nurse are sorely taxed. To combine nursing arts with empathy and understanding implies professional status neither quickly nor easily attained. Like certain soldiers who have enormous pride in their regiments, perhaps we should have some special insigne for those who see the possibilities in cancer nursing, something that says, "I'm in chronic disease nursing, one of the most difficult spots of all!"

THE WORDS WILL COME

How do we talk to our patients? What do we say when they tell us their pain is increasing? Here, again, if we listen they may be helpful to us; we may learn how to make them comfortable. To brush their complaints aside with a routine "It'll be better tomorrow" is not worthy of us. Could we say instead, "Tell me just how you feel. Perhaps together we can think of a better position for you," or "I know you had a bad night. Will you let me try something new (I'm speaking here of nursing measures, of course) and tell me if it helps?" Then your patients know you are sincerely interested. Assured by your manner, some of their tensions decrease, their sedatives are more effective, and their pain is reduced.

In nursing we have a profound need to comfort, to clarify, to expatiate through words. One reason for this is very simple—juxtaposition. Nurses are, most often, the professional people who are *there*. In cancer nursing the art of communication is especially vital. Patients who know their diagnosis often want to discuss what Browning called this "last, great adventure," and a frequent question is, "Nurse, am I going to die?"

The concern of nurses over this query does them credit; that they are unsure of themselves in this sensitive area is not strange. The answer is, of course, that there can be no standard reply. Each patient has a different background, feelings, and aspirations—what satisfies one will harass or mystify another. Because we are all unique, each question deserves an individual response.

What we must do first, before we can talk about imminent death, is to know how we ourselves regard it. Our patients need comfort and courage, and in the absence of a spiritual adviser, surely this is our province. If we find this topic fraught with fear and horror then we can offer little better than gaudy bravado or a quick change of subject when it is mentioned. Neither is helpful.

Is it the cessation of all we know that we fear? Many of us have already lived through more harsh experiences than death, and some of us, in times of deep anguish, have wished for death as preferable to the heavy loads life imposed upon us. Surely to the old and friendless, to the suffering, to parents who have shared the dishonor of their children who committed cruel and senseless crimes, death must come as a friend. Although we cannot control its timing, few of us would want to live forever.

Nothing is more certain than that death will some day come to all of us. Does this knowledge make it so much harder to bear, so impossible even to contemplate? Perhaps this advance notice is something precious, a time to be closer to loved ones, to be more aware of beauty, to cherish friendships, to forgive old grudges, to experience more vividly every nuance in life and feeling.

Those last months may be a sort of second chance for the patient who now realizes there are no more years to squander, that this is a period to put home and business in order, to say or do the kind things he has deferred in the past. That many patients afflicted with cancer have found courage and serenity in their last months of life we know from reading—in the prospect of death the present assumed a new meaning.

This adjustment is expressed in a sonnet written by a doctor who was doomed with leukemia, beginning:

Now is death merciful. He calls me hence
Gently, with friendly soothing of my fears
Of ugly age and feeble impotence
And cruel disintegration of slow years![1]

---

[1] Hans Zinsser's sonnets.

If we are very sure of our own feelings, if we have some central core of philosophy to rely on, then this is reflected in our manner with patients. The precise phrases we use, when we have empathy, are not important. We need not learn a speech, for the words will come.

WISDOM IN HONESTY

When desperately ill patients are concerned about themselves is it really helpful to tell them they are progressing? Whether or not they know the diagnosis, most of them realize from the physical signs that the situation is grave. A nurse need not be a crepe hanger if she answers the doleful comment "I guess I'm terribly sick," "You *are* sick. That's why I'm here to help you." Her exact words are not nearly as important as her manner, her voice, the expression on her face. If these are sympathetic, if she radiates warmth, if she has empathy for her patient, the words will be acceptable.

How do we feel about the woman down the hall who is doing beautifully after a hysterectomy but who is determined to run every nurse she sees to a shadow? She may be one who has always been plain, who has never been loved, whose life has never been interesting or rewarding to her. Now she is the center of attention. Doctors listen when she speaks, she receives flowers and cards, she has been the central figure in the drama of surgery. She simply can't resist prolonging her day in the sun. She is the eternal child who calls "Mother—watch me!" As nurses, let us be big about this. Let her have her ball.

Have we considered the age of most of our cancer patients? It is predominantly a disease of the middle or later years. Now it is a human trait to cling to the delusion that we are indestructible. While we are young we never consider ourselves in the role of grandparents, and until the very end of our lives we reject the idea subconsciously that we shall die. Yet midway in life we are forced to conclude that our eyes and our joints have changed. This time of failing physical powers often is accompanied by other distresses—we aren't as sure as we were of our jobs, of the success of a marriage, we no longer plan ahead with the old verve, we no longer dream the dreams of youth.

Our patients often receive the diagnosis of cancer in their middle years when life is no longer at its first high peak. This is the reason why some of them defer the physical examination that might have revealed their condition earlier. They simply don't feel up to the trip to the doctor's, or to making the arrangements. This is a time of increased interest in the body, and that is with good reason, for life is often threatened then. Women may become morbidly interested in symptoms as their families leave home and they find themselves without role or purpose.

Knowing this, it is not always enough to tell a patient after a physical examination, "You do not have cancer." He may need interpretation and help of a different type, based on wide knowledge of his whole background. Perhaps, one day, cancer detection clinics will add this to their existing functions.

WOMEN, NOT ANGELS

Sometimes nurses are revolted by the nature of the service required by cancer patients. This is understandable. Who could say it is pleasant to care for the noxious geyser that so unexpectedly spouts from a colostomy? The last dressing has scarcely been adjusted when the whole sticky mass once again clings to the sheets, the nightgown, the pubic hair. Of course this tries the nurse's patience—but it is much worse for the person who endures it. When revulsion is replaced by compassion, when we think, "What can I do to help?" instead of "Poor me!" we are functioning on a high level.

Cancer nursing is often tiresome and discouraging. We find it irritating or even infuriating at times, for we are women and not angels. But it is deeply rewarding to give service to those who are suffering; it is a privilege to be close to people who need us so desperately. There is both beauty and excitement in this work, and in the discovery of it we become worthy of man's great heart and brain; without this appreciation and response the spinal cord would be sufficient.

Reading 54
Adaptation of the Spouse and Other Family Members to the Colostomy Patient
Ruth B. Dyk
and
Arthur M. Sutherland

DISCUSSION

"Home is the place where when you come they have to take you in." The family has universally been recognized as the agency for protection of the aged and infirm and the care of the sick. This basic function is true of all cultures, though the manner and extent of care have varied at different periods and within different cultures [3]. Discussing the value of the family in the adaptation of the ill person in our own culture, Richardson states, ". . . on the basis of experience with our families; without some sort of unified family life the possibility of individual adjustment is remote" [4].

The medical profession tends to assume that posthospital, convalescent care will be automatically undertaken by the family and that emotional needs will also be adequately met. Unfortunately, these assumptions are not always justified. The care that family and spouses can give may be very limited, not only by real deficits, but also by the nature of the relationship within the family.

The nature and quality of family care is determined by the nature and quality of the preoperative relationship. The operation and its residuals merely introduce new factors that must be integrated into a continuum of existing relationships. The family's response to the patient's needs does not occur in a vacuum. It is profoundly modified by the longstanding relationships between its members and the patient. The operation does not set up new relationships superseding all others.

Moreover, the meaning of the operation or its residuals to each family member is an important determinant of his response to the patient's needs. There may be strong feelings of disgust or revulsion at the colostomy and its function, or fear of cancer, or a more diffuse disgust at body mutilation. Fragile relationships can thus be seriously disrupted. Strong preoperative relationships can usually overcome even strong negative feelings. The meaning of the operation and its sequels must be integrated into a dynamic relationship among the patient, the spouse, and the members of the family.

The nature of the family's response postoperatively is consistent with its attitudes during the time of onset of symptoms, the visits to the physician, and the surgical experience. One should be able to predict the extent of nursing care or emotional support to a patient that will be available from a family member, especially the spouse, from behavior and expressed feelings during the early phases of treatment. The quality of the relationship remains consistent throughout the sequence of the whole experience. The form of the expression of the relationship is related to the specific phase of the total sequence.

Supportive spouses help and encourage their mates to seek and accept adequate and prompt medical care. They conceal their fears and sometimes the diagnosis and minimize the dangers of surgery. The needs of the patient take precedence over their own. They make or help to make practical arrangements for hospitalization. When the patient returns home, they put no limitation on the quality and extent of the care they give, and the patient's comfort takes precedence over their own. Much effort is directed to maintaining the patient's self-esteem.

Exclusion by the patient of the spouse from significant participation in any phase occurs mainly in those marriages in which the feelings between the marital partners appear to be ambivalent or lukewarm. Such patients are usually men. Exclusion seems usually to be based on expectations of inadequacy of response or of rejection. The spouse can not be relied on to meet dependent needs. Rather than test the limits, which are foreseen as very constricted, such patients portray themselves as not needing care, as being "independent." The pattern of exclusion or of permission of only minimal or restricted help continues throughout the entire sequence.

Such marital unions appear to be "facade" marriages. It is very difficult to determine the actual quality of the marriage, because the interviewer is presented with idealized versions of great defensiveness. The facade as a rule must be preserved, especially by men, who appear to accept the responsibility for the success or failure of marriage, apparently based on feelings in part related to adequacy of earning power.

Spouses who are not excluded, yet fail to participate in the early phases of the experience, give little help in the later phases. Physical illness of the spouse is often associated with emotional incapacity to take an active part in planning or to sustain the patient. Emotional incapacity may exist without physical incapacity. In either case, the patient can expect only minimal help from the spouse, but not rejection. Such patients are usually women who as a rule receive help in some degree from other members of the family.

In contrast to the men, these patients complain of the lack of help and of the weakness of their husbands. They present no facade, are far from defensive, and are explicit in portraying their husbands as ineffective, inept, generally incapable, and usually life-long failures. The chronic failure to provide adequate financial support is the most frequent focus of complaints. As a rule, these patients portray themselves as the dominant, effectual member of the marriage.

Some spouses, both men and women, are overtly hostile and do not participate in any phase. They are frank in their demonstrations of hostility. Not only do they give no help, but postoperatively they may add to the patient's difficulties. In such marriages there has been a long history of overt antagonism and mutual recriminations.

There is an interesting variant of hostile and rejective spouses that can easily deceive the physician. The patient is often dilatory in seeking treatment. Indifferent during the period of early symptoms, these spouses become insistent, threatening, and coercive once the seriousness of the disease becomes apparent to them, usually through medical pressure. They are active in making arrangements. They give the appearance of great interest and solicitude for the patient in the early phases, but their subsequent behavior reveals the true nature of their feelings. They give minimal or no help postoperatively and are frankly hostile and rejective. Their preoperative interest in the patient seems only to be concerned with preservation of utility values or to prevent themselves from being handicapped by sick spouses. Antagonisms throughout the marriage and hostility postoperatively are so overt that the initial interest does not appear to be a reaction formation to guilt for hostility.

Almost all patients are discharged home before the perineal wound is healed. As a rule their preoperative vigor has not been completely regained. They have not as a rule standardized their irrigating practices. Urinary incontinence is often present. Few patients can afford professional nursing care and only for the occasional patient can visiting nursing services cover all nursing contingencies. The greater part of nursing care must of necessity come from the family. Such care includes cleaning the perineal wound or helping with the act of irrigation, often done nude, and other acts of direct body care.

Not all spouses are able to give such body care. The sight of the colostomy and of the perineal wound, and the direct and protracted contact with feces and the violated body arouses such revulsion that the spouse may not be able to give body care. Some of these feelings are shared by the patients themselves, who express beliefs that such body care would be beyond that which could be expected of any except inured professional personnel or a partner in a marriage of long standing.

No spouse who is hostile, indifferent, or excluded from participation in the preoperative phase of the illness can be relied on to give such body care. The quality of the relationship between the patient and the spouse in such cases is rarely sufficient to overcome the disgust and revulsion aroused in the partner. On the other hand, those spouses who have demonstrated their real interest and concern in the patient during the preoperative phase are usually able to overcome their own feelings and give intimate, direct body care, including management of the perineal wound and aid in the act of irrigation.

The nature of the preoperative sexual relationship between male patients and their wives is a surprisingly accurate guide to the ability of the latter to give body care. Whenever wives of male patients were able relatively easily to accept sexual union preoperatively, body care is usually given and accepted. Only rarely, and then under stress, is body care given when the preoperative sexual rapport has been poor. Often the colostomy must be concealed from the wife and body care is out of the question.

In those marriages in which the preoperative sexual rapport was good and body care given freely postoperatively, the interest of the partners in each other throughout marriage appears high and does not deteriorate in the stress of their mutual learning to live with the colostomy. These marriages give evidence of having been based on mutual trust, dependence, and affection, and these qualities are intensified after surgery. During the convalescent period the balance of interdependence shifts heavily to one side and the patient appears dependent, perhaps unduly so, on the ministrations of the spouse. As a rule, this imbalance is temporary and subsequent events may show that the patient is fully able to accept, in turn, the dependent demands of the spouse. In all these marriages the partners are free in their expressions of admiration and praise for each other. They appear sure that their trust in each other is well founded, that their dependent needs will always be met, and that they will not be isolated by unacceptability.

Those marriages in which the sexual rapport has been poor and in which body care is withheld after surgery appear to have been largely unions where expectations for marriage have not been fulfilled. There are often histories of longstanding bickering and tension. In these, the men complain rather regularly of the sexual frigidity of their wives and the lack of nurturance and affection, and the wives complain of their husbands' low earning power and failure to provide as expected. Postoperative deprivation of earning power or invalidism is not easily tolerated and may be rewarded by wives with cessation of sexual intercourse. This has been observed elsewhere [2]. Female patients withdraw readily from intercourse and increased friction results. When the husband continues to provide, he may express beliefs that his life is being shortened by the rapacity of his wife.

Such marriages rarely improve through the impact of major illness or extensive surgery. Where relationships have been poor before these events they almost always deteriorate. They militate against the recovery of the patient's psychological health and tend to perpetuate psychological invalidism.

Revulsion at and rejection of the spouse's mutilated body, now "like a beast," which precludes both sexual activity and body care, is far more common in wives than in husbands. Men appear to be far less affected in their sexual and bodily relationships to their wives by the colostomy. The preoperative acceptance of sexual relations by women patients does not determine whether they receive body care postoperatively. When there has been a warm personal relationship between the spouses despite sexual "frigidity," she may expect to receive body care. Whenever the relationship has been hostile, which regularly includes sexual "frigidity" on the part of the wife, she can neither expect nor accept body care from her husband. He may continue, nevertheless, to demand sexual activity until she refuses, usually with expressions of fear of further injury to her body.

The sexual implications involved in giving and accepting body care are further suggested by the patients' preference for receiving such care from spouses and by the exclusion of children, particularly those of the opposite sex. The intimate nature of the body care precludes its being given by those persons with whom a sexual relationship is tabooed. Reluctance or refusal to expose the body to their children may also be based on the fear of appearing ugly and old, and so being rejected.

Other types of care, such as the assumption of obligations for support or maintenance, are often considered inappropriate for children. There was a general consensus that even adult children should be shielded from the parents' misfortune and that they should not be handicapped by being burdened. To some patients, assistance of any variety may be intolerable. Such attitudes are prevalent in our culture, in which value and esteem are based on maintaining independence and in which dependence creates fears of rejection or abandonment.

This basis for esteem holds true especially for men who are, in fact, regarded as failures if they cannot rely on themselves and be relied upon for support. But even for women, to whom dependence is both culturally and psychologically more acceptable, loss of esteem may be greatly feared if the parent-child relationship is reversed. Care by a daughter signifies to them a loss of control and status. It represents the oncoming of old age and the possibility of rejection and isolation. The necessity for care by children or other forms of dependence may bring into focus prematurely the problem of unacceptability and loss of esteem common to an aged or aging population.

Unfortunately, it cannot be assumed that the spouse is able to meet the emotional and physical needs of the patient or even remain neutral in the patient's attempts at adjustment. Illness in a husband or wife does not automatically call forth the best efforts in the spouse. Rather, it is a serious threat to the dynamic equilibrium of the relationship between them. How this relationship is modified by serious illness is dependent on the multitude of factors that have gone to form it and are currently active.

The patterns of adaptation to illness and the colostomy evolved by the patient are never independent of this relationship, which shapes even minute details in those patterns. It is, therefore, a powerful force for good or evil. The spouse is often the key to the patient's success or failure in adapting himself to his disability.

REFERENCES

1. Anshen, R. N. (ed.): *The Family: Its Function and Destiny.* New York, Harper & Bros., 1949.
2. Ginzberg, E.: *The Unemployed.* New York, Harper & Bros., 1943.
3. Kluckhohn, C.: Variations in the human family, in Anon.: *The Family in a Democratic Society.* Anniversary Papers of the Community Service Society of New York. New York, Columbia University Press, 1949, pp. 3-11.
4. Richardson, H. B.: *Patients Have Families.* New York, The Commonwealth Fund, 1945, p. 268.

5 Sutherland, A. M., Orbach, C. E., Dyk, R. B., and Bard, M.: *The psychological impact of cancer and cancer surgery.* I. Adaptation to the dry colostomy; Preliminary report and summary of findings. *Cancer,* **5**:857-872, 1952.

Reading 55
A Dynamic Approach to the Ileal Conduit Patient
Sister M. Agnes Clare Frenay

Dynamic patient care considers the motivational forces affecting the patient's behavior. It seeks to discover the reasons for his actions, interactions, and reactions in an effort to direct them into wholesome and socially acceptable channels. The nurse who is aware of her own feelings and motivations is more likely to control and utilize them therapeutically in her approach to the patient. Through her understanding of his problems and needs which are reflected in his behavioral responses, she is able to change impersonal care into a loving, individualized service to the sick.

Biological processes, altered by disease and surgical intervention, tend to disturb the dynamic balance between the forces of body and mind. Before the nurse can assist the patient in restoring this balance to a state of normalcy, she must understand his condition, the surgeon's operative goals, and her own role in promoting his recovery.

The patient undergoing surgery for ileal conduit is in great need of dynamic nursing care. This operation is done to divert the urine away from an incapacitated bladder to an isolated ileal segment which promptly channels it through a cutaneous stoma into an ileostomy appliance.

Diagnostic evaluation consisting of a series of cystoscopic examinations and urograms must provide convincing evidence that bladder damage is irreversible and salvage of the upper urinary tract from recurrent ascending infection can only be accomplished by surgery. In neurological patients, cystometrography usually reveals a spastic bladder with high intravesical pressure and low volume. Candidates for an elective ileal conduit may be children with congenital sacrospinal cord lesions such as meningocele, myelomeningocele, or spina bifida, or they may be adults in the most productive period of life with neurogenic bladders and incontinence due to cord injury or neurological disease, or victims of vesical carcinoma with or without exenteration surgery [1].

Reprinted from *The American Journal of Nursing,* vol. 64, no. 1, pp. 80-83, January 1964.

When the patient with a neurogenic bladder is a child, incontinence is often a cause of severe psychological trauma which affects his personality development adversely. Ridicule and merciless teasing by playmates because of his urinous odor are experiences not easily forgotten. The nurse who cares for the child undergoing surgery for ileal conduit must make allowance if he seethes with hostility, screams unreasonably, is boastful or self-centered or tacit, diffident, and withdrawn. To her, this is a child with a real problem, engaged in a conflict between his innate need for recognition and the crushing realization of his inadequacy. Does he not use this behavior mechanism to force recognition and obscure his inadequacy by boasting and aggressiveness [2]? Or if his behavioral responses reveal asocial tendencies, are they not the result of unhappy experiences and a growing sense of rejection? The understanding nurse makes a special effort to capture the child's love through her genuine interest in his welfare. But she also acts with firmness when it is necessary to set limits to his behavior.

When ileal conduit is performed during the preschool age before undesirable behavior patterns have been firmly established, the child's psychological development may progress normally in years to come.

Adults undergoing surgery for ileal conduit are likely to have been troubled with a neurogenic bladder resulting in progressive incontinence for years. The cord injury or the onset of a neurological disorder, such as multiple sclerosis, may have occurred a decade or more previously. To this type of patient, surgery for ileal conduit means coping with another difficulty in the hope of getting rid of troublesome symptoms. His psychological preparation for the operation is comparatively simple.

PREOPERATIVE PREPARATION

The surgeon usually discusses the operative procedure and the expected outcomes with the patient, while the nurse further explains what was not understood and seeks to banish his doubts. The patient should know preoperatively that he will receive nothing by mouth for days. He should be impressed with the importance of deep breathing and coughing to ventilate his lungs and clear them of secretions. He must understand why he will have a nasogastric tube, continuous intravenous infusion, and an ileostomy appliance after surgery. This type of information, couched in language which he can comprehend, helps him to accept the treatment and to cooperate fully in trying moments. Knowledge engenders understanding, and understanding is the motivating force which stimulates cooperative efforts.

To establish a therapeutic relationship, the nurse must have rapport with the patient and inspire him with confidence. No matter how brave he is, he will fear surgery. The fearful patient needs more anesthetic and is more prone to develop shock than the relaxed patient who takes the inevitable in stride. Trust in God, in the skill of the surgeon and anesthesiologist will help him to overcome his feeling of insecurity.

Another vital concern is family interaction. The excited wife who rushes to the patient's bedside before he is taken to the operating room is likely to revive anxiety and apprehension in the patient who is about to feel the benefit of the premedication. The nurse, cognizant of the dynamics of emotional responses, includes the family in the preoperative psychological preparation in an effort to save the patient such a traumatizing experience. She realizes that relatives, too, are under tension. They need the support of an understanding nurse, particularly during the long hours of waiting while the patient is in surgery.

The operation for ileal conduit presents a major crisis in the patient's life. Therefore, throughout the patient's stay, dynamic nursing care must consider his psychosocial, spiritual, and physiological needs. The patient must be aware that his recovery and return home are hastened by his cooperation. Family living will be easier, social and occupational relationships more normal, and the odorous stigma of incontinence removed. Looking toward the achievement of these goals, he will be motivated to pay the price of short-lived pain and distress. His behavior will be then goal-directed and adjustive, not governed by blind impulses or frustrations.

During the patient's hospitalization, there is a reduction of gratification of basic needs. Perhaps for the first time in his life he is unable to satisfy his hunger. He is given a low-residue diet a few days before surgery, then liquids only, and finally nothing by mouth before and after surgery.

To cleanse the intestinal tract, the patient receives cathartics and enemas as needed. Enteric bacteriostatic agents such as succinylsulfathiazole (Sulfasuxidine) and neomycin sulfate virtually sterilize his bowels.

The dynamic approach to the patient is easier when the nurse has a good understanding of the surgical procedure. The details of the present method of ileal conduit have been evolved through the ingenious work of Eugene M. Bricker, professor of clinical surgery, Washington University. Essentially, it includes a dissection and mobilization of the ureters, isolation of an ileal segment, end-to-end anastomosis of the ileum, transplantation of the ureters to the ileal segment and creation of an external stoma or ileostomy for urinary drainage [3]. To perform this operation the proximal portions of the ureters must be free from cicatricial lesions [4].

Although the bladder has lost its functional capacity following an ileal conduit procedure, it is only removed in the presence of vesical carcinoma and uncontrolled bladder infection. The ileal conduit is, of course, a passageway or channel and *not* a reservoir for urine. Through constant peristaltic action, the urine entering the isolated segment moves toward the ileal stoma and passes to the exterior without being stopped by a sphincter mechanism. This prompt evacuation prevents urinary stasis in the ileal segment and its associated sequelae: hydronephrosis and pyelonephritis.

POSTOPERATIVE CARE

During the immediate postoperative period the physical aspects of dynamic nursing care take precedence. The patient is in dire need of intensive care. Communication is essentially nonverbal. The nurse's calm and competent manner, and her all-absorbing interest in his comfort and well-being, give him a feeling that he is in good hands. Her occasional word of encouragement affords him emotional support and wins his cooperation.

Assuring Adequate Drainage

The nurse's primary concern is now to maintain the adequacy of the newly created urinary drainage system. Before the patient left the operating room, a plastic ileostomy bag was glued to his skin around the stoma to receive the urine. This temporary appliance was attached by a plastic tube to a collecting bag placed far below the level of the isolated loop to encourage urinary evacuation by gravity. Normally, ileal segments empty more completely with the patient in the supine or right side-lying positions. After the blood pressure has stabilized, the patient may be placed in a semi-Fowler or sitting position to stimulate effective drainage.

To prevent urinary stasis, the nurse should check the plastic ileostomy appliance for an accumulation of urine frequently and, if necessary, manipulate the bag so it will evacuate. This is of primary importance in the prevention of postoperative complications resulting from pathogenic bacterial growth in stagnant urine and ureteral reflux leading to renal damage. In the presence of infection, an overproduction of mucus by the inflamed ileal mucosa may cause occlusion of the stoma with partial or complete blockage of urinary outflow. If the nurse is unable to remove the mucus with a cotton pledget, the physician should be notified before back pressure results in ascending infection. Interference with proper drainage may also be due to kinking of the ileostomy bag or its compression when the patient is accidentally lying on it. To avoid these difficulties, the adequacy of the drainage system should be checked each time the patient's position is altered.

The temporary ileostomy appliance is fragile and easily torn. Whenever a soiled ileostomy bag has been removed, the skin around the stoma is cleansed with acetone and then painted with tincture of benzoin to protect the skin and facilitate adherence of the new ileostomy bag. Before this bag is applied, the film covering the square adherent surface is peeled off slowly and the small round patch removed around the perforated line. The opening is then cut larger to fit the size of the stoma. The adherent surface is pressed around the stoma and held in place for a minute to seal the bag to the skin.

Instead of using a temporary ileostomy appliance, the surgeon may prefer to drain the ileal segment for a few days with a Foley catheter which is connected by plastic drainage tubing to a collection bag below. This type of drainage permits the nurse to irrigate the ileal conduit to remove mucus from the isolated segment.

Gastric Suction

A basic principle in the postoperative care of the patient with ileal conduit is to keep the intestines absolutely quiet until the ileal anastomosis has sufficiently healed. This is accomplished by eliminating the patient's oral intake and initiating intermittent gastric suction preferably under low pressure. The nurse checks the functional adequacy of the suction machine as well as the type and amount of gastric fluid aspirated. To keep the Levin tube open, the nurse disconnects it from the machine about every hour and irrigates it with a saline solution.

Fluid and Electrolyte Balance

Surgery for ileal conduit interferes with normal homeostasis, since the oral route of satisfying the basal requirements of food and drink is denied the patient. In addition, gastric suction tends to disturb the acid-base equilibrium by withdrawing hydrochloric acid from the stomach and to induce hypokalemia by lowering the potassium level. This deficit may be accompanied by alkalosis. Consequently, a carefully planned regimen of intravenous fluids becomes imperative in the postoperative care.

To detect any evidence of biochemical imbalance, the patient's serum electrolytes of sodium, potassium, and chloride as well as the carbon dioxide combining power are checked daily. These laboratory findings offer guidance in the choice of parenteral fluids which not only must help the patient maintain a nearly normal water and electrolyte balance, but also provide nutrition and sometimes antibiotic therapy. Renal function is likewise a primary concern since it tends to be depressed after surgery and to disturb the fluid and electrolyte metabolism. As a prophylactic measure mannitol may be added to the first postoperative venoclysis to stimulate the glomerular filtration rate. A 24-hour coverage of 3000 cc. intravenous fluids is usually considered adequate, and should be regulated so that the patient receives 1000 cc. of the infusion within each 8-hour period.

It is important to understand how ion concentration can affect the dynamic balance of the mind and body. As in the case of potassium ions, the stress associated with serious operations partially explains the frequency of hypokalemia. The patient in a state of potassium depletion experiences extreme exhaustion due to the lack of potassium, especially in muscle cells. The feeling of utter debility gives him the impression that his condition is poor, his operation a failure, and his hopes for a brighter future are shattered. His frustration hinders his adjustment and blocks his motivational tendencies and his will to live. Fortunately, with the judicious administration of potassium chloride, hypokalemia can usually be avoided.

However, metabolic alterations and hormone activity may lower the potassium concentration in a way not yet clearly known. If hypokalemia occurs, the nurse's understanding of the patient's psychophysiological responses to potassium depletion may help her in using the dynamic approach effectively. She should convince her patient that his feeling of exhaustion is temporary, and he will respond well to treatment in time. Her words of encouragement will help motivate him to accept his condition more realistically and continue his cooperative efforts.

On the first postoperative day, the patient is allowed to walk a few steps and sit in the chair. Early ambulation raises his morale and improves urinary evacuation. The activity schedule is gradually increased as the patient's bodily strength returns to normal.

After several days or a week postoperatively, the patient's bowel sounds return and gastric suction is discontinued. He is permitted to take 30 cc. water every hour and, if tolerated, clear liquids. The diet is gradually increased.

POSSIBLE COMPLICATIONS

With meticulous surgery and expert nursing, complications will be few. A stricture of the ileostomy opening may necessitate manual dilatation and catheterization of the ileal conduit for removal of residual urine.

Irritation of the skin adjacent to the stoma rarely occurs. If it does, it may be complicated by Monilia infection, which responds well to Mycostatin ointment.

A distressing sequela is a dynamic ileus, a condition usually relieved by decompression of the distended bowel by the Miller-Abbott tube. Equally troublesome are intestinal obstruction and a leak of an ileal anastomosis. When symptoms arise, an intravenous urogram is made followed by retrograde study of the ileal conduit.

A Foley catheter with a 5 cc. balloon is inserted into the stoma, and under fluoroscopic guidance the ileal segment is filled with a diluted Hypaque solution. Three roentgenograms are obtained to demonstrate the emptying ability of the ileal segment and the status of the uretero-ileal anastomoses [7]. Intravenous urograms are repeated monthly to provide continuity of care after discharge from the hospital.

Minimal hydronephrosis occurs frequently after surgery and is usually transient in character. When it becomes progressive it is a matter of grave concern. Recurrent and persistent pyelonephritis is a dreaded complication and requires prolonged chemotherapy.

THE HOLISTIC VIEW

Sometimes the nurse is so completely absorbed in carrying out a multiplicity of orders related to the operation that she focuses her attention on the ileal conduit, an isolated segment of a whole, instead of on the patient as a person and a member of a family. He wants to be accepted and cared for in his entirety. As soon as he has sufficiently recovered from his surgery, his physical, emotional, and spiritual needs become determinants of his behavior.

The patient who has been struggling for years to preserve his muscle function at its maximum capacity wants exercise. Since the patient knows that lack of exercise will rapidly increase his disabilities, he develops fear, anxiety, and tension. He may feel a sense of frustration and helplessness or rebellion at the prospect of further interference with normal activities. If his tensions cannot be expressed, his body will find a way of expressing them. It is well known that tensions and emotional reactions exert a powerful effect upon body chemistry and physiology. The patient may have diaphoresis, a rise in blood pressure, pulse, and respiration rate, and increased urinary drainage. His behavior will reflect his emotional tension. He may appear irritable, depressed, and fatigued or demanding, attention-seeking, and full of complaints.

This imbalance of the forces of body and mind is avoidable. The nurse who listens to the patient attentively provides him with opportunities for emotional release. When he expresses his fears and anxieties, she not only gains a better understanding of her patient, but also offers him highly effective therapy. This insight serves as a foundation for her holistic approach, which attempts to meet all the patient's needs with emphasis on those that loom high in his own estimation.

The nurse's role is one of guidance and psychological support. Whatever the patient's problem is, she encourages him to do his own thinking and find the solution for it.

For the paraplegic it undoubtedly means the preservation of his muscle power through exercise within the limits of his functional capacity.

For a housewife with multiple sclerosis whose psychological needs for affection and belonging have been stifled by the indifference and neglect of relatives, the problem is one of family interaction. Feelings of resentment and hostility harbored for years are too deeply rooted to be banished by the efforts of the nurse during a few weeks' hospitalization. The odorous stigma which made the patient socially unacceptable before her surgery for ileal conduit is rarely the only barrier to family cohesion. If her long-term illness has made her regressive, egocentric, and irritable, or if she pays little attention to her personal appearance to make herself attractive to others, it is not surprising that mutual affection between her and her family has grown cold. The nurse who understands the dynamics of human behavior can motivate the patient and encourage the family to grow in thoughtful consideration of the patient's needs. However, she must realize that attitudinal changes develop slowly and only if nurtured by insight and good will. The nurse may not see the results of her efforts, but the good seed she has sown is likely to bear fruit long after the patient has returned to her home.

Then there is the patient with ileal conduit for localized carcinoma of the bladder who may be grateful for the gift of life that has been bestowed upon him anew. The less fortunate victim of widespread metastatic involvement of the pelvic organs and exenteration surgery tends to be little concerned with his ileal conduit since he considers it only a fraction of a severely traumatizing experience. The nurse's dynamic approach should be individualized yet positive, invigorating, and wholesome, motivating the patient to face reality in an effort to adjust to his condition and preserve his mental health. If she has gained insight into the psychological background of his personality by listening carefully and observing his family interaction, she will understand her patient. To foster an optimistic attitude does not mean to minimize the patient's problems or deny their existence. The tactful nurse knows when a comforting word is feasible or when it is better to help the patient face the truth courageously.

The nurse who administers dynamic patient care helps the patient cope with the stresses of surgical intervention and also assists him to complete his rehabilitation. The nurse taught him early during his hospitalization measures of health conservation and intelligent self-care. He knows the importance of a high water intake in the prevention and control of urinary infections. He is well aware that the ileostomy appliance must be emptied frequently to prevent pooling of urine in the ileal segment. Since he has observed how the permanent appliance has been cemented to the skin adjacent to his stoma and learned how he can keep it clean and free from odor, he feels secure in assuming its care. He returns home, accepted by his family, and restored to nearly normal living.

REFERENCES

1 Straffon, R. A., and others. The ileal conduit in the management of children with neurogenic lesions of the bladder. *J. Urol.,* **89**:198-206, February 1963.
2 Schneiders, A. A. *Personal Adjustment and Mental Health.* New York, Holt, Rinehart and Winston, 1959, pp. 209-211.

3   Bricker, E. M. Substitution for the urinary bladder by the use of isolated ileal segment. *Surg. Clin. N. Amer.,* **36**:1117-1130, August 1956.
4   Flint, Lloyd, and Colock, B. P. Technique of ileal conduit for ureteral diversion, in *Surgical Practice of the Lahey Clinic.* Philadelphia, W. B. Saunders Co., 1962, p. 695.

Reading 56
Early Carcinoma of the Breast
Carol A. Gribbons
and
M. A. Aliapoulios

Carcinoma of the breast is the leading cause of death among Caucasian women in the United States who are between the ages of 39 and 54. It strikes them in their prime years as mothers whose children are requiring maximum supervision and guidance, or in their busiest years as career women [1].

There are approximately 68,000 new cases of cancer of the breast each year in this country. Early detection and treatment are mandatory, and are the responsibility of both patients themselves and the medical profession. Most masses of the breast are discovered by the patient, while others are found in the course of routine physical examination.

The first step in diagnosis is a complete history, including a history of the patient's family, because statistically there is an increased incidence of breast cancer in families of persons who have breast cancer, compared to the general population. If a woman has nursed her children for more than three months, she has decreased her risk of developing cancer of the breast. Likewise, breast cancer is significantly less frequent in married women who have borne children than in single nulliparous women. Previous pelvic—especially ovarian—surgery and the use of hormones or oral contraceptives are investigated.

A careful physical examination comes next. In addition to the size of the mass, other ominous signs include skin dimpling, ulceration, fixation to the skin or underlying pectoral muscles, and enlargement of axillary, supraclavicular, and cervical lymph nodes. Metastases to bone, lung, liver, or elsewhere also are looked for.

Any mass in the breast should be treated as a potential cancer until

Reprinted from *The American Journal of Nursing,* vol. 69, no. 9, pp. 1945-1950, September 1969.

proved otherwise. New methods have greatly increased the early detection of cancer. One such method is mammography, the soft-tissue x-ray of the breast: it demonstrates breast masses and aids in identifying those that may be malignant. But mammography is a gross diagnostic procedure, and the carcinoma must be large enough to be visible against the background of glandular tissue. It is safe and utilizes low-beam x-ray. Although it is not a substitute for physical examination, mammography may be useful for screening large or diffusely lumpy breasts, since a small carcinoma can frequently be distinguished radiographically, yet missed clinically [2].

Another diagnostic method is the conventional Pap smear, which is valuable if there is nipple discharge or breast ulceration. Thermography utilizes the principle of infrared emission as a direct function of surface temperature to distinguish the increased vascularity of breast carcinoma. This can be graphically portrayed on photographic films. Xeroradiography, on the other hand, applies the principles of x-ray and Xerox in order to provide a quicker and more detailed method of breast mass identification. However, these are newer diagnostic techniques which are available in only a few medical centers.

To any woman, a mastectomy is a major insult and carries with it an emotional impact that is "out of all proportion to the loss of function and tissue involved" [3]. Reassurance should come from all medical personnel, with the realization that, for every six to eight patients who have biopsies, one cancer is found. Early excisional biopsy is most important from both a diagnostic and an emotional standpoint. But because of these statistics, it is our belief that, unless the patient specifically asks, we should not go into the postoperative implications of extensive surgery until after such surgery is done. The physician is obligated to mention, but not to belabor, the necessity for removing the breast if a diagnosis of cancer is made histologically.

The preferred method of diagnosis is by excisional biopsy in the hospital, while the surgeon awaits the frozen section results and then proceeds with mastectomy if it is indicated. Some physicians favor needle biopsy of the mass. This procedure is helpful only if it reveals cancer or fluid with complete disappearance of the mass. The most confusing diagnoses involve patients who have diffuse, nodular, fibrocystic disease. These patients require close follow-up, whether or not a biopsy is performed.

In cancer of the breast, the location and the size of the mass are important prognostically. Medial lesions have a less favorable prognosis than lateral lesions, because they drain directly into the intrathoracic lymphatics. Nodal involvement increases the chance of distant metastasis. There is a clear correlation of five-year and ten-year survivals with the size of the tumor and the extent of lymph node involvement, and only a partial correlation of survival to location and histologic type [1].

TYPE OF SURGERY

The choice of simple versus radical versus super-radical mastectomy for carcinoma of the breast depends on many factors. These include the extent of the original lesion as well as the skill and convictions of the individual surgeon. Many skilled surgeons, however, perform only simple mastectomies (retrieving easily obtainable axillary lymph nodes without removing the pectoral muscles) and follow this with x-ray treatment if lymph node involvement is demonstrated by the pathologist [4].

Simple mastectomy is the operation of choice in very sick and feeble patients for reasons of expediency. This procedure is also done occasionally to remove any foul ulcerating mass that is disturbing to the patient, as well as making radiotherapy more likely to be effective for this patient. Certainly, McWhirter's results with simple mastectomy followed by irradiation have been quite good [5].

Prophylactic simple mastectomy, though rarely done, should be considered in women who have had previous contralateral breast cancer, in those with an extremely strong family history of breast cancer, or if repeated benign breast masses have caused important anxiety.

The more conventional approach to breast cancer without widespread metastases is the radical mastectomy. For patients who have lesions that are discovered early, this offers a five-year survival rate of 80 to 90 precent, which is difficult to improve on. In addition, it indicates the extent of lymph node involvement, which is important prognostically to the physician as well as the family, and is helpful in planning further treatment. In a radical mastectomy, the axillary lymph nodes as well as the breast and the pectoral muscles down to the chest wall will be excised.

Super-radical mastectomy—radical mastectomy plus dissection of the internal mammary lymph nodes—offers excellent cure rates, although the concept has not gained widespread approval [6]. Candidates for this procedure are those who have a high risk of internal mammary metastases and those whose infiltrating breast cancer arose in the medial and central portions of the breast. Even though the five-year survival rate is good, this surgery demands great skill, and its chief proponent cautions that "the extended operation is a more difficult procedure than the classical radical mastectomy and should be performed only under ideal circumstances" [7].

PERSONAL SUPPORT

In all patients, it is extremely important that the psychologic care be started before surgery. We believe that this is chiefly the physician's responsibility, since he is the one who must allay the patient's fears about the disease and its prognosis [8].

From this point on, the nurse and other health team members who come into contact with the patient must exert every effort to instill confidence and minimize anxiety. The nurse should assure her patient that she has time to discuss any problems that may be troubling her. Such discussions should be straightforward and yet they must be compatible with the patient's ability to face reality.

Enlisting the intelligent cooperation of the husband is of considerable help in minimizing postmastectomy depression. During this trying period, he may have difficulty displaying love without pity, while trying to be cheerful in the presence of his wife.

The religious needs of some patients are quite often their deepest needs. For such patients, the clergyman provides the kind of encouragement and support to both the patient and her family that is obtainable from no other source.

We believe that nurses, usually but not always, are best suited for giving postoperative advice and instruction, so at our hospital, the tumor service has added a nurse to coordinate the activities of all patients with malignancy. The nurse follows the patients in the hospital and in addition sees the patients when they return to the clinic for postoperative visits.

EARLY POSTOPERATIVE CARE

When a woman who has a breast mass is admitted, the nurse sees her preoperatively for the purpose of establishing a relationship and allowing her to express any anxieties she may have. The patient also has the assurance that someone she knows will follow her postoperatively. The same nurse sees the patient in the recovery room, which reinforces the patient's confidence.

After radical mastectomy, the patient needs the same care as any surgical patient, plus a great deal of emotional support. She will have a pressure dressing on for two or three days which constricts her chest, so the nurse assists her to cough by placing her hands on each side of the patient's chest. She must be encouraged to cough deeply and to take deep breaths at frequent, regular intervals. Breathing exercises will aid in full return of respiratory function. Once the pressure dressing is removed, the patient will have more mobility.

On the day of surgery, intravenous feedings are administered. If the I.V. is in the hand on the operated side, it may add to the patient's discomfort and limit her range of motion. She should be given medications freely as needed because the pain can be quite severe, and if she is not medicated, she is apt to lie perfectly still and listless in order to minimize her pain.

During surgery, the surgeon may insert a spring-loaded portable suctioning apparatus (Hemovac) or other drainage tubes to help drain the serosanguineous fluid that collects under the skin flaps. Such drainage allows the patient more freedom of movement and reduces the need for constant reinforcement of pressure dressings. It is left in place for two or three days, depending on the amount of drainage. The Hemovac should be partially inflated to insure maximum drainage, and the amount drained recorded with the output.

The patient is most comfortable in a semi-Fowler's position with a pillow placed under the arm on the operated side. This helps prevent lymphedema which may occur postoperatively due to lymphatic obstruction. Otherwise, when she is sitting or lying and her arm is not resting on a pillow, the arm could be supported by a sling. Changing the position of the arm from inward to outward rotation will limit shoulder pain and help prevent limitation of shoulder motion [9,10]. This positioning should be done whenever the patient is lying on her back. The affected arm should be placed at right angles to her body, with the elbow flexed and the palm down. She can then be helped to move her arm to outward rotation by moving her arm and shoulder back against the bed so that her palm is up.

The nurse encourages the patient to use her operated arm as much as possible after the first few days. She is encouraged to maintain good posture and not to hold her arm close to her body. She should use her operated arm to wash her face, comb her hair, brush her teeth, and feed herself until formal exercises are begun, which should be between the fifth and sixth postoperative day. Exercises are modified depending on the nature and extent of skin grafting.

RECOVERY

Early in the period of convalescence, it is desirable to interest the patient in prostheses and brassieres. The nurse who sees the patient every day can assess when the patient is ready to see models of available prostheses.

Prostheses

It is very important to wear a garment that is comfortable and fits properly. The breast form is made to correspond exactly to the shape of the opposite breast. Artificial breasts, filled with liquid, polyethylene, or air, have been designed to simulate the natural breast more exactly in weight and mobility. The patient may be fitted and wear a prosthesis because it maintains her sense of balance and keeps the body in alignment; if the patient's shoulders are not in good alignment, there will be a strain on her back. It is also important to be fitted as soon as possible after the physician gives permission, because if a long period of time is allowed to elapse, the patient will tend to protect her arm and develop poor posture, making a proper fit much more difficult.

As a temporary measure and while the patient is in the hospital, she is encouraged to adjust her regular bra, so that she does not get started in the habit of poor posture. A pad filled with some soft material, such as lambswool or cotton batting, can be constructed and sewn inside the bra. One end of the pad is attached to the center front of the bra, bringing the fullest part of the pad across the incision. The other end is attached to the back of the bra. Any space between the bra cup and the pad can be padded with loose cotton.

Another temporary method of adjusting the bra is to baste a sanitary napkin or other large cotton pad to the inside. The gauze ends of the napkin can be pinned near to the center front of the bra, so that the broad filler of the pad lies smoothly across the incision, cushioning the underarm area.

Any of these pads should be changed daily to avoid matting. To avoid pressure on the shoulder from the brassiere strap, the shoulder strap on the affected side should be lengthened by adding a few inches of elastic. In order that the temporary bra will not shift and ride up, especially during exercise, a V-shaped piece of elastic can be added to the lower edge of the bra and fastened to the garter belt [11].

Meanwhile, the choice of exactly the right prosthesis is very important, and the patient should be shown what is available, the cost involved, and where it may be purchased. The proper care and the handling of the prosthesis should be discussed with the patient. She will want to know how long it will last. This depends on its care and use, but generally it will last from two to three years; sometimes, up to four years.

Some of the newer forms (Identiform, Tru-Life) require only that a loose-fitting cotton packet be sewn into whatever bra, foundation garment, or bathing suit the patient already has.[1] Care should be taken when the wearer swims in salt water or chlorinated water, as the material can be damaged.

Prostheses are also available through some small order companies. Padded bras with removable inserts may be purchased inexpensively in most department stores. The patient can adapt these to meet her needs by removing the pad from the natural breast and placing the two pads together on the operated breast to insure more fullness.

---

[1] Listings of local dealers can be obtained from "Tru-Life," S. H. Camp & Co., Jackson, Michigan, and from Identical Form, 17 West 60th Street, New York, N.Y. 10023, as well as from catalog houses such as Sears, Roebuck.

For proper fitting of a bra or prosthesis, the patient should take a cardigan sweater with her, which she can put on backward. The sweater fits snugly and will help her judge what looks proportionate.

Many patients feel that they will never be able to participate in swimming or beach activities. Jantzen and Cole of California, Sandcastel, Sinclair, and Camp make bathing suits that patients can wear and look feminine in without feeling self-conscious.

"Reach to Recovery"

"Reach to Recovery is not a club, not group therapy—its purpose is to return the woman who has had a mastectomy back to normal as quickly as possible, by helping her with her psychologic, physical, and cosmetic needs."

This is the philosophy of Mrs. Terese Lasser, a championship golfer who had a radical mastectomy herself in 1952. Because of what she went through in finding her own way back to recovery, she and her husband, the late J. K. Lasser, started the "Reach to Recovery" program. Today the program is supported solely by the American Cancer Society. It has chapters in all 50 states and in several other countries.

Upon authorization of the attending physician and on request from a nurse or social worker, a volunteer—another woman who has had a mastectomy—visits the patient in the hospital and teaches her temporary comfort measures and exercises. The volunteer also gives the patient a ball on the end of a string and a rope for exercises, a temporary prosthesis (a bra pad filled with Dacron), the Reach to Recovery Manual, and her telephone number.

For comfort when she first walks about in the hospital, the patient is taught to use an underarm rest. A roll about 18 inches long and 6 to 8 inches in diameter may be made of Turkish towels or newspapers, placed under the axilla on the operated side as close and as high as is comfortable, and then tied, over a soft pad, on the opposite shoulder.

For the full-breasted woman who feels off balance when she walks, the unoperated breast may be supported in a sling that is pinned over a soft pad on the opposite side, near the clavicle.

The name "Reach to Recovery" stresses that the basic principle of all exercises is, of course, to reach. At first, the patient merely squeezes the rubber ball with her hand. Gradually, she tries to throw it farther away each day.

The patient can also strengthen her hand and forearm by resting them on a table where she has sheets of newspaper that she crumples and discards, one by one.

Standard position for all the exercises is standing with head erect, arms at sides, and feet hip-width apart. It is better to exercise in low-heeled shoes or bare feet and, at first, in front of a mirror, if possible. The patient is taught to keep her arms straight at the elbow and close to her ears. She should start her exercises slowly and do them for short periods, initially.

The patient should also observe in her mirror the alignment of her shoulders, and make a conscious effort to square her shoulders by rolling them back while keeping the arms down. This is relaxing and also helps fill out the hollow that often occurs just below the shoulder. After a while, her posture may be better than ever before.

Two of the several other Reach to Recovery exercises are described here. In the wall climbing exercise, the patient stands, feet well balanced, resting her forehead against the wall. She then reaches up slowly along the wall, trying every day to reach farther above her head, keeping her arms close to her ears, and marking with pencil or tape the highest reach each day.

In one of the Reach to Recovery exercises, the patient tosses a rope or a triple-thickness length of bandage with large knots at both ends over the shower rod or any other rod or hook placed about seven feet high. While seated, she pulls back and forth, starting down with the unoperated arm. She gradually works up to repeating this 25 times a day—at first doing it five times each in the morning and evening.

Reach to Recovery tells the patient not to have her blood pressure taken or to have injections given in her operated arm. If lymphatic drainage is sluggish, she should also protect herself from infection by avoiding cutting her cuticles and by using waterproof gloves when gardening.

The program also keeps up-to-date lists of appropriate bathing suits and offers detailed information about prostheses, including the suggestion that a patient can make her own weighted breast form by filling material of the right shape with birdseed, rice, barley, or other grain.

On invitation, Reach to Recovery gives programs for nurses and other personnel responsible for the care of patients. Their lectures describe reactions of patients, exercises, and prostheses, and demonstrate the use of elastic, pressure, and pneumatic sleeves.

Arm Swelling

Because of the nature of the surgery the lymphatic channel is disrupted, and the patient should be told how to deal with swelling of the operated arm if it occurs. In most cases, elevating the arm on a pillow will reduce swelling. It may also be necessary for her to elevate the arm over her head while she sleeps. For persistent swelling, a lymphedema sleeve or hand gauntlet (both are made by Jobst) can be prescribed. As the swelling is reduced, a smaller sleeve or gauntlet will become necessary so that maximum pressure will be applied at all times. This controls the edema for almost everyone. Best results are obtained when gravitational exercises are done while wearing the sleeve. Surgery for persistent lymphedema has been done in other centers to restore lymphatic drainage, but this is not favored at our institution.

Radiation

If the patient is to receive radiation therapy, she may experience a great deal of emotional stress because this raises the question of incurability. The surgeon, radiologist, and nurse can help answer some of the questions which arise because of the need for this further treatment.

The patient should be taught to protect the irradiated skin with a thin layer of lanolin, to wash the skin gently, and to avoid harsh, drying soaps.

Returning Home

After discharge, the role of the family in restoring emotional tranquility and aiding in her rehabilitation is of tremendous significance to every patient.

When the patient returns home, she can soon substitute simple household chores for the exercises she was performing in the hospital. The basic exercises may be abandoned as soon as the corresponding household activities are substituted. Activities at home that will put the patient's arm and shoulder through complete range of motion include sweeping, vacuuming, pulling out and pushing in drawers, mopping the floor, washing windows, raising windows, hanging clothes, and buttoning a blouse that fastens in the back [11]. She is encouraged to begin slowly and then gradually to increase her physical and social activities as recommended by the physician.

We have incorporated some of this information into a booklet, *Helpful Hints after Breast Surgery,* which we give to patients to take home. Some patients are also interested in the Reach to Recovery Foundation, a program of the American Cancer Society. It is a voluntary service to aid patients who have had a mastectomy. If called, one of its members will visit the patient in the hospital, demonstrate exercises, give advice on prostheses, and help plan her rehabilitation at home.

REFERENCES

1. Moore, F. D., and others. *Carcinoma of the Breast.* Boston, Mass., Little, Brown and Co., 1968.
2. Egan, R. L. Mammography. *Amer. J. Nurs.,* **66**:108-111, January 1966.
3. Clark, K. Rehabilitation and the cancer patient, in *Handicapped and Their Rehabilitation,* ed. by Harry A. Pattison. Springfield, Ill., Charles C Thomas, Publisher, 1957, pp. 293-296.
4. Crile, George, Jr. *Biological Consideration of Treatment of Breast Cancer.* Springfield, Ill., Charles C Thomas, Publisher, 1967.

5 McWhirter, R. Simple mastectomy and radiotherapy in treatment of breast cancer. *Brit. J. Radiol.,* **28**:128-139, March 1955.
6 Urban, J. A. Surgical excision of internal mammary nodes for breast cancer. *Brit. J. Surg.,* **51**:209-212, March 1964.
7 Urban, J. A. What is the rationale for an extended radical procedure in early cases? in *Current Cancer Concepts Multidisciplinary Views: Carcinoma of the Breast,* ed. Philip Rubin. New York, American Cancer Society, 1969, pp. 11-12.
8 Lewison, E. F. *Breast Cancer and Its Diagnosis and Treatment.* Baltimore, Md., Williams and Wilkins Co., 1955, chaps. 7, 13, 18.
9 Bouchard, R. *Nursing Care of the Cancer Patient.* St. Louis, C. V. Mosby Co., 1967.
10 Smith, Genevieve W. When a breast must be removed. *Amer. J. Nurs.,* **50**:335-339, June 1950.
11 American Cancer Society. *Help Yourself to Recovery.* New York, The American Cancer Society, 1957.

Reading 57

Psychological Impact of Cancer and Its Treatment IV—Adaptation to Radical Mastectomy

Morton Bard
and
Arthur M. Sutherland

DISCUSSION

The psychological experience of mastectomy for the patient consists of three phases. The first is the *anticipatory phase,* during which the patient anticipates injury and consequent interference with previously achieved adaptation to life. The second is the *operative phase,* in which the anticipated injury takes place. The third phase can be designated as the *reparative phase,* since it is during this postoperative period that the patient attempts to re-establish her previous adaptation by a variety of techniques. During each phase a sequence of reality events and emotional reactions is constantly in process for each patient.

The removal of a breast is a terrifying experience for any woman. It has an enormous impact that begins at the very moment she discovers the first symptoms and continues throughout the course of treatment and convalescence.

Reprinted from *Cancer,* vol. 8, no. 4, pp. 670-672, July-August 1955.

Unfortunately, knowledge of the patient's responses to other and totally different situations of stress in the past is not very helpful in understanding or predicting her response to the stress of having cancer of the breast. Each stress experience has a very specific meaning; thus each patient will respond to a given stress in accordance with the specific meaning it has for her. Consequently, the only useful guide to the patient's ability to handle anxiety is to determine the meaning of the radical mastectomy to her.

Fear of death in the operation and the probability of therapeutic failure, the violation of the beloved body, the loss of sexual attractiveness can all serve as the primary focus of anxiety. It is the physician's obligation to determine the source of anxiety prior to attempts to deal with it.

Renneker and Cutler maintain that the patient's initial problem "is that of protecting the breast; only later does she begin protecting her life." We do not agree. The focus of anxiety varies greatly in each case and at different times in the same case. Only individual psychological evaluation can determine the underlying fear. The same authors have also stated that "one method of easing acceptance of amputation is to indoctrinate the woman preoperatively with the concept of her breast as a danger to her future. This causes a shift in thinking away from the breast as a prized possession toward viewing it as a foreign body that threatens life."

It must be extremely difficult for a woman to dissociate herself from an emotionally significant organ and objectively view it as a thing apart. The function of the breast as an organ and its importance in female psychosexual development signify its vast implications in the emotional life of any woman. Apparent calm may mask inner turmoil that knows only temporary bounds and may explode as late as the convalescent stage.

It is doubtful that it will ever be possible to develop an absolute and infallible plan to apply uniformly in the relationship with any cancer patient. The most fruitful approach is for the physician or surgeon to focus entirely upon the patient's feelings and attitudes, thus establishing a significant relationship with her. The establishment of a warm and supportive relationship must precede any effort to give information to the patient. If such a relationship *has not* been established, factual discussion or even being, as Renneker and Cutler suggest, "humanly factual" may well result in emotional disorganization. "Facts" communicated by a person perceived as hostile and punitive are infinitely more threatening than those "facts" given by a person regarded as protective and friendly. Acute anxiety, to which a distant or hostile person invariably contributes, rather regularly results in gross distortions of "fact." Indeed, a warm supportive relationship will often be sufficient to sustain the patient and make long "factual" discussions unnecessary.

Paradoxical though it may seem, a supportive physician or surgeon may find the patient ventilating hostility and resentment directed towards him.

The patient feels secure enough in the relationship to release the suppressed feeling. The physician or surgeon should meet this test of trust by acceptance and understanding. When the medical authority becomes impatient and angry, the patient's anxiety increases and fantasies of retaliation at the hands of the powerful physician or surgeon result.

The experiences of the radical-mastectomy patient during hospitalization vitally influence her subsequent ability to resume her usual functioning after her return home. Much of the fear and tension during hospitalization can be greatly modified by the sincere interest of her physician and surgeon. When a psychologically valued organ is threatened and removed, the patient requires constant reassurance. If a patient is left to face the surgical experience and hospitalization unaided, psychogenic invalidism may develop and continue long after the disease itself has ceased to be the primary focus of professional interest and concern.

A long time after discharge from the hospital and after the experience is no longer so fresh in memory, most women report that they cannot rid themselves of the constant feeling that they "will never be the same again." Often, intensive inquiry on this point reveals that, despite "good adjustment" or "acceptance" of the physical loss, a psychological wound remains, which these women are convinced will never heal. These feelings are quite inaccessible to confirmation by casual conversation or superficial observation.

Other authors have pointed out that the loss of a breast constitutes a blow to femininity. While undoubtedly true in a very general sense, it must be emphasized that femininity varies in its meaning to each woman, and threats to it evoke a host of dissimilar responses.

Another reported finding is that exaggerated emotional reactions may be expected to occur in young women still able to bear children, whereas milder reactions occur in older, postclimacteric women who have had husbands and children. They have had real proof of their femininity and are now not so desperately in need of the symbol. We have been unable to confirm this finding in our experience and have seen profound depressive reactions in still married women whose reproductive life was over and who have had children. The breast acquires individual meaning to each woman based upon her resolution of fears pertaining to the achievement and maintenance of heterosexuality and motherhood. However this meaning is integrated, it remains active throughout life. Integrative resolutions and adaptive resources related to feminine function and self-worth do not mysteriously disappear with the hormonal change at the menopause. The impact of breast amputation will depend less on a woman's age than upon the character adaptations disrupted by it.

No matter what her age, the mastectomy patient, in common with any patient subjected to multilative surgery, is often the prey of profound hypochondriacal feelings, and a belief may be established that an irremediable injury has taken place that renders the whole body unable to function as vigorously as before and leaves it vulnerable to further injury. For the older patient, mastectomy may signal the onset of old age, uselessness, and decrepitude.

It has been said that the "mature" woman will have less reaction to mastectomy than the "neurotic" woman with an abnormal investment of emotion in her breasts. If the mature woman is defined as one who has less reaction and therefore has a "normal" investment in her breasts, then this statement is circular and must obviously be true. Unfortunately, the impact of mastectomy, as of other mutilating surgery, cannot often be predicted prior to the event.

The rather moralistic fashion of dividing personalities into the mature and immature, the normal and the neurotic, seems to have less and less meaning as our understanding of the dynamics of adaptation deepens. These appear more and more to be abstract entities better designed to fit into theories than to describe real people. They add nothing to our understanding of dynamic processes. The emphasis should be placed on understanding the *meaning* of the specific experience to the individual patient in his total life adaptation rather than on an abstract personality type that can withstand any experience abstractly regarded as stressful.

Planning for the use of a prosthesis is an integral part of patient management. The physician and surgeon should have information available regarding the most recent prosthetic developments and counsel their patients about where they can be obtained. Many patients are under the impression that a prosthesis cannot be worn until healing is completed, and they therefore unnecessarily restrict their social activities. A good prosthesis can be worn even over a small dressing. Some patients become virtual recluses during the immediate postoperative period because they do not know that prostheses can be used.

One difficulty experienced by patients after removal of the breast is the sense of physical imbalance or of being "crooked." This sensation may contribute greatly to hypochondriasis or convictions of injury and thus increase or prolong the period of invalidism. A good prosthesis aims to restore sufficient weight to the operative side and bulk to the axilla so that the imbalance is compensated.

The physician or surgeon should not hesitate to avail himself of the help of other disciplines in his efforts to aid the mastectomy patient. The psychiatrist can provide valuable insight into the patient's problems and add greatly to the physician's knowledge of his patient and the ease of management. The social worker can also render valuable assistance in tangible concrete services to the patient in reality problems. In addition, she can also provide continuing emotional support. Of course, the nurse who has continuous contact with the patient is a powerful force in the patient's early efforts to adapt to the experience. Furthermore, as a woman she provides the patient with an object for testing reality and for working out unconscious feelings. Consequently, the nurse who has understanding of the patient's emotional needs and who can act in accordance with this knowledge serves as a powerful impetus in the rehabilitative process.

REFERENCES

1. Bard, M.: *The Relationship of the Personality Factor of Dependence to Psychological Invalidism in Women Following Radical Mastectomy.* Unpublished Ph.D. thesis, New York University, 1953.
2. Chadwick, M.: *The Psychological Effects of Menstruation.* New York, Nervous and Mental Disease Publishing Company, 1932.
3. Dyk, R., and Sutherland, A. M.: *Psychological Impact of Cancer and Its Treatment: V.* Impact of extensive surgery on the family. (To be published.)
4. Mead, M.: *Male and Female: A Study of the Sexes in a Changing World.* New York, William Morrow & Co., Inc., 1949.
5. Menninger, K. A.: *Somatic Correlations with the Unconscious Repudiation of Femininity in Women. J. Nerv. & Ment. Dis.,* **89**:514-527, 1939.
6. Renneker, R., and Cutler, M.: *Psychological Problems of Adjustment to Cancer of the Breast. J.A.M.A.,* **148**:833-838, 1952.
7. Silverberg, W. V.: *Childhood Experience and Personal Destiny: A Psychoanalytic Theory of Neurosis.* New York, Springer Publishing Co., Inc., 1952.

Reading 58
Laryngectomy

Elizabeth Ford Pitorak

Sitting in silence and writing rapidly, Mr. J. put down his innermost feelings. When he had been told he had cancer and would need a laryngectomy, he had become depressed and questioned whether life without a voice would be worthwhile. He had gone so far, he wrote, as to take a pistol from the dresser drawer. Looking up at me, he put his forefinger to his head as one would to

Reprinted from *The American Journal of Nursing,* vol. 68, no. 4, pp. 780-786.

denote shooting oneself. As we communicated, he indicated that now, several days postoperatively, he no longer wanted to take his life.

Several weeks later, Mr. J. visited the ward and with pride attempted to say "hello" with his new "voice." Mr. J. is but one example of many such patients. Unfortunately, not all of them share their deep feelings and concerns with their nurses.

There are approximately 30,000 persons with laryngectomies in the United States, and more than 2,000 laryngectomies are being done each year. Cancer of the larynx occurs most often in white males at about the sixth decade of life. The ratio of male to female is 13 to 1, which means that the patient is generally the breadwinner of the family and in an age bracket when finding a new type of employment is difficult [1].

Some of the predisposing factors to cancer of the larynx are such irritants as cigarette smoke, alcohol, and noxious fumes. Over 75 percent of these patients are smokers.

This disease is usually classified as intrinsic or extrinsic. The former is a term used for carcinoma of the glottis or anterior commissure, those folds of mucous membrane, hard, white, shiny, and glistening, which make up the true vocal cords. Approximately 60 percent of all cancers of the larynx arise from the glottis, and, unlike those tumors which arise from surrounding structures, they rarely metastasize; but when they do, it is to the cervical lymph nodes and late in the disease. Therefore, hoarseness persisting longer than two to three weeks should be investigated by a physician. Surgery is the treatment of choice. Ackerman and del Regato note that "Left to themselves carcinomas of the endolarynx will . . . occlude the air passage and necessitate a tracheotomy" [1].

The extrinsic classification is used for those lesions which arise outside of the larynx—laryngeal wall, false cord, laryngeal ventricle. These tumors usually are not discovered until they have spread beyond the point of excision. Common symptoms are a "lump in the throat" or pain due to ulceration. Because the true vocal cords are not involved, hoarseness does not develop until late in the disease, not until the muscles at the base of the tongue—which also raise the larynx—are involved and the tongue becomes fixed. The treatment of choice is radiotherapy and surgery. The five-year survival rate is about half that of patients with intrinsic disease [2].

Tuberculous lesions, laryngoceles, polyps, and papillomas are often mistaken for carcinoma, but biopsy through indirect laryngoscopy will confirm a diagnosis.

SIGNIFICANCE

The possibility of losing one's voice can be terrifying, since the voice is our primary means of communication. It is through our inflections and the words we choose that we express our emotions—anger, affection, happiness, sadness. Melody, rhythm, and range add a very personal quality through which we can recognize a person even when we do not see him. After a laryngectomy, all these are lost. The patient must begin again and the voice he acquires is, at best, foreign to him and mechanical sounding. It is this the patient must face and this to which he must adapt.

In addition to concern about losing his voice, the patient facing a laryngectomy fears the cancer itself, with its possibility of recurrence, and the prospect of a painful lingering death. No wonder some patients are thrown into a state of panic and depression; no wonder others avoid or deny the diagnosis. A typical reaction, with tears, disbelief, anger, expressions of hopelessness and hostility, is, "Why did this happen to me?" A well-known physician, who is a laryngectomee, says that when he was told that his biopsy showed cancer, he walked to a nearby field in tears, tears not of grief or self-pity, but of annoyance and anger that such a thing should be happening to him. He was furious. But following this initial response, he was able to collect his thoughts and make the necessary operative arrangements [3]. Not all patients will regain control so rapidly. Some will continue to be angry and depressed, blaming themselves, especially if their fear of the diagnosis had kept them from seeing a physician earlier. Others see cancer as a disease acquired as punishment for real or imagined wrongdoing.

The fear of this surgery is normal: fear of anesthesia, of bleeding, of mutilation, of castration. To men the loss of the larynx—the Adam's apple—is often associated with losing their manhood.

These feelings can be dealt with best when the patient can express them, but then the climate must encourage discussion and the opportunity must be available. Establishing this is part of the nurse's responsibility as she admits the patient to the ward and prepares him for surgery.

PREOPERATIVE CARE

Preoperative teaching should reflect consistent philosophy. Close collaboration between nurse and physician keeps the nurse informed about the medical plan for care and makes the physician aware of the nursing care plan. The nurse, thus, has a basis from which to work and clarify any misconceptions the patient may have.

Certain types of information about what will happen postoperatively are appropriate for most patients: the suctioning process, methods of communication to be used, feeding methods. If the family is included in the preoperative teaching they too will know what to expect and they can offer information about the patient that will be useful to the staff. If it is impossible for one nurse to do all the teaching, a detailed care plan which includes what has been taught and what is yet to be taught needs to be developed, a plan that everyone can understand, one which lists the goals to be attained and the approaches to be used.

Knowledge of the patient's position in his family and society and his relationship with his peers and family members will help personnel understand how this illness will affect him and what it may mean to him. Good interviewing techniques will help establish a rapport which will lead him to express his concerns. Because he will not be able to communicate except in writing during the first few weeks postoperatively, he needs an opportunity to verbalize his fears before surgery. At this time the nurse must find out whether he can read and write in English, or in another language, or perhaps not at all. For the patient who cannot write, alternative methods of communication will need to be planned with him for use postoperatively.

Some physicians have a laryngectomee visit a patient preoperatively. There are both pros and cons to this. Some patients have refused to have surgery after seeing the stoma and hearing a laryngectomee's "voice." For others, seeing someone who has learned to cope is tangible evidence that they, too, can survive and they, too, can learn to speak again.

POSTOPERATIVE REACTIONS

The immediate postoperative period is a particularly frightening time because the patient cannot talk, and he is trying to adjust to a new way of breathing. Following a total laryngectomy there no longer is an opening from the mouth into the trachea. Instead, the trachea is sutured to an opening in the neck forming a permanent stoma. The patient is depressed or apathetic. He feels helpless, tearful, even suicidal. He may have deep resentment. Subconsciously, the surgeon is seen as the injuring agent, but since he is visualized as being too powerful to attack, the resentment is directed to those in the immediate environment: the nurse or his family. His resentment may take the form of complaints, demanding attitudes, or overt hostility; nothing is right from the time taken to answer his light to the way procedures are performed [4,5].

During this time the family needs much support. If they have not been warned what to expect, they can be confused and easily upset by the patient's emotional responses. Often they are not sure whether to encourage or discourage communication.

COMMUNICATION

The problems of communication are frustrating for patient, staff, and family. If an "intercom" system is in use, a note on the answer board should remind all the staff that the patient cannot talk and they must go into his room to answer the call light. It seems simple enough to ask a patient to write his communications, but for a considerable number of patients, writing and spelling at this time is no easy task. Deciphering a patient's notes carefully will prevent the frustration of misinterpretation. A magic slate is useful so that conversation can be erased. If paper is used, it should be destroyed in the patient's sight at the conclusion of the conversation. Many times these notes contain material which is personal and not intended for everyone to read.

Writing can be a long slow process, and it is tempting to finish a sentence for the patient. Avoid this. Instead, sit down and give him time. Laryngectomees often say that when they are in a group the conversation ends before they have had time to finish writing their remarks. Then they become frustrated, and begin to nod and smile in silence to avoid slowing the conversation.

Questions that have a "yes" or "no" answer will not give a patient an opportunity to express such feelings as anger by underlining words or printing words larger, or writing heavily with a pencil. Given the opportunity, it is not uncommon for patients to write about their concerns with cancer and with dying.

Some laryngectomees say that they can whisper, but their whispering is difficult for most people to understand. Patients who whisper also tend to develop mannerisms that are difficult to discontinue when esophageal speech is learned.

Unknowingly, visitors and staff make a patient uncomfortable when they chatter because of their own discomfort with silence. And because the patient cannot talk, he is often treated as if he were deaf or demented; everyone shouts at him!

What about the patient who is unable to read or write? Cues can be taken from the expression in his eyes, his facial movements, his gestures. A reed type of electric larynx is available and could be used in the immediate postoperative period if all other methods fail. But since this instrument is bulky and makes a whirring sound when it is in use, it should be the instrument of choice only for patients who have difficulty in learning esophageal speech or for the frail and elderly. However, an estimated 40 percent of laryngectomees successfully rely on such a mechanical aid to enable them to carry on their work and to converse at home.

When talking to a laryngectomee about the loss of his voice, it is helpful to talk to him in terms of it being a temporary loss since he will be learning a new method of speaking. Also, one must be careful not to instill negative attitudes when referring to esophageal speech; words must be chosen with care. The thought of belching back air, for example, may be repulsive to some people.

SUCTIONING

A patent airway is necessary to maintain life. The laryngectomee, therefore, will have a permanent tracheostomy with a laryngectomy tube, a cuffed tracheostomy tube, or no tube. Most nurses are familiar with the technique for suctioning a tracheostomy; however, a few additional points are important. The laryngectomized patient must be suctioned nasally as well as tracheally since he can no longer blow his nose. With his trachea connected to an opening in his neck, air cannot be forced from his lungs through his nose—the way we "blow" our noses. Nasal and tracheal catheters should be kept in separate containers to prevent contamination of the tracheobronchi. Or better still, fresh sterile catheters should be used each time the patient is suctioned.

Suctioning should be firm but gentle.[1] Rough, careless suctioning will tear the mucosa and lead to hemorrhage and edema of the inner trachea wall. A vented, or Y, connector should be used rather than a straight connector. If a straight connector is used and the catheter is clamped off with the fingers before it is inserted into the trachea, maximum build-up of negative pressure is applied to the lungs suddenly when the catheter is unclamped. Another way to prevent build-up of negative pressure in the lungs is to have the external diameter of the catheter no larger than half the internal diameter of the trachea [6].

For most patients with a laryngectomy tube in place, a size 14 catheter is appropriate. The catheter should be moistened with normal saline before it is inserted because a dry catheter will damage the mucosa of trachea and bronchi. Suction is not applied until the catheter is in place; otherwise, suction is pulling air and mucus out while the catheter is being pushed in, an antagonistic action which will damage mucous membrane. The catheter can be inserted 6 to 8 inches until an obstruction is met, then pulled back slightly, and suction applied. When the carina, the bifurcation of the main bronchus, is touched the patient will cough. A 360-degree rotating motion of the catheter between thumb and forefinger as it is removed will prevent pulling on the mucosa. Further "grabbing" of the mucous membrane can be avoided by releasing the suction periodically as the catheter is removed. Ramming the catheter back and forth in the trachea will only cause additional trauma.

If it is necessary to go into the left and right main stem bronchi, the patient should be instructed to turn his head in the opposite direction of the bronchus to be suctioned, with his chin tilted toward the shoulder. It is always easier to go into the right bronchus—larger than the left, which goes

---

[1] See *Respiratory tract aspiration* (programmed instruction supplement), *The American Journal of Nursing*, **66**:2483–2510, November 1966, for pointers on suctioning technique.

off at a sharper angle. Most patients can be aspirated as long as 15 seconds before being given a rest of up to 3 minutes. Depending upon individual readiness, a patient can be taught to suction himself as early as the second postoperative day, but not all patients will be willing or able to suction themselves this early.

Catheters which are not clean, unhygienic technique, and trauma to the mucosa of the trachea are often precipitating factors in tracheal infection. With destruction of the epithelium there is production of a purulent exudate with more than the usually expected normal crusting [7].

The inner cannula needs the same care as a tracheostomy tube. Crusts sometimes form at the base of the laryngectomy tube. Usually they can be removed with forceps or by having the patient cough them out. In rare instances, the crust is so large that it is necessary to remove the complete laryngectomy tube. A laryngectomee once told me that one of the most frightening experiences he had had in the hospital was an episode involving an obstructed tube. Apparently the nurses had not removed and cleansed the inner cannula routinely; it became encrusted, and the patient went into respiratory distress. But as soon as the inner cannula was removed, he was able to breathe normally.

Net gauze—a 4- by 4-inch gauze square, but with no cotton inside that could be aspirated—is used to protect the skin around the laryngectomy tube.

Air breathed by a laryngectomee goes directly into the trachea without first entering the nose where normally it would be moistened. Therefore, some artificial means of humidification has to be provided. A dry laryngectomy tube with minimal secretions is a sign of too little humidification.

There are several methods of providing external humidity: a collar can be fitted over the trachea and connected to a Mistogen unit, a moistened piece of gauze can be hung over the stoma, or a vaporizer can be run in the room. Usually by the time the patient is discharged, he needs these only when normal humidity drops.

Because air is not breathed through the nose, nasal secretions are not absorbed; rhinorrhea occurs. This, plus cough and the secretion of mucus, tends to reinforce the patient's belief that he has a cold. This is very frustrating and patients need frequent gentle nasal suctioning. In time, the body gradually adjusts to the altered physiology, and the symptoms diminish or completely disappear [8].

POSTOPERATIVE ROUTINES

There's a potential dead space under the skin flaps following a laryngectomy. Catheters, inserted under these flaps and connected to either a Gomco or a Hemovac, a small plastic apparatus which creates its own suction, will impede the accumulation of fluid. In addition, a pressure dressing over the flaps can be used to further prevent accumulation of serous fluid or a hematoma. Such wound catheters are removed approximately three days postoperatively.

Elevating the head of the bed 30 to 45 degrees facilitates breathing and prevents pull on the sutures. It is the position of maximum comfort. At first, when the laryngectomee changes position in bed or sits up, the nurse should support the back of the patient's neck with both hands or teach the patient to do this. Without such support, laryngectomees say they feel as if their heads will "fall off."

In contrast to many other surgical procedures, there is minimal postoperative pain. In the process of making the skin flaps, sensory nerve endings are cut. These take approximately six months to regenerate. However, patients will complain of headache, sore throat, and generalized discomfort from the nasogastric tube. They will also experience pain when swallowing. Thus, at first, it is more comfortable for the patient to expectorate saliva instead of swallowing it. Frequent oral suctioning helps too.

Most laryngectomees will have a nasogastric tube for feeding purposes for approximately 7 to 10 days. This tube will prevent fistula formation by removing stress on the pharyngeal suture line from swallowing and by decreasing the possibility of contaminating the suture line.

Tube feedings start with dextrose water, skim milk, or orange juice and gradually progress to a blenderized house diet. The fluids should be given at room temperature to prevent nausea and abdominal cramps. In some institutions patients are taught to do their own tube feedings, but the ability of each patient to do so must be considered first.

In some instances, patients might be given fluids by mouth on the first postoperative day, especially if synthetic sutures with an uninterrupted suturing technique are used and drainage is provided from the skin flaps by catheters connected to a Hemovac [9].

COMPLICATIONS

The most common complications are atelectasis, pneumonia, carotid artery rupture, fistula formation, and stoma stenosis. Atelectasis and pneumonia can usually be prevented by proper suctioning the first few days postoperatively, adequate humidification to prevent crusting, and regular cleansing of the tube. Carotid artery rupture may occur with patients who have had radiation therapy or radical neck surgery which leaves insufficient protective tissue over the artery. If the artery does rupture, application of direct pressure is the emergency treatment. Fistula formation is usually prevented with the use of suction under the skin flaps to remove old blood and secretions. Stoma stenosis results from extensive infection, fibrosis, or fistula.

The laryngectomee faces many changes in his life because of the altered physiology. These involve activities of daily living as well as speech therapy. Rehabilitative measures are begun in the immediate postoperative period and continue throughout hospitalization, through his transition home, and thereafter, too.

He will always have problems in relation to humidity, especially in dry weather. Many patients wear a metal screen attached to a knitted bib covering the stoma. As the exhaled air hits the metal, it condenses, thus providing humidity. Small amounts of mucus coughed up can be left to dry on the bib, also providing some humidity.

Bath time can provide humidity. If a tub bath is taken, the curtain should be pulled around the tub so that maximum moisture is retained in the air. For safety's sake, the drain should be kept partly open to prevent water coming high enough to enter the stoma. In the bath, the patient should keep a towel around his neck; when washing his face, he should use a mirror, both as precautions against water getting into the stoma.

A shower with an adjustable nozzle is an ideal way to provide maximum humidity. The stream should be adjusted so that it is chest high. To protect the stoma, a special shower cover can be used or a wash cloth can be held between the teeth with one end hanging down as a shield.

During the winter months, room humidity should be kept at 40 to 50 percent, slightly higher than that in the average home. If the heating system causes room air to be particularly dry, it might be necessary to install a humidifier or to place containers of water in the various rooms in the house.

Humidity is a problem in the summer as well, especially if the laryngectomee is in an environment where an air conditioner is in constant use. A room humidifier will counteract the air conditioner's normal dehumidification.

PRECAUTIONS

The laryngectomee who uses a safety razor should be cautioned about the danger of cutting his neck without knowing it. This area will be numb until nerve endings regenerate—approximately six months. Precautions should be taken to prevent the inadvertent entrance of shaving lather into the stoma. If aerosol shaving cream or toilet water gets into the trachea, severe coughing results, which can be frighteneing and uncomfortable.

Water-soluble lubricants, mineral oil, baby oil, or Vaseline can be applied to the skin around the stoma to prevent cracking. Leaving any of these on for 10 minutes will permit dried mucus to be removed quite easily.

Laryngectomees are prone to halitosis and crusting of the tongue. They can control these discomforts by brushing the tongue gently with a soft toothbrush and by frequent use of an oral astringent.

Since a laryngectomee can no longer blow his nose, mucus must be removed manually from the nares. A damp cloth can be used to clean the nostrils. The laryngectomee also cannot blow, suck on a straw, sip soup, gargle, or whistle because he can no longer force air from his lungs out through his mouth or nose, or force air through his mouth to his lungs.

Certain other changes take place because air is no longer breathed through the nose. For example, patients complain that they have lost their sense of smell. However, Ritter found that laryngectomees can smell just about as well as the normal person if fragrances are sprayed directly into the nares [10]. Initially, patients also complain of loss of taste, much of which is actually smell. But over a period of months, they cease complaining. Either they accommodate or become hypersensitive to smells to meet their own needs. Some laryngectomees have said that they can taste when they learn to speak.

Laryngectomees are afraid that they will suffocate at night if the bed covers get up around their necks. They need to be told that they will automatically turn if they have an insufficient respiratory exchange. If the stoma tends to collapse or is not large enough to provide sufficient air during sleep a laryngectomy tube may need to be inserted at night.

Cloth handkerchiefs will decrease the amount of dust which the laryngectomee breathes. Pieces of paper tissue can also be inadvertently aspirated into the trachea and bronchi on inspiration.

The laryngectomee's frequent cough is a protective mechanism which prevents mucous plugs. The tracheobronchial tree attempts to compensate for the lack of normal nasal humidification by secreting excessive amounts of secretions. Expelling these secretions causes the excessive cough. As the months pass, the tracheobronchial mucosa undergoes metaplasia to a more squamous type of epithelium which is compatible with dry air, and when this occurs the excessive mucus and cough diminish.

The male patient can expectorate the secretions through the stoma even when wearing a shirt and tie. If the second button on the shirt is removed and sewn onto the button hole, an opening is left through which a handkerchief can be inserted to remove mucus. Some patients become distressed by this because it draws attention to the fact that they are neck breathers—another adjustment problem. Some patients learn to treat this as they would the normal wiping of the nose.

Crust formation can be a constant problem for some patients. Tweezers, forceps, and a handkerchief can be used unless the crusts are large and adherent. Applicators or fluffy materials should not be used as they could be aspirated into the lungs. Occasionally, crusting becomes so severe that a patient has to be bronchoscoped.

The stoma should be covered with a knitted bib to prevent coughed-up mucus from being sprayed or a foreign body such as an insect from getting into the trachea. But equally important is the psychologic necessity to cover the stoma. Men can wear ascots, turtle-necked sweaters, or shirts with neckties. The shirt usually needs to be one to one and one-half sizes larger than that worn before surgery. Women can wear high-collared blouses, turtle-neck sweaters, scarves, or a large necklace.

Most laryngectomees do not have to wear a laryngectomy tube once the stoma has become an adequate size—about six to eight weeks postoperatively. However, some patients may have to wear it part of the time, and some, constantly [11]. The laryngectomy tube should be scrubbed with soap and water and soaked in alcohol each day. To insert it the patient should breathe in, hold his breath, insert the tube, and then breathe normally. His head should not be hyperextended, as this narrows the stoma.

The patient should know that if he drinks alcohol the amount of secretion from the trachea will decrease, that he will be sensitive to dust and smoke, and that recurrent bronchitis may occur. But, in general, except for preventing water and other foreign bodies from entering the stoma, his activities need not be restricted. One laryngectomee, for example, inadvertently slipped into water over his head while docking a boat. By thinking quickly and flexing his neck so that his chin covered his stoma until he could get his head above water, he saved his own life.

Any type of work where dust or other irritants are inhaled will require precautions, such as a mask or several thicknesses of gauze over the stoma. The laryngectomee who works in a noisy environment where he is required to give directions to others can use a megaphone. However, where he works and what he does will depend on whether he learns esophageal speech or uses an electronic larynx. Many types of employment require the use of both hands simultaneously, precluding the use of the electronic larynx, which needs to be held against the throat. A patient's general physical condition and his ability to do heavy work will also affect employment. The social worker, patient, nurse, and doctor, together, can help him in determining what kind of work he can do.

A considerable number of these patients have to change employment or take a reduction in pay. One survey showed that 67 percent of laryngectomees received a reduction in salary, and 28 percent lost or changed their jobs [12]. Policies about employing laryngectomees are often based on a lack of information about laryngectomees' health, work capacity, and speech ability.

The laryngectomee, like other persons, may at some time need emergency care. Any person found unconscious and needing resuscitation should be examined to determine whether he is a neck breather. Respiratory resuscitation of a laryngectomee calls for mouth-to-stoma technique, or infant-size face-mask-to-stoma, instead of mouth-to-mouth. Some persons wear a Medi-Alert tag stating they are neck breathers. Other types of identification which are helpful are windshield stickers and billfold identification cards.

Speech therapy, is, of course, the most important rehabilitation need. The speech therapist's intensive work with the patient is not begun until the operative area is completely healed. It should then continue until speech is learned or therapist and patient decide that the effort will not be productive. Not all laryngectomees can learn esophageal speech, and some will not have the motivation to do so. Persons who live alone and have very little verbal stimulus frequently do not learn this type of speech. These are the persons who should acquire electronic devices so that they do not have to spend their lives in silence.

REFERENCES

1. Ackerman, Lauren V., and del Regato, J. A. *Cancer,* 3d ed. St. Louis, Mo., C. V. Mosby Co., 1962, p. 440.
2. Nealon, T. F., Jr. (ed.). *Management of the Patient with Cancer.* Philadelphia, Pa., W. B. Saunders Co., 1965.
3. Long, P. H. On having a cancer. *Med. Times,* **87**:1192-1195, September 1959.
4. Nahum, A. M., and Golden, J. S. Psychological problems of the laryngectomy. *J.A.M.A.,* **186**:1136-1138, Dec. 28, 1963.
5. Sutherland, A. M. Psychosocial aspects of cancer: psychological impact of cancer surgery. *Public Health Rep.,* **67**:1139-1143, November 1952.
6. Rosen, Michael, and Hillard, E. K. Effects of negative pressure during tracheal suction. *Anesth. Analg.,* **41**:50-57, January-February 1962.
7. Conley, J. J. Diagnosis and treatment of encrustations in the trachea; their relation to radical surgery of the head and neck. *J.A.M.A.,* **154**:829-832, Mar. 6, 1954.
8. Reed, G. F. Long-term follow-up care of laryngectomized patients. *J.A.M.A.,* **175**:980-985, Mar. 18, 1961.
9. Saunders, W. H. Techniques in laryngectomy to minimize postoperative complications and permit immediate feeding. *Ann. Otol.,* **72**:431-440, June 1963.
10. Ritter, F. N. Fate of olfaction after laryngectomy. *Arch. Otolaryng.* (Chicago), **79**:169-171, February 1964.
11. Scott-Brown, W. G., and others (eds.). *Disease of the Ear, Nose and Throat,* 2d ed. London, Butterworths, 1965, vol. 1.
12. Gardner, W. H. Laryngectomees (neck breathers) in industry. *Arch. Environ. Health* (Chicago), **9**:777-789, December 1964.

Reading 59

Speech after Laryngectomy

Sol Adler

As one man pointed out after a laryngectomy, "If you lose your voice, you may find a few compensations. You can't argue with your wife; you don't have to bother with telephone pests; and you'll never talk yourself out of a job or into trouble." But most speechless persons want to learn how to talk again. After all, speech is the primary means whereby social relationships are achieved and maintained, and its loss seriously threatens a person's sense of security, adequacy, and acceptance.

Approximately 2,000 laryngectomies are performed in this country every year, mostly on men over age 50. Whether the cause is disease or accident, laryngectomy produces a grave crisis for the person who now finds himself unable to speak.

Anyone who helps provide care for such a patient needs to be informed about the nature of his problems, and equally well informed as to what he or she can do to help. A speech correctionist, of course, is best equipped to help such a patient. But when one is not available, or even if he is, the nurse must also share in the speech reeducation responsibility.

Rehabilitation for the laryngectomee involves: (1) the mental and emotional preparation of the patient for the operation and the recovery period; (2) speech reeducation; and (3) guidance in solving the practical problems of living without a larynx.

EMOTIONAL PREPARATION

Since each person reacts to crisis in his own fashion there is really no one set way to prepare all patients for what is to come. In some instances the surgeon provides the psychologic help, but he may call on a speech correctionist to do the preoperative counseling. At other times, this duty—in whole or in part—may fall to the nurse. Whoever does it, the primary objective is to minimize, beforehand, the patient's alarm when he regains consciousness and finds that he cannot speak or even whisper.

Significant points that should be included in the preoperative discussions are: (1) an explanation of the operation, (2) discussion of postoperative feelings, (3) preparation for loss of speech, and (4) discussion of normal production of speech. The main thing is to try to give the patient some

Reprinted from *The American Journal of Nursing*, vol. 69, no. 10, pp. 2138–2140, October 1969.

insight into what is going to happen so that when he wakes up and finds a sizable hole in his neck, he will at least know that it is supposed to be there.

He needs to be prepared, too, for the way he is likely to feel and react after the operation—especially the postoperative depression so likely to occur. If a patient knows that these feelings are normal and to be expected, he may be less upset about them. It goes without saying that he should also be prepared for his loss of speech. He should be instructed to communicate with his doctors, nurses, and family in the early period after the operation by writing, and he should be cautioned to avoid any early attempts at speech.

The preoperative period is also a good time to give the patient some simple but essential facts about how speech is produced in the human body. He can be shown by description and illustration, for instance, how speech sounds are normally produced. This can be done by placing appropriate degrees of obstruction in the way of a stream of air that is directed outward through the pharyngeal, oral, and nasal cavities.

In normal speech, sound is produced by modifying the respiratory process. When the moving column of exhaled air reaches the larynx, it is obstructed by the adducted vocal cords, which are forced to vibrate and produce sound. The sound is then carried into the pharyngeal, oral, and nasal cavities, where it is modified into vowels and consonants by means of resonation and articulation.

But when the larynx is extirpated and the trachea attached to the neck, the air column is diverted away from the resonators and articulators. Without a column of air moving through them, they cannot form the sounds of speech and, consequently, phonated speech and most of whispered speech are lost.

During these preparatory discussions, though, it is usually better to discuss only the mechanics of normal speech and wait until the patient has experienced its loss before introducing him to the problems of producing a second voice. The tone and quality of an artificial larynx or esophageal speech are not nearly so appealing to one who has a normal speaking voice. Only after the need to communicate has become urgent is the patient able to look forward to learning to use this new voice.

The patient needs assurance, however, that although he will lose his ability to speak and to whisper, there are several methods by which he can soon reestablish communication. Probably he should be told first about the artificial larynx, along with its advantages and disadvantages. He is likely to find esophageal speech more attractive, however, and its general character should be explained without burdening him preoperatively with the details and with the problems of its production.

This general information is to reduce the patient's anxiety about being permanently speechless and to create confidence that should he fail with one method, others are available to him.

SPEECH REEDUCATION

Speech therapy should not be started until the muscles and mucous membranes are well healed and no longer tender. This is for the surgeon to decide.

The therapy usually begins with a review of the mechanics of speech production as it occurs when the larynx is present. Then the patient can be told the modifications that the operation made in the speech organs. Assets rather than liabilities should be stressed, by pointing out to the patient that much of his speech apparatus has not been altered at all and that his operation did not affect many of his previous speech habits and skills.

The patient should understand, for instance, that although his larynx has been removed, his lungs are still intact, and the trachea now leads to the opening in the neck through which he breathes. Since he can no longer use his nose, mouth, or throat for breathing, he must learn to substitute other structures for his missing ones. In so doing, he learns to speak with a new voice.

Although artificial devices are available to help laryngectomees speak, most persons prefer to talk without them. There are two natural speech-forming methods: esophageal and pharyngeal.

ESOPHAGEAL SPEECH

Esophageal speech is usually attempted first, and the chief requirements are patience and determination on the part of the patient. If at all possible, he should have an opportunity to meet and to hear a successful esophageal speaker. If such a speaker is not available, however, the patient could listen to a good phonograph record or tape recording of esophageal speech.

Although esophageal speech is considered to be the most efficient method, it differs from normal speech in its hoarse, low-pitched, and often belchlike quality. The patient may find these features objectionable if he attempts to evaluate them before he loses his voice.

It is not imperative that the nurse be able to produce esophageal speech, although it is desirable. But whether she can or cannot, she does need to be thoroughly familiar, for teaching purposes, with the principles.

The patient must learn to swallow air into the upper part of the esophagus and immediately force it back. As it passes the narrow throat muscles, it is made to pulsate, and a belchlike sound, similar to that of a vowel, is produced.

When the patient belches, and if he concentrates on it, he can develop a kinesthetic awareness of what is going on and learn more quickly, perhaps, to imitate the movements voluntarily. Drinking Cokes or any carbonated beverage will usually help the person who cannot belch voluntarily. If such beverages are used, however, it should be only in the initial therapy sessions and only to help develop a kinesthetic awareness of this new speech process.

The important thing is for the patient to learn to control the air at the upper opening of the esophagus since, in essence, the opening of the esophagus functions as a substitute for the vocal cords. These sounds from the esophagus are then molded into speech by the mouth in the usual way.

The patient does not really "swallow" air in the ordinary sense; as a matter of fact, air taken into the stomach cannot be released easily for speech. But the removal of the larynx increases the space in the neck available to the esophagus and permits it to expand to accommodate the air necessary for speech production. It may be that this is why a laryngectomee learns to use esophageal speech more easily than someone learns when he is not a laryngectomee.

If the patient tries to whisper or to speak before speech therapy, he may develop habits that will impede his progress in esophageal speech production. In this so-called "buccal" or "pseudowhispered" speech, the patient builds up air pressure in his oral cavity and then overarticulates to produce a crude whisper, which is rarely intelligible and is hardly useful for communication. Some patients, however, inadvertently discover this phenomenon and continue to use it, despite the frustration and physical strain that accompany it.

The person learning esophageal speech must also learn to inhibit breathing while speaking. If he does not, the noise of the air turbulences produced in the tracheostomy tube during breathing are not only unpleasant and distracting but will mask the still weak sounds of esophageal speech produced in the mouth and throat. Considerable practice is necessary to learn how to inhibit expiration during speech.

The steps in learning esophageal speech are outlined on the next page [Levels of Esophageal Speech]. Through the entire process the patient must never cease to practice. He will find it easier to talk in the afternoon and at night than in the morning. No laryngectomee is in his best voice in the morning, but his speech gets more distinct as his voice builds up during the day. He can slip in practice sessions at frequent intervals. When he is driving to work in the mornings, for instance, he can open his mouth and vocalize on "ah" or other vowels.

PHARYNGEAL SPEECH

The pharyngeal method is the second way of producing postlaryngectomy speech. The individual locks air in his throat by using the tongue and its muscles, thereby eliminating the necessity of swallowing air deep in the esophagus. Often the patient learns esophageal speech first and uses it until he learns to establish an easy flow of air into the mouth and nose and has developed the necessary muscles so that enough pressure for vocalization can be built up.

He locks the air in his throat by placing the tip of his tongue centrally against the lingual side of the lower gums and arching the tongue so that its center touches the roof of his mouth, just as if he were making the "k" sound. By pushing the arched part of the tongue hard against the velum and forward, he will feel a slight thump in the throat. When this occurs, he must make a sound immediately or the locked-in air will be lost.

Once the patient can control air in this way, he proceeds to vocalize in esophageal speech.

LEVELS OF ESOPHAGEAL SPEECH

1 *No esophageal sound production—no speech* Little or no attempt at verbal communication is made. The patient communicates by writing and may attempt pseudowhispered speech.

2 *Involuntary esophageal sound production—no speech* The patient is able to produce an esophageal sound involuntarily as the indirect result of swallowing air (common belch).

3 *Voluntary sound production part of the time—no speech* At this stage, the patient can produce an occasional esophageal sound after great effort. A therapy session may result in only one or two voluntary sounds.

During later aspects of this stage, some sounds may be produced which contain modulation and some simple differentiation of vowels. This level is characterized by inconsistency of production, with involuntary sounds appearing more frequently than the voluntary.

4 *Voluntary sound production most of the time—vowels differentiated, monosyllabic speech* At this stage, muscular control for sound production is close to satisfactory. The patient begins this level with the ability to produce voluntary sounds in an undifferentiated way, but he soon starts to make different vowel sounds and then proceeds to the production of several monosyllabic words. He will find that of all the sounds he had once been able to make, the "h" sound is the only one impossible for him now. Example: "Hello, how are you?" will be, "Ello, ow are you?"

5 *Esophageal sound produced at will—single-word speech* The patient is now able to produce esophageal sounds whenever he wishes. The effort is almost always rewarded. The attempts have little or no continuity; but single words, especially short ones, are easily distinguishable by the listener.

6 *Esophageal sound produced at will with continuity—word grouping* The patient is able to group words in short phrases. The significant thing at this level is the continuity of production, even though it takes constant, conscious effort.

First he tries two words in one breath, and the mark / indicates stopping for breath. The patient will say, "One, two / three, four / five, six / seven, eight / nine, ten," or "A, b / c, d / e, f / g, h / i, j / . . ." He can now work on polysyllabic words and relies on speech entirely, with no more communication by writing.

Emphasis is now placed on breath control. The therapist gives the patient material to read, which is marked where the patient is to swallow air. The patient is told to swallow air at every / and say the hyphenated combination as one word: "/ Nine / / brown / hens / ran / out / of / the-barn / into-the-rain." "/ The-kitten / cannot / run / into / the-garden."

7 *Automatic esophageal speech* Once the patient has reached this level, he speaks with continuity and without thinking of swallowing air. His speech is rapid, automatic, and produced without effort. Although hoarse-sounding and lacking in volume, it is naturally and easily produced.

ARTIFICIAL LARYNX

There are two kinds of artificial larynx: one mechanical, one electric.

The mechanical larynx is a metal cylinder containing a reed. It has two rubber tubes, one at either end. The patient places one tube in his mouth, the other over the tracheostomy opening. Air coming from the neck sets the reed vibrating and produces a sound similar to that of a toy horn. The mouth forms this sound into words.

The electric larynx is a mechanical box similar to a flashlight, containing batteries and a vibrator. The patient holds the vibrator against the side of his neck, and its vibrations are utilized by the articulators to form a type of speech that is fairly monotonous.

TRACHEOSTOMY HYGIENE

A final and important task for the patient is to establish satisfactory mental and physical hygiene in order to live comfortably with his laryngectomy. Once he learns the proper management of the tracheostomy tube and the tracheal fistula, he will have greater security. If he uses gauze under the tube, he should be told to change it as often as it becomes soiled.

The adjustment and redesign of shirts and dresses and the use of small, gauze, tracheal napkins with neckbands are details which make for more comfortable living. As soon as possible after the operation, a man should begin wearing a collar and tie. The knot is placed above the neck opening and the second button is left open, so that the opening into the trachea can be reached easily. The buttonhole can be sewed up and the button sewed over the closed buttonhole, so that the shirt appears to be buttoned.

Some men wear custom-made shirts or have regular shirts altered to raise the collar so that the button and complete collar are above the trachea opening. The distance between the first and second buttons is increased. Some prefer bow ties, so that the opening can be reached easily.

Women can wear colored scarves or costume jewelry to conceal the opening.

The patient may have been accustomed to smoking. This may be forbidden for some reason by the doctor, but speech therapy does not necessarily mean that the patient must give up smoking.

The patient will note that he does not taste and smell as well as before his operation, but he can be reassured that gradually and spontaneously these sensory functions will recover.

Since the air passing into the lungs through the tracheostomy tube or fistula is not warmed nor filtered by the nose and throat, the patient will experience some inconvenience from the secretions that accumulate in his trachea. He must be taught how to clear his trachea inconspicuously when in a social situation.

He will also find that speaking is difficult in noisy environments. With help, he can learn how to manage his conversation and his position in relation to the listener so that he can be heard and understood without unusual effort.

Excitement, embarrassment, or any other unsettling emotions will make speaking more difficult, since generalized relaxation is so important in mastering the use of the second voice.

The successful development of a "second voice," most patients soon realize, means the difference between leading active, useful lives or spending the rest of their days completely mute. This is their motivation—but they need encouragement, instruction, and help in learning to speak again after laryngectomy.

Reading 60

Milieu Design for Adolescents with Leukemia

Joel Vernick

and

Janet L. Lunceford

Some persons might view a cancer nursing unit as one in which an atmosphere of dread and fear prevails. This atmosphere does not surround our twenty or more adolescent patients over a period of a year with leukemia on the Chemotherapy Service of the National Cancer Institute. For these children with all the normal adjustment problems of teenagers, the problems of adjusting to a hospital, and anxiety about impending death, we established an environment in which these adolescents could feel they were understood as persons. Our program, milieu management, is similar to those developed in residential treatment of emotionally disturbed children.

The Children's Program of the Cancer Nursing Service includes patients from the ages of 9 through 21 years. Every child in this age range admitted to the Leukemia Service is automatically part of the program.

Our program is based on the philosophy that the patient is helped more by being able to talk about his fears and anxieties and problems—including the possibility of death—than by dealing with these problems alone.

Anyone has difficulty responding to many questions that adolescents ask about their progress and their conditions, especially the question, "Am I going to die?" Our emphasis on frank discussion does not mean that we would give an affirmative answer to such a question. Rather, all professional workers in the unit are encouraged to offer children an opportunity to talk about the matters that worry them, and this includes death. At the same time, we stress that children should be told there is always hope and that the medical team is doing everything possible to get them well enough to return home.

The more a patient knows about his own condition and progress and those of his friends and other patients on the floor, the less anxious he becomes. Of course, all anxiety is not dissipated. But our goal is the freeing of anxiety in as many areas as possible to enable the patients to function more productively.

FUN AND RESPONSIBILITIES

We are concerned with creating an atmosphere to meet, to the highest degree possible, the physical, emotional, and social needs of the patients. Though afflicted with a fatal illness, patients are encouraged to function as normally as possible. They themselves prefer to be treated as they were before they became sick. The oft-used maxim, "treatment of the whole patient," is an actuality and not a fantasy.

The patient activities program provides weekly movies, Friday night bingo, traveling stage shows, gym activities, arts and crafts, band concerts, and the like. Occupational therapy is another program that provides varied activities to maintain maximum functioning of patients. Bedside programs are offered by occupational therapy where necessary. Children have many picnics and cookouts, go swimming at the local pools in the summertime, visit local points of interest, and make trips to the drug store.

A child might require a wheelchair to get to and from the station wagon. We might decrease the number of occupants of the car to accommodate the wheelchair. Trips are sometimes scheduled by the social worker, sometimes by group decision, and sometimes they are just such spur-of-the-moment ideas as, "Let's go out for a pizza." The physician's permission is needed for a child to make trips outside the hospital.

When physically able, the children are expected to attend school, which is housed in the building. They are responsible for keeping their rooms neat, and we expect them to adhere to rules about hours, use of TV, and so forth. We encounter many of the problems in establishing authority and discipline that parents normally encounter.

These levels of authority are inherent in the roles of the staff nurse, the social worker, the head nurse, and the physician. If a problem arises, one or more of these persons discusses it with the child involved. For example, if a patient refuses to attend school, we make efforts to help him find his own way through his resistance. In some situations, the head nurse follows up such an interview by one of her nurses. At times, when we think that the touch of greater authority is indicated, the physician supplies it.

INTERVIEWS WITH CHILDREN

The social worker holds individual and group interviews with the children. They discuss their feelings about their illness and decide how to discuss leukemia with their friends, relatives, and teachers. On rare occasions these group interviews are formally scheduled. The social worker is on the nursing unit for the entire working day and the nursing staff are also always available, giving children many opportunities for discussions with them. In addition, trips, while providing enjoyment for the children, also serve as occasions when all subjects are open for discussion.

When youngsters' questions about leukemia require the answers of a physician, we arrange for the chief pediatrician to meet with the patients.

Food for teen-agers is important. At one point, a group was in quite a state over the food. Informal group sessions were held, and the social workers suggested a get-together with the dietitians. A meeting was attended by eight teen-agers, the head nurse, the social worker, the head dietitian, and the dietitian responsible for our floor. The patients were able to suggest some changes in the daily menu. They also accepted the fact that some of their suggestions were not practical.

When the social worker interviews a child or a group in a patient's room, it is understood (as discussed at weekly team meetings) that any nursing personnel who enter the room are welcome to become involved. The group might be discussing the death of a patient, and the social worker will say to the nurse, "We were just talking about Penny." This draws her into the discussion. The exchange during such interviews is therapeutic for all—staff and patients.

HELPING PATIENTS TALK

To free a patient to talk about himself, his friends, and death, staff members must understand the serious predicament of the patient. This is crucial. The best way to communicate this understanding is to answer questions truthfully. One can be friendly, cheerful, and cooperative, but this is not the same as helping the patient with the basic problems at hand—mainly, the fear of dying and death.

However, we recognize that all nurses cannot agree to or feel free to discuss such matters. Particularly at the outset of our program, there was much resistance. The general attitude expressed verbally and non-verbally was: The less these problems are discussed, the less upset the children will be. Also, some nurses thought milieu management would cost them time needed for physical care of patients.

We decided, therefore, that all nurses on the unit need not become involved. At one of the team meetings, the choice was put to the nursing staff as follows: Those who were willing to discuss such matters with the children could, and support would be provided for them. Those who wished to avoid such subjects were to inform a questioning child that someone else would talk with him, and then to tell the head nurse or the social worker the child had questions.

The more individual and group interviews the social worker held with the children, the more staff nurses could see that, contrary to their earlier belief, such action did not upset the patients. Rather, more healthful emotional functioning resulted. Gradually, some of the nursing staff adopted this approach. An important aspect of this process was the weekly team meetings and informal discussion, in which the social worker discussed interviews held with the children. Conferees focused their attention, not only on the problems of the children, but also on the difficulties of the staff in adapting to the problems.

Nurses also realized that the "extra" work was something that they could accomplish during such routine activities as giving medications and taking temperatures. As some staff members exhibited willingness to talk, patients were able to communicate more readily on a meaningful level.

It is interesting to note that the patients did not take our word about encouraging them to ask questions. They tested staff members. Rapidly, they determined which staff members would answer and which would be evasive or not tell the truth and they put all staff members in either of two categories. Thus, those on whom the patients knew they could rely for honest discussion were the ones with whom they established closer relationships.

DEATHS OF FRIENDS

Despite the diversions and activities that the hospital personnel provide, the adolescent never escapes from the omnipresent knowledge about leukemia and his impending death. He is with others who have the same disease from remission to the terminal state. He soon becomes sophisticated about the actions of the staff and the equipment associated with terminal care—the oxygen equipment, the hypothermia machine, and the electrocardiograph. He also knows that the patients nearest the nurses' station are usually the most seriously ill.

Nurse B. was in the nurses' station with the head nurse when C., aged 13, approached and asked if a certain patient had died. Miss B. became momentarily flustered. Afterward, she said, "It was very hard for me to answer the question. However, I was almost at once convinced that I should tell her the truth, and so I did."

Another patient, T., age 13, approached Miss V. and asked, "Did something happen last night?" Something had happened. T.'s friend had died.

One way to deal with such a round-about question is to feign a misunderstanding of the true question that is being asked. Miss V., however, revealed insight and sensitivity. She said, "Do you mean, did somebody die last night?" Then they discussed the impact of it on T.

While these are only two examples which indicate several stages of intellectual and emotional development when the stimulus for learning is present, many more could be cited. However, it also needs to be pointed out that there were those on the nursing staff who were unable to involve themselves in such an emotional area, and in the final analysis, each person has to resolve such problems in the manner best suited to his own intellectual and emotional adjustment.

Section D

Geriatric Conditions

The concept of rehabilitation in geriatrics may seem incongruous to the person who sees old age as an insidious process which is irreversible and final. There are two facets to rehabilitation in nursing which challenge such a concept. One is that rehabilitation begins with prevention. The second is that each person has a right to perform at his highest potential. Nursing has much to contribute to the aging patient if both concepts are kept in the forefront while planning nursing care. Aging of tissue may be irreversible, but many of the concomitant effects are not. For the sake of organization it is well to divide the effects of aging into loss of sensory reception, loss of motor ability, or ability to respond to one's environment, and a third area which cannot be anatomically defined, loss of spirit. This last area has been given various names: courage, spunk, grit, and nerve. They all refer to the indomitable human spirit which responds to the environment and is frequently labeled motivation.

The need to survive will bring many patients to nursing care. Lack of the strength or will to perform the tasks of nourishing the body to provide for its activity or to care for its elimination needs are two events which precede asking for nursing care either in the home or institution. When one has maintained competent control over essential tasks over the time of one's life span, it is not easy to surrender this control to strangers.

The needs which Maslow called needs for belongingness, love, and self-esteem can create almost insurmountable problems for the aged. For those who are ill, the difficulty in maintaining identity is heightened by being cut off from normal family, neighborhood, and peer relationships. Loss of control over one's body functions, loss of privacy, subjection to intrusive procedures, and exposure of the body increase loss of self-esteem. Attitudes of the nurse, physician, and other helping personnel may deepen the loss as they work at the patient rather than with him. They may give depersonalized autocratic treatment and fail to prepare the patient for what to expect, or what is expected of him. At best his psyche will be damaged; at worst, he may have to refer to his identification band to know who he is.

The well-made nursing care plan emphasizes the right of each patient to be the best person he is capable of being, to participate in his own decision making, to act independently and to use his physical and mental powers at their highest potential.

Providing safety for the aged is often done at cost to the total person. Safety measures are not downgraded, but each one should be evaluated as to its first purpose—to protect the institution or the patient. The actual effect of the measure should then be estimated. An example is the side rail on an elderly person's bed. Patients frequently climb out of bed around the rail, risking falling in a difficult and narrow space when adequate night lighting and the customary bed height would enable the patient to be independent in a far safer manner. Again, it is institutional policy to put eye glasses in a safe place to prevent breaking, while the aged fumble in a nearly sightless state to find their way about. It is suggested that plastic lens be substituted instead, and the patient be allowed to have his glasses readily available.

The equation given in making the nursing care plan is especially important in planning care for the aged. This equation is:

$$\text{Patient's resources} + \text{Nursing care to supplement or complement} = \text{Whole person or an independent person functioning according to society's expectations}$$

This chapter is devoted to providing assistance to the nursing practitioner in planning her care. If properly planned, rehabilitation is built in as one of the dimensions in both prevention and in restoration procedures. The assessment of the patient's resources reflects losses of sensory and motor function, and it should include the substitutions and adaptations which the patient has been able to make if these losses have been gradual. As shown in the section on loss of sight and hearing, gradual loss allows for gradual adjustment while sudden loss is overwhelming. Assessment of the human spirit and its part in rehabilitative planning is influenced by the quality of interaction between the family and helping personnel.

It is significant that in the articles which follow so much is written about taking *time,* and overcoming the effects of depersonalization. It seems reasonable to assume that depersonalization is more easily prevented than overcome. Equations for geriatric nursing care become:

Patient's resources + Protected environment = Whole person
   and/or
Patient's resources + Time = Whole person
   and/or
Patient's resources + Assistive devices = Whole person
   and/or
Patient's resources + Repersonalization = Whole person

Principles which underlie such care which will lead to (1) keeping the geriatric patient in the mainstream of life by maintaining or creating interests which will occupy his leisure time, (2) preserving or helping him regain his normal range of motion, (3) preventing him from feeling unproductive and inadequate and helping him maintain the greatest degree of independence. The patient expresses his own feelings about this:

> They say "swallow this" or "turn around" and I'd be confused—not understand what was wanted and then something would be done to me. It made me feel indignant because I wasn't participating of my own volition . . . being done to, instead of doing with.[1]

Never underestimate the patient's own resources, or the possibility for restoring resources which are dormant due to a crushed human spirit.

> There is no one to know if I am dead or alive. What happens to me, if I sleep, if I cannot eat, cannot sleep? No one knows. It doesn't matter. Life is finished. I have only the grave.[2]

---

[1] Doris Schwartz, Barbara Henley, and Leonard Zeitz. *The Elderly Ambulant Patient.* New York: MacMillan, 1964, p. 293.
[2] Ibid., p. 294.

PREVENTION IN REHABILITATIVE GERIATRIC NURSING

Keeping the patient in the mainstream of life and helping him maintain his present abilities seems such a simple task that the nurse who is skilled in intensive nursing care might overlook it. With the present day nurse staffing patterns, highly important preventive nursing tends to be replaced with task-oriented nursing which is geared to the administrative need to get the job done. Depersonalization may be caused through default rather than ignorance, but the effect is the same. The person who is "done to" rather than "done with" soon loses the ability to participate through either physical losses or losses of motivation. Depersonalization occurs as a result of interaction which does not consider the patient as an individual with human feelings, but tends to treat the patient as an object for procedure. Depersonalization can be prevented through social interaction of the quality which respects the individual as a human.

The equation:

Patient's resources	+ Nursing care	= Whole person
becomes		
More care may eventually	+ Diminished patient	= Whole person
become	resources	
Lack of human resources	+ Total physical care	= Person in a
(human vegetables)		totally dependent state

Amburgey has written an intriguing article reflecting her understanding approach to the problems of the aged person who suffers from sensory loss or who is transferred to a new and confusing environment. Instead of expecting adjustment from the patient in a strange world, she supplements and complements his own resources.

The equation for care in this instance is:

Patient with	+ Nursing	= Whole or independent person
reduced resources	innovations	

The patients in Amburgey's modified environment are assisted to perform at the highest potential through assessment of their resources and supplementation. The patients were observed to note conditions which cause stress and anxiety. These were used as the basis for making the modifications which allowed the patient to maintain his independent existence. The described orientation to a new unit is one of the high points of the article. The importance of taking *time* is stressed. The challenge to every nurse to try a little harder, to make one more attempt, is present as Amburgey says that devising specific measures to maintain a patient's self-integrity calls for creativity, patience, understanding, and consistency on the part of the nurse.

Particularly important in this preventive phase of rehabilitative geriatric nursing is the component of *time*. The nursing assessment may indicate patient resources which are adequate to meet his needs in his protected environment, but at a diminished rate of activity. He can act, if allowed to proceed at his own pace. Pacing is referred to over and over again in the articles which follow as one of the most important principles to be used in caring for the geriatric patient.

In order to prevent the patient from becoming the human vegetable or totally dependent person in a previous equation, the patient must be allowed to use his remaining abilities at his own rate of activity. It is much easier to hurry through a procedure than to wait for the slow individual to accomplish it himself—the young and skillful aide buttons the housecoat in a few seconds while the patient would have taken several minutes. But the patient loses not only the fine finger coordination required for dressing himself, he also loses the human spirit that motivates him to be independent and leads to his self-esteem. It takes time to lead the weak patient from the bed to the bathroom, but only seconds to place a bed pan. Again, the loss is manifold.

Stone has studied the behavior of the aging person and analyzed various responses which he makes to helping personnel. One of the most important and salient characteristics of his behavior is the time needed to perceive. Appropriate responses can be made only when the person has perceived adequately and accurately.[3] Self-pacing is simple yet immeasurably valuable if it allows the older person to communicate and to participate in his own affairs. Alertness and orientation are maintained; apathy is postponed. Assessment of the patient's ability to sense and react to reality is the first step in the nursing process. Planning appropriate action is based on an accurate assessment and keen observation of the effects of each nursing intervention by testing it for its worth. The principle which underlies the entire article is *"Older persons have slowed perception and reactions, but they still have them and will keep them only if they are used."*

---

[3] Sensory perception is studied through sensory deprivation at this time. John P. Zubek (ed.), *Sensory Deprivation, Fifteen Years of Research,* Appleton-Century-Crofts, New York, 1969, contains a wealth of information from research on healthy subjects which can be extrapolated to the geriatric patient in a changed environment or in a state of decreased sensory stimulation. A number of cases of patients with eye surgery necessitating patched eyes reveal that the problem of sensory deprivation caused changes in the patient's ability to act appropriately and other evidence of profound disturbance. See especially article 10 by C. Wesley Jackson, which summarizes and analyzes the clinical studies in "Clinical Sensory Deprivation: A Review of Hospitalized Eye Surgery Patients."

Inappropriate nursing plans and implementation may go back to administration and its policies regarding staffing, task orientation, custodial versus rehabilitation care and a lack of the long-range view. Long-range views and human development are communicated as policies down through channels from the decision-making level of administrative hierarchies. If the decision is to keep patients clean and nourished—to care for survival needs only—human needs versus task-oriented nursing care becomes academic. Prevention is a costly procedure which shows no immediate profits on the balance sheet. It pays off over the long run, but if immediate goals are the only consideration, there is probably no time to wait for the patient to use his own failing resources in a meaningful way and to maintain his self-esteem.

Principles underlying preventive care for the geriatric patient stress supplementing and complementing the patient's own resources, never replacing them. Scrupulous attention is given to maintaining human dignity and self-esteem. To prevent depersonalization it is imperative to maintain the personality intact. The present and future must be linked to the past. The patient's identity both as a name and as a person must be used constantly by those who work with him. His work, hobbies, friends, relatives and pets are important links. When the nurse tells the patient her name, she in effect utilizes one of the best and more direct ways of orienting him to his strange environment and tells him that a specific individual will be giving him personal attention.[4] The patient who awakens at night with confusion and anxiety is reassured when he hears the familiar name and realizes more quickly where he is. The rules of common courtesy are used in every interaction. They serve as a buffer to the unavoidable indignities which the individual suffers when he surrenders control.

The need for keeping the patient informed as to his own care must be repeated over and over. He must have a part in the decision making about himself if he remains a person instead of a passive and helpless human vegetable. Social interaction on any plane is to be preferred to the silence of being ignored. Patients use quarrelsomeness and contrariness as measures to

---

[4] Primary nursing as the nursing which is based on one nurse–one patient nursing assessment and planning is an ideal which is realistic for the geriatric patient. This is described by Marie Manthey, Karen Ciske, Patricia Robertson, and Isabel Harris in *Nursing Forum,* vol. 9, no. 1, 1970. For the geriatric patient whose care is extended through time, it is possible for the primary nurse to make and maintain contact with her patient. A few minutes a day will reassure the patient that his nurse is concerned about his welfare. With one nurse responsible for planning care and evaluating, the patient receives a personalized form of nursing which may prevent the deterioration that can occur when a change to a different environment or change of circumstances is necessary. The primary nurse assesses the patient on admission, plans his care with others, and maintains continuous followup throughout the patient's stay. This is not private duty nursing (although private duty nursing is primary nursing); it is responsibility by one nurse for the overall planning and contact with the patient. The patient knows who his nurse is and on whom he can rely for care.

get attention when the other means fail. Quarrelsome roommates may love each other dearly and feel abandoned when separated. Such a relationship may maintain the patient's sense of autonomy over some part of his life.[5]

Charles has searched the literature for the characteristics of the older patient and the adaptations which must be made on the basis of these. He has divided these into sensory and motor changes, calling attention to the losses that occur and some of the nursing interventions which augment the patient's own deteriorating function. As in the Stone article, "Give the Older Person Time," emphasis is laid on the necessity for pacing action to the rate which allows participation by the older person. Particularly important is the area on learning ability. The aged have much learning to do and at a time when their sensory and motor powers are limited. Nursing care can be based on the information contained in the principles for learning. Principle no. 1 seems to be "Never hurry or push the learner." The principles in caring for the elderly person in a way to preserve his self-esteem seem to be the basic principles for learning and adjusting. The loss of resiliency must be taken into consideration in making long-range plans.

That which is not used is lost, but that which is used grows in strength and accuracy. For maintaining the highest potentiality of the patient it is necessary to supplement his resources but never substitute for them. Nothing less than maximum involvement in his own affairs will prevent depersonalization.

RESTORATION IN REHABILITATIVE GERIATRIC NURSING

The problems of the geriatric patient can be roughly divided into three categories:

1 Loss of ability to sense one's environment
2 Loss of one's ability to respond to one's environment (usually thought of as motor loss, although it may be dependent upon no. 3)
3 Loss of motivation or the desire to react meaningfully with one's environment, whether physical or social

---

[5] In Zubek, (ed.), *Sensory Deprivation*, Chapter 11 by Seward Smith—"Studies of Small Group Confinement"—describes studies of able-bodied younger men in such circumstances as simulated spaceships, underwater laboratories, Antarctica expeditions, and other instances of isolation for small groups. Behavior in such circumstances is beginning to fall into predictable patterns, one of which is the phenomenon of withdrawal rather than expressed aggression to the people with whom one is confined. This suggests that the bickering of two persons in a small room in a hospital or nursing home may represent healthier behavior than the passive behavior which is much more acceptable to staff. The lack of mobilization in an extended care unit may be comparable to the limited mobility found in the Antarctic. The reader who is interested in developing this idea is referred to the chapter indicated and further to the studies which are cited in the supplemental bibliography.

Problems are rarely clean-cut packages with defined boundaries; they usually interlock and influence one another. The problem of motivation cannot be isolated from the other two. For this reason this chapter on rehabilitation in the nursing care of the aged is dependent upon other sections of the book. It is necessary to refer to other sections to avoid repetition. Sections which apply to the geriatric patient include the following:

1 Rehabilitative nursing care of the blind
2 Rehabilitative nursing care of the deaf
3 Pain considerations
4 Rehabilitative nursing care of the patient with bowel and bladder problems
5 Rehabilitative nursing care of the patient with stroke
6 Rehabilitative nursing care of the patient with arthritis
7 Rehabilitative nursing care of the amputee
8 Rehabilitative nursing care for the patient with cancer

It is obvious that a considerable portion of the content of this text is included in the above. Nursing of the aged is a very challenging type of nursing care, and it demands a very wide range of knowledge and nursing skills. No two geriatric patients are alike, and nursing care for each must be personal and individual. The nurse who cares for the geriatric patient will find it necessary to be abreast of the research and knowledge in the medical-surgical nursing field as well as in the specialized field of geriatric nursing.

One area which is lightly touched upon should be stressed. This is the need for leisure-time activities to fill the unlimited time of the geriatric patient. Is this nursing? One might question whether or not the nurse, as the person recognizing the need, should be able to fill it, or should ignore it. It is a full-time task in an institution which has a number of elderly patients. The nurse must interpret the need to administration and in some cases to the community. Clean, well-fed, rested patients stare at the wall in a state of apathy. Schwartz found that elderly patients with as high as eight chronic conditions have considerable capacity for creative recreation if opportunities are provided.[6] The great blocks of uncommitted time need to be filled with some laughter and satisfying activity, preferably with others or in a group, to prevent the frustration, boredom, and inertia which come with loneliness. In a crowded lobby of a nursing home, an aged mother told her son, "There is no one to talk to." Planned sensitive recreation and leisure activities can overcome such a problem. In Sink's article "Remotivation: Toward Reality for the Aged," one person's efforts in helping the aging patient to enjoy more meaningful living snowballed as its success was shown. Depersonalization appalled the young nurse who studied Robinson's *Remotivation Techniques:*

[6] Schwartz et al., *The Elderly Ambulant Patient,* op. cit.

A Manual for Use in Nursing Homes,[7] and she developed a process for repersonalizing. Perhaps the greatest outcome was the use of the techniques by the nurses' aides in actually caring for patients so that many were reached who were unable to attend a group meeting. Community involvement resulted when young people came into the home and participated in the group process.

The physical trauma becomes mental trauma when the elderly person foresees a period of helplessness and further dependency, loss of self-esteem, and financial burden. It is easy to understand why this condition may be associated with confusion and psychotic reactions. Personality changes which increase the estrangement of staff and patient can be predicted and prevented with well-planned care by the staff and family. Current theories of disengagement and its effect on the sick role may have important implications for the elderly patient who is incapacitated for any reason, but particularly so for the person who is aged and suffering from a fracture of the femur.

Francis starts rehabilitation nursing care of the patient with internal hip fixation with good preoperative care. Two components are emphasized: time and enjoyableness. Untrustworthy support will prevent patient effort, and it is basically patient effort which reduces the period of immobility. The patient must trust the people who assist him into a new activity.

Alba and Papeika describe the nurse's role in preventing circulatory complications which arise with a fractured hip. Although this is stated in relation to a specific entity, the problem is the same whenever and for whatever reason the elderly go to bed and remain immobile. The pathophysiology of thrombus formation is that of aged blood vessels and pressures, or lack of movement which provides the milking action on the veins. Mobility of the patient would seem the easy answer, but the factors pointed out in the article by Francis focus on the realities of the situation.

A series of photographs is devoted to assisting the patient with ambulatory devices. These assistive devices are used in maintaining mobility for the patient with injury to weight-bearing limbs, especially the older with fracture of the femur. Successful use of ambulatory aids can facilitate final recovery, or it may lead to a condition short of full recovery. The pictures furnish a simple guide to the most common movements needed to rise from a sitting position, stand, walk, and finally sit again. When a physical therapy department is not available, the nurse must be aware of the use of the walker, and she can learn by actual practice as she uses it herself.

---

[7] Alice M. Robinson, *Remotivation Techniques: A Manual for Use in Nursing Homes.* Philadelphia, Pa.: Smith, Kline and French Labs, n.d.

In the final selection Sebrell discusses many facets of geriatric nutrition. He points out the significance of the build-up of nutritional deficits and indicates the cultural problems inherent in the tastes and preferences of the elderly. So seemingly prosaic a problem as losing one's teeth can have very serious nutritional effects among the elderly due to related attitudes and perceptions. Sebrell suggests that the nutrition problems of the aged are very similar to those of other age groups, ". . . for the aged . . . are just people who have lived a little longer than the rest of us."

Reading 61

Environmental Aids for the Aged Patient

Pauline I. Amburgey

Few experiences are worse than being lost, not knowing what is where, or what comes next. Many elderly persons find themselves in this distressing situation—the former professor who suddenly realizes that he is lost in a hospital ward, the grandmother whose lifetime outlet has been physical activity until a fractured hip immobilized her, the fastidious old gentleman whose awareness may be so blurred by medication during hospitalization that he soils himself.

The nursing goal for these elderly people must be to help them cope as normally and independently as possible within the limits of their disabilities. With this approach, disabilities or deficits that appear irreversible may be overcome gradually, at least to some extent. There are practical environmental aids such as modification of the physical plant and of the activity program which can assist even disoriented ambulatory persons to negotiate their surroundings more successfully. Basic lighting is a case in point. Since many older people have impaired vision, more and brighter lights may help. And because night and darkness often contribute to disorientation, night lights are important in rooms, halls, and bathrooms.

Specific visual aids such as signs direct all of us but, for some confused patients, the inconspicuous letters on ordinary signs are not enough. Substituting bold, black, ten-inch lettering on a contrasting pale background for the usual three-inch lettering not only makes reading easier but may also catch the attention of the preoccupied patient. To the person who has sensory aphasia, a printed sign usually is meaningless, but he may still associate colors. If the bathroom door is painted white, perhaps he can learn to find his way there provided the nursing staff will help him make the color association.

One hospital developed a color coding program for confused elderly women whose deficits were considered permanent. Each patient was given an identification bracelet of colored, ceramic beads. A matching colored placard was attached to her dormitory door, and a matching colored table mat and vase were placed on her dining table. With practice, some of these patients learned to find their way, independently, to their rooms and to the dining area.

Reprinted from The American Journal of Nursing, vol. 66, no. 9, pp. 2017–2018, September 1966.

When both men and women are housed in the same unit and must distinguish the correct bathrooms, a large, black silhouette of a man or woman superimposed in sharp contrast on a white door may help them reach the right bathroom by associating color, figure, and sign with a specific place.

Relatively simple structural changes in the physical plant provide environmental assistance and assurance. Closed or possibly locked doors will protect disoriented patients from wandering into areas where they might be injured. Half doors make certain rooms inaccessible, but still allow patients to look in as they walk by. Many can make the appropriate association from what they see—tables set with dishes and silverware will suggest eating and this room as the place where they will dine. A half door to conference and staff rooms reassures the patient that the nursing staff is close at hand since he can see them as he passes by.

Personal belongings are environmental aids whose value is sometimes overlooked. Any patient's possessions, but especially those of the aged, are constant reminders of his identity and individuality, and often help him relate to his surroundings. If he looks into a room filled with beds and sees on one of them a bathrobe which he recognizes as his own, he may well be reassured that this is his bed and here is where he will sleep.

Another source of stress for patients with memory deficits and shortened attention spans is decreasing competence in the activities of daily living. Every patient always should be encouraged to do whatever he can for himself even though this may be very little. Simplification or modifications of clothing can enable many patients to maintain a degree of self-sufficiency. For example, Velcro fasteners instead of buttons may enable a handicapped person to dress himself.

There is a variety of possibilities for adapting routines for those patients who respond slowly. Instead of rushing to do something for a patient, the nurse should consider that perhaps all he needs to accomplish a task is more time to prepare for it and more time to perform it. Let him know what is coming next by supplying him with cues or hints. He may be able to follow a schedule of regular activities if it is printed on a blackboard and if supplementary verbal announcements call his attention to an approaching event. Sometimes placing an article connected with a particular activity within his visual field will help him complete an activity with greater ease. Even such a simple chore as getting ready for breakfast involves a number of steps. He wants to dress. Are his clothes placed where he can see them? He should wash, brush his teeth, and comb his hair. Are his toilet articles conspicuously placed in the bathroom?

For some patients, special instruction for each activity must be repeated at intervals, but the courtesy of allowing them time to prepare and time to perform should still be observed. At mealtime, a series of announcements—"Lunch will be ready soon," "Lunch will be ready in five minutes," "It's time to eat now"—may start even the markedly debilitated patients moving toward the dining room.

Perhaps a patient needs assistance with only part of a task—let him feed himself the "finger foods" even if he can't manipulate a fork and knife. Perhaps he can dress himself if his clothes are laid out in proper sequence or if he is handed each garment separately. Pacing activities in measured steps so that the patient can keep up also fosters self-care. Explanation of a procedure in slow, distinct, short sentences, with repetition if necessary, will lessen the anxiety connected with uncertainty and encourage him to move ahead at his own speed. But if he still is struggling to comprehend the meaning of the nurse's first direction and she is rattling off a second one, his bewilderment will be compounded.

A new environment means an adjustment to all of us. Elderly persons sometimes function less well or become disoriented when they are transferred from one ward to another or from a hospital to a nursing home. Pacing the change in a logical sequence may make the move less traumatic. For instance, if a person in a geriatric admission ward is ready for transfer to another area, he should be informed that soon he is to move and be given a reason for the move. He should hear about the place where he is going and what to expect. On another day he should be taken to his new ward, shown around, and introduced to patients and staff. If he is severely disabled physically, the nursing staff from his future ward should visit him in the admission area. On still another day he might have lunch on his new ward and perhaps join in its activities. When finally he is transferred, this ward may no longer seem "new" because he finds himself in familiar surroundings with acquaintances, not strangers.

The environmental aids and human consideration discussed here are not limited to the ambulatory aged, but apply quite as much to all geriatric care. The acutely ill patient in a general hospital, for instance, often experiences disorientation. Although he may not have to find his way about since he is at bed rest, he does need to be as active as possible during his illness to hasten recovery to his former level of independence. Even when a person's condition is deteriorating steadily, maintenance of as much self-sufficiency as he desires for as long as possible is probably the best care the nurse can offer him. Perhaps he cannot wash his face, but could dry it if given adequate time. Completing even a fraction of a task will bolster his sense of competence and make his illness more bearable.

Nursing the disabled, aged patient calls for a myriad of specific measures to preserve his integrity. Devising them calls for creativity, understanding, consistency, and patience on the part of the nurse.

Reading 62
Give the Older Person Time
Virginia Stone

Gerontology is a young and explosive science, even though the people it studies are old. This science, concerned with the process of aging and with special emphasis on old age, provides knowledge about psychologic, biologic, and sociologic relationships—many of them of a normal, nonpathologic nature. It is in this growing body of knowledge that the nurse can now find a sounder foundation for the practice of gerontologic nursing.

Research findings indicate that older people have special needs due to the process of aging, and some of these needs call for a nursing approach that differs from the approach needed for other age groups. Among them is the need for a different "pacing" of nursing care.

Society today is geared to a fast pace of living, yet old age is distinguished by a general slowing in the timing of behavior. In other words, the phenomenon of slowing is characteristic of senescence. "To pace" can imply to run, to slow down, since this is what is happening to these older persons. It is this phenomenon of slowing that should influence the gerontologic nursing approach; the nurse will need to modify her pace if the older person's needs are to be met in a way that is satisfying to the patient.

The timing of behavior in old age has been most often studied from psychologic and physiologic frames of reference, and the research has usually been conducted on animals or apparently healthy older people. Knowledge of the effects of illness on behavioral timing is therefore scanty, but it is a reasonable assumption that illness, in most instances, would tend to slow the processes even more.

Psychologic research has clustered around the familiar process of the stimulus-response mechanism. Though the basic theory has stood the test of time, the functioning of the process in old age is still a mystery. The process itself has three major components: the stimulus, the processing of information, and the response. The nurse originates many of the stimuli, and she

Reprinted from *The American Journal of Nursing*, vol. 68, no. 10, pp. 2124-2127, October 1969.

also has the opportunity to evaluate the appropriateness of the response. In computer language, the output depends on the input. The challenge to the nurse is to use herself therapeutically so that her stimuli will produce the desired responses.

TIME TO PERCEIVE . . .

How well the patient perceives the stimulus is a major influence on the strength with which it comes through and on the patient's response to it, and two important determining factors in his perception are his visual and auditory ability.

Light, for instance, needs to be intensified as the size of the pupils of the eyes decreases. When illumination is low, the older person has increasing difficulty in recognizing objects. Thus he might object to eating by candlelight because "I just can't see what I'm eating." Or another patient may be slow to grasp a medicine container that is offered; when he does, after struggling valiantly to see the object, he may easily spill the contents.

Diminished auditory perception may also delay reaction time or influence the response. Two factors need special consideration: the pitch of the speaker's voice in relation to the patient's hearing threshold, and the ability of the patient to discriminate between different sounds of speech. A response may be delayed because the older person did not hear nor discriminate and, therefore, has difficulty in processing the information.

In relation to the stimuli, then, the nurse should evaluate the older person's perceptual ability and modify or pace her nursing approach so as to make optimum use of, or to raise, the person's level of perception. For instance, for those older persons who have difficulty with speech discrimination, speech paced slowly enough to permit clear enunciation of syllables will give the person time to comprehend and process the information.

The intercommunication system between the nurses' station and the patient's unit distorts the voice to the point where the older person may find it difficult to understand. If the older patient presses the button and a disembodied voice replies, "Yes, can I help you?" he can become so confused that in attempting to reply he forgets his reason for ringing the bell and fails to make his need known. Therefore, when an older person is institutionalized, the nurse should test the call system with the patient to determine if he can hear and discriminate speech coming to him in this way. Sometimes the nurse can get around the difficulty by modifying the pace of her own speech. If this doesn't work, a different call system should be used.

A good example of the nurse's role in stimuli production and response evaluation is reported in a research project, "Expanded Speech and Self-Pacing in Communication with the Aged" [1]. The authors describe the use of expanded speech when caring for the aged with speech discrimination difficulties. They say that speech should be just expanded out more in time: that is, truly slower. No other verbal stimuli should be given until the person has responded to what has already been said. The rate of pacing is, therefore, determined by the time needed for responses.

Faulty perception, whatever the cause, frequently leads to an inappropriate response. And these inappropriate responses may cause the person to be labeled uncooperative, confused, or even senile.

TIME TO RESPOND . . .

The older person's reaction time is slower, and he takes longer to make decisions. Moreover, as the amount of information associated with the decision is increased, the time required to come to a decision is proportionally increased.

The older person compensates for his diminished mental and physical capacity by taking a longer time to perform [2]. If provision is not made for this, the accuracy of the performance will probably be affected. Thus the older person who is learning to stand again after illness or incapacitation may be capable of doing this, provided he is given enough time to compensate for the slowness of his reactions. As one 80-year-old man said, "I could stand if they would just give me time."

TIME TO LEARN . . .

Much geriatric nursing practice includes teaching. These older patients need to learn how to use such new devices as walkers, hearing aids, or wheelchairs, and they need to be informed about their own changing health care needs. Therefore, the nurse must understand the learning processes of older persons. They *can* learn—but it takes longer.

In one study of learning ability it was demonstrated that older people could, in fact, respond fairly rapidly when given sufficient time; but, when this time was reduced, they were less likely to respond at all [3]. Older people are known, too, to feel a need for accuracy. Therefore, they must understand exactly what is expected of them before they will attempt to do it.

TIME TO MOVE AND ACT

Physiologic as well as psychologic changes contribute to the slowing-down process. Muscular weakness is common, for instance, and this, along with the increasing arthritic stiffness of the joints, affects the older person's mobility. Many, however, have made outstanding adaptations to their restricted movements, and the nurse needs to be aware of these adaptations.

One elderly woman with long-standing arthritis in both hips had learned to adapt to her misery by sitting in a chair rather than lying in bed. She had had many illnesses at home and throughout all of them had remained in the wheelchair during the day. She carried out limited exercises of all her joints and even walked a little.

When she had to be hospitalized because of an acute illness, however, she was placed on complete bed rest. She begged to be allowed to sit in a chair because she had so much discomfort when lying down, and, because of her pleading, some viewed her as a cantankerous old woman. They changed their attitude, though, when they eventually became aware of this patient's ability to adjust to treatment when she was sitting more comfortably in a chair.

Circulatory changes may also dictate a slower pace with the elderly. For instance, the sudden drop of blood pressure that quite commonly occurs when an older person rapidly changes his position from lying to sitting or standing may cause momentary loss of consciousness or giddiness. The nurse should therefore realize that when the older person is transferred from bed to chair he needs to sit on the side of the bed for a period of time before proceeding to the chair; or, after sitting in a chair, he should get up slowly.

Simple nursing procedures can become so routinized that it is easy to overlook adaptations that might be helpful or necessary for the older people. Take the routine back rub, for example. When the older person is asked to turn on his side or back, one has first to be sure that the stimulus—the verbal request—was received. Then the patient must be given enough time to process the information and, finally, to respond to it. And the nurse must remember, in making this seemingly simple request, that the patient's physiologic processes are slowed down—he needs time to move his old and stiffened joints. If any part of this process is hurried, the patient may reject the nurse's offer to make him comfortable. Often he just smiles and says, "Don't bother."

Similarly, the older person may turn down an opportunity to go to church or a social function because of the time it takes for him to groom himself properly. He is uncomfortable when he is hurried. An aging person can be motivated and often is already motivated—but he must be given time to reach his goals.

I cannot understand why it is often believed or assumed that the chronically ill and aged need less nursing care time than other patients. For optimum care, the nurse must pace her behavior to accord with the patient's timing and this calls for a general slowing down. The more accurate the pacing, the higher the level of care and the greater the amount of time necessary.

The findings from gerontologic research reported here are indicative of the ever-increasing body of knowledge in this area upon which quality nursing care for our senior citizens can and should be based. And there is a need to test more of these findings and determine their applicability to nursing. As this process proceeds, the body of knowledge specific to gerontologic nursing will expand, and care for geriatric patients will be adapted more accurately to their specific limitations and needs.

REFERENCES

1 Panicucci, Carol L. Expanded speech and self-pacing in communication with the aged, in *ANA Clinical Sessions (Papers), American Nurse's Association, 1968, Dallas.* New York, Appleton-Century-Crofts, 1968, pp. 95-102.
2 Birren, J. E. (ed.). *Handbook of Aging and the Individual.* Chicago, Ill., University of Chicago Press, 1959, pp. 609-610.
3 Eisdorfer, C., and others. Stimulus exposure time as a factor in serial learning in an aged sample. *J. Abnorm. Soc. Psychol.,* **67**:594-600, December 1963.

Reading 63
Outstanding Characteristics of Older Patients
Don C. Charles

Is there any reason for treating older patients differently from middle-aged or younger ones, other than those reasons dictated by specific illness or disability? Obviously, the older patient *is* different, simply by virtue of his having a great many years, of having an aged body, of having left most of his peers behind.

He may, however, be quite unwilling or unable to accept these differences himself. Some years ago, I inquired of a colleague of retirement age, "When did you first begin to feel old?" At first, he looked puzzled, and then annoyed as he snapped, "I haven't ever felt that way yet!" I was young and naive and would know better now than to ask the question.

Yet it was not many months later that the same man complained to me that he was old, that nobody wanted him around, that he wasn't any good

Reprinted from *The American Journal of Nursing,* vol. 61, no. 11, pp. 80-83, November 1961.

for anything. Which of his protestations should I have believed? Actually, both statements were accurate. The second one was made after he had retired and had suffered a serious illness.

These responses suggest something of the degree to which health and the immediate environmental situation affect the older person. Having relatively little time left to live, he often finds it difficult to take a long and hopeful view when misfortune—illness, accident, loss of loved ones—strikes him.

To the young person the elderly patient's tenuous hold on life may suggest that he has little to live for. I remember the surprise—and faint disapproval—in the voice of a young woman when she told of asking a nice, white-haired old lady in confidence at what age women ceased being physically interested in men. "You'll have to ask someone older than I, my dear," was the reply.

Old people *are* different from young ones, and thus they do require different care. But, like young people, they are still individuals with needs and desires and with some of the means for satisfying them. Knowing some of the ways in which older patients differ from younger ones in their physiological and psychological functioning may be helpful. Following are some of the most noteworthy age changes and some suggestions for helping patients adapt to them.[1]

SENSORY AND PERCEPTUAL FUNCTIONS

We are constantly bombarded by stimuli of many sorts: noises, lights, colors, odors. Our sense organs—eyes, ears, nose, skin, inner ears—detect these stimuli and transmit impulses to the appropriate brain centers for interpretation. The latter process of getting meaning out of experience is what the psychologist calls perception. As people age, the efficiency of both the information-gathering and information-interpreting functions declines somewhat.

Vision

Some age changes are well known: the decline of acuity, speed of focusing, and accommodation in near-point vision. Less familiar, perhaps, is the fact that breadth of the field of vision narrows several degrees from middle to old age. The matter of light and vision is of practical concern to the nurse. With increasing age, adaptation to darkness deteriorates.

Thus, it is most important that older patients not be faced with the necessity of going from lighted rooms into dark hallways, bathrooms, and the like. High levels of illumination are needed for tasks which demand good

---

[1] For a comprehensive evaluation of research evidence on the psychological aspects of aging, see James E. Birren (ed.), *Handbook of Aging and the Individual*, University of Chicago Press, 1960.

acuity—craft work or reading, for example. Each 13-year age increase requires approximately doubled light intensity.

This combination of narrowed field, slower perception, reduced acuity, and need for high illumination suggests that elderly ambulant patients need careful supervision, especially at dusk or at night, if they are to get about safely.

Auditory Perception

While everyone suffers some high-frequency hearing loss in the adult years, most people retain fairly good hearing for speech sounds throughout life. However, with age there is increasing evidence of deafness in the sound range of the human voice. After age 75, about 2 men out of every 10, and 1 woman out of 10, suffer from noticeable deafness. The result is increased difficulty in hearing speech.

Patients are sometimes unaware that they are not perceiving accurately some vowels or consonants or are unwilling to admit their lack of understanding. Therefore, the nurse, as a matter of course, should speak slowly, enunciate clearly, and check to see if she is being understood, especially when instructions for medication or self-care are being given.

Even the presence of a hearing aid is no guarantee of hearing. It may be turned off, intentionally or unintentionally, or it may be malfunctioning. I know one elderly, deaf woman who habitually keeps wornout batteries in her instrument, saving her good set for church and special social occasions.

Body Perception

By this I mean an awareness of the body's position, its status, and functioning. There is a steady loss of pain sensitivity after the age of 50. This might seem at first to be a good thing, and, indeed, some elderly people apparently do not suffer as much as their disorders would suggest.

However, loss of pain sensitivity is dangerous. Older people, without apparent awareness, not uncommonly suffer fractures, bruises, or other damage to the body, which should have medical attention; the nurse needs to keep alert for symptoms of such damage, even though she has no report of an accident.

There is some loss of kinesthesia, perception of movement of body parts. Of greater concern is the loss of sense of balance, apparently owing to changes in the inner ear. Many of the falls suffered by elderly people are not a product alone of weakness or poor muscular control, but a lack of awareness that the body is off balance until it is too late to recover.

For this reason, even patients who are not particularly feeble need stair and hallway railings, grips by the tub, and other appropriate supports. Some will require canes or a nurse's guiding arm.

The loss of ability to adapt quickly to temperature changes is well known. Older people thrive on a constant temperature and require frequent changes of covers or wraps when the temperature fluctuates.

MOTOR SKILLS

In discussing motor performance, we must consider several processes: sensing and decision-making in the brain and central nervous system and responding.

Sensory functions were discussed previously. Decline of muscular strength is continuous after the twenties. It is selective. Loss of back strength, for example, occurs early and is quite rapid, while good hand strength is retained into quite old age. Accompanying the decline of strength is decline in capacity for continuous exertion, necessitating more attention to rest periods to avoid excessive fatigue. The implications for convalescent patients and those undergoing occupational therapy are obvious.

The general slowing down of responses in older people is familiar to all of us. While some slowing occurs in the peripheral (sensory and muscular) apparatus, the significant change occurs in the central nervous system. Thus, it is not sensing or responding that is so difficult for aged people, but rather *deciding how to respond.*

This is especially marked in complex performances, in unfamiliar tasks, and where the stimuli are presented too rapidly or in an irregular fashion. Apparently, there is a tendency to overlap the organization of one act or movement with the previous one, resulting in jerky and piecemeal performance.

To get the most efficient motor functioning from the older patient, therefore, one must structure the situation so there is sufficient time for planning in his central nervous system. This may be accomplished by presenting instruction or information slowly, allowing time for him to get set, by using rhythmic stimuli when possible, and especially by avoiding hurried, confused, or emotion-laden orders.

It is interesting to note that motor functioning in familiar tasks declines little, if at all, provided that the skills have been exercised regularly. The older person may steer an automobile, knit, or repair a watch as efficiently as he did two or three decades earlier, while less difficult but new tasks may be done clumsily and inefficiently.

LEARNING ABILITY

Most nurses are teachers, although they may not think of themselves in this way. Some—certain public health nurses, for instance—teach in formal training situations. Most of the nurse's teaching, however, takes place incidentally as she goes about her duties in the sick room and the ward. Old patients have a great deal of learning to do—learning to master new prosthetic appliances, learning to approach familiar tasks in new ways as heart, limbs, or muscles fail to respond as they once did.

The nurse is likely to be the professional person in most intimate and frequent contact with the elderly patient as he attempts to acquire these new skills. Even more difficult is his need to learn new understanding of himself, to change his attitudes toward many things. Thus the nurse needs an answer to the familiar question, "Can you teach an old dog new tricks?"

Research evidence suggests that the most appropriate answer to this question is, "Yes, if you have the time to teach him and he has the desire to learn." In other words, old people still learn, but the importance of time, teaching techniques, and motivation increases with age.

It was once supposed that intelligence reached a peak in the teens and thereafter declined steadily and with an increasing rate. Current evidence to the contrary suggests that at least some people continue improving in ability into middle age and perhaps beyond. Unquestionably, however, the older person does differ from a younger one in his learning characteristics. His loss in speed has been alluded to earlier. This is only one facet of his learning behavior, of course.

To say that he becomes less efficient is true, but only partially so. His loss is relatively slight in areas which are familiar through his everyday experience. However, he becomes steadily less efficient if he is forced to reorganize old familiar material in new and strange ways.

His memory, too, deteriorates. Here again, old and often-repeated material is retained at a relatively good level, but new and especially strange and unfamiliar material is lost readily. Thus, an elderly woman may remember the details of a recipe used for her daughter's wedding cake many years ago but becomes hopelessly confused about the name of a drug prescribed for her or about the name of a disorder her physician mentioned.

Another well-known characteristic of the thinking process of old people is rigidity. Tasks requiring quick changes of "set"—expectation or readiness to respond in a certain way—are usually not performed well. Under stress, the older person tends to repeat himself even though it is apparent to himself as well as others that what he is doing isn't working. He may even regress to a bit of behavior that was successful in the past.

In the little country town where I grew up, there were still a few older farmers driving horses when I was a child. I remember the account of one, reluctantly converted to an automobile, shouting, "Whoa! Whoa!" and pulling on the steering wheel as he crashed through a store front.

Deterioration in the organizing function of the brain leads to some failures in logical thinking. When pressed to solve too-difficult problems, the older person is likely to retreat into discussion of extraneous material rather than provide logical inferences from evidence.

Perhaps it should be noted at this point that the discussion of deterioration refers to ways in which persons become less efficient in their learning and reasoning as they grow older. One should not infer that all old people are rigid, illogical, forgetful, and so on. There are tremendous differences in individuals in rate of deterioration, and, obviously, current level of functioning is relative to the original peak level.

There is at least one psychologist, for example, who is producing stimulating and scholarly books although he is past 90. I have no doubt that he functioned more efficiently in the 1890's when he took his doctor of philosophy degree than he does today, but his work is currently more creditable than that of many younger men in the field.

Most older persons, unlike the scholar just mentioned, are not high achievers. There is a tendency to sit back, to relax, to let things go as they will. Too, physiological conditions may affect drive or ambition. For whatever reason, a major problem with older learners is motivation. Before learning can occur, there must be some desire to learn, some perception of reward for making the effort.

The nurse who is trying to help elderly patients acquire new ways will have to be skillful in making learning seem intrinsically rewarding and satisfying. Praise, recognition of even a little progress, encouragement, and patience are essential.

To summarize teaching techniques with older patients:

1 Use every motivating device at your disposal; praise and recognition are of greatest importance.
2 Keep materials in the context of the familiar as much as possible. Relate new experiences or materials to familiar ones, especially in the early stages of learning.
3 Assume that a great deal of time will be spent in any learning situation. Never give the impression of pushing or hurrying the learner, regardless of your own need to get the job done.
4 Help the patient understand the task; he may be unable to perceive the relation of parts of the task to the whole.
5 Keep stimulus and response together when demonstrating or explaining.

ADJUSTMENT

It would be unrealistic to attempt to treat the broad topic of adjustment of aged people in so brief a space as this. There are, however, some points that should be noted.

In general, the adjustment of healthy individuals resembles their adjustment at an earlier period of life. Behavior is relatively consistent over a period of time for reasons of both genetic and environmental continuity. However, there is a continuing loss of life-enjoyment, of feelings of self-confidence and usefulness, and a general loss of zest.

There is, in addition, a loss of what might be called resiliency. Stress of any kind causes more anxiety and elicits a greater reaction than was true at an earlier age, and recovery is slower. The youthful person generally expects to recover from illness or disability, to be as good as new again. The aged person is only being realistic when he recognizes that he won't be new again.

One frequent manifestation of this realization is hypochondriasis. In many older persons, normal aches and pains are magnified, excessive attention is directed to digestive and eliminative functioning, and exaggerated reports of sleeplessness are made. Most of us know inactive older persons who nap happily in the daytime and then complain bitterly of sleepless nights. Only time for acquaintance and familiarity will enable the nurse to distinguish which symptoms have an organic basis, which are serious, and which trivial. The family's reports are not always reliable, either.

The real adjustment problem of age lies in apathy and futile resignation. One bit of evidence of this is the close relationship between age and suicide. But depression does not need to proceed to the extreme of suicide to be harmful to the patient. Loss of the will to live can be as fatal psychologically and physically as more direct forms of self-destruction.

Obviously, formal psychotherapy with neurotic or depressed patients is not considered the forte of the nurse. She may, however, play a role in prevention. Both overconcern with bodily health and a loss of will to live may be aggravated or even instituted by a common condition—boredom. There is accumulating evidence that deprivation of stimulation, literally from birth to old age, is a cause of psychological malfunctioning.

It is highly desirable that old people experience as stimulating an atmosphere as possible and that they continue to do as many things as their condition allows. It is especially important to keep this need in mind when caring for patients in nursing homes or in working with those who are chronically ill and bedfast.

Elderly men and women, with all their crotchets, can be rewarding patients. Their philosophies, occasional wry humor, and accounts of their experiences are often enjoyable to the listener. By keeping in mind their psychological needs and capacities, the nurse will help them retain dignity and self-respect. She will encourage them to use and, thus, to maintain their remaining skills and abilities. Her reward will be not only a virtuous feeling of altruism, but the satisfaction of pleasanter and more cooperative behavior in patients.

Reading 64

Remotivation: Toward Reality for the Aged
Susan Mary Sink

This article is an account of my experiences as I tried to understand and meet the many needs of aged, mentally ill patients in a nursing home. At the time I was a senior nursing student who, because of personal circumstances, had been forced to withdraw temporarily from the school.

Saint Luke's Infirmary is located in Centralia, Washington. The physical facility, formerly the city hospital, has an occupancy which varies from 60 to 85 patients. Patients live mostly in private or double rooms on three floors. About 90 percent of them receive state aid; half of the patients are ambulatory or semiambulatory and, as would be expected in this type of institution, most of them are on tranquilizing drugs.

The home is operated by the Sisters of Charity of Providence, three of whom are registered nurses. The rest of the nursing staff is typical of many nursing homes—middle-aged women with limited or no previous training, but the need to work to help support their families. The turnover among this group is high, and this has handicapped long-range projects.

When I came to Saint Luke's, I was not given a job description, but I was told that I was to assist Sister Melece, an R.N., in caring for 30 women patients on the first floor. Making patient care assignments and helping with care as needed were my chief responsibilities. I was also encouraged to plan recreational and occupational therapy activities.

A feeling of inadequacy engulfed me as I began to observe the complexity of the job and the various unmet social and psychological needs of most of the patients. Having just come from Seattle University School of Nursing, I had lofty ideals of "personalized patient care," and not having had any extensive experience with aged or mentally ill patients, I was overwhelmed: What and how could I do for them?

One of the problems was the diverseness of these patients. There were, for example, about a dozen retarded patients who, because of their inability to live in an open society, had sought the security and protection of institutional living. They obtained a small income from the home for part-time, menial work. Many had spent years in state-operated institutions for the retarded. The home also shelters relatively young patients with such chronic conditions as multiple sclerosis, Parkinson's disease, and stroke. The largest

Reprinted from *Nursing Outlook*, vol. 14, no. 8, pp. 26–28, August 1966.

group of patients are those aged persons who do not have a home to go back to and are physically unable to live by themselves.

During my "free" hours I sought to understand the problems at work. I had brought some textbooks and an assortment of nursing notes from my former classes, and I found an abundance of past issues of *Geriatrics* in the basement of the home. As I read and searched in print for comparable situations, I began to compile a list of the difficulties I was encountering:

1 Because there are so many different types of patients I don't know how to begin an organized approach toward meeting their needs.
2 No one seems really interested or has the time to provide needed therapy.
3 There seems to be so little communication between patients, and between patients and staff.
4 Many of the patients seem so apathetic. They just sit in their chairs all day and look out of the window.
5 The staff do not treat the patients like persons. Seldom do they speak directly to patients, call them by name, or encourage them.

Boiled down, it was: depersonalized institutionalization aggravated by senility. Depersonalization is a disease, though it is doubtful that it would be found in medical or nursing texts under that title. What can be more degenerative than passive behavior, excessive dependency on others, social isolation, and refuge in custodial care institutions? Many of our older citizens are afflicted with one or more of these symptoms, especially when they have spent many years of their lives in mental institutions. Perhaps one can honestly say that these institutions in the past have aggravated this "roleless role."

State mental hospitals frequently release their geriatric patients to nursing homes. This transfer is made either because intensive treatment or the kind of custodial care offered in these institutions is no longer needed or beneficial, or because financially speaking, the cost to a state for nursing home care is considerably less.

To me, the obvious solution to the problem was repersonalization, but not so obvious was how I would go about implementing a repersonalization program.

Help came in the form of two of my former nursing instructors who observed the situation at first hand, offered some practical advice, and gave me some more literature, including the manual *Remotivation Technique: A Manual for Use in Nursing Homes.*[1] The instructors, who had used remotiva-

---

[1] Robinson, Alice M. *Remotivation Technique: A Manual for Use in Nursing Homes.* Philadelphia, Pa., Smith, Kline & French Labs., n.d.

tion technique in several psychiatric nursing situations, suggested ways for me to try it in mine. Particularly pertinent, I thought, were the five steps of remotivation technique: (1) the climate of acceptance; (2) a bridge to reality; (3) sharing the world we live in; (4) an appreciation of the work of the world; (5) the climate of appreciation.

Literally borrowing ideas, principles, and program procedures from the manual, I began the organization of groups. I personally visited the patients I did not know well and checked all the available information, such as medical, social, mental, and physical records. When the opportunity presented itself, I talked with the families of patients. Some of my inquiries concerned the patient's former interests, hobbies, occupations, and living localities, and earlier personality. In short, I grasped any bit of information that would help me to know and understand the patient as an individual. I asked patients' relatives what they thought their son or mother or daughter would like while living at Saint Luke's, and the responses were encouraging and informative. Many of them thought their relative "could do more," and wanted him to do "something other than sit around all day."

With the aid of the nursing supervisor, I selected ten women patients. Then I went to each of those selected and invited her to come to the recreation room downstairs that afternoon for a little "social hour." The initial invitation met with five refusals, such as "I've never been down there before"; "If Mrs. Waldon is coming, I won't!" I hated to push, but felt these refusals were born of fear of the "unknown," feeling "out of place," or just plain "indifference." I insisted pleasantly—jesting with one, encouraging another, until they all accepted.

The first meeting was held during the Thanksgiving season, a time I realized had once brimmed with activity for many of them. One by one, they came and assembled around the large table in the recreational room. Their sex was about the only thing they had in common, but there were two who could "carry the ball" in conversation.

Step one, the "climate of acceptance," was enacted. As I circled the group, I spoke individually to each one. "Isn't this a colorful autumn day?" "Your hair looks no nice, Josephine, when it's curled and combed like it is now." "How is your grandson?" I was struck by the way each seemed to perk up with this bit of personal attention.

The four remaining steps of remotivation technique then fell into line. They listened and responded—especially when they recalled their past activities at Thanksgiving time. Quite by accident, two of the group discovered that they came from the same town in Minnesota. (Since that time, these two women have made frequent visits to each other's rooms, reminiscing about things back home.)

At the end of the hour, I asked the group if they would like to come again. Responses ran from a bored, indifferent "Well, maybe" to a "Oh, yes! It's so good to get out of my room!" I had explained to them the general purpose of the meetings, emphasizing that I would welcome their suggestions for future meetings. I wanted them to be actively involved and not just passive joiners who would come just because a bell rang for another meeting. Then I asked what they wanted to name our group and how often we should meet.

Responses to this query came in abundance. Mrs. Saunders, a woman with multiple sclerosis, suggested: "Why not call ourselves the 'Sample Meeting?' I used to belong to a church group who met in different members' homes, and every member brought some goods and samples to work on for the church while there. And," she continued, "because each of us brought something and worked together we were successful in helping one another and others." Miss Backet, a sweet little spinster, then suggested with real enthusiasm, "Let's do call ourselves the Sample Club; I've always just loved clubs!" So by general agreement we became the Sample Club. Obviously this title was more meaningful to them than something like the "remotivation technique meetings." Different titles—same program. We decided to meet twice a week in the afternoons. I told them I would post the exact dates and times on the newly installed bulletin boards which had been placed on each of the three floors.

Some of the other topics we covered in ensuing meetings were: Christmas carols, women's fashions, the beauty of flowers, canning vegetables and fruits, and death.

Perhaps one might question the prudence of discussing death in a group such as this one. I felt apprehensive about even broaching the subject, and yet, I felt an inner urgency to do so since many of the patients had so often talked of or implied feelings about wanting to die. Some had openly expressed, "I came here to die." Another reason for presenting this topic was that one of the major responsibilities of the home's personnel is to help patients prepare themselves for death.

I began the meeting on death with a reading from the Old Testament—Psalms 129 and 22. There was so little response when I closed the Bible, I felt like singing a requiem for the meeting itself. There were downcast eyes, straight-lined, closed mouths, frequent changes in posture—in short, a deep sadness seemed to fill the air. Then I proceeded with the fourth step: "appreciation of the subject."

Hesitantly, haltingly, the women then began to reveal their thoughts about death. "I guess death is a time everybody has to meet." "I hope my life will be my ticket to a good death." "I don't like to think about it—but I often do. It's so unknowable." "Sometimes I feel bad about wanting to die, but there's nothing to live for now." "If it weren't wrong, I would like to kill myself now, but I have to keep going until God takes me." For the first time in any of the sessions, the women began to question one another as to how they felt about death. They talked about what life after death might be like, how they wanted to be reunited with their husbands and loved ones, and what they expected heaven to be like.

Then the conversation lagged, so I asked them how they could prepare themselves for death and how they could help one another meet and accept it. No one answered. I wondered whether this question was too personal. Then Josephine, a woman who had frequent epileptic seizures, said: "One way could be by loving one another here on earth, being kind, overlooking the 'odd' qualities in one another." (Was Josephine pleading for herself?) Others in the group agreed that being good to one another now would make it easier to die, that they would not have so much to regret. Their making death a part of living came as a surprise to me. I felt relieved and happy about it. After the patients had talked further about how they could treat each other better, the meeting ended—a success!

Anyone who has worked in a nursing home is aware that the constant bickering and pettiness among patients is distressful not only for the patients but also for the personnel. The week following the discussion on death, the staff noticed a new thoughtfulness among the patients, evidenced by such little remarks as "Let's wait for Mrs. Adams before we go on the elevator. She's afraid to go on that contraption alone."

There is a Chinese proverb which says: "One stout pole cannot support a house alone." I, too, needed more support,, and it came in two ways. The first was in the person of a fellow worker, Mrs. Hall, a 50-year-old woman who had reared five children and had an especially warm, concerned attitude toward the elderly and infirm. I explained the technique to her and asked if she would be interested in helping me with it. (Of course, I had cleared this proposal beforehand with the administrator, who had readily complied with my plan.) After attending some of the Sample Club meetings and studying the remotivation technique, Mrs. Hall organized her own group, composed of men and women.

My second source of help was a group of ten young girls who lived in the neighborhood. These seventh- and eighth-graders organized a volunteer group and voted to call themselves the Cheeries because, after having seen and socialized with the patients at the home, they felt they could help best by being cheerful. This positive, simple philosophy provided an effective approach to some of the obvious problems created by depersonalization.

In time the Cheeries proved to be good leaders in the remotivation program. Besides their youthful enthusiasm, they were full of ideas and methods of introducing different subjects for the meetings. Many belonged to Campfire and Girl Scout groups. The activities and the attitude of brotherhood fostered by these organizations prepared the Cheeries to be successful with the patients. They have weekly Saturday morning group sessions with the patients.

One of their group meetings failed disastrously, however. The topic was "dancing," and when these youngsters demonstrated the "Watusi," the older folks were lost. When Mr. Gangly suggested they do the "Lindy Hop," or the "Cake Walk," the Cheeries just looked puzzled. It became apparent that the chasm of time between these two age groups was too wide to bridge. The meeting came to a close rather abruptly when Mrs. Smith declared she didn't approve of such dancing (I'm still not sure whether she meant the "Lindy" or the "Watusi"), and resolutely left the room in her wheelchair. They had learned their lesson. Thereafter, all topics were scrupulously inspected for meaningfulness for the patient.

A more positive factor in the Cheeries' contribution is the ability to follow up. For example, when a patient remarked that she had formerly been interested in knitting, one of the Cheeries brought her a gift of yarn and a set of knitting needles. Again, after the nearly blind Mrs. Cass mentioned in a meeting how she had always enjoyed walking in the woods, the Cheeries started to regularly take her for walks in the nearby park and neighborhood. She often returns to Saint Luke's with a collection of leaves or flowers that a Cheerie has gathered for her to touch and smell. These examples could be multiplied many times.

The future looks brighter than it did on my first day at Saint Luke's. We now have a sewing club, bingo parties, the BPC Club (Birthday Preparation and Celebration), and a single group which meets in the recreation room or the chapel. Plans are under way to organize still other groups and to reorganize the present ones and add variety to them. Also, in the future, we hope to take part in a remotivation technique workshop in order to deepen and improve our approach.

In addition to the changes brought about by these group activities, there have also been changes in approach to nursing care. Some of the nurses' aides who attended one or more of the meetings have been stimulated to use a simplified motivation technique while actually caring for patients, then bringing the technique to the bedside. For example, when entering a room, they greet the patients by title and name (step one), and seek to initiate objective, pleasant conversation. The former problem of depersonalization has been alleviated to a marked degree by the introduction of motivation.

Reading 65
Nursing the Patient with Internal Hip Fixation
Sister Maria Francis

Although Ambroise Paré recognized fracture of the femoral neck almost 400 years ago, and despite the many advances of internal fixation, this injury still is difficult to treat. It will remain a problem until aseptic necrosis and nonunion can be lessened. Proper reduction, accurate and adequate internal fixation, and conscientious pre- and postoperative care are vital to these patients.

In our present society, with its longer life span, many a senior citizen's appearance and activity belie his chronological age. But osteoporotic, degenerative processes have crept into his skeletal framework insidiously, unnoticed until the day he slides on the scatter rug, stumbles over the grandchild's toy, or slips on a newly polished floor. Because osteoporosis has weakened the lamella of the femoral neck with its supportive calcar femorale, such trivial accidents may cause a subcapital fracture in the upper end of the femur.

A recent study of 296 patients with intracapsular fracture of the femoral neck furnishes some clues to help the orthopedic nurse view her patient in clearer perspective. Of these 296 patients the method of injury was learned for 279: of the 253 fractures which resulted from minor accidents, 187 occurred indoors and 66 outdoors; only 26 patients experienced severe accidents. Another significant finding was a history of concurrent diseases. Among these 296 patients, 137 had a recognizable cardiac lesion: 39 were arteriosclerotic, 91 hypertensive, and 7 rheumatic; 62 patients had no abnormal heart condition but a host of other medical problems. These were so pronounced in 32 individuals that they were semi-invalids before sustaining the hip injury. Only 97 had no definable medical difficulties and were

Reprinted from *The American Journal of Nursing*, vol. 64, no. 5, pp. 111-112, May 1964.

healthy at the time of accident. Obviously, then, the orthopedic nurse receives a patient who has not only a hip fracture but often a medical disease.[1]

PREOPERATIVE NURSING CARE

Ideally, the patient is admitted to the hospital directly from the radiology department because this eliminates painful moves from ambulance to bed to stretcher to x-ray table and back to bed again. The hour of admission initiates the beginning of rehabilitation. The patient is placed in bed on an orthopedic mattress or on one with boards between mattress and springs to provide firm support. During the 48 to 72 hours which may elapse before surgery, the nurse can do much to reassure and prepare her patient. First, she should evaluate his particular requirements. Since he probably is elderly, and perhaps is having his first hospital experience, she should explain the usual hospital life to him—mealtimes, how to use his signal bell, visiting hours, the various doctors and technicians whom he will meet, and perhaps the average progress for patients with similar injury.

She should introduce her patient to his self-helper, the over-head trapeze. Learning to assist himself in necessary movements will bolster his self-sufficiency. When he finds that by grasping the bar and using his "good" leg he can raise himself comfortably on to the fracture bedpan, he is saved both embarrassment and discomfort. Also, if this simple procedure is mastered soon after admission, it may eliminate the need for an indwelling catheter after operation. Patients actually have become dehydrated and undernourished for no reason other than their aversion to bedpans. With the trapeze, too, the patient can raise himself from the pillow or help turn to a more restful position. The by-product of this activity—exercise of the large muscles of his chest and arms—will stimulate deep breathing, important now but far more essential after surgery.

Mealtime is the nurse's opportunity to acquaint her patient with the art of eating from a position which, at first, seems anything but comfortable. She patiently assists him to manipulate himself into the most comfortable position possible. The older he is, the longer this will take, but it is time well spent if it adds enjoyment to his meal.

Fluids and diet as tolerated can be encouraged because these patients with hip fractures have little, if any, gastrointestinal distress either before or after fixation. In selecting foods, one emphasizes proteins and vitamins and, above all, considers each individual's chewing powers! It is not wise to

---

[1] Banks, H. H. Factors influencing the results in fractures of the femoral neck. *J. Bone Joint Surg. (Amer.)*, **44**-A:931-964, July 1962.

spoon-feed elderly patients unless they are extremely helpless or senile. But if a patient does require complete feeding, the graceful manner of the nurse affects his appetite more than one would imagine. Usually, kindly supervision or slight assistance will insure adequate and enjoyable nourishment. The nurse must strive to help her patient maintain his independence even if it is only in choosing Jello or pudding.

A comfort factor for any sick person, but one that deserves special attention among orthopedic patients, is skin care. If traction is used, frequent inspection of the affected limb and of any parts indirectly involved is a "must" for assuring unimpaired circulation. Bathing, massage, and positioning to relieve pressure are vital to prevent decubiti. The heels must be watched for redness or blister. As prophylaxis, a small blanket may be placed under the leg from below the knee to the ankle.

POSTOPERATIVE CARE

Those general practices of orthopedic nursing already highlighted grow in importance during the postoperative period. They are supplemented with careful execution of such procedures as change of body position with exercise of the unaffected parts, safeguarding of the fixation immobilization as determined by the particular surgery, and ambulation when it is ordered.

Implementation of these three measures varies according to the type of fixation used. The nurse should know the distinctions between the procedures customarily employed in two of the most favored treatments, immobilization by use of a hip prosthesis or by Smith-Petersen nail.

Usually the surgeon specifies the details of immobilization. His choice depends on the degree of stability of the hip joint which he found during surgery. If he employed a prosthesis for internal fixation, he directs the nurse to use one of the following methods of immobilization:

1   Arrange sandbags on each side of the entire leg so that it is in neutral rotation and abducted at approximately 20 to 30 degrees.
2   Use an antirotation boot to maintain stable position of the extremity. In some cases he advises abduction at the same time.
3   Place in skin or skeletal traction—for very unstable hips only—and suspend extremity in a Thomas splint and Pearson attachment which supports the leg from the knee down.

Exercise of the affected limb, either active or active-assisted, frequently is begun about the second or third, or the seventh or eighth postoperative day, but the specific time depends on the joint's stability. The nurse should turn her patient on his unoperated side, for a short time only. Pillows between his legs will prevent adduction and rotation.

Ambulation commences from five days to six weeks after surgery, again with consideration of the hip joint stability. If full weight bearing during ambulation is prescribed, the nurse should encourage her patient to discard his walker when he can.

If the Smith-Petersen nail is the fixation device, postoperative nursing care is simpler.

Immobilization, if used at all, is of short duration because hip motion is encouraged as soon as the patient can cooperate. He is turned from side to side as early as the first day. On the second or third day, he should be helped out of bed and into a chair for a brief period. However, even though this person with a nail fixation exercises much sooner than one with a hip prosthesis, all weight bearing on the operated side is prohibited for at least three to six months. But, once again, time is variable, dependent upon the patient's condition and the surgeon's judgement.

The nurse should make a patient's move from bed to chair as natural as possible. First, the bed is lowered either by removing its casters or using the high-low mechanism. Second, she assists him to the edge of the bed so that he can place his feet on the floor. She encourages him to wear shoes from the start for proper support. The sitting position is maintained for five or ten minutes. When he stands, the nurse adjusts his robe length to prevent tripping. Constantly having to lift his robe would prolong the fear and apprehension so often entertained about walking.

The patient's chair should have a framework of utmost stability but simple design, a back which is either solid or has vertical slats extending nearly to the seat, to which the back joins at a right angle, arms sufficiently wide to serve as "rests" and "push-ups," seat width proportioned to his size, depth that provides room for his thighs to rest comfortably without popliteal pressure, and height that permits his feet to rest on the floor with his legs nearly perpendicular to his thighs.

Two factors affect his acceptance of this big step forward to recovery—time and enjoyableness. The sitting-up period must be kept short, 30 to 45 minutes at the most, and taken two or three times daily at intervals appealing to the patient. This arrangement prevents the overfatigue, discouragement, the real aversion to further trials which one very long period often causes.

The nurse directs every effort toward helping her patient enjoy this exercise so that he anxiously anticipates its repetition. For the avid reader, she locates paperback books because of their light weight. She can secure a strong piece of cardboard over the chair arms and challenge him to defeat her or an imaginary opponent at cards, checkers, or Scrabble. He may like to write letters or prefer to eat his lunch in this more familiar sitting position. Any project which will not be too great a strain is worthwhile if it keeps him contentedly out of bed. Many patients of this age group are satisfied just to relax while spinning yarns or sharing each other's experiences.

The orthopedic nurse should realize that her personal contributions to her patient's happiness deserve an equal rating with her technical proficiency. Since victims of hip fracture have an average age of nearly 70 years, it is quite evident that the very best nursing skills must be accompanied by an understanding approach if geriatric patients are to resume their lives with the most physical dexterity and emotional independence. The nurse's aim as she positions, turns, and encourages her patient, and plumbs her own ingenuity to arouse his interests, is to hasten his return to normal living. Although her words cannot be those of St. Peter, "Rise up and walk," she can sincerely say with him, "Such as I have, give I thee . . ."—compassion and understanding.

Reading 66

The Nurse's Role in Preventing Circulatory Complications in the Patient with a Fractured Hip

Immaculata M. Alba
and
Janice Papeika

It has become increasingly apparent that even in this scientific day and age, nursing intervention in the areas of prevention of illness and rehabilitation still has not become an integral part of the nursing care plan. The concern we feel regarding this lack of intervention on the part of the nurse has been one of the reasons for writing this paper.

When a person is immobilized for any length of time, as with a fractured hip, a process begins the outcome of which the nurse can to a certain extent predict and control. Nursing care becomes dynamic when the nurse makes meaningful and knowledgeable intervention to restore the patient to his former state of health. Static nursing care enhances the stasis to which the patient is already predisposed. It is the objective of this paper to suggest nursing care measures designed to prevent stasis and its resulting complications. Keeping in mind that stasis affects all body systems, the complications of the circulatory system will be emphasized here, and since most patients with fractured hips are elderly, the particular needs of this age group will be taken into account.

Because the nurse may be caring for a patient at any time during his recovery, it is important to institute the most effective preventive measures appropriate to the point where she begins. For example, the nurse caring for the patient in the immediate postoperative phase has responsibilities that may vary somewhat from those of the nurse who begins caring for a patient who already has signs and symptoms of complications.

THE PATHOPHYSIOLOGY OF THROMBUS FORMATION

The chief complication with which we are concerned here is thrombus formation. Preventive nursing care is enhanced when the nurse is aware of the pathophysiologic changes leading to thrombus formation.

Newton's first law of motion states,

> Every body perseveres in its state of rest—unless it is compelled to change that state by forces impressed thereon.

Although Newton was not referring to fracture patients, the point is just as appropriate here. When the body is at rest the metabolic needs are reduced, causing a reduction in all body processes. In the circulatory system, this means that cardiac output is diminished. However, the blood volume does not diminish appreciably, and the venous system, acting as a reservoir, tends to become filled. The middle layer or media of the veins contains less elastic and muscular tissue than that of the arteries, so that the veins collapse when empty and do not retain their shape.

Forces which affect the flow of blood through the vessels may be summed up as follows: (1) shape of the vein; (2) straightness of the vessel; (3) muscular activity; (4) viscosity of the blood; (5) gravity; and (6) changes in the size of the lumen of the vessel.

Contraction of the muscles in the extremities facilitates the compression and the valves are arranged so that direction of flow can only be toward the heart. Therefore, each time a person tenses his muscles, blood is moved toward the heart. When a patient is immobilized, the muscle "pump" is not in operation and stasis occurs.

The Influence of Age

Stasis, disease, dehydration, and roughening of the vascular endothelium are conditions which may be found in the elderly—even those without an orthopedic condition—all caused either by microorganisms, surgery, or trauma, and all can cause intravascular clotting. In addition, this kind of patient is likely to have one or more chronic diseases which will further decrease his reserve and place an additional burden on his capacity to adapt. This simply means that his body is less able to cope with situations placing stress on his functional capacity.

Senescence brings about fibrotic changes in the vascular system as in the rest of the body. Fibrotic tissue replaces some of the elastic tissue in the media and causes decreased venous return. The veins become dilated and tortuous and the blood cannot move as fast around these curves.

The Effects of Trauma

Trauma usually precedes a fractured hip, and the need for surgical intervention to obtain optimal bone union and alignment carries with it the possibility of infection. These factors may destroy the integrity of the vascular wall. Immobility during this time, both preoperatively and postoperatively, predisposes the patient to stasis.

When the rate of blood flow is slowed, cells tend to leave the center of the blood vessels, where they are normally concentrated, and move toward the periphery where they come in contact with the vascular walls. Normally, the intima and platelets are mutually repulsive, each being negatively charged to prevent intravascular clotting. However, a damaged wall loses its charge and attracts platelets. The platelets, adhering to the vessel wall, trigger off the clotting mechanism. Leukocytes and large numbers of platelets gather at the site of adherence. The thrombus at this point is not firmly attached and can become an embolus. Clinical evidence of blood flow disturbance and inflammation usually are not present at this stage but may be anticipated at a somewhat later time.

Within the vessel, part of the thrombus is attached at the point of origin. The remaining portion floats freely within the lumen. It becomes adherent when contact is made with the vessel wall, and thus the lumen becomes obstructed. Vasospasm from irritation further constricts the lumen, flow is impeded, and more coagulation takes place. The involved veins reveal edema, degeneration of smooth muscle fibers, and proliferation of fibroblasts. Because of this fibrotic process the valves become thickened, scarred, and completely functionless. Venous walls become sclerotic and their lumens become tortuous and irregular. Permanent disturbances in the hemodynamics occur.

Causes of Embolization

Theories which may explain the embolization of a thrombus suggest that any sudden increase in venous pressure, such as may accompany coughing, sudden motion, and straining at stool, may cause part of the thrombus to break away from the wall, becoming an embolus. Excessive clot retraction occurring in chronic anemia, which is often present in the elderly, because of longstanding poor nutritional habits, or in anemia following surgery, may also tend to loosen the clot from the vessel walls and permit it to be dislodged by the passing stream of blood.

THE NURSE'S ROLE IN PREVENTION OF THROMBOSIS AND EMBOLUS

It would appear that the nurse must act as the "forces impressed thereon" in Newton's first law if she wishes to change the patient's "state of rest." It will undoubtedly fall to the nurse to plan with the physician those nursing measures that will prevent these complications.

Gluteal and quadriceps setting exercises are valuable supplements to the usual range-of-motion exercises because they are easy to perform, painless, and can be done without much supervision. Footboard walking is another easy feat for the patient to perform on his own, once it is explained to him. The use of an overhead trapeze or rope attached to the foot of the bed allows the patient to actively exercise the upper extremities and trunk and gives him more independence. The trend toward early ambulation with help can be included as a factor of major importance. Deep breathing exercises, coughing, and turning should still be considered essentials in preventing stasis in the pulmonary vascular bed.

In view of the relative lack of elasticity of the veins and the structure and function of the valves, position plays an important part in venous return. The patient may usually be turned from side to side and the legs may be elevated to promote flow toward the heart. As mentioned earlier, changes in the size of the lumen affect blood flow. When the vessel is compressed, blood cannot flow through readily. The straighter the vessel, the less resistance to flow. Constant flexion of any joint must be avoided since it causes compression and subsequent pooling of blood. Use of the Gatch bed, pillows or rolls under the knees, or other positions causing flexion should be approached with caution.

Properly used, elastic stockings provide support for tired, sagging veins. The stockings must be of the correct size and must be removed at least once every 8 hours, so that they do not act as a tourniquet. If edema, mottling of the skin, numbness, tingling, or cold feet occur, the stockings should be removed at once. The patient's subjective signs may be the first clue a nurse has that something is wrong.

Since dehydration increases the viscosity of blood, adequate hydration is necessary to prevent intravascular clotting. Thus the forcing of fluids assumes prime importance and cannot be minimized.

Securing the Patient's Cooperation

Patients having reparative surgery of the hip do not willingly accept turning, no matter how lofty the goals of the nurse. The discomfort of the patient is probably the chief reason meaningful nursing intervention is not undertaken. Even the most knowledgeable and technically competent nurse may often be deterred from doing what she knows to be best—in this case turning and moving the patient to prevent the complications that she knows may begin to appear postoperatively.

Several approaches to this problem that we have found helpful include administering analgesics a half hour before attempting to reposition or exercise the patient, and preparing the patient preoperatively for the exercises and movements that will be expected of him after surgery. Careful, clear explanations before attempting to move him and the provision of sufficient assistance will all be of help in reducing fear and pain. The nurse should also enlist the cooperation of family members to provide the emotional support so necessary during times of stress.

Above all, the nurse must know her patient: she must recognize his limitations, aid him to set goals for himself, and allow him to set the limits of his capabilities, and then support him in his attempt to meet these goals.

We strongly maintain that the nurse, who spends more time with the patient than anyone else, is in a far better position to prevent circulatory complications of the fracture patient than any other member of the health team.

REFERENCES

Beland, Irene L., Read, Esther H., Ronan, Jane F., Passos, Joyce, and Martin, Nancy: *Clinical Nursing—Pathophysiological and Psychosocial Approaches.* New York, The Macmillan Co., 1965.

Beeson, P. B., and McDermott, W. (eds.): *Cecil-Loeb Textbook of Medicine,* 11th ed. Philadelphia, W. B. Saunders Co., 1963.

Harrison, T. R.: *Principles of Internal Medicine,* 4th ed. Blakiston Division, McGraw-Hill Book Co., 1962.

Reading 67
Tips on Using Crutches, Canes, and Walkers
Charles D. Bonner
Jack Hofkosh
Robert H. Jebsen
Charles Neuhauser

Text reprinted from "Tips on Using Crutches, Canes, and Walkers," *Patient Care*, pp. 17-51, October 1968. Copyright © 1968, Miller and Fink Publishing Corporation. All rights reserved. (The photographs appearing in this article are similar to, but not identical with, the ones in the original article.)

Figure 67-1. **WALKERS: Standing up**

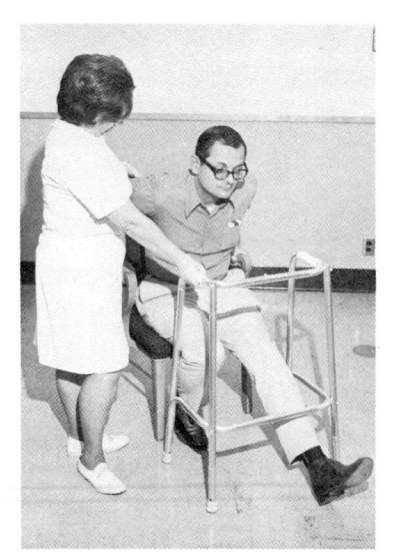

A. After surgery for a broken left hip, this man is learning how to stand with his walker. He sits on the front edge of the chair, which will help him bring his center of gravity over his right foot. Notice that his right foot is slightly under the chair, which helps him straighten his knee.

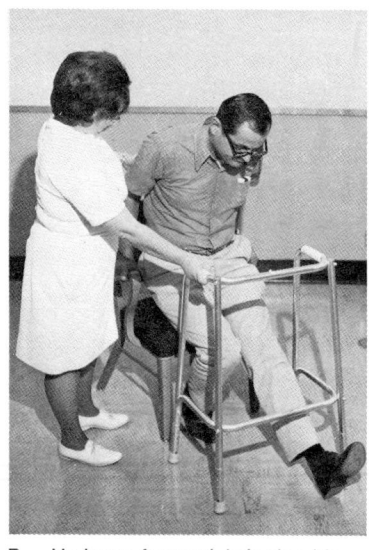

B. He leans forward, bringing his head forward, and pushes down on the armrests with his hands.

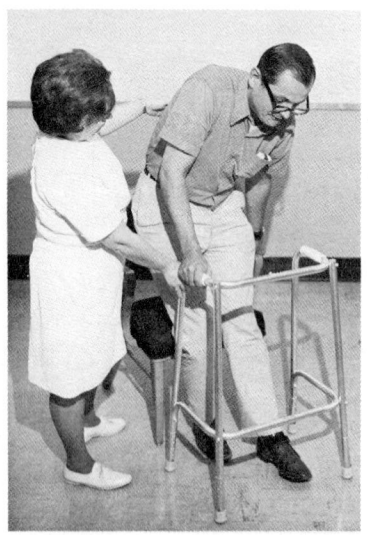

C. He moves the hand opposite the injured leg to the walker and shifts his weight forward onto his strong leg.

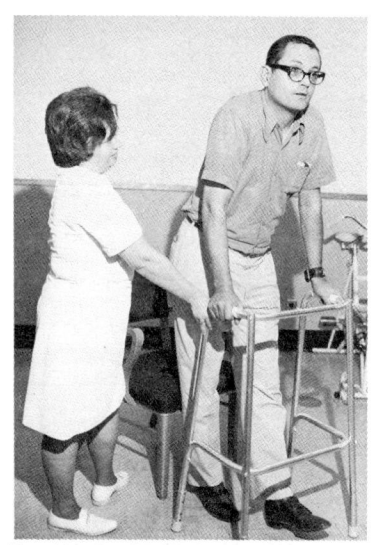

D. He stands erect.

530

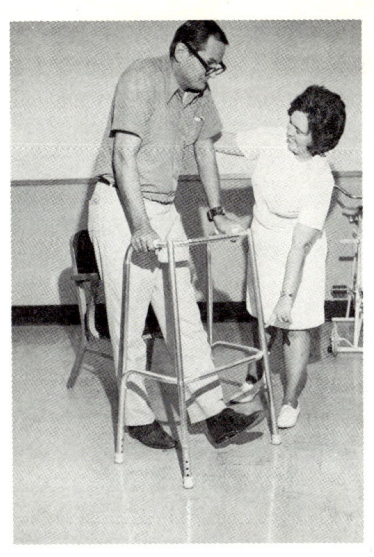

A. "Keep your heel off the floor as you stand up," the nurse cautions the patient. Notice that his elbows are slightly bent when he stands in one place.

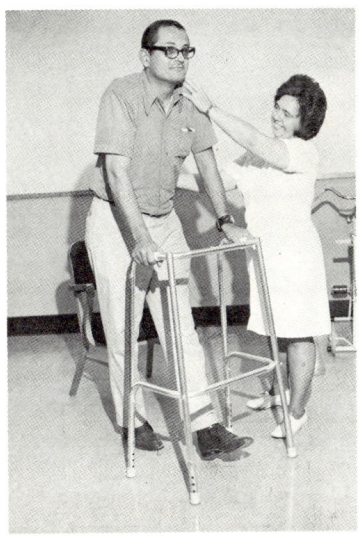

B. He places the walker 8-10 inches ahead.

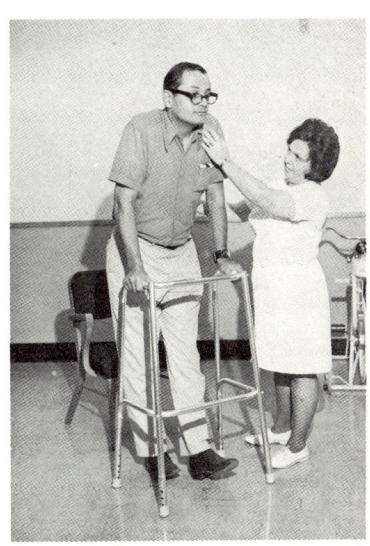

C. He straightens his elbows to swing himself forward to the walker.

531

Figure 67-3. **WALKERS: Sitting down**

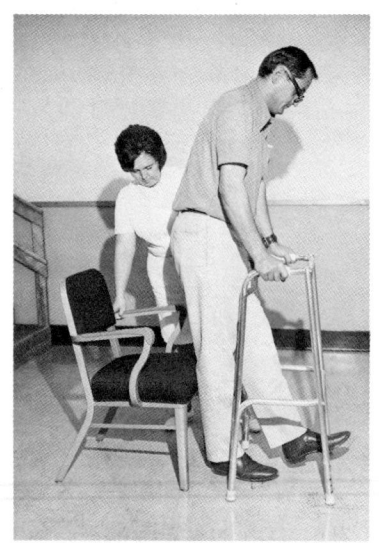

A. "Be sure the back of your strong leg is against the chair before you sit down," warns the nurse.

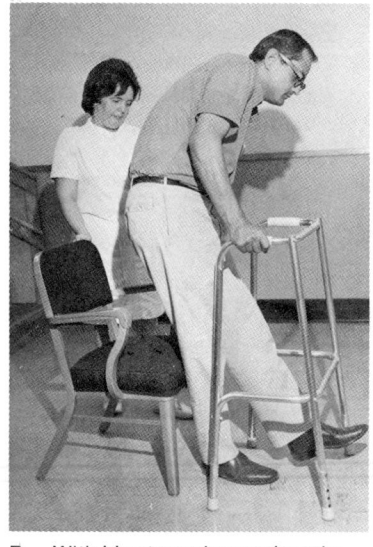

B. With his strong leg against the chair, he puts his opposite hand on the chair arm.

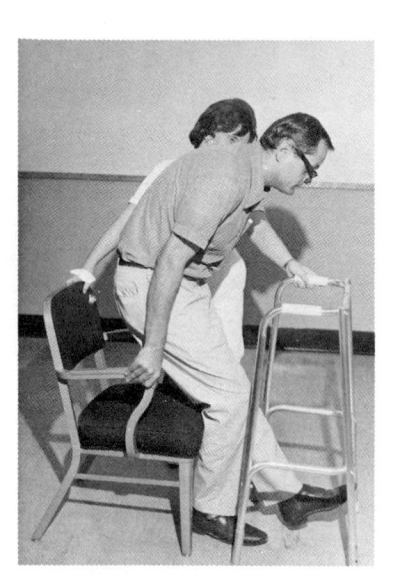

C. Then he places his right hand on the right chair arm and leans forward as...

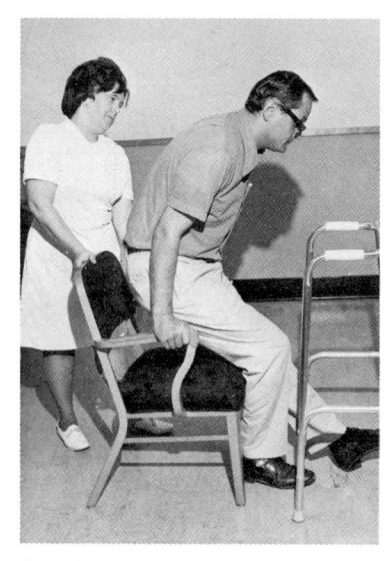

D. He gently lowers himself onto the chair. He is instructed to avoid low chairs and to use chairs with arms whenever possible.

Figure 67-4. **AXILLARY CRUTCHES: Standing**

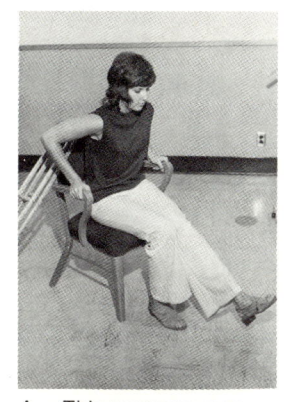

A. This young woman keeps her crutches handy by hooking them on the back of the chair. To stand she slides forward in the chair, with the foot of her strong leg slightly under the chair.

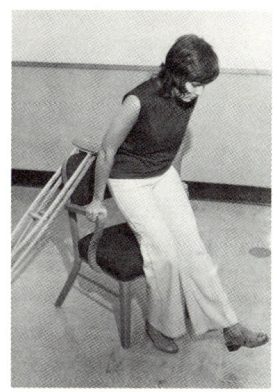

B. She pushes down against the armrests and leans slightly forward as she stands.

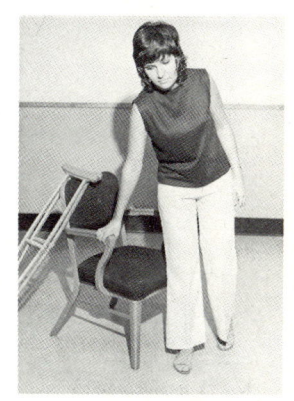

C. She pivots on her strong right foot.

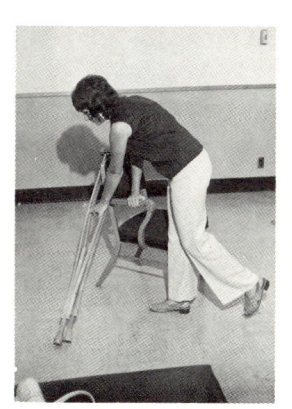

D. Placing both hands on the armrest, she picks up both crutches with the one hand.

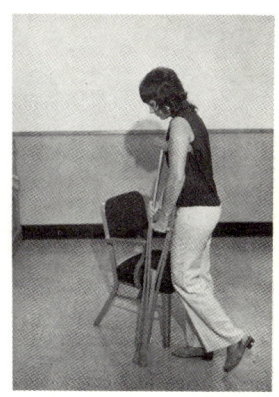

E. She then places both crutches under one arm before shifting one crutch to the other arm.

533

Figure 67-5. **AXILLARY CRUTCHES: Sitting down**

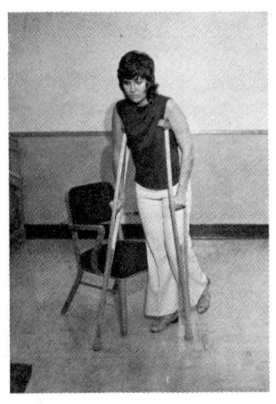

A. As the young woman approaches the chair she moves her strong leg in close to the chair.

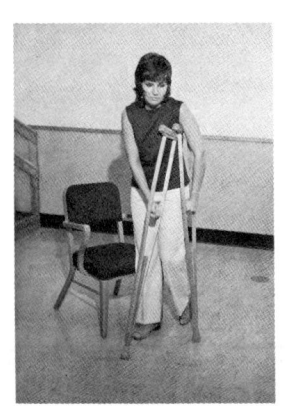

B. She then places both crutches under her left arm.

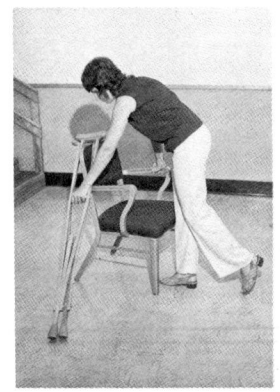

C. Placing her right hand on the left arm of the chair, she hooks the crutches on the back of the chair.

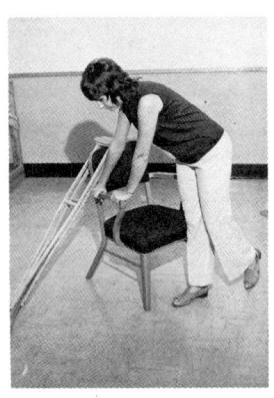

D. Now she pivots on the right foot.

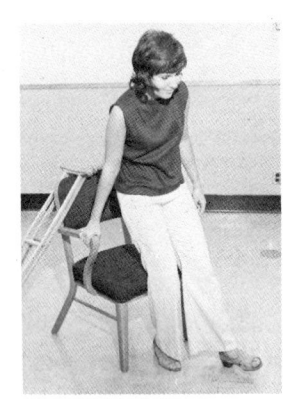

E. Placing her right leg against the chair, she brings her right hand around to the right chair arm.

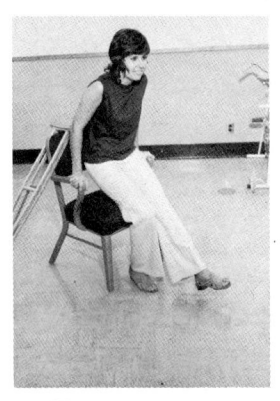

F. She gently lowers herself into the chair.

Figure 67-6. **AXILLARY CRUTCHES: Going upstairs**

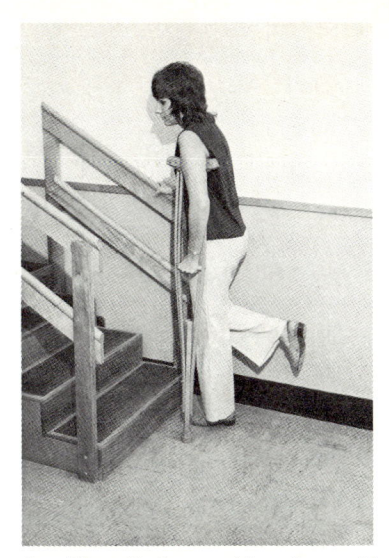

A. "Up with the good leg, down with the bad." Since she cannot put any weight on her left leg, she uses her crutches and the handrail to support her weight.

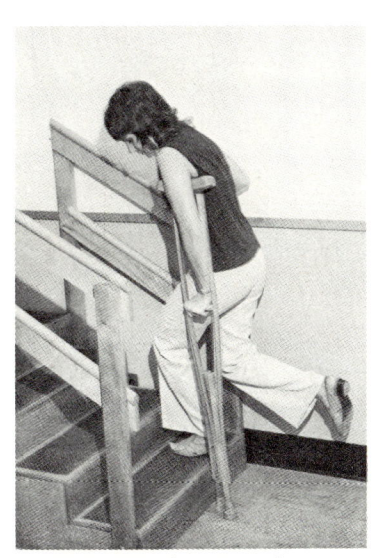

B. She swings her strong leg up.

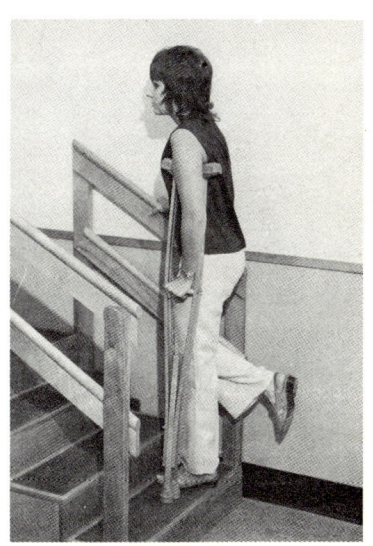

C. Then she lifts her body weight by straightening her strong hip and knee as she would for normal stair climbing. Leaning forward helps in straightening a weakened "strong knee."

535

Figure 67-7. **AXILLARY CRUTCHES: Coming downstairs**

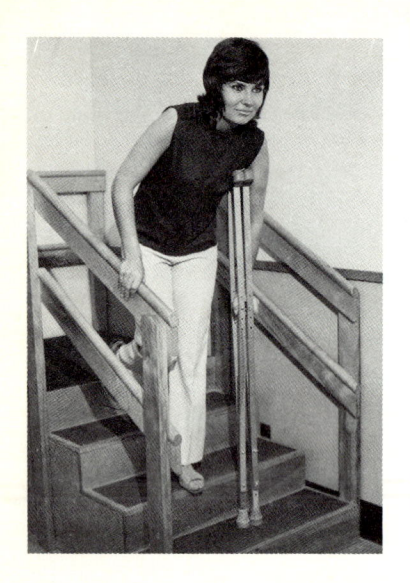

A. "Up with the good leg, down with the bad—for going down too." With her crutches on the strong side going down, she keeps the stronger left leg on the step above as she moves her crutches down a step.

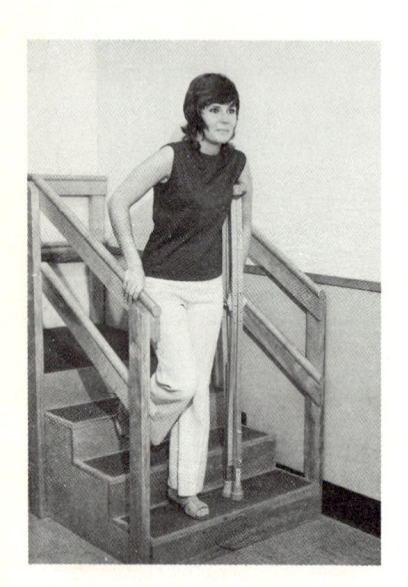

B. Then she brings her leg down. Notice that she keeps her head and shoulders back to keep her center of balance from pitching forward. The rule "up with the good leg, down with the bad" holds for curbs too. Two crutches are used instead of crutch and rail.

Reading 68

It's Not Age That Interferes with Nutrition of the Elderly

W. Henry Sebrell, Jr.

Malnutrition in the elderly is already a clinical problem of some significance, but it is really beginning to be fully appreciated by the medical profession. As their numbers increase, the elderly will need more and more help and guidance from the health professions, more careful search for the responsible factors, and more individual attention in advising on diet and eating habits.

If the elderly patient has a nutritional problem, his difficulty could be some nutritional error peculiar to the aged, but this possibility becomes increasingly remote as we learn more about geriatric patients and their needs. "Geriatric nutrition" deals mainly with the results of a lifetime accumulation of bad habits, mistakes, accidents and disease and very little with the physiological changes which accompany aging. Search for the source of the difficulty should be in other directions, with the answer most likely to be found in certain specific aspects of his life pattern that distinguish the elderly from younger individuals.

Almost all elderly patients can assimilate well. There may be minor changes in digestion that can be attributed to age, although these differences in the life pattern may have a profound effect on diet and eating habits. It is in this field that we can offer the most help to the enfeebled, discouraged, malnourished geriatric patient.

In the first place, it is important to remember that the elderly patient is living in a world totally different from the one he was born into. This has important nutritional implications because eating habits are established early in life and they tend to persist. We relish most the foods we were given as youngsters and we do not always find it easy to enjoy strange flavors, odors, and textures in foods new to us.

Studies by many authorities in the field of nutrition have confirmed the early establishment of food preferences. Many current observations also attest the difficulties arising when attempts are made to alter diets. Furnishing wheat to some groups in India, starving because of lack of rice with which they are familiar, creates problems in acceptance. Japanese soldiers taken prisoner during World War II not only did not like the food offered by their American captors, they actually were made ill when they first tried to eat it.

It is no wonder that the elderly patient tends to dislike many modern

Reprinted from *Nutrition Today*, vol. 1, no. 2, pp. 15–18, June 1966.

processed foods. To him they just don't taste the same as the foods that were obtained from the family garden and prepared in the farm kitchen. To the elderly, food and its preparation used to be more interesting, enjoyable, even exciting, than it is now.

A study in food preference, using citrus products, gave interesting confirmation of the importance of early experience. A group of elderly patients were offered a choice of reconstituted frozen orange juice, freshly squeezed orange juice, and a fresh orange. Preference was for the whole orange, with fresh prepared juice second and the reconstituted juice third.

This becomes highly significant when the following facts are considered: (1) No one in our society who has passed military draft age had frozen orange juice as a baby. (2) No one beyond high school age established his food preferences at a time when frozen foods were on the market. (3) No one over grammar school age formed his eating habits when frozen dinners were available to shoppers. The elderly individuals most likely chose the whole orange because that was the only way they could get oranges when they were in their formative years.

A serious factor affecting eating habits of the elderly is that of dentition. A high percentage have lost their own teeth, and the quality of dentures varies greatly. According to the United States Public Health Service, more than 22 million people in the United States wear dentures. Many have never learned to use them for adequate mastication. It was formerly the practice of many dentists to await gum healing after extractions before fitting dentures. The patient who had become accustomed to a mouth without teeth found the new plates intolerable. The result is that many of our present elderly patients wear their dentures in their pockets more than in their mouths. Some have not been able to afford proper dental care, with the result that their dentures do not fit well. These factors have a profound effect on their food selection. They tend to avoid some foods of importance in good nutrition simply because they cannot use them and maintain mouth comfort.

A striking example of this type came to our attention recently. This was a case of pellagra in a woman who lived in a flat not far from the Medical Center. She was in her seventies and a bit senile but the difficulty arose because she had lost all her teeth. She was living almost exclusively on corn meal mush because she couldn't chew much of anything else that suited her taste.

Many elderly people reduce their consumption of meat. We say they seem to have lost their taste for meat but this is probably not true. They just can't eat it with comfort. The same thing applies to many fruits and vegetables. The intestinal tract is thus deprived of the bulk it needs in order to keep its production-line type of activity working properly. Sluggishness thus induced, plus inadequate grinding and poor mixing for exposure to digestive enzymes, accounts for much of the malnutrition and constipation plaguing the aged. Their nutritional apparatus is not out of order. It is handicapped, and does not get a chance to function.

Some elderly people are deprived of an important stimulus to appetite and the enjoyment of food because of a diminished sense of smell. It is possible that this loss may also interfere with full secretion of saliva and other digestive fluids. A considerable portion of food enjoyment is derived from the sense of smell, and if it is decreased, some of the old pleasure is missing. More importantly, the psychic stimulus which starts the flow of saliva and gastric digestive secretions is lost. Some authorities believe that function of the chief and parietal cells of the gastric mucosa tends to decrease with age. Diminished secretion of hydrochloric acid has been observed. Whether this is due to atrophic change in the mucosa or to inadequate stimulus is not known.

The deficiencies due to aging need not be a factor in malnutrition; if the digestive apparatus is given a chance to operate normally, most healthy older persons can probably utilize their food about as well as their grandchildren.

Factors that are entirely exogenous are brought into the picture by the socio-economic status of the elderly patient. The clinician who is trying to help the elderly patient with a nutritional problem cannot afford to overlook the contents of his shopping bag. Most elderly people live on retirement incomes. They shop for cheaper foods. This usually results in a grocery shopper's shift to the left—to carbohydrate and away from protein. They need meat, fish, poultry, milk and eggs, but potatoes are cheaper.

Another factor entirely unrelated to nutritional physiology is the fact that many of these patients live alone. They may or may not like it but there is little doubt that it has an influence on the way they prepare their meals, if indeed they often bother to prepare an appetizing dinner, let alone breakfast and lunch. They may even lack facilities for the proper preservation and preparation of food.

It may well be that the only companion of the lonely old person is malnutrition. Loneliness is no stimulus to good eating. We tend to enjoy our food more when we share it with others, particularly at pleasant social affairs. It's doubtful that there ever was a lonely epicure.

Physical handicaps can interfere seriously with efforts of the elderly to obtain adequate meals. Arthritis, Parkinsonian tremor and other infirmities are serious deterrents to the activities associated with preparing meals, and sometimes even with eating.

Alcoholism should not be dismissed lightly in discussing problems of any age group. When it exists in the elderly, it may produce numerous difficulties, but one of its chief effects is to raise another barrier to proper food intake. The result may be manifest in one or more significant deficiencies.

We are certain that beriberi, pellagra and scurvy occur in many of our big cities. They may result from other disease processes but many of these cases result from the factors discussed above. We see deficiency diseases at the Medical Center but do not regard their prevalence in New York as unusually high. The trained eye would probably pick up a similar picture in almost any large city in America. These conditions have *not* disappeared from the United States, in spite of the widely held belief that they have.

What is most disquieting about this situation is the fact that many of these diseases are overlooked or misdiagnosed because we have become less alert to their possibility. Early manifestations are not observed because they are not looked for or because the signs and symptoms of early deficiency disease have been forgotton. The possibility of such deficiencies should be kept in mind whenever an elderly patient is examined.

There may be mineral deficiency as well as vitamin lack. Iron intake may be inadequate, or there may be poor absorption, with the result that the patient suffers iron deficiency anemia. Calcium is more apt to be low because of low intake rather than poor absorption. In recent years it has been recognized that chronic calcium undernutrition and the associated negative calcium balance are important factors in the osteoporosis that so frequently plagues the aged.

Since demineralization of bone in osteoporosis may be the end result of prolonged negative calcium balance, it is reasonable to assume that higher calcium intake from middle age onward would be desirable and should be recommended. Milk and milk products are, of course, the best source of dietary calcium but should be advised on an individual basis only. Butter fat has been indicated as an etiologic factor in hypercholesterolemia. Therefore, in cases of hypercholesterolemia, skim milk products are preferred.

The possible role of nutrition in the aging process has been left out of this discussion intentionally because so little is known. It may be that a lifetime of adequate nutrition will have some influence on longevity. As matters now stand, we have been able to achieve a striking increase in life expectancy at birth but not very much in the elderly. Maximum length of life is not much more now than it was in 1900. What we are seeing is an approach toward the maximum by a vastly increased number of people who have been able to escape the former killers of the younger years.

We *do* know that after adolescence age has very little influence on nutritional requirements. For all we can see, the older individual responds to proper protein nutrition in about the same manner as a younger person. Furthermore, some studies have indicated that there is no difference in the ability of old or middle-aged men to adapt to changes in the protein level of their diets. Indeed, it has been shown that, if given a diet high in protein, old men retain nitrogen and exhibit a remarkable ability to increase their protein reserves. This process appears not to be influenced by androgen administration. Quantity may have some influence, but reduction in quantity may be secondary to the many factors introduced by the changed pattern of life as discussed above.

As a result of the multiplicity of these factors, and the many variations in life pattern, it is essential that each case be treated on an individual basis. It is folly to believe that elderly patients can be lumped off as a homogeneous collection of units and each given a piece of paper with the same diet list printed on it.

Every aspect of the patient's life should be investigated. In addition to the history of indigestion, constipation, flatulence, specific food intolerance, and other evidence of digestive malfunction, the other factors should be noted. Does the patient really enjoy his food? What sort of diet did he have when he was a youngster? Does he remember dishes that he enjoyed more than others, and does he ever see them now? Does he live alone? Does he prepare a well-balanced meal for himself or is one prepared for him? Can he eat a steak in comfort? How much milk does he use? Does he use the vegetables and fruits that supply his needs for vitamins? Does he have nasal congestion interfering with his sense of smell? Who does the grocery shopping? What comes home in the shopping bag? And what is the most frequently used method of food preparation?

Careful inquiry into the influence of the life pattern may solve many nutritional problems for the aged, who, after all, are just people who have lived a little longer than the rest of us. They really aren't as different as we might think, and they react to the conditions under which they live just about the same way we would if we traded places with them.

Modern medical science has done much to help the aged over illnesses against which they were defenseless not so long ago. Nutrition is only beginning to come into its own as a scientific discipline, and its importance for the well-being of the elderly is just beginning to be recognized. We hope that our growing insights into the relationship between health and nutrition and the special nutritional problems of the elderly, combined with leap-frogging advances in food science and food processing, can be used to make man's later years vastly more enjoyable and productive.

Part Five

Alcoholism and Drug Abuse

Section A

Alcoholism

The great majority of disabilities are problems principally to the patients themselves, and, in a lesser but still significant extent, to their families. Problems of addiction, however, are rapidly approaching the dimensions that reflect a national crisis. The etiology of this contemporary phenomenon is both manifold and complex. To the extent that cause and effect can be unraveled, meaningful preventive programs can be established. Many times, however, the nurse's first encounter with a patient will not be in the time period when preventive measures are indicated, but rather at the time when the patient is a full-fledged alcoholic or drug addict. At any rate, it is crucial that the nurse be alert and responsive to the trends in order that she can take appropriate rehabilitative measures of either a preventive or corrective nature.

    The preventive approach is illustrated by Potter in her description of an industrial program for alcoholism. She properly stresses the thorough and careful steps to be taken along the way in order to enlist the cooperation of necessary resources at hand.

Epp provides valuable orientation for the nurse as to the kinds of behavior to be expected from new alcoholic admissions, and she suggests a number of nursing procedures in order to bring about some semblance of cooperative response from the patient.

The article by Quiros makes many suggestions that are faithful to the promise of the title "Adjusting Nursing Techniques to the Treatment of Alcoholic Patients." She draws verbal pictures of the most crucial aspects of the nursing of alcoholic patients. She describes the medical care and points out the essential relationship necessary to successful rehabilitation. Listening to the patient is portrayed as a particularly important aspect of the treatment.

Reading 69

The Nurse's Role: In the Prevention and Control of Problem Drinking

Helen L. Potter

If I were to choose one basic bit of advice from my own experience to pass on to an industrial nurse about to venture forth toward an alcoholic program, it would be simply, *Don't Get Discouraged!* Comparatively speaking, other problems of health education are nonexistent. The road to achieving an effective and applicable In-Plant Program is paved with many and severe disappointments. A once well-organized, smoothly functioning health education and accident prevention program suddenly becomes a chaotic maze. You, the industrial nurse, are suddenly engulfed in a bombardment of rebuttal, rejection, stumbling blocks, and stone walls. *Why??* The answer is obvious. You have walked out into the sunlight with the most controversial illness of our time. Each individual has his own ideas about alcoholism and how it should be dealt with, and feels it his "bounden" duty to expound at length on the subject.

This is a chance to test your salesmanship. Before any ground work can be laid you must sell the idea that alcoholism is an illness and must be treated as such. Your first duty is to furnish accurate information about the nature of alcoholism and its treatment, stressing always the importance of early detection and referral. The initiation or development of an alcoholism program in industry depends upon the unreserved collaboration of management, the medical and nursing staff, and community resources. If you are fortunate enough to have a full-time plant physician, such a program should be easily implemented after it meets his approval. Everyone will respect his judgment and back his recommendations. However, if you are a nurse working alone, your problems will be many, many more and varied.

DEVELOPMENT OF POLICY

Perhaps the best way to convey my message to you would be to relate my own experiences in the development of a formal policy to initiate treatment for the problem drinker. In the division of the corporation in which I am employed, we have a minimal problem with problem drinking. However, the primary function of the medical department is preventive medicine, the key

---

Reprinted from *The American Association of Industrial Nurses Journal*, pp. 14–16, October 1965.

to success being to stop the illness before it has a chance to start. Therefore, the program on alcoholism was approached much the same as any other health subject. For example, we have a very active and rigid tetanus immunization program, yet, to my knowledge there has never been a case of tetanus in the plant. The company is not willing to wait until a large percentage of our employees come to the medical department with "locked jaws." They want to prevent such an occurrence. So it is with alcoholism; prevention is the order of the day. The primary goal of the medical department is health education—to promote safety attitudes and good health habits with the ultimate goal of decreasing injuries on and off the job and eliminate as much absenteeism as possible. The relationship of mental health, accidents, and absenteeism is realistically accepted at our plant. Good mental hygiene is the foundation for improving safety attitudes and health habits. Our alcoholism information program was included as a portion of our mental health program.

To begin with, I was sent to the Florida School of Alcohol Studies to gain as much knowledge of the illness as possible and learn what community resources existed in this field. On my return, we launched forth in all directions. Our local Personnel Manager, Division Medical Direction, and I visited the Florida Alcoholic Rehabilitation Program in Avon Park to observe "in-hospital" treatment of the alcoholic, and the local out-patient clinic in Jacksonville for an indoctrination in treatment of the ambulatory patient. We began the education of our employees with the showing of a series of films carefully chosen and reviewed for the purpose of giving authentic information on the illness in an inoffensive manner. [The films, for your information, were: "Anger at Work," "Mr. Finley's Feelings," "Age of Anxiety," parts I and II (this is the actual interview of the Drs. Menninger by Walter Cronkite), and "To Your Health."] We were able to provide a constant flow of well-chosen literature and to distribute it to employees through the plant. It came from the F.A.R.P., and the members of the staff at the Center were most helpful with advice and assistance.

IN-PLANT TRAINING

Now it was time for the Supervisory Training Program in the plant. Allan Dana, Industrial Consultant, F.A.R.P., provided this for us. When the training program was completed, all employees had a clear understanding of the plant program and how it was to be used. Mr. Dana assisted us in defining the specific administrative, medical, and nursing policies and establishing a procedure for implementing these policies. After another series of revisions, the Procedure Manual emerged tailored specifically for our needs. We are pleased and proud of the end result, and will always be grateful to F.A.R.P.

for the endless and tireless efforts in assisting us. The manual specifies guides in early detection and process in referral for treatment of problem drinking, pointing out where the responsibility lies.

There is no fool-proof formula for setting up any phase of health education, but there are points applicable to all industrial nurses:

1 The nurse must have the respect and cooperation of management, the industrial physician, the employees and the local labor union.
2 She must familiarize herself with community resources.
3 Whether an employee is mentally ill or not, the nurse must have a knowledge of human behavior and be unbiased and open-minded in her opinion.
4 Competency in effective programming is equal only to the industrial nurse's knowledge and its appropriate application.
5 Remember that your attitude shows and the problem drinker will sense it.

The industrial nurse is, indeed, in an enviable position to play a significant role in the alcoholism program in industry, as well as other departments of health education. Anticipation of illness and prevention at the nucleus of our economic society is her responsibility; the working man is the most vital, yet most often neglected man, healthwise. Classes are set up nationwide for child care, maternal care, immunization, etc., but there is nothing for the working man, the most vital cog in the wheel of civilization. If he is not educated on the job, then he is ignored. I hope that eventually there will be some sort of health program wherever people are working, regardless of size of establishment or number of employees. Until then, those of us who are fortunate enough to be included in this fascinating world should utilize every effort and take advantage of every available community resource to promote the health, safety, and productivity of the employee.

RESULTS

At this point, the question in most of your minds is, "How well is your program functioning?" To this I will answer, "Surprisingly well." No doubt, as time goes by it will have to be amended or perhaps even discarded and started all over again. This is not failure. Rather, this is success. The effort has certainly reduced the stigma associated with alcoholism, which is one of the most desirable results. I have had multiple inquiries from other industrial plants who have now begun setting up similar programs for their employees. Local hospitals, ministers, doctors, law enforcement officers, nurses, and teachers have begun to come seeking knowledge and help for problem drinkers. If we can get these people interested enough to discuss the problem openly, then surely our program is successful.

There is a final thought I would like to leave with you—*Unless you are really sincere about this program, don't start it!* If you really are interested in such a program, then prepare yourself. Be sure you are working with the approval and guidance of your Medical Director. Get well acquainted with staff at clinics, local AA groups, clergymen interested in the drinking problem, local physicians and nurses knowledgeable and interested in the problem drinker. You will find it necessary to call for help from each one of these people if your program is to be successful. Check with your local hospitals to see what facilities they have for treatment. Analyze your plant situation. Do not think that you can get a store-bought, mail-order-type program that will be effective. It will be up to you as the industrial nurse to initiate the program. It will also be a personal failure for you if the program fails. Know yourself. . . . Know your company. . . . Know your community. . . . Then proceed. Follow up, evaluate. Ask yourself: Is business being conducted more efficiently? Is there a better employee-employer relationship? Is there less absenteeism? More productivity? Fewer accidents? What is the union's attitude toward me, as well as the program? Have I made a contribution to community health?

SUMMARY

Don't expect immediate acceptance and results. Our program represents almost two years of preparation, trial and error. It is still a constant challenge. Once you begin, you cannot let up. If you do, the framework will fall flat on its face. So, get yourself well prepared and make contact with knowledgeable and understanding people in the field. Your compensation will be the inner satisfaction of seeing the results.

Reading 70
Nursing the Alcoholic

Mary Lane Epp

Why do people act as if an alcoholic, when drunk, is different from any other drunk person? A drunk man or woman is not usually dangerous; in fact, it is unusual to find more than one out of about 300 who is obstreperous. Most of us have encountered people who have had too much to drink at a party; sometimes they have to be handled rather deftly to avoid a scene. An alcoholic is simply a drunk person who has got drunk too often, and for

Reprinted from *The Canadian Nurse*, vol. 61, no. 8, pp. 618–620, August 1965.

too long a time. But he is not unconscious, and he is painfully aware of your attitude. He knows whether you are disgusted, sympathetic, impatient, tolerant, angry, or amused.

Any patient going into any hospital is frightened and ill at ease for several days; an alcoholic is even more frightened. He does not know what treatment he will receive, but he does know that he is going to suffer the pangs of withdrawal. This increases his basic feelings of insecurity and anxiety. Since his fear may boil over into anger, he must be treated very carefully. It is essential that personnel maintain a calm, pleasant, and unhurried manner. Like most persons, the alcoholic reacts favorably to a smile of welcome on admission.

Perhaps one of the "musts" in successful treatment of the alcoholic is a sense of humor. Of course, you must be careful to laugh *with* him, not *at* him. He knows that he is not at his best—to put it mildly—and you must be careful to protect his dignity as much as possible. In protecting his dignity, you help to keep the situation on a definite level of acceptable behavior. Jocular remarks about his state are not acceptable. Try not to notice his slurs, fumbles and stumbles any more than you would a disability such as an artificial limb or a glass eye.

You *don't* tell the alcoholic what to do, you *ask* him. Sometimes a patient will say, "You can't make me do anything." You agree, "I know I can't, but you will, won't you? Please?" If you are being pleasant and kind, he doesn't want to spoil this. Your knowing exactly what you want him to do exerts pressure on him. Once you have suggested something, wait quietly and he will usually follow your suggestion.

For instance, you are admitting the patient and you want him to go to his room, get undressed and into bed. If he is able to walk alone, you let him follow you, as gentlemen do, and carry his own bag. You get his pajamas out, taking a quick look at the same time for a bottle or pills. He may want to sit on the side of the bed and smoke; more than likely, he'll want you to light his cigarette and to have one with him. If you smoke, do so. Sit down and enjoy it and start getting acquainted with him.

When a person is intoxicated, his thinking is slowed down. Attempts to hurry him make him confused and angry. Besides that, he wants to look you over before he makes himself quite defenceless by taking off his clothes. Some patients expect to have their clothes "locked up" as soon as they take them off, so their reluctance is understandable. They will be surprised and pleased when you hang their garments in the closet in their room.

If a patient becomes delirious, it sometimes helps to remove everything, except his pajamas, so that he can be more easily persuaded to remain in his room. I can remember one patient who always arrived on a stretcher, completely anesthetized with alcohol. The only way we could keep him in hospital until he "dried out" was to remove the bottoms of his pajamas and wet them. We found this would keep him in bed because he'd once had an "involuntary" prior to admission and had had no dry replacement!

Finally, the preliminaries are over, the cigarettes are finished, and you stall lighting up again. "Let's get you into bed, first—the doctor is coming and he wants to examine your chest." You may have to help by quietly getting shoes, socks and jacket off, talking all the while about the weather, or some equally inconsequential subject. If a patient is very drunk and refuses to have his clothes removed, let him lie down as he is and cover him with a blanket. Time will sober him up and he will be sick, shaky and most cooperative in a few hours. The longer he sleeps without a sedative, the better, since the addition of a sedative to an unknown quantity of alcohol can cause a dangerous degree of anesthesia.

Some patients use foul language. This is unpleasant, of course; but if you can accept it in a matter-of-fact way, as part of nursing alcoholics, it will raise your status with the patient. He may remember how he behaved on admission, but he will be ever so grateful if you forget and pretend that he was a perfect gentleman. After all, the nurse is only a target for the abusive patient; he does not know you, so it cannot be anything personal. Maybe he is enjoying the ability—often encouraged by alcohol—to express himself toward women: he will swear at you, confide in you, or ignore you, as he chooses. There is always the possibility that he is in a "blackout" and literally will remember nothing. The people around him have no way of knowing whether or not he is suffering from this strange type of amnesia caused by alcohol.

Most patients think that "tapering off" is the ideal way to withdraw from alcohol, and they want to get started on this right away—with the first drink being served immediately. Tapering off might work with heroic effort on the part of both staff and patients; but it takes a much longer time, and often bogs down completely with the patient demanding more and more whisky at shorter and shorter intervals. The nurse becomes a bartender, and the patient gets drunker instead of drier. Usually, the patient knows that he has had his last drink before he enters. Many, however, ask for one last drink—just in case—and the best way to counter this is to say, "Well, you came here to stop drinking, didn't you? I will get you something else."

Sweetened water flavored with fruit juice is good; pure fruit juice in large quantities is liable to be irritating to his probably inflamed gastrointestinal tract. Another beneficial drink is a high-protein powder mixed with milk or dried skim milk and water. However, the condition of a patient's liver has to be taken in account before encouraging this drink. The majority of alcoholic livers are affected to some extent, and have become fatty and enlarged. Any signs of liver failure, such as swelling, jaundice, etc., contraindicates the use of the protein drink.

Alcohol has a diuretic action and sometimes a patient has to be restrained from trying to remedy too quickly the situation caused by prolonged drinking. He may start to vomit if he drinks or eats too much, too soon. Some patients are so dehydrated on admission that they require intravenous fluids.

Most alcoholics dislike being dirty or having anyone else see them that way. Some go to a great deal of trouble getting bathed, shaved and changed before coming to hospital, intoxicated though they may be. Others, of course, are too drunk and sick to care, and arrive in a rather pitiful condition. It is much easier to change the sheets than to bathe an intoxicated, resentful patient; besides, he is too sick to be bothered and needs to rest and sleep. It isn't as if he is going to stay in his admission state very long. By the next day he will be scrubbing himself like mad and hoping you haven't noticed how much he needed it.

There are, however, a few patients who are careless about personal hygiene. This is usually an indication of organic deterioration due to prolonged use of alcohol, or a more or less severe type of underlying personality disorder, e.g., schizophrenia.

Sometimes a patient is brought quite reluctantly to the hospital. He is literally dragged, pulled, pushed, or carried, or he may arrive strapped to an ambulance stretcher. You can imagine that the patient who arrives under these circumstances is usually disturbed and fighting mad. The best way to handle him is for all the men who have been fighting with him to get out of sight as quickly as possible and leave him alone with the nurse, who is quiet, gentle, and waits patiently for him to calm down. A man will not hit a nurse, even when he is drunk. Admittedly, this patient is not going to be too cooperative in following through with treatment. However, it is usually possible to get him sobered up so that he will not kill his wife or become involved in a fatal car accident—this time. He may even buy the whole program! You never can tell.

A beginning must be made. We must not wait for the patient to choose to come for treatment. Sometimes preparation for his committal to a provincial mental hospital, with a choice of other hospitals, is necessary. The patient may choose, not if he will do something about his drinking, but what he will do. In the long run, recovery from addiction is the granddaddy of all "do it yourself" programs, because no one can make anyone else stop drinking. One can only help.

An effective program consists of at least a three-week period of lectures, films, interviews after the sobering up and withdrawal have been achieved. A two-year follow-up period of weekly lectures, letters, and telephone calls is initiated after discharge.

One of the gravest dangers of continuous heavy drinking is organic brain damage. This, of course, automatically rules out the new learning which is necessary in changing to a life without alcohol.

Women alcoholics seem to have more difficulty in accepting the disability of alcoholism. They cannot forgive themselves for being "alcoholic," let alone the things they may or may not do when they are drinking. They seem to feel at a terrible disadvantage when admitted to hospital in an intoxicated state. Some will proceed to try the patience of the nurses to the limit—they are weepy, demanding and noisy. Perhaps, being women, nurses expect more of them; and the patients, being women, hate to have other women who are spick and span see them and judge them. Certainly the utmost tact and kindness is required, even though the patient remains resentful and uncommunicative. After a few days of gentle care, she will probably respond to at least one of the nurses. She will soon be beautifully groomed and often very smartly and tastefully dressed. This change in appearance often is truly dramatic. Women alcoholics are often excellent, even obsessive housekeepers; sometimes they claim that they never neglect their homes, even when drinking.

The stigma of alcoholism is much worse for women than for men. The relatives feel this too, and often protect the drinker, partly for their own sakes, till organic brain damage has occurred.

As is true in any situation, not all people in hospital are compatible with all others. We accept this sorting-out and choosing process. Good nursing care establishes good rapport with an alcoholic, the same as with any other sick patient. Since this person is actually sick, not just drunk, we must forget the drunk part of it, even though we may feel it "serves him right" because it is self-inflicted. It helps to remember that our culture tolerates the use of alcohol; that an alcoholic has got into trouble with it because he was unaware of the dangers involved, and because it did something special to relieve his tensions and anxieties. There is always the belief, even if the dangers are known, that "nothing can happen to me."

In an on-going program, the patient will continue to turn to the nurse he has chosen to talk out problems, to receive reassurance or a pat on the back when revisiting the clinic. If a person who already feels inadequate and inferior commits a grave social error, his need for approval becomes almost pathological. The nurses, because of their continuous contact with patients, are faced with the greatest responsibility in restoring, to some extent, the wounded ego by attention and praise. For instance, any patient likes to be told he looks better, but you should try to be specific: "Your eyes are clear today"; or, to a lady, "I like your hair-do." But do not say it unless it is true. Remember the man in the film "Lost Weekend" as he scrutinized himself in the mirror? That was a very realistic touch. An alcoholic knows how he looks, but he likes you to mention it—if you can say something comforting.

If you explain to a patient that you will be able to give him a medicine that will help to ease his withdrawal pangs, but that he will probably have to suffer some discomfort, he is usually patient and cooperative. He expects to suffer, even though he would rather not. Alcohol is a depressant and the body has been functioning as if it had a brake on. Suddenly, alcohol is cut off (the brake is released) and a speeded-up state prevails. This leaves the patient restless in the extreme, agitated, tremulous; he simply cannot sit or lie still. Sedatives will help tone down his agitation since they have an effect similar to alcohol. If we give too much sedation, it will make him feel as "good" as the alcohol did. Not only will withdrawal be prolonged, but the patient may begin to suffer from the excess of the medicine, just as he did from an excess of alcohol. Tranquilizers seem to be more effective than barbiturates.

We must remember that many patients change their addiction from alcohol to pills, or to some other central nervous system depressant, e.g., chloral hydrate or paraldehyde. For successful rehabilitation, it is imperative that alcoholics stop trying to change the way they feel by putting something in their mouths. They must learn to trust and talk to other people about themselves. Understandably, this takes a bit of doing; and some cannot learn. Their early experiences with people have damaged the possibility of such relationships permanently. These persons will obtain various kinds of drugs in some way, and have recurrent bouts with alcohol.

Surprisingly few alcoholics develop delirium tremens (d.t.'s) during withdrawal from alcohol. If this condition frightens the staff as much as it frightens the patient, then the treatment is usually deplorable. Withdrawal generally reaches its peak on the third day, and the patient may start hallucinating. (This is probably preceded by sleeplessness or restlessness for approximately 24 hours; increased sedation is essential at this time.) He is in a pitiable state, tremulous and literally "scared out of his wits." Many hear threatening voices, cursing them for things they have done, perhaps telling them they would be better off dead, and that they had better kill themselves. In obeying this suggestion, one patient broke a window and then cut himself with the broken glass; others have tried to jump out of windows. But with a nurse in constant attendance, these things cannot happen. Even though the patient does not recognize the nurse in his delirium, he is reassured, comforted and not quite so frightened if she is with him.

Occasionally, the nurse needs to "play-act" at this stage. The patient may hand her an imaginary leash and ask her to walk his dog—which she does—up and down the room; or he may think that he has a bottle and glasses and is pouring drinks. He will hand her a non-existent glass, like a child playing house. One patient, who was an interior decorator, proceeded to paper his room. He went through all the motions, swearing at the incompetence of his non-existent helpers and expecting the nurse to hand him his tools. He even stood up on the bed to paper the top part of the wall. He didn't do any harm and, finally, collapsed on the bed, and went to sleep.

The patient with delirium tremens needs sleep. Sedation is doubled or tripled, and the intervals between doses are reduced. If such large doses of sedative are continued, they can produce their own symptoms of restlessness and delirium, a form of idiosyncrasy to excessive amounts of the drug. Then your patient is worse off than before. Common sense must, therefore, prevail. After you have given enough sedation to floor an ox, you stop, and put up with the restlessness and roaming. The delirium seems to run its own course. Eventually, the patient will go to sleep for such a long time that you will begin to worry about him. Let him sleep. Never mind food, fluids, or bladder. His sleeping changes from a twitching restlessness to a relaxed, untroubled sleep, and he eventually awakens in his "right mind."

Some patients hallucinate without being disoriented; they know they are just "seeing things" and will describe them graphically. Sometimes auditory hallucinations occur without delirium. In certain patients, the hallucinations continue for several days even though the patient is ambulatory, is socializing with other patients, is eating at the table, and sleeping—with considerable sedation—at night.

For some unknown reason, delirium tremens and hallucinations are usually worse at night. Sometimes a patient will complain of nightmares before he goes into delirium; at other times, the nightmares are as close as he gets to delirium. At times, the patient believes that the hospital staff is going to hurt him. He feels that he must get away. In this case, the nurse accompanies him. When the patient realizes that the nurse is not going to be left behind, he will usually turn back. One man flagged a taxi and went to his home, accompanied by his nurse. His relatives reassured him, and they all returned to the hospital, where the patient remained.

For these patients, alcohol has gradually become the most important thing in life. At the same time, it has been slowly changing from a helpful substance to a hurtful one. Education is necessary to help him understand why he found it helpful in the first place; to make him aware of the subtle, inescapable change that has been taking place, and what can be done about it. Then there is the long period, at least two years, during which time the new ideas are being put to use with varying degrees of success, in terms of emotional ease and adjustment to reality.

It is important for the patient to relieve his tensions by means other than the use of drugs or alcohol. One way is for him to learn the act or technique of relaxation, which he can begin to practice a few days after admission. This demonstrates to him that he can learn something new to help control his life.

Some alcoholics are benefited by treatment with LSD-25 (Lysergic Acid Diethylamide). As an adjunct to psychotherapy, this drug, for unexplained reasons, seems to help people re-live intense emotional experiences, no matter how far back into childhood or infancy these may be. Patients carefully selected by interviews and extensive psychological testing are taken off any drugs they may be receiving a day or so before they have LSD-25. They are permitted only clear tea or coffee the morning of the treatment. The drug, LSD, is in the form of a tablet taken by mouth. The starting time of the reaction varies greatly, in fact, the whole performance is a very individual sort of thing. In an hour or two the patient may tell you that the wall is advancing and receding; he may cry or laugh, or get violently angry; he may talk or be perfectly quiet.

The reaction goes on for several hours and the patient needs someone with him all the time. The nurse can play an important supportive role. After four to six hours, a sedative, such as Largactil, is usually given, since the drug LSD is a strong stimulant and the patient needs to rest. He will remember all of his thoughts and will need to think about them in order to make the whole experience useful.

Several patients have told me, with positive sincerity, that they went through the birth experience under LSD and felt angry or frightened. Perhaps the mother communicates her fear and anguish to the baby. It seems that sometimes a tiny infant can experience intense feelings of extreme loneliness and fear. And we sometimes treat them as if they are nothing more than little bundles to be fed and changed!

If anxiety—which may eventually lead a person to alcoholism—originates in infancy, it would seem logical that we should start a preventive program against addiction at the very beginning of life.

Reading 71

Adjusting Nursing Techniques to the Treatment of Alcoholic Patients

Alyce Quiros

Many nurses despair at meeting the problems of hostility, masochistic need for rejection, and excessive dependency expressed by the problem drinker. And there is much reason for inexperienced workers to be anxious about their ability to meet these problems.

There is no need for such anxiety or hesitation, however, when the nurse understands what is really involved in the patient's behavior and how

Reprinted from *Nursing Outlook*, vol. 5, no. 5, pp. 276–279, May 1957.

her role determines the relationship between them. We meet this and other problems at the San Francisco Department of Public Health Adult Guidance Center, an alcoholic clinic.

The problem drinker's indirect plea for help led to the clinic's establishment. In 1949 a clinic was started at the county jail in San Bruno, and because it was the only available treatment for alcoholics, many persons submitted to voluntary arrest in order to receive help there. Later, the staff decided that treatment could be more effective outside a punitive setting, and in 1951 the Adult Guidance Center was established as a voluntary outpatient clinic at its present address.

In the five years I have been working there, we have treated some 6,000 persons. Anyone is eligible for treatment who is a resident of San Francisco, comes to the clinic voluntarily, recognizes that he has a drinking problem, is willing to do something about his drinking problem, and shows evidence of being able to use constructively the clinic services we offer.

Statistically, the median clinic patient is 44 years of age, is or has been married, has two children, is above average in intelligence, and has had a high school education. He belongs to the lower middle class—the semi-skilled labor group or above, and his average weekly income is $74.25.

Although I have referred to our median patient as "he," one fourth of the patients we treat here are women. According to the Yale alcohol studies, there are more than 80,000 problem drinkers in San Francisco—or about one in every six adults.[1] Problem drinking is rated as the number four public health problem in the United States.

SOCIAL WORK

On the clinic team at the Adult Guidance Center are doctors, nurses, psychiatric social workers, and psychologists. A new patient is seen first by the psychiatric social worker and given a "screening" interview to determine his eligibility.

This contact is very important in establishing rapport with the patient who, for the first time, may come to realize that someone is really "on his side." Frequently during this interview, even though he may have been forced to come to the clinic through threat of divorce, loss of job, or a similar reason, he may decide that he does have a drinking problem and would like help. If eligible for treatment, he is given an appointment for an interview during which the social worker elicits a history of his problem, explains the different clinic services, and attempts to create a harmonious relationship between clinic and patient. This is reinforced through the polite and under-

[1] Keller, Mark, and Efron, Vera. Alcoholism in the big cities of the United States. *Quarterly Journal of Studies on Alcohol*, **17**:63-72, March 1956.

standing approach of secretaries, nurses, and other staff members. As one of our patients remarked, "I can't be so bad if healthy people treat me this way. There may be hope for me after all."

MEDICAL CARE

Next, the patient is seen by the doctor for an evaluation and the prescription of any medical treatment which may be indicated. Sometimes our patients are very ill, and their initial drinking may have served as an anesthetic to relieve unbearable tensions. Later they may continue drinking because of the temporary relief alcohol seems to give them from such physical symptoms as severe tremors, nausea, vomiting, and diaphoresis—all effects of prolonged drinking. Medical treatment can relieve these symptoms and enable the patient to recover without further use of alcohol.

Mephenesin [3- (ortho-toloxy) -1,2-propanediol] and similar preparations relieve the tremors; viscious xylocaine (a-Diethylamino-2.6-aceto-xylidide) anesthetizes the gag reflex and gastric mucosa, and when it is followed by some of the Dramamine (beta dimethyaminoethyl benzohydryl ether 8-clorotheophyllinate) preparations, or by chlorpromazine hydrochloride, nausea and vomiting may be combated. Barbiturates are used usually for sedation and to induce sleep, but only for the first few nights because we know that our patients have a propensity to addiction. All these medications are given for the acute withdrawal state; other medications may be given as a supportive measure either on an emergency or long-term basis. Patients may receive intramuscular injections of vitamins or adrenal cortex, and the new tranquilizing drugs are used when long-term sedation is desired.

NURSING

After the doctor's interview, the nurse sees the patient and gives him the prescribed medications. He receives only enough to last until he is seen the following day. Usually each new patient is seen daily for five days and the frequency of his visits is decreased gradually until he is on a monthly visit basis.

On his first visit, or any subsequent visits, depending on his degree of illness and receptivity, the nurse will discuss certain health measures with him. These will include such matters as diet, sleeping habits, and a yearly chest x-ray. Her discussion depends on how ill he is and how receptive he is to such discussions.

We find that the patient's diet usually is very poor. Breakfast, if any, may be a sweet roll and coffee, lunch a sandwich, and dinner mostly starch. Such diet regimen may well leave him with a "let down" feeling in midmorning or afternoon and increase his chances of drinking at this time. If he has been drinking for a long time, it is highly probable he did not eat during the drinking period and his body is depleted of protein and vitamins. In order to supplement this, we give a high-protein milk preparation with honey.

The nurse also discusses certain dietary abuses. These patients frequently have a lowered tolerance for coffee, and excessive use of it in their already nervous state will aggravate tremors and interfere with sleep. The alcoholic patient may eat candy in large quantities in an effort to handle his anxieties in much the same way that he turned to alcohol. It is not uncommon for him to eat a pound or two of candy at one time. This causes a rapid rise in blood sugar with a subsequent rapid fall, leaving him weak and shaky.

We must use special discretion in discussing this, however, so that we do not become a "depriving mother." We must remember that he is already attempting to give up alcohol, and this is very difficult. In discussing diet, we give the necessary information but leave the decisions about food up to him.

We encourage our patients to have a chest x-ray once yearly, and we have an average of approximately one patient a week who must have repeat x-rays because the picture often shows suspected tuberculosis or bronchogenic carcinoma.

We have ample opportunity to carry out the important job of teaching. As soon as the patient is sufficiently recovered, routine medical orders are written and the nurse follows through with the patient. Part of his clinic treatment entails his attending a series of six orientation lectures and discussions, and the doctors, nurses, psychiatric social workers, and psychologists take part in these.

During that time when the patient's clinic contact is with the nurses, we must be constantly aware of what is happening to him, and we refer him back to the doctor if he is feeling upset, under greater stress, or tells us (or indicates otherwise) that he might drink.

If he has been drinking, he needs medication other than that which he has been getting. He may have an urgent problem that he would like to talk over in detail with someone else, in which case we refer him to the doctor or psychiatric social worker. We may find that he does not have a place to stay or food to eat. Our social workers work closely with Alcoholics Anonymous affiliates and the Salvation Army in making food and lodging arrangements. We also are able to refer him for individual or group psychotherapy when this seems indicated.

SPECIAL ASPECTS

There is an even more important phase of nursing in the alcoholic setting than what I have described earlier; I shall call it relationship therapy. This is a therapeutic nurse-patient relationship in which we try to understand the patient and our own feelings about him as an alcoholic person. In so doing we are able to guide him toward a more mature stage of emotional development.

Often the alcoholic is a product of rejection; very often he comes from a broken home. His parents either rejected him by neglect, or to counteract their desire to neglect him, they may have gone to the other extreme and overprotected him. In any event, he was not able to grow and mature normally, and regardless of the cause he is still looking for the love and understanding he has missed, and, therefore, is living on a somewhat childlike emotional level. He wants to be told what to do, yet resents being told. Paradoxically, he will attempt to force the nurse into the role of the familiar parent, and he will constantly test her to see if she is really interested in him or if this is just a facade.

> Mr. S. would pick a time when the waiting room was crowded to capacity, then, following treatment, he would stand in the door obstructing my exit and start asking me questions. That he knew the answers was evidenced by his answering them himself.
> Being quite human, my immediate response was one of irritation. Realizing this, I asked myself, "What does this person really want?" and I began asking him questions that expressed my interest in his health and feelings. At this, Mr. S. would make a hasty retreat from the room.
> Even though he wanted understanding and treatment, the situation in which he was receiving it was relatively unfamiliar to him and caused anxiety which he could not handle. He returned many times after my initial expression of interest, and he said that he felt that this was the one place where people were interested in him. I had responded to the testing trap he had set in the right way to be helpful.

Mr. S. showed the insecurity that is shared by all our people. In asking me questions which he could answer, he was able to elevate himself to a more secure position, and had I been less anxious I would have sensed what was occurring much sooner than I did.

Many times the patient will attempt to induce anxiety in those surrounding him—doctor, social workers, nurses, friends, or spouse. If he is able to make another person anxious, then he can *temporarily* feel superior and be relieved of his anxiety. He has evidence that someone else is willing to carry his burden. We see this frequently in a marital situation in which the nonalcoholic spouse does all of the worrying, accepts all responsibility, and thus leaves the drinking partner without sufficient anxiety or need to work out his own particular problem.

All too often workers tend to overidentify and oversympathize with the nonalcoholic spouse and, instead of giving real help, perpetuate the tension-arousing situation. We have to recognize that sometimes the nonalcoholic spouse finds it emotionally necessary to be the martyr; often he, or she, married an alcoholic from an unconscious need to boost his or her own ego by contrast.

In some cases, where we have given the nonalcoholic spouse psychiatric help, he, or she, has been able to recognize how his, or her, own problems or needs have aggravated the partner's drinking. Once aware of this, the nonalcoholic spouse was able to expend energy aiding the healthy part of the alcoholic's personality rather than abetting the sick part of it.

Sometimes, after we have had one or two interviews with the nonalcoholic spouse, the alcoholic patient has stopped drinking without ever making any visits to the clinic. Because we have not followed up these cases, it is impossible to say how many of them remained permanently abstinent, but certainly a new level of mutual understanding had been introduced into the marriage relationship.

The nurse attempts to strengthen the well part of the alcoholic. For example, Mrs. E. would come into the clinic acutely intoxicated and with a bottle in her purse. If the nurse had become angry and punitive, the sick part of the patient would have been strengthened, her sick need to be rejected would have been fulfilled. By contrast, when the nurse said, "We believe that you are here because you want help, but you are making it difficult for us to help you," this appealed to the well or positive part of the patient. She was then better able to make a choice.

In our contacts with the alcoholic patient we have to be cautious not to overidentify with him in his progress or his relapses. Naturally our hope is toward his abstinence. If we are overly solicitous, however, he will sense our anxiety through our expressions of joy at his improvement, or our disappointment if we see signs of relapse. The patient may even lie to us in his anxiety to obtain our approval; he may become upset if he senses that we do not have the stability that he himself lacks; or he may drop out of treatment rather than gain our disapproval.

Under these demanding circumstances, some nurses may experience emotional upheavals and find the work too upsetting to continue in it. We find it helpful to keep in mind the numbers of persons with this chronic illness, and to remember that the course of any illness is rarely one of steady improvement. Relapses may occur in alcoholism just as they may with any other chronic disease. We also become anxious about medical and surgical patients whose attitudes or behavior in some way are upsetting and threaten their recovery—perhaps a patient with a gastric ulcer or diabetes does not follow his diet, or a cardiac patient refuses to stay in bed—but we do not give up medical nursing.

Another reaction nurses have to alcoholic or other noncooperating, chronically ill patients is that of the authoritative mother, and the patient may respond to this while we are at his side. If we are to be helpful on a lasting basis, however, we must understand that the patient's not cooperating is because of some special need. He is as confused about his behavior as the nurse may be, and understands it even less. Again, sympathetic questioning is usually sufficient to get some understanding of what is going on and enable one to guide the patient toward more constructive and cooperative behavior.

Many times our patients try to manipulate us into telling them what to do. Mr. R. would come into the clinic to tell us about his girl friend, who insisted that they go to bars together. He would sit there quietly sipping Cokes while she drank highballs, and he would become upset by the liquor around him. He was even more upset by her lack of consideration. Through such questions as "I don't think that is right, do you?" or "What should I do?" he attempted to involve the nurse in his problem and have her make a decision. If she had done so, she would have taken responsibility that was his—and she would have been responsible for its success or failure. This would have deprived him of an opportunity to use his own judgment and accept the consequences. Just listening often helped him reach the answer himself and gain self-confidence and pride.

LISTENING AND REFERRING

Because many patients have exaggerated fears of what other people will think of them, and fears that they may be "crazy," we use great care in talking with them to avoid such words as psychiatrist and psychotherapy. These patients can accept well a simple statement such as, "You seem to have a problem that you need help with. Do you wish to talk it over with someone here?" This is much less frightening than saying, "Do you want to talk to the psychiatrist?"

If patients are in psychotherapy, the nurse must work closely with other members of the staff so that the treatment is as consistent as possible. Different approaches to his treatment might well leave the patient as confused as the child with a permissive mother and a strict father. And like the child, he may exploit such a situation.

Some patients build up strong positive feelings toward the nurse which are especially helpful when they are receiving medical treatment only. Patients in psychotherapy, however, often attempt to bring their problems to the nurse. If they verbalize their anxieties to her outside the psychotherapy hour, the problems become diluted and the patients fail to work on them in the proper setting—which is with the psychotherapist. It is difficult for some nurses to refrain from trying to do something more than listen and refer patients to the right person, but it is most important that they should.

Sometimes one's own feelings and attitudes can interfere with proper treatment. If one feels that to refer a patient for psychotherapy is unfriendly or insulting, it will be difficult to make such a referral. This usually is based on a misunderstanding and fear of what psychotherapy really implies.

If a nurse takes a moralistic attitude, a feeling that "he could stop if he only wanted to," implying that the patient is drinking just to be "bad" or "irresponsible" rather than because he is sick, the patient senses this. He probably will respond by feeling even more guilty and angry with himself because the nurse's attitude has confirmed what he already feels about himself.

The nursing care of the alcoholic person must be based on acceptance and firmness, like a good mother's, as well as on understanding. We attempt to nurture responsibility in our patients by encouraging them to keep their appointments. Without these limits, they might feel that we were not interested in them at all. Some who were, accidentally, not given a return appointment have left treatment. Many times the patients may request or demand certain medicines or quantities of medicines that have not been ordered. We respond with "the doctor is giving you what he feels is best for you," which expresses our interest and yet sets certain limitations.

Often our patients will test us by seeking limitations just as a child tests its parents. Recently this need for limitations was portrayed in a cartoon depicting the furniture piled high in the middle of the living room. Two children are standing on top, and one turns to the other and says, "My God, why doesn't someone stop us before we kill ourselves?"

As good parents, those of us working with alcoholic patients must guide them until they no longer need our help. Miss Peltenburg, our chief psychiatric social worker, was once asked, "Do you hold your patient's hand?" She replied, "Yes, and we let go finger by finger."

Section B

Drug Abuse

That the United States has a drug problem—users and nonusers alike—is scarcely news. Drugs, of course, whether recognized or not, are the problem for the users. The users, in turn, are part of the drug problem for the nonusers. In a much broader context drugs are a problem for everyone. Sometimes from a concerned, preventive standpoint, as with one's own young children or students; sometimes from a conceptual problem, as with Mr. Middle-class America who suffers from the generation gap as youngsters talk and sing in words and about things to which he is not tuned in. Again, sometimes our concern is a late but necessary concern, that of trying to rehabilitate the user who has lost control. The nurse might well have an important role in all phases of a program to ameliorate the deleterious effects of improper drug usage. There is no doubt, however, that she will encounter the user in a hospital situation where her initial ministrations may be in a crisis situation. Such contacts can be expected to increase in the future, until, one hopes, the Weltanschauung of youth turns its restless eye elsewhere to find diversion or fulfillment.

One of the predictable concomitants of the proliferation of drug usage in our country is the development of rehabilitation programs specifically for those addicted to drugs. The articles dealing with rehabilitation nursing vis-à-vis the drug problem for the most part are descriptions of specific hospital or agency programs. These descriptions provide models that should prove useful and practical, and they provide general information about drugs as well.

Van Dusen and Brooks give valuable suggestions about dealing with the drug user. Their ideas are derived from experience with youthful drug addicts in the well-known Awareness House Training Center in Tucson, Arizona.

The article by Ramirez describes a program for the rehabilitation of the drug addict that provides step-by-step suggestions. He places considerable emphasis on orderly procedure based on a wealth of experience. For example, disregard of some of the cues patients themselves provide can lead to ". . . haphazard mingling of patients at different stages of rehabilitation, (which) is distinctive for all patients."

The article by Pearson deals with a program utilizing methadone as a substitute for more dangerous drugs. The basis and rationale for the programs are described in detail. As described by Pearson, the utilization of methadone by itself is not the equivalent of rehabilitation. Accompanying the gradual switch from heroin to methadone is intensive and meaningful counseling.

Reading 72
Treatment of Youthful Drug Abusers
Wilson Van Dusen
and
H. Bryce Brooks

Our work brings us into close contact with thousands of young drug abusers. We will epitomize here what would be of most use to physicians.

PATTERN OF DRUG USE

For a long time, youthful drug abuse was confined to lower-class delinquents who used marihuana and narcotics. For reasons too complex to go into here, drug abuse has spread like wildfire among young persons from ages 10 to 25. We have met with youths in many schools. It is no longer a surprise to find that half the young people in a high school and 20% to 30% of those in junior high and grammar school have experimented with dangerous drugs. The pattern of development is fairly consistent. It begins with marihuana and volatiles (glue sniffing, gasoline, hair spray, PAM, and so on) and graduates to LSD and then to amphetamines, barbiturates, and even heroin. This pattern is true in all socioeconomic groups and in all qualities of family background. Drug abuse is now most common in the middle and upper classes.

Youth has a culture of its own, as reflected in dress, rock music, language, marked influence on each other, and even similarity of social-political outlook, but the culture has shifted toward drug usage. Threats of arrest prove useless. Education on the dangers of drugs is useless, except perhaps in grammar school. Commonly, high school teachers have students in the classroom who are obviously "high" or somnolent on drugs. This is not exaggeration or a simple fad that will pass. Drug use is still increasing, and its use is extending downward into grammar school. Some 10 to 20% of public school children may be considered drug-dependent, with more than half of all youths experimenting with drugs. The much-debated innocence of marihuana looks less innocent as time goes on. Besides the disturbances that occur with the regular use of marihuana alone, it is an easy introduction into the company of drug abusers and to other drugs. The physician who is aware of this drug culture can be of significant help, although his role is not the most central one.

Reprinted from *Modern Medicine*, July 27, 1970, pp. 74-76. The authors are affiliated with Awareness House Training Center, Tucson, Ariz. They wish to acknowledge the help of Dr. Edward Quass, Mendocino State Hospital, Calif.

Young people are interested in trying virtually anything that might produce interesting psychic effects. Some youngsters raid the medicine cabinet for pill parties, where pills are dumped into a bowl, mixed, and taken indiscriminately. Participants then sit around describing the effects they get.

The doctor can be of help by following these suggestions:

1   Prescribe only needed quantities of barbiturates, amphetamines, sleeping pills, tranquilizers, or analgesics.
2   When prescribing these drugs to parents, caution them to hide the pills. You need not impute blame to their children. We are in an age when these pills are widely misused and should not be handy to everyone.
3   Do not put prescription pads around so they can easily be stolen.
4   Destroy disposable hypodermics. Many young "needle freaks" use just the needle attached to an eyedropper.
5   Be alert to tricks that call for more psychotropic, mood-altering pills. Some young people even have a PDR and can come up with a definitive list of symptoms. Physical symptoms are lacking, though.

It is estimated that 50% of all amphetamines (speed) used illegitimately comes from legal sources. Young people more readily take pharmaceutically marked pills than bathtub medication, and physicians are major unwitting contributors to the use of these illicit drugs.

CARE OF THE BAD TRIPPER

Most young people who have a "bad trip" on drugs try to keep it to themselves and to friends. Their fear of authorities and of parents finding out makes them likely to describe a bad trip as some other illness. We have heard hair-raising accounts of bad trips that were treated by other young people, using whatever medicine was on hand. In some instances, friends had to resort to artificial respiration.

The bad tripper is someone who has taken drugs that alter perception, thought, and feeling to such an extent that the individual is frightened. LSD, for instance, is a psychic amplifier that can cause a little fear to be magnified into all-out life-or-death panic. Other people around the bad tripper appear to have distorted faces and intentions. When confronted with such an individual, the first step is to find a quiet, sheltered environment. Send away those who are anxious, but keep at hand friends who are supportive. Bad trippers are very suggestible, so make use of this. Get the patient to sit or lie down and establish calm and rapport. It is important to know what was taken and how long ago. A question like "How long ago did you drop it?" is more likely to get an honest answer than "What seems to ail you?" The patient may be disoriented, but he is more inclined to admit drug use if the physician implies that he knows about it. Find out what drug was taken. What was taken and how long ago leads to the greatest reassurance the patient can have—the rediscovery that he has taken something which has changed how he feels. Use repeated reassurance that the drug changes how he feels and that the effects will wear off; such reassurance may be necessary many times to get the bad tripper to calm down. The patient will pick up assurance from those around him, and his own self-control will return. He may then react better to a light conversation around real things. "It is 3 P.M., so you must be past the main drug reaction. You are coming down. Guess you missed school today. Do you have a job?" The majority of bad trippers have been talked down by friends who have been through the drug reaction themselves.

The physician will be inclined to abort the drug reaction by using other drugs. We do not recommend this unless a clear medical emergency occurs. For one thing, one cannot be sure what drug or drugs were taken. Many users take more than one substance. If the drug is black market, it could contain unknown substances such as atropine, heroin, strychnine, rat poison, and so forth. For instance, most black-market mescaline and psilocybin turn out to be something else. A few deaths have occurred by giving chlorpromazine (Thorazine) for LSD, not knowing the LSD contained atropine. Bad trippers come up with the most colorful and bizarre symptoms. Often they will feel they are dying or losing their minds, or they may have a panicky preoccupation with something that seems quite fanciful. But the only real medical emergencies are convulsions, unconsciousness, cessation of respiration, or withdrawal symptoms.

By direct suggestion, the bad tripper can be taught self-control and gain from the experience. A sympathetic, attentive person may show him that others care and condition his attitude toward the helping professions. In any event, other drugs only shorten the time it takes to come down, and the use of a hypodermic on a frightened, disoriented person can be a further trauma.

Normally, a person can be talked down in ten to fifteen minutes to the point where he will relax and wait for the other drug effects to pass. When a subject is brought in handcuffed by the police, the matter is more difficult. Fear may have been compounded by rough treatment. In these instances, we have kept the police out of the room and established a contract for good behavior before the handcuffs are removed. From there on, the procedure is as described above.

Because friends and ex-drug users are so successful in talking down a disturbed subject, the physician may want to establish that there is no medical emergency and then turn over to others the main job of talking down and baby-sitting an anxious subject. Bad trips are most likely to occur on weekends and holidays when the physician may want to be elsewhere. Since many larger communities have an emergency phone service, free clinic, or other drug abuse service staffed by people who have dealt with hundreds of bad trips, he may want to refer the case to them and remain on call if needed. Or he might talk down a bad tripper and then leave him with a trusted friend to act as a temporary nurse.

If medication is to be used, the best results we have seen have been with diazepam (Valium), 10 mg. three times a day, for either LSD or amphetamine intoxication. For marked paranoid symptoms, acetophenazine maleate (Tindal), 20 mg. three times a day, is helpful. True physical addiction to barbiturates is somewhat rare, but withdrawal can lead to fatal convulsions. In these individuals, we have seen the best results with pentobarbital, given until intoxication occurs, followed by systematic withdrawal from that known dosage. For heroin withdrawal, methadone given over a two- to three-day period is the method of choice. The recently withdrawn heroin addict is such a whining, demanding, manipulative person that most would leave this treatment to experts.

CONCLUSION

Those of us working close to the drug scene are not sanguine about the future. A fairly large proportion of young people may have their lives and their social productivity altered by drug use, and drug dependency may come to outrank alcoholism. However, most of the other trends of today's young people do look useful. Although successful approaches are known for every aspect of drug abuse, most involve changes in the culture of youth itself that are not easy or simple to implement.

The physician will find that he is expected to know about this new drug scene. He will also find he is one of a host of concerned groups and agencies. Because of his traditional leadership in matters relating to drugs, his support of others' efforts will be particularly influential and appreciated.

Reading 73
Help for the Addict

Efren Ramirez

I have been intimately concerned over the past seven years with the problem of drug addiction. By offering a new, comprehensive approach to its treatment and prevention, I hope to begin reversing the trend of failure in coming to grips with this growing human tragedy.

Reprinted from *The American Journal of Nursing*, vol. 67, no. 11, pp. 2348-2353, November 1967.

How serious is the narcotics problem? In New York City alone, where 50 percent of all addicts in the United States live, the 1966 central Narcotics Register listed 35,000 known active heroin users. But for every known addict, there probably are three whom we do not know. New York City police reports show that between 1963 and 1964 there was a 75 percent increase in criminal arrests of admitted narcotics users under the age of 16 years, and a 95 percent increase in arrests for violating the narcotics law by young persons between the ages of 16 and 20. Goods stolen by addicts to pay for drugs in New York State alone are estimated at 500 million to a billion dollars a year.

These figures suggest the overwhelming size and scope of this problem of addiction, the tremendous human suffering and waste it causes, and the failure of previous methods to make even a small dent in its tough surface. My approach is based on the hopeful findings of a five-year demonstration project in the Commonwealth of Puerto Rico. Of the first 124 drug addicts who were graduated from this program, only 7, or 5.6 percent, had become re-addicted during the 3½ special year follow-up period. These encouraging results—almost a total reverse of the relapse rate which has been close to 92 percent in federal institutions and over 70 percent in the most advanced experimental centers in the United States—seemed to warrant using the Puerto Rican project as a model for treating addicts elsewhere. The New York City program, known as OCAP from its placement under the Office of the Coordinator of Addiction Programs, was established in July 1966.

OVERVIEW

Basic to our model is the fact that all persons who succumb to drug use, in my observation, have certain character disorders in their psychological makeup. I believe that the addict's successful recovery from these disorders involves three simultaneous processes: behavioral conditioning, attitude modification, and emotional and vocational maturation.

Drug abuse is a symptomatic behavioral complex in response to a kaleidoscopic combination of intrapsychic, interpersonal, and impersonal factors impinging on a human being. Almost every addict *chooses,* sometimes gradually, sometimes abruptly, to join the drug scene as a way of coping with his particular mosaic of impinging influences. To do this, he disengages himself from the main stream of his social environment and seeks an engagement, partial or complete, in a psychopathic subculture. This subculture may be as obvious as the minority group ghetto, or it may exist almost invisibly.

To recover such disengaged persons requires the construction of a sequence of changing subcultural settings and institutions which move the addict in small steps from the extreme of the severely psychopathic subculture toward the opposite extreme, the subculture of individual choice, or the subculture which offers him the maximum chance to achieve his potential. Our model reproduces this sequence of changing environments. By gradually and productively engaging in each progressive setting, the patient modifies his behavior, step by step, and increases his capacity to function adequately in the society of his choice without having to resort to drugs.

The process of recovery takes an average of two to three years, in three easily definable phases. The first one, induction, emphasizes behavioral conditioning. It lasts an average of two to three months and is primarily a training process that engages the raw, unmotivated drug addict in the "street" (the "street" can be located in the open community or in a correctional or involuntary commitment facility), and carries him through a gradual detoxification that may be completed in a day-treatment center or in a hospital ward. The clean addict is then challenged to make a demonstrable commitment to the long-term treatment which will lead to his eventual rehabilitation.

The second phase, treatment, requires an average of 8 to 10 months. Here total milieu therapy is employed to modify negative attitudes and to reinforce productive attitudes in both patients and staff members. In this way, the second phase is used not only to treat patients but to train staff members. Treatment carries the patient from the point where he decides upon long-term rehabilitation to the stage where his overall consistent behavior with peers, staff, relatives, and neighbors earns him recognition by all of them that he is a contributing citizen rather than a social parasite. At this point, he is discharged to the next and last phase of rehabilitation.

This third phase, re-entry, lasts about a year, and comprises five steps. Its name was suggested by a rehabilitated addict when he said, "Going back home is almost as tough a job as the astronaut's re-entry into the earth's atmosphere." Re-entry provides three main services: (1) an evaluation of the success of phases I and II through observation of the total behavior of the re-entry candidates; (2) the use of trained parapsychiatric manpower (the re-entry candidates themselves) to aid and complement the professional staff in the different stages of phases I and II; and (3) the all-important opportunity for the ex-addict to confirm his rehabilitation to his own satisfaction by tackling more and more demanding emotional, vocational, and social tasks.

After he completes this phase, the ex-addict is certified as rehabilitated. He is now a free agent and may choose either to stay with the program as an employee, if he qualifies in equal competition with others, or to do other work. He is eligible for vocational training, individual treatment and counseling, and educational opportunities sponsored by the program. At the same time, he agrees to cooperate with any follow-up procedure which may be required for research purposes.

INDUCTION

Induction, by far the most difficult phase, is accomplished in three distinct stages: "the street" encounter, "the half-way in" service, and final detoxification. The encounter is best handled by a certified ex-addict or by a re-entry candidate of levels four or five in a storefront office or equivalent setting in a neighborhood of high drug incidence. This office, known as a community orientation center or COC, is managed by a paid member of a supportive community organization, RARE, which is composed of addicts' relatives and potential employers. The COC is a readily available, confidential office within the community where immediate referrals can be accepted. The addict who comes here is engaged, together with other street addicts, in attitudinal confrontation groups—encounters—where his behavior is explored by his peers. He is stimulated by daily contact with a successfully rehabilitated ex-addict, the community orienter. He is encouraged by both the orienter and his peer group to cut down his use of narcotics as proof of his stated desire for cure. (At this stage, we do not listen to what the addict *says,* but to what he *does.*)

Over half of the addicts encountered in this way immediately begin the long haul of rehabilitation and come regularly to the COC as directed. Most of the others eventually become engaged, in proportion to the success of those before them. Effectiveness of induction, at this earliest stage, is also proportionate to the absence of professionals from the COC. The raw addict relates only to persons who understand addiction, and, in his opinion, only another addict can know what he feels.

The half-way setting, which is a day-evening care center, or DECC, accepts addicts referred by the community orienters from the COCs clustered around it. Continuity of service between COC and DECC is maintained by the community orienters. These staff members, ex-addicts at level five of re-entry, work in their communities during the afternoon and early evening and at the DECC during the morning. This integration of professional and ex-addict staff provides a favorable environment—not quite "street," not quite hospital—for further induction of the incoming addict.

The DECC simulates, as far as possible, a hospital environment. This gives the inductee a prehospitalization opportunity to learn to discipline himself so that the professional staff in the next setting, the hospital, can be truly a treating and not a disciplinary staff. While he is making this adjustment, the addict has vital transitional support from his community orienter and other ex-addicts. By staying in the DECC from about 9:00 A.M. to 10:00 P.M., the addict is separated from his endemic environment most of his waking hours. An ever-increasing number of addicts complete their physical detoxification before admission to the hospital.

By December 1966, all addicts in the Puerto Rican project were achieving detoxification in the DECC and doing so without using opiate substitutes. Detoxification becomes less and less a withdrawing from drugs and more and more a cleaning up of the addict's mind.

Nurses and occupational therapists are the backbone of patient services in the DECCs, and nurses and occupational therapists provide a full-time service, whereas other staff members perform their important functions on a part-time basis. Both nurses and occupational therapists are of major influence in stimulating attitudinal change in addict-patients. Fundamental to this change is helping patients to accept authority and undertake responsibility for increasingly larger tasks.

The nursing staff cares for the patients' physical health, supervises them in housekeeping and operational chores, and, in order to fill the inductee's entire time, programs such activities as frequent peer group encounters with ex-addicts and staff, area maintenance, responsibility for discipline, and elimination of isolationist recreations like watching TV, reading comic books, and daydreaming. Occupational therapists teach patients specific crafts such as painting and carpentry, and give prevocational training in punctuality, caring for tools and equipment, and completing projects.

By being constantly discouraged in his psychopathic behavior and concomitantly reinforced in productive behavior, the inductee gradually is helped to change his manipulative, acting-out, and irresponsible conduct so that he may profit from the coming phase, hospital treatment. If no hospital is available for completion of his induction, some addicts can be treated in another setting.

The OCAP Program
(Average Length Is 2 to 3 Years)

Phase I		INDUCTION, averages 2–3 months
	COC	Community Orientation Center, site where raw addict is first encountered; storefront office in open community or involuntary commitment facility; staffed by ex-addicts known as community orienters; administered by RARE
		RARE Community organization, Rehabilitation of Addicts by Relatives and Employers, 11 chapters now active
		AWARE Community organization, Addiction Workers Alerted to Rehabilitation and Education; persons interested in addiction but not related to an addict; 11 chapters active
	DECC	Day-evening care center or "half-way in" setting; addict begins and sometimes completes detoxification process; staffed by professionals and ex-addicts
	MPDW	Mental and physical detoxification ward in regular, closed, medical facility; addict completes detoxification, prepares for full in-patient treatment; staffed by full health team and ex-addicts

The OCAP Program Continued

Phase II   TREATMENT, averages 8–10 months
           Therapeutic community   Free-standing facility such as Daytop Village or psychiatric unit modified for communal living; staffed by professionals and ex-addicts; addict begins to assume real responsibility for self, family, and community

Phase III   RE-ENTRY, averages 12 months
           Re-entry house or, for some, the family home
           Re-entry house   Supervised residence operated and managed largely by ex-addicts who take increased responsibility for addicts in Phase II as they progress through five levels:

             Level I   Clinical aide in MPDW, works a 6-hour shift daily

             Level II   Clinical assistant in DECC, works 7-hour shift daily

             Level III   Full-time therapeutic aide in a therapeutic community

             Level IV   Assistant community orienter in COC

             Level V   Community orienter

At completion of Level V, ex-addict is certified as rehabilitated; may apply for employment in OCAP program or return to open community.

The inductee who goes from the DECC to a mental and physical detoxification ward, or MPDW, enters a regular, closed, medical facility which serves about 25 addicts at any one time. A basic medical staff of physicians, nurses, and occupational therapists cares for the residual medical problems associated with completing his detoxification. Supplementary, part-time social workers, psychologists, ex-addicts, and others help him to solve the problems awakened by his drug-free status, and to make the long-range commitment necessary to benefit from the treatment experience.

How long he stays on the MPDW depends on his own capacity to respond, the thoroughness of his previous induction, and the admission flow to the detoxification and treatment wards. Slower patients may be reclassified, return to the DECC for further induction, and then re-enter the MPDW. Decisions to reclassify or promote patients are made by an interlocking evaluation committee including members of the corresponding services.

TREATMENT

Treatment, the second phase, takes place in a residence which incorporates the basic elements of a "therapeutic community." In a hospital, this can be achieved by modifying a regular psychiatric ward to provide communal living for about 40 persons at a time. The staff of professionals and ex-addicts provides patient care, and the patients take a larger and larger part in their daily affairs as their capacities grow. A single psychiatrist, with one psychiatric resident as his trainee, heads the ward. During this stage, the patient makes marked attitudinal strides through deep, consistent exploration of his own character. During frequent peer group discussions and confrontations with professionals and ex-addicts, he reassesses his own role in life and begins to assume real responsibility for himself, his family, and community. He becomes able to "feel" again. Addicts close to the end of treatment so often develop gastric hyperacidity that a request for Gelusil is a distinct sign of improvement!

The chief therapist meets three times a week with each of four groups of 10 patients. With professional and ex-addict colleagues, he classifies patients according to their functional and attitudinal status. Diagnostic labels are not used. All therapy groups, ward work, and maintenance responsibilities are organized in strict relation to patients' functional capabilities.

Each group therapy session is observed by different staff members who then meet with the same group to discuss in more detail those aspects which relate to their disciplines. For example, the nurse discusses with the group the interpersonal aspects of staff-patient relationships; the occupational therapist gears his activities to the developments in therapy; the social worker dwells more profoundly on the family's part in the patient's treatment; the teacher employs teaching methods and materials which complement the team's efforts; the ex-addict brings the whole thing to a more "gut" level; and the religious counselor makes his advice pertinent to the on-going therapy.

Weekly evaluation meetings, attended by the entire treatment staff and directed by the chief therapist, focus all these therapeutic activities on patient progress and needs. If therapy is sufficiently intensive, about one patient a week is evaluated as fully treated and graduates to the next phase. Continuity of care is guaranteed by part-time assignment of the Phase II treatment personnel as re-entry supervisors.

RE-ENTRY

Although their basic treatment has been completed, patients still face the crucial transition from an isolated, supportive environment to everyday life in the communities where they became addicted. To prepare for their return, most ex-addicts go to a re-entry house. This is a supervised residence in which they themselves perform most of the operation and internal organization, aided by professionals and trained ex-addicts. Here, too, the nurse and occupational therapist provide essential services. Some ex-addicts are able to live at home while still participating in the re-entry program, in which they achieve emotional and vocational maturation through further group confrontations, orthodox psychiatric treatment, vocational training, and professional schooling.

Re-entry's five levels consist of increased work responsibility with addicts in earlier stages of the plan. At level one, ex-addicts are assigned to one of the four six-hour work shifts a day, seven days a week, as clinical aides in a detoxification ward. At level two, ex-addicts work about seven hours daily as clinical assistants to the staffs of day-evening care centers. At level three, they become full-time therapeutic aides in a therapeutic community. Here they participate and, in some cases, lead the tri-weekly intensive group sessions. By level four, ex-addicts are ready for work in the open community. They begin by assisting the community orienter. At this point, ex-addicts are eligible for certification. Once certified, they can depend on the official backing of city and state authorities in their efforts to find employment and a respected place in their communities.

ESSENTIALS FOR SUCCESS

The actual settings for this three-phase course of rehabilitation may vary considerably in location, size, physical facilities, and even staffing patterns. For example, the encounter stage for addicts entering under the New York state program may be at Riker's Island; for others, the store-front office; the therapeutic community may be a 30-bed unit at Beth Israel Hospital or the Daytop Village group of 200 ex-addicts on Staten Island.

Experience has proved, however, that some elements are basic to the effectiveness of each stage in relation to the others. The first essentials are appropriate functional assignments and segregation of services. Haphazard mingling of patients at different stages of rehabilitation is destructive for all patients. Therefore, the status of each patient must be carefully identified and even more carefully matched with the service which is most beneficial for him. A patient's failure to function adequately at any level must not be handled by punishment but rather by his reclassification to the level where he can perform successfully.

This, of course, requires another basic element, a very close working relationship between the staffs of the different facilities within the chain of rehabilitation. An interlocking staff is one means to achieve structural continuity. Another way is to develop shared training programs for the staffs of the various facilities. Either process, or ideally both, coupled with steady dialogue at the executive level, can gradually evolve criteria for standardization and coordination. These criteria, through the help of civic and governmental authorities, can become public policy.

CORE CONCEPTS

In translating our theoretical model into practice, these key concepts have emerged as the irreducible core of the system:

Help, in the context of this program, does not mean allaying the addict-patient's anxieties by giving him a false sense of his own potentialities, or letting him escape from situations with which he feels he cannot cope. For example, the inductee is not protected from the consequences of his behavior if the police pick him up for stealing or other crime after he enters the program. "Help" means bringing him head-on, through group or individual confrontations, with a clear picture of his *own* makeup. He must face both the interpersonal factors—his relationships with fellow human beings and their institutions—and the impersonal, or those forces which are largely independent of human action. If this sort of help is consistently offered, the patient has little choice but to grow, regardless of his limitations.

Professional attitude refers simply to helping patients face themselves and reality in this fashion. *Professional,* in this program does not imply the particular skills of a staff member—as a psychiatrist, nurse, or ex-addict—or of a fellow patient, but specifically this person's ability to help the patient into a profound understanding of his own being.

Responsibility, central to this program's existential approach, means the ability to face reality directly and to respond to it positively. To the extent that a person can accept responsibility for his life, he becomes a free moral agent. This freedom cannot be imposed from outside the person. It is developed from within and it forms the basis of freedom in the community and in society.

Our recognition of the addict's responsibility to order his own life is a direct departure from the traditional approach to sociopathic personality disorders. We believe that it is precisely this element in our philosophy which has contributed most to the success of the Puerto Rican project and to the progress of the 2,000 addicts now engaged in the New York City program. Of these 2,000 about three-fifths now are underoing induction, one-fifth are in treatment, and one-fifth are re-entry candidates.

Authority, at the core of interpersonal relations, is a power which can be delegated to someone else, as contrasted to responsibility—the ability to respond—which cannot. The tension between authority and internal responsibility is one of the strongest propellants toward forward movement in the therapeutic community because when one encourages a patient to assume responsibility by granting him authority, one stimulates him to grow as a person.

This process works most dramatically during group confrontation, where participants constantly are challenged to attempt harder tasks and surmount increasingly difficult problems. It is important that the authority figure or challenger—whether he is a psychiatrist, ex-addict, or another patient—strikes the correct balance between the degree of responsibility the patient is asked to assume and his ability to assume this much responsibility. If he is asked to perform tasks that are beyond him, he may suffer destructive anxiety; if he is under-stimulated, he may become bored and lose interest.

The therapeutic community, as conceived here, is one whose interpersonal relationships promote human growth within the boundaries of impersonal, unchangeable reality on the one hand, and personal, constitutional limitations on the other. Growth occurs through the authority-responsibility relationships which evolve in continual individual and group confrontations.

In so far as the general community can be made therapeutic, true social development occurs. Communities which are most therapeutic show the strongest immunity to disruption and are, in themselves, the best preventives to drug addiction. In our program, for instance, we have established 11 community groups of addicts' relatives and employers (RARE) and another 11 local groups (called AWARE) made up of interested citizens who are not related to addicts but are working with them.

Another extension of the "therapeutic community" is to local institutions such as schools in order to enrich teacher-pupil, teacher-parent, and teacher-supervisor relationships by improving the authority-responsibility balance between each. The teacher-pupil relationship succeeds best when the teacher constantly stimulates the student to grow. The method—individual or group confrontations—is applicable to any given behavioral problem. Through training, a teacher can understand and use this concept of interpersonal relationships in dealing with his students.

In applying this model to an ever-widening field, we have encountered that particularly painful and frustrating response, resistance to change. This response is strong—some changes we ask threaten long-cherished assumptions. Resistance to change is not abnormal, of course, not a symptom of illness and maladjustment, but it is clearly a debilitating force when pitted against attempts to solve human problems.

If resistance is interpersonal, it reflects the individual's difficulty in accepting responsibility for his own life. This resistance we expect to find in the street addict before he has been offered the possibility of rehabilitation. Intrapersonal resistance also characterizes those who form the culture surrounding the addict and exist in monotonous, constant dependency. Interpersonal resistance indicates difficulties in coping with authority relationships. This typifies the attitudes, prevalent in many communities, which permit people to turn their backs on the drug addict when they are the very ones who could wipe out the conditions which foster his addiction.

The progress of the community prevention program, like that of the addict rehabilitation program, can be measured by the extent to which resistance has been allayed. The three steps in this process are facing the initial resistance, working through this resistance, and finally, cooperating toward common goals. It is man's responsibility, whether he is an addict, a psychiatrist, a politician, or any other member of the species, to examine his basic attitudes and to cultivate those which will enable him to take a responsible part in the world around him.

Reading 74
Methadone Maintenance in Heroin Addiction:
The Program at Beth Israel Medical Center
Barbara A. Pearson

Only pennies a day are needed for freedom from the shackles of heroin addiction—pennies for methadone. Methadone is a synthetic narcotic which, unlike heroin, does not produce euphoria, sedation, or a distortion of behavior in a tolerant individual. The basic goal of the methadone maintenance treatment program (MMTP) is to rehabilitate the hard-core heroin addict by providing him with a daily dose of methadone to block the euphorigenic potential of heroin.

The founders of the methadone maintenance program at Beth Israel's Bernstein Institute, Dr. Vincent P. Dole and Dr. Marie Nyswander, first hit upon the idea of methadone maintenance during their studies of the pharmacologic effects of opiates on the metabolism of the body. Their hypothesis was that a "basic cause of a continued narcotic addition is a drug hunger or craving created by a metabolic deficiency as a result of opiate abuse" [1]. The regular daily administration of methadone satisfies this physical craving or drug hunger of heroin addiction.

Methadone is an addicting drug. However, there are three main advantages in substituting methadone for heroin. First, it is possible to slowly build an addict up to a stable dose between 80 and 120 milligrams of methadone per day. Secondly, although methadone is a potent analgesic for the nontolerant individual, at a stabilization dose, it produces no euphoric effects in the drug-tolerant heroin addict and, in fact, blocks the euphoric effect of heroin [2]. Finally, methadone is longer-acting than heroin. Its 24- to 38-hour duration, as opposed to the 2-hour effect of heroin [3], permits the addict to take methadone on a fixed schedule every 24 hours [4].

Reprinted from *The American Journal of Nursing*, vol. 70, no. 12, pp. 2571–2574, December 1970.

Methadone is believed to be sufficiently free from toxic or dysphoric effects to permit its use in continual treatment. Thus far, medical and psychometric tests have disclosed no definite signs of untoward effects except constipation. Some patients have complained of temporary insomnia and occasional impotency when they first begin taking methadone. Also, some increased diaphoresis may be noted. However, mental and neuromuscular functions appear unaffected [5].

The methadone patient who is hospitalized in a general hospital is able to receive, and should be given, analgesics similar to those given to any nonaddicted patient. In fact, the methadone patient may need a slightly higher dose of analgesics. Because of the narcotic-blocking properties of methadone, the methadone patient will not become readdicted to potent analgesics if he receives his daily methadone dose. The only analgesic which should not be given to a methadone patient is Talwin. Talwin is an opiate antagonist. It blocks the effect of methadone and causes a methadone patient to go into withdrawal [6].

Methadone is administered orally. It is usually mixed in Tang or a fruit juice to mask its bitter taste. Oral administration helps to eliminate the psychologic association with syringes or a "set of works" and, in fact, with the ritual of "shooting up."

Admission to the methadone program is completely voluntary. Prerequisites are few: New York City residency, an age minimum of 18, and at least a two-year history of opiate mainlining. Preference is given to addicts who have been unsuccessful in previous attempts at heroin detoxification. The major ingredient on the patient's part is motivation! Addicts with "mixed addictions," such as barbiturates, amphetamines, or alcohol with heroin, may be ineligible. Rarely are those with severe psychiatric disorders accepted [7].

The methadone program at Bernstein is divided into three phases. The patient is started on methadone in phase I. The dosage is slowly and progressively increased until the patient become stabilized, that is, when he reaches his individual maintenance blockage level. At this point, the patient will feel neither a drug hunger nor the euphoric effects of heroin should he "shoot up." This process takes about three to six weeks. It may be done either on an outpatient basis or an inpatient service on a closed, unlocked hospital unit.

Once a patient has reached his stabilization level he is transferred to phase II, an outpatient department. He visits the department daily to receive his methadone. As he assumes more responsibility he may be given medication to be taken at home which reduces the number of times he needs to visit the clinic. As in phase I, the patient in phase II leaves a urine specimen on each visit to be tested for the use of methadone and for the abuse of opiates, quinine, barbiturates, and amphetamines.

Phase II is a time of major adjustment and transition for the patient. His life-style must be altered and his ties with the addict subculture severed. Frequently the patient's only friends are other methadone patients who share similar problems. Many of the patients are handicapped by their lack of education, training, or job skills and by their criminal records. This is the time when support and encouragement are of utmost importance. During phase II, patients lose some of their idealism as the reality of society and its prejudices against the heroin addict and ex-addict come to light.

Patients in phase III are those who are considered by staff to be stable, productive members of society. At least a year on phase II and the absence of any drug or alcohol abuse are prerequisites for phase III. All of these patients are employed, attending school, or managing a home.

In all three phases, doctors, nurses, counselors, social workers, and vocational counselors are readily available to the patient. An integral part of the multidisciplinary team is the research assistant, a rehabilitated addict who is a methadone patient himself. His knowledge of both the addict and the square worlds provides valuable insight to both staff and patients.

THE METHADONE NURSE

The role of the methadone nurse is much more than that of a licensed person who dispenses methadone. The methadone nurse is the one who is in continual contact with the patients. Frequently, she represents the "normal," a model of the square that a patient can use as a reference in his interactions with nonaddicts.

She is in an ideal position to detect subtle changes in a patient's appearance, behavior, and attitude by combining her observations with her knowledge of the patient's background and his present situation and with her understanding of the manifestations of various drugs. For example, Jack, a patient in his early thirties, drives a taxi at night and usually comes to the clinic for his medication when he finishes his shift at 8:00 A.M. Because of fatigue, he may look as if he has spent the night abusing barbiturates. If the nurse was not aware of Jack's situation, she might have associated his tired movements, rumpled clothes, stubby beard, and bloodshot eyes with barbiturate abuse instead of fatigue.

When the nurse does observe signs of drug abuse, she shares this with the rest of the staff and acts upon it after discussing the incident with the patient. In their discussion of the drug abuse, the nurse makes an effort to determine what triggered the acting out and to explore how the patient felt about the incident.

It is not unusual for a patient to experiment with drugs during phase I of the program. During this period, he may take some heroin out of curiosity to test the methadone or he may feel he needs it as he is being built up to his maintenance level. It is most important that the patient trust the staff enough to tell them when he takes drugs and how much; it is also important for the staff to be nonpunitive. A punitive attitude destroys trust and sets up a barrier that may prevent the patient from sharing further and future problems. Talking about the incident in private helps the nurse to establish rapport with the patient. She is interested in knowing the circumstances which led up to the abuse, how further incidents can be prevented, what the patient wants to achieve for himself, and how the staff can be instrumental in helping him achieve these goals.

Health teaching constitutes a large part of the nurse's interaction with patients. Addicts are just as ignorant about their physical makeup as the general nonaddict population. For many, old wives' tales and home and street remedies constitute their only medical information. Because the common cold and heroin withdrawal have similar symptoms (rhinitis, tearing, generalized malaise), the nurse may encounter difficulty in helping the patient to understand that the most effective treatment is aspirin, fluids, and rest—not more methadone.

Long, hard years of addiction have conditioned addicts to associate the slightest discomfort or anxiety with a need for more drugs. Frank, a patient in his late twenties, had just entered therapy with one of the methadone program psychiatrists and was experiencing stress and anxiety. Although his dose was within the upper limits of a maintenance dose, he constantly complained that his medication was not holding him, that is, the dosage of methadone was not sufficient to stabilize and to maintain him in a "normal state" midway between euphoria and withdrawal. Intellectually, he could reason that methadone was not his problem, but emotionally he could not. He had been conditioned to exhibit symptoms of withdrawal whenever personal discomfort became intolerable.

The pleas for a medication increase are often cries for help with emotional and psychological problems. In such instances, listening to, and talking with, the patient is more therapeutically valuable than an appointment with the doctor or brushing off the patient's cries of nonsense.

Amenorrhea in female opiate addicts is a fairly common health problem. Thirty-five-year-old Sally confided to me that she had been experiencing severe nosebleeds over the past several weeks. In the course of the conversation, she revealed that she had not menstruated for 14 months. Until we discussed the menstrual cycle in general terms, using an illustrated chart, Sally had assumed that her nosebleeds originated in the uterus and that this blood was finding an outlet through the nasal passages.

Nutritional teaching is another important function. The addict on the street usually has a very poor diet. He would rather get high than eat. When he is high he does not think about food; when he is "coming down" from his high, his only concern is getting money for his next fix. It is not unusual for a patient to gain weight rapidly in the methadone program. He may eat out of boredom, restlessness, or anxiety and stress. Lack of exercise may also be a factor. It is the nurse's responsibility to be aware of fluctuations in a patient's weight. A rapid weight loss may be an indication of the use of diet pills or amphetamines.

One patient, Beth, gained 60 pounds since her admission to the program. Accustomed to the demanding street life, she found housekeeping in her studio apartment took little effort. Lacking employable skills, having a long criminal record, and being fearful of the ever-present threat of rejection, she had little motivation to seek employment. Her days were spent watching soap operas and nibbling. She found a job as a cook's helper, but this only added to her weight problems because she was constantly tasting the food. Beth's attempts at dieting were futile and she became understandably discouraged. A discussion of her reducing methods revealed that her regimen included 15 containers of yogurt a day in addition to meat, vegetables, and fruit. After going over her eating habits, the methadone nurses emphasized the positive aspects of her diet, recommended nutritious additions, and pointed out subtractions.

Many patients are on a low-sodium diet to control hypertension or edema in their extremities. The methadone nurse must take the patient's financial status, cultural eating habits, and availability of foods into consideration in planning a low-sodium diet that the patient can follow. In dispensing diuretics and hypertensive drugs, she must do so with discretion and full awareness of possible toxic effects to prevent and detect possible mismanagement and abuse of these drugs.

The principles and techniques of psychiatric nursing are tightly woven into the interactions of the methadone nurse. The patients come from a wide range of socioeconomic and cultural backgrounds. There are few who fit into the stereotyped picture of a junkie. At times it is difficult to remain consciously aware that the patients were once heroin addicts, who survived because of deceptive appearances, manipulation, and cunning. Most patients resemble anyone else in a crowd.

Some of the patients have schizophrenic tendencies; many exhibit personality defects and difficulty in social adjustment. For years, drugs had helped them allay feelings of depression, inadequacy, alienation, and frustration; they provided an avenue for the resolution of aggression, anger, and tension. When a person begins to fully experience these normal feelings, pent-up emotions are let loose. The nurse and the rest of the staff are there to help the patient deal with these feelings.

A great number of the patients have difficulty with their sexual identity. They misinterpret many actions because of their past experiences, fantasies, and interruption of the maturation process. Male patients often think that the only way of expressing appreciation is to ask the nurse for a date or to try to kiss her. Saying "no" without rejecting the patient can be tricky, especially when negative responses can be interpreted as personal rejections.

The staff is also there to help the patient cope with the prejudgment and prejudice of society against addicts. These attitudes tend to reinforce the addicts' feelings of inadequacy, futility, worthlessness, and criminality; make his hope and motivation for help more remote; and intensify his feelings of hostility and alienation.

It is a very difficult and trying experience in self-control and nonjudgment for the methadone nurse to prevent her own attitudes and prejudices about addiction from entering her relationship with the patients. This is especially true when a patient "slips" or "fouls up."

Joan, for instance, was a methadone patient who turned to barbiturates whenever anxiety and stress became too much for her. A crisis in her home life inevitably provoked an episode with "goofballs," causing weeks of absenteeism from her job. When her intake of pills reached the point of an imminent overdose, Joan would be placed in the hospital to be slowly and safely withdrawn from the barbiturates. Several weeks later she would emerge from the hospital, drug free, her physical health restored, with a resolve to remain that way. Suddenly, months later Joan would appear in the methadone clinic sedated, with lame excuses of fatigue, plus all of the obvious manifestations of barbiturate abuse. After several hospitalizations it was difficult for both the staff and Joan to have confidence and trust.

Patience, understanding, and compassion are essential in work with addicts and ex-addicts. Constant self-evaluation and a pooling of staff knowledge and insight into each patient is vital in warding off the negative, pessimistic attitudes which may creep in. It is easy for these attitudes to be reinforced by the unresponsiveness of many heroin addicts to rehabilitation. The patient himself must be ready and willing to climb to the next step in his rehabilitative process and the nurse must recognize and accept this.

For many heroin addicts, the methadone program is the life preserver thrown into their murky quicksand. There are always some patients, however, who are not ready to assume responsibility for their actions even after they have been stabilized on methadone. Once on methadone, they find that they have lost the crutch of euphoria which provided them with relief from physical and psychological discomfort; the prospect of dealing with the world and with society overwhelms them. Naturally, they are apprehensive and insecure. Some of the patients retreat to other drugs, such as amphetamines and barbiturates, in order to try to regain a high and an escape; some turn to alcohol. The staff works closely with these patients on a one-to-one basis to try to establish their self-confidence and self-esteem. They attempt to channel the patient's interests from a preoccupation with drugs and a clinging to the familiar street life and addiction subculture to more productive, socially acceptable outlets.

Fortunately, the majority of methadone patients make it on their own, with only the help of methadone. Eighty percent of the persons admitted to the methadone program become self-sustaining, functioning, contributory members of society. They have found in themselves the motivation and strengths needed to shake the shackles of heroin addiction.

REFERENCES

1 Joseph, Herman. Heroin addiction and methadone maintenance. *J. New York Probation Parole Offic. Ass.,* **1**:18-40, Spring 1969.
2 Dole, V. P., and Nyswander, Marie E. Rehabilitation of heroin addicts after blockage with methadone. *New York J. Med.,* **66**:2011-2017, Aug. 1, 1966.
3 Martindale, William, in R. G. Todd (ed.), *Extra Pharmacopoeia,* 25th ed. London, Pharmaceutical Press, 1967, p. 794.
4 Sells, S. B. *Rehabilitating the Heroin Addict.* Report of the Institute on New Developments in the Rehabilitation of the Narcotic Addict, held at Fort Worth, Texas, February 16-18, 1966. Washington, D.C., U.S. Dept. of Health, Education, and Welfare, 1966.
5 Dole, V. P., and Nyswander, Marie E. Medical treatment for diacetylmorphine (heroin) addiction. *JAMA,* **193**:646-650, Aug. 23, 1965.
6 *Physician's Desk Reference to Pharmaceutical Specialties and Biologicals.* Oradell, New Jersey: Medical Economics, 1970, p. 1481-1482.
7 Beth Israel Medical Center, Morris J. Bernstein Institute. *Methadone Maintenance Treatment Program.* New York, The Center, n.d., p. 8 (pamphlet).

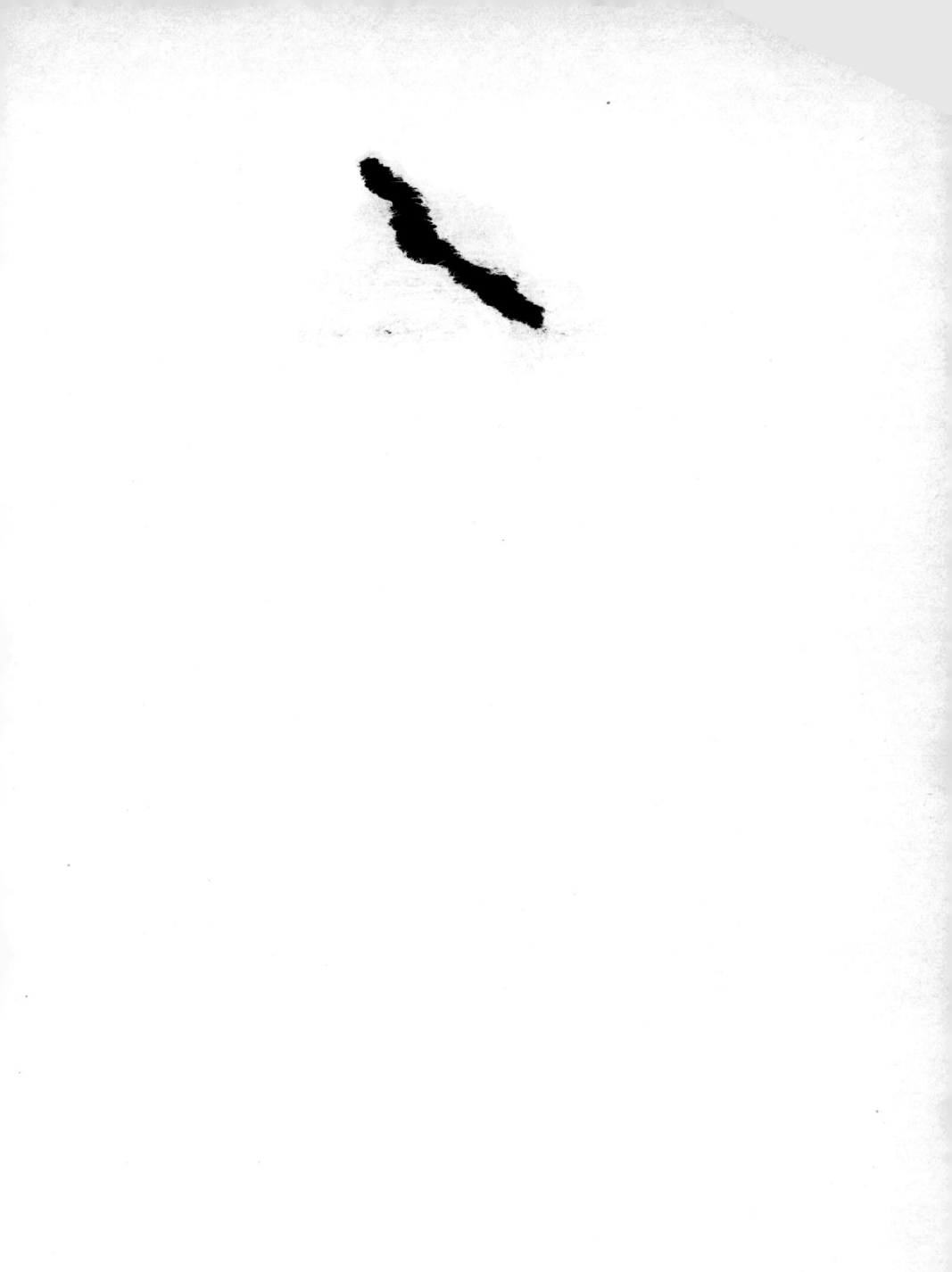